American Heart Association

Monograph Series

Cardiovascular Applications of Magnetic Resonance

Edited by

Gerald M. Pohost, MD

Director, Division of Cardiovascular Disease and
Center for NMR Research and Development,
University of Alabama at Birmingham,
Birmingham, Alabama

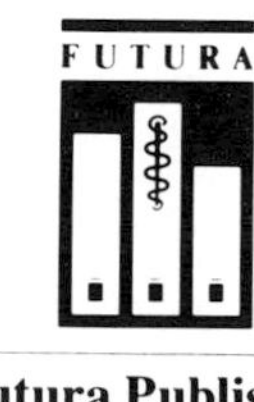

Futura Publishing Company, Inc.

Mount Kisco, NY

Library of Congress Cataloging-in-Publication Data

Cardiovascular applications of magnetic resonance / edited by Gerald Pohost.

p. cm.—(American Heart Association monograph series)

Includes bibliographic references and index.

ISBN 0-87993-548-0

1. Cardiovascular system—Magnetic resonance imaging. 2. Heart—Nuclear magnetic resonance imaging. 3. Nuclear magnetic resonance spectroscopy. I. Pohost, Gerald M.

[DNLM: 1. Cardiovascular Diseases—diagnosis. 2. Cardiovascular System—anatomy & histology. 3. Magnetic Resonance Imaging. WG 141C2667]

RC670.5.M33C365 1993

616.1'07548—dc20

DNLM/DLC

for Library of Congress 92-48279

CIP

Published by
Futura Publishing Company, Inc.
2 Bedford Ridge Road
Mount Kisco, New York 10549

LC #: 92-48279
ISBN #: 0-87993-548-0

Printed in the United States of America.

Printed on acid-free paper.

Contributors

Leon Axel, PhD, MD Department of Radiology, Hospital of the University of Pennsylvania, Philadelphia, Pennsylvania

Robert J. Bache, MD Departments of Medicine, Biochemistry, Radiology and the Center for Magnetic Resonance Research, University of Minnesota Health Sciences Center, Minneapolis, Minnesota

Sanford P. Bishop, DVM, PhD Department of Pathology, University of Alabama at Birmingham, Birmingham, Alabama

Paul A. Bottomley, PhD, General Electric Research and Development Center, Schenectady, New York

Thomas F. Budinger, MD, PhD, University of California at Berkeley, Berkeley, California

Gary R. Caputo, MD Department of Radiology, Associate Professor of Radiology and Bioengineering, University of California, San Francisco, California

V. P. Chacko, PhD Johns Hopkins School of Medicine, Baltimore, Maryland

Barry L. W. Chapman, PhD CNMR Laboratory, University of Alabama at Birmingham, Birmingham, Alabama

Michael A. Conway, MB, MSc MRC Biochemical and Clinical Magnetic Resonance Unit, John Radcliffe Hospital, Headington, Oxford, England

Gregory B. Cranney University of Alabama at Birmingham, Center for NMR Research and Development, Birmingham, Alabama

Louis J. Dell'Italia, MD The University of Alabama at Birmingham, Department of Medicine, Division of Cardiology, Birmingham, Alabama

Albert de Roos, MD Department of Diagnostic Radiology, University Hospital Leiden and the Interuniversity Cardiology Institute of the the Netherlands, The Netherlands

Jan A. den Hollander, PhD Center for NMR Research and Development, University of Alabama at Birmingham, Birmingham, Alabama

Hans-Joseph Deutsch, MD Klinik III fur Innere Medizin, der Universitat zu Koln, Germany

Joost Doornbos, PhD Department of Diagnostic Radiology, University Hospital Leiden, The Netherlands

Chris Doumen, PhD Department of Cellular and Molecular Physiology, The Milton S. Hershey Medical Center, The Pennsylvania State University College of Medicine, Hershey, Pennsylvania

Charles L. Dumoulin, PhD General Electric Research and Development Center, Schenectady, New York

Jerzy Duszynski, PhD Department of Cellular and Molecular Physiology, The Milton S. Hershey Medical Center, The Pennsylvania State University College of Medicine, Hershey, Pennsylvania

Robert E. Edelman, MD Director, Magnetic Resonance Imaging, Beth Israel Hospital, Boston, Massachusetts

André C. Eichenberger, MD Radiology Department, MR Centre, University Hospital, Zurich, Switzerland

Gabriel A. Elgavish, PhD Division of Cardiovascular Disease, Department of Medicine, University of Alabama at Birmingham, Birmingham, Alabama

Matthias Friedrich, MD Herzzentrum der Universitat Erlangen, Erlangen, Germany

Arthur H. L. From, MD Departments of Medicine, Biochemistry, Radiology and the Center for Magnetic Resonance Research, University of Minnesota Health Sciences Center, Minneapolis, Minnesota

Walter A. Fuchs, MD Radiology Department, MR Centre, University Hospital, Zurich, Switzerland

Christopher J. Hardy, PhD General Electric Research and Development Center, Schenectady, New York

Charles B. Higgins, MD Department of Radiology, University of California, San Francisco, California

Bob Hu, MD Division of Cardiovascular Medicine, Department of Medicine, Stanford University, Stanford, California

F. Mark H. Jeffery, PhD Mary Nell and Ralph B. Rogers Biomedical Magnetic Resonance Center (Department of Radiology), University of Texas Southwestern Medical Center, and Dallas Veterans Affairs Medical Center, Dallas, Texas

Markus Jungehülsing, MD Klinik fur Nuklearmedizin der Universitat zu Koln, Germany

Emanuel Kanal, MD Director, MRI, Department of Radiology, University of Pittsburgh, and Pittsburgh NMR Institute, Pittsburgh, Pennsylvania

Heinrich, Kolem, MD SIEMENS AG, Bereich Medizinische Technik, Erlangen, Germany

Hideo Kusuoka, MD Division of Cardiology, Department of Medicine, The Johns Hopkins University School of Medicine, Baltimore, Maryland

Kathryn F. LaNoue, PhD Department of Cellular and Molecular Physiology, The Milton S. Hershey Medical Center, The Pennsylvania State University College of Medicine, Hershey, Pennsylvania

Ting Y. Lee, PhD Department of Radiology, St. Joseph's Health Care Centre and University of Western Ontario, London, Ontario, Canada

Nadja M. Lesko, MD Northern Hospital of Surry County, Mt. Airy, North Carolina

Kerry M. Link, MD Department of Radiology, Bowman Gray School of Medicine, Winston-Salem, North Carolina

Steve P. Loehr, BA Department of Radiology, Bowman Gray School of Medicine, Winston-Salem, North Carolina

Peter R. Luyten, PhD MR Application Department, Philips Medical Systems, Best, The Netherlands

Albert Macovski, PhD Magnetic Resonance Systems Research Laboratory, Department of Electrical Engineering, Stanford University, Stanford, California

Craig Malloy, MD Mary Nell and Ralph B. Rogers Biomedical Magnetic Resonance Center (Department of Radiology), Department of Internal Medicine (Division of Cardiology), University of Texas Southwestern Medical Center, and Dallas Veterans Affairs Medical Center, Dallas, Texas

Eduardo Marban, MD, PhD Division of Cardiology, Department of Medicine, The Johns Hopkins University School of Medicine, Baltimore, Maryland

Graeme C. McKinnon, PhD Radiology Department, MR Centre, University Hospital, Zurich, Switzerland

Jeanie B. McMillin, PhD Department of Pathology and Laboratory Medicine, The University of Texas Health Science Center, The Medical School at Houston, Houston, Texas

Craig Meyer, PhD Magnetic Resonance Systems Research Laboratory, Department of Electrical Engineering, Stanford University, Stanford, California

Moriel NessAiver, PhD Picker International, Highland Heights, Ohio

Dwight G. Nishimura, PhD Magnetic Resonance Systems Research Laboratory, Department of Electrical Engineering, Stanford University, Stanford, California

Lambère J.M.P. Oosterwaal, MD MR Application Department, Philips Medical Systems, Best, The Netherlands

Ronald Ouwerkerk, PhD MRC Biochemical and Clinical Magnetic Resonance Unit, John Radcliffe Hospital, Headington, Oxford, England

John Pauly, PhD Magnetic Resonance Systems Research Laboratory, Department of Electrical Engineering, Stanford University, Stanford, California

Dudley J. Pennell Royal Brompton National Heart and Lung Hospital, London, United Kingdom

Ronald M. Peshock, MD Departments of Radiology (Division of MRI Research) and Internal Medicine (Cardiology Division), University of Texas Southwestern Medical Center at Dallas, Dallas, Texas

Gerald M. Pohost, MD Director, Division of Cardiovascular Disease and Center for NMR Research and Development, University of Alabama at Birmingham, Birmingham, Alabama

Frank S. Prato, PhD Departments of Nuclear Medicine and Magnetic Resonance and Biophysics, St. Joseph's Health Care Centre and University of Western Ontario, London, Ontario, Canada

George K. Radda, DPhil, FRS MRC Biochemical and Clinical Magnetic Resonance Unit, John Radcliffe Hospital, Headington, Oxford, England

Nathaniel Reichek, MD Director, Noninvasive Laboratories, Hospital of the University of Pennsylvania, Philadelphia, Pennsylvania

Roxann Rokey, MD Department of Internal Medicine, Section of Cardiology, Baylor College of Medicine, Houston, Texas

Guy Salama, PhD Department of Physiology, University of Pittsburgh, Pittsburgh, Pennsylvania

Rolf Sauter, PhD SIEMENS AG, Bereich Medizinische Technik, Erlangen, Germany

Saul Schaefer, MD Division of Cardiovascular Medicine, University of California, Davis, Sacramento, California

Monika Schneider, MS SIEMENS AG, Bereich Medizinische Technik, Erlangen, Germany

Udo Sechtem, MD Klinik III fdur Innere Medizin der Universitat zu Koln, Germany

Frank G. Shellock, PhD Tower Imaging, Los Angeles, California

A. Dean Sherry, PhD Mary Nell and Ralph B. Rogers Biomedical Magnetic Resonance Center (Department of Radiology), University of Texas Southwestern Medical Center, Dallas, and University of Texas at Dallas, Richardson, Texas

Robert G. Shulman Department of Molecular Biophysics and Biochemistry, Yale University, New Haven, Connecticut

Peter Theissen, MD Klinik fur Nuklearmedizin der Universitat zu Koln, Germany

Chun Y. Tong, MsC Department of Biophysics, St. Joseph's Health Care Centre and University of Western Ontario, London, Ontario, Canada

Robert Turner, PhD Laboratory of Cardiac Energetics, National Institutes of Health, Bethesda, Maryland

Kamil Uğurbil, PhD Departments of Medicine, Biochemistry, Radiology and the Center for Magnetic Resonance Research, University of Minnesota Health Sciences Center, Minneapolis, Minnesota

S. Richard Underwood Royal Brompton National Heart and Lung Hospital, London, United Kingdom

Arnoud van der Laarse, PhD Department of Radiology, University Hospital Leiden, and the Interuniversity Cardiology Institute of The Netherlands, Utrecht, The Netherlands

Ernst E. van der Wall, MD Interuniversity Cardiology Institute of the Netherlands, Utrecht, The Netherlands

G. Wesley Vick II, MD, PhD Department of Pediatrics, Section of Cardiology, Baylor College of Medicine, Houston, Texas

Gustav K. von Schulthess, MD, PhD Radiology Department, MR Centre, University Hospital, Zurich, Switzerland

C. A. von Weymarn Radiology Department, MR Centre, University Hospital, Zurich, Switzerland

Peter G. Walker Cardiovascular Fluid Dynamics Laboratory, School of Chemical Engineering, Georgia Institute of Technology, Atlanta, Georgia

Bang Wan, PhD Department of Cellular and Molecular Physiology, The Milton S. Hershey Medical Center, The Pennsylvania State University College of Medicine, Hershey, Pennsylvania

Samuel J. Wang, MS Magnetic Resonance Systems Research Laboratory, Department of Electrical Engineering, Stanford University, Stanford, California

Robert G. Weiss, MD Division of Cardiology, Johns Hopkins Hospital, Baltimore, Maryland

Richard E. Wendt III, PhD Department of Cardiology, Baylor College of Medicine, Houston, Texas

Richard D. White, MD Head, Section of Cardiovascular Imaging, Division of Radiology, Cleveland Clinic Foundation, Cleveland, Ohio

Karsten Wicklow, MS SIEMENS AG, Bereich Medizinische Technik, Erlangen, Germany

Gerald Wisenberg, MD, FRCPC Department of Medicine, St. Joseph's Health Care Centre and University of Western Ontario, London, Ontario, Canada

Ajit P. Yoganathan Cardiovascular Fluid Dynamics Laboratory, School of Chemical Engineering, Georgia Institute of Technology, Atlanta, Georgia

Jiangi Zhang, MD, PhD Departments of Medicine, Biochemistry, Radiology and the Center for Magnetic Resonance Research, University of Minnesota Health Sciences Center, Minneapolis, Minnesota

Preface

Magnetic resonance imaging and spectroscopy are relatively new technologies that hold great promise for application to the cardiovascular system. Clinical magnetic resonance approaches are already being routinely used to evaluate the morphology of the great vessels, heart chambers, and in the basic science laboratory, to evaluate certain aspects of myocardial metabolism. The present monograph was developed to determine the present and future utility of magnetic resonance approaches as applied to the assessment of the heart and blood vessels.

The first half of this monograph is devoted to imaging and the second half is devoted to spectroscopy. The monograph will provide timely information of a basic and clinical nature on magnetic resonance spectroscopy and imaging and their applications to the cardiovascular system. It should be an asset to the scientist, physician, and health care professional.

Taken to its optimal utility, magnetic resonance methods using a single instrument should ultimately provide a "one-stop shop" for the clinical assessment of the cardiovascular system. Thus, within the next few years a single system could be developed to allow assessment of chamber and great vessel morphology and function, quantitation of flow through normal and abnormal orificies (eg, aortic valve and ventricular septal defect, respectively), arterial morphology both within and outside the vessel (including the coronary arteries), evaluation of myocardial perfusion at rest and/or during stress or pharmaceutical-induced vasodilation, and assessment of myocardial metabolism to evaluate tissue viability. If one "stop" could provide such a plethora of relevant information, it could obviate the need for numerous other modalities and help in our quest for containment of medical care costs. This is the promise of magnetic resonance.

Gerald M. Pohost, MD
Chairman, Council on Clinical Cardiology
American Heart Association

Contents

Section 3: Safety Issues

Section 1

Magnetic Resonance Imaging

Part 1

Cardiac Morphology and Function

Chapter 1

Magnetic Resonance Imaging of the Cardiovascular System

S. Richard Underwood and Dudley J. Pennell

Magnetic resonance imaging (MRI) has advantages over other imaging techniques that include the absence of ionizing radiation, high-resolution images with a large field of view, and tomographic acquisition in any plane. Magnetic resonance imaging has been used widely for assessment of the brain, spinal cord, and other static organs such as the joints for almost 10 years, but has only recently found a clinical role in the cardiovascular system. The developments that have made MRI more suitable for the heart include tomographic acquisition in any desired plane (Figures 1 to 3), accurate cardiac chamber volumes at any phase of the cardiac cycle, accurate measurements of blood velocity and flow, noninvasive angiography, and the promise of myocardial perfusion imaging following injection of paramagnetic contrast agents. Rapid imaging techniques such as ultrafast gradient-echo imaging or echo-planar imaging have decreased image acquisition time to between 30 and 500 msec, and it appears that real-time MRI will soon be feasible.

Anatomy

The Aorta

The aorta is seen particularly well because of its size and relative immobility, and because there is natural contrast between the wall and moving blood. Magnetic resonance imaging is useful in the diagnosis of many aortic diseases (Figure 4).[1]

Dissection is readily detected and its extent can be seen, including the involvement of other vessels (Figure 5). The entry and exit points are more difficult to localize, but aortic regurgitation is readily detected and quantified. Although an adequate assessment of the coronary arteries is not obtained, this is not always necessary preoperatively, and invasive investigation can be avoided with a

From Pohost GM (ed.), *Cardiovascular Applications of Magnetic Resonance.* Mount Kisco, NY, Futura Publishing Co., Inc., © 1993.

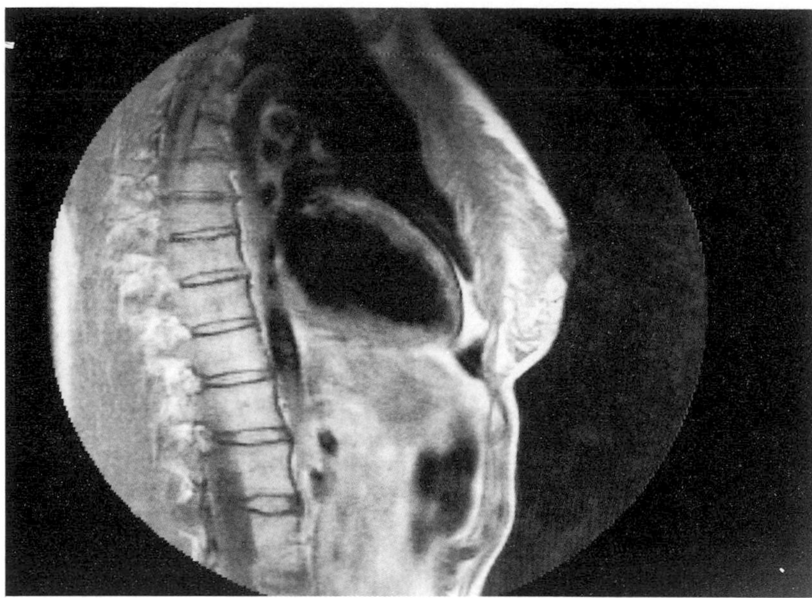

FIGURE 1. *Normal vertical long axis. The oblique vertical long-axis plane is acquired from the transaxial plane with a vertical plane offset by the leftward angulation of the left ventricle.*

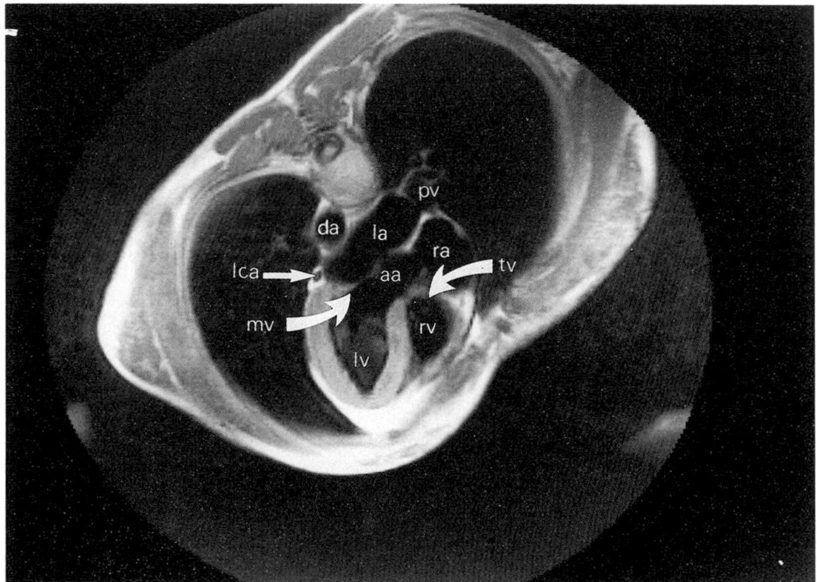

FIGURE 2. *Normal horizontal long axis. This double oblique plane is found from the vertical long axis with an off-horizontal plane angulated according to the downward inclination of the left ventricle. This spin-echo image shows the left ventricle (LV), left atrium (LA), mitral valve (MV), right ventricle (RV), right atrium (RA), tricuspid valve (TV), aortic outflow tract (AA), pulmonary veins (PV), descending aorta (DA), and left coronary artery (LCA).*

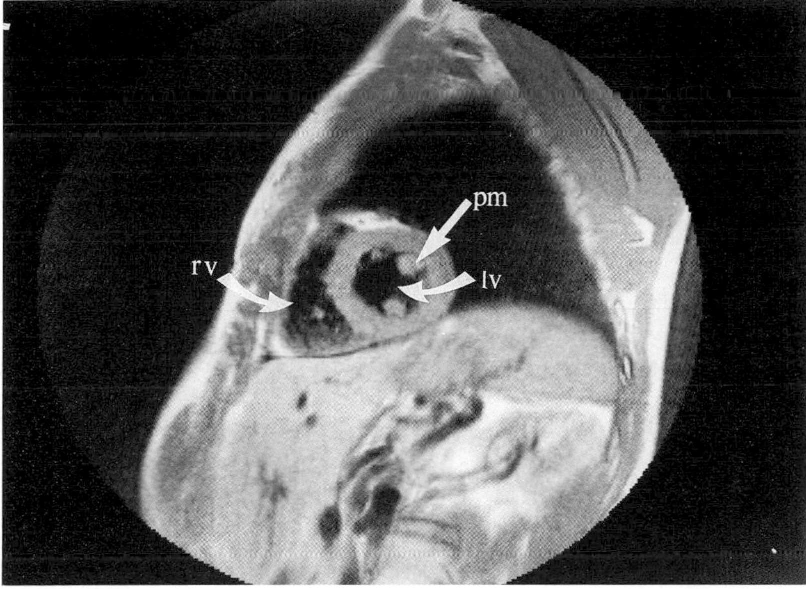

FIGURE 3. *Normal short axis. This plane is perpendicular to both the vertical long axis and the horizontal long axis. In this spin-echo image, the right ventricle (RV) is seen below the sternum and the left ventricle (LV) appears in circular cross section. The papillary muscles (PM) are also seen. This plane is well suited to wall-motion studies.*

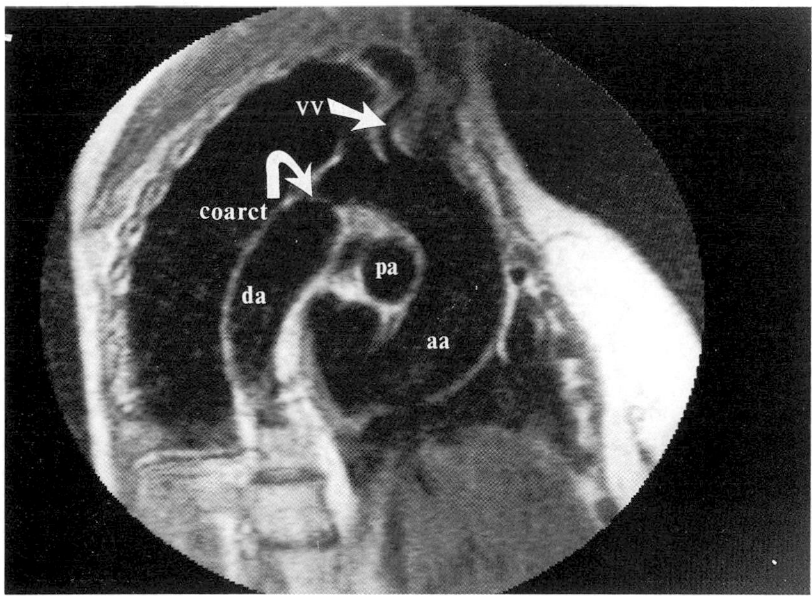

FIGURE 4. *Aortic coarctation. A spin-echo image in an oblique plane is shown that encompasses the entire thoracic aorta. The ascending aorta (AA) rises from the aortic valve and the arch gives off vessels to the head and arms (VV). In the proximal portion of the descending aorta (DA) a shelf is seen at the site of coarctation (Coarct). The pulmonary artery (PA) is adjacent.*

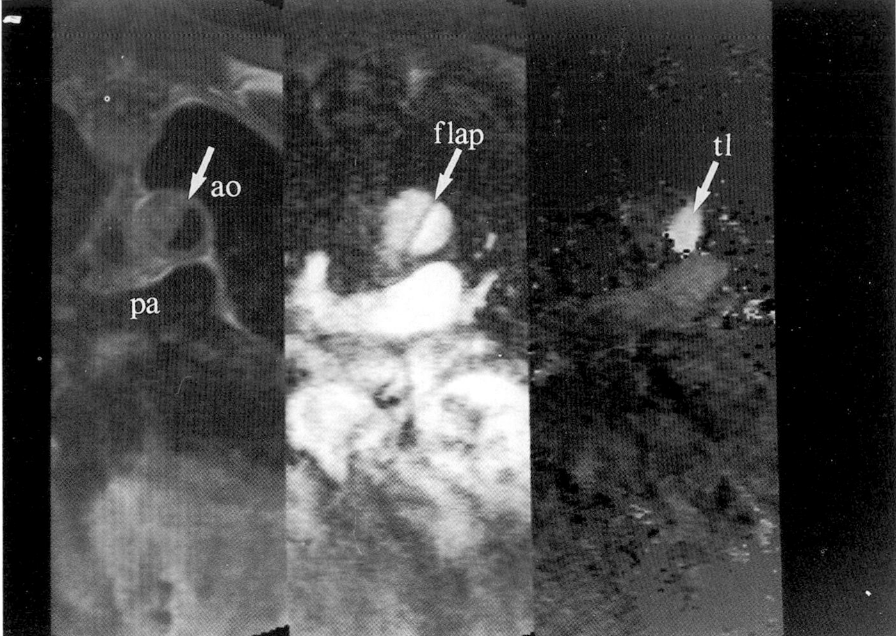

FIGURE 5. *Aortic dissection. Three images are shown in the coronal plane with the arch of the aorta (Ao) seen in cross section above the pulmonary artery (PA). The spin-echo image (left) shows high signal medially in a false lumen (arrow). The gradient-echo image (center) shows the dissection flap (flap) and high signal from blood in both the true and false lumens. The velocity map (right) shows rapid flow in the true lumen (TL) but no flow in the false lumen.*

combination of echocardiography and MRI.[2] Magnetic resonance imaging is at least as sensitive as x-ray computed tomography[3] and has the advantages of oblique plane acquisition and no contrast injection requirement, but it is more difficult to image sick patients with the current generation of scanners. Comparison of MRI with transesophageal echocardiography in the detection of dissection showed equivalent sensitivity, but significantly higher specificity and superior detection of thrombus formation for MRI.[4] Cine sequences that give high signal from blood and lower signal from thrombus are very helpful, and the ability to measure velocities in the two lumens provides additional functional information, such as whether the false lumen is required to supply vital organs.[5]

Other aortic abnormalities that are well seen by MRI are aneurysms, coarctations, abscesses, and inflammatory disorders and it is ideal for the follow-up of patients with Marfan's syndrome.[6]

Congenital Heart Disease

This is another area where invasive investigation can be avoided in selected cases. Because of the quality of the images and the wide field of view unhindered by limitations

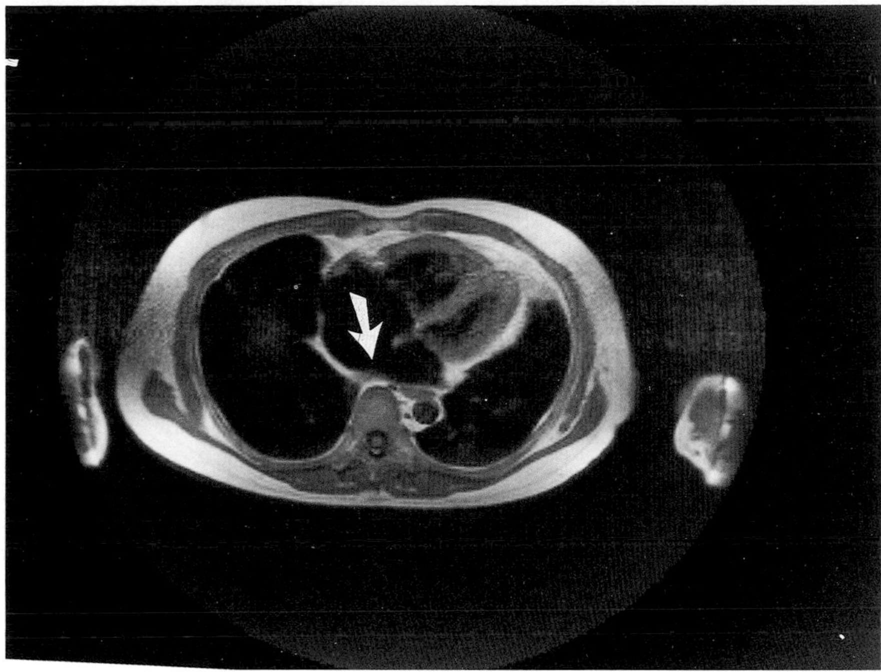

FIGURE 6. *Atrial septal defect. A secundum defect of the atrial septum is seen (arrows) and the right heart is dilated.*

of acoustic windows, MRI has a clear advantage over echocardiography. The acquisition of contiguous slices allows clarification of even the most complex problems.[7]

Magnetic resonance imaging is also useful in detecting pulmonary artery abnormalities[8] and in the detection of ventricular[9] and atrial septal defects (Figure 6).[10] The strength of MRI in the assessment of septal defects is not so much in detecting the lesion, which will usually have been found by echocardiography, but in assessing its functional significance by the direct measurement of the Qp/Qs that is achieved by measuring flow in the aorta and main pulmonary artery. Abnormalities of the atrioventricular valves are also well seen.[11]

Magnetic resonance imaging is particularly valuable in assessing patients with congenital heart disease after surgery because distortion of the anatomy, scar tissue, and the location of surgical conduits make diagnostic echocardiography difficult.[12] Magnetic resonance is also able to assess right ventricular function and tricuspid competence in these patients.[13]

Thrombus and Tumors

A common reason to refer a patient for MRI is to assist in the diagnosis of intracardiac filling defects. Tumors of the heart and surrounding structures are well demonstrated (Figure 7),[14] but with the possible exception of lipomata (high signal)

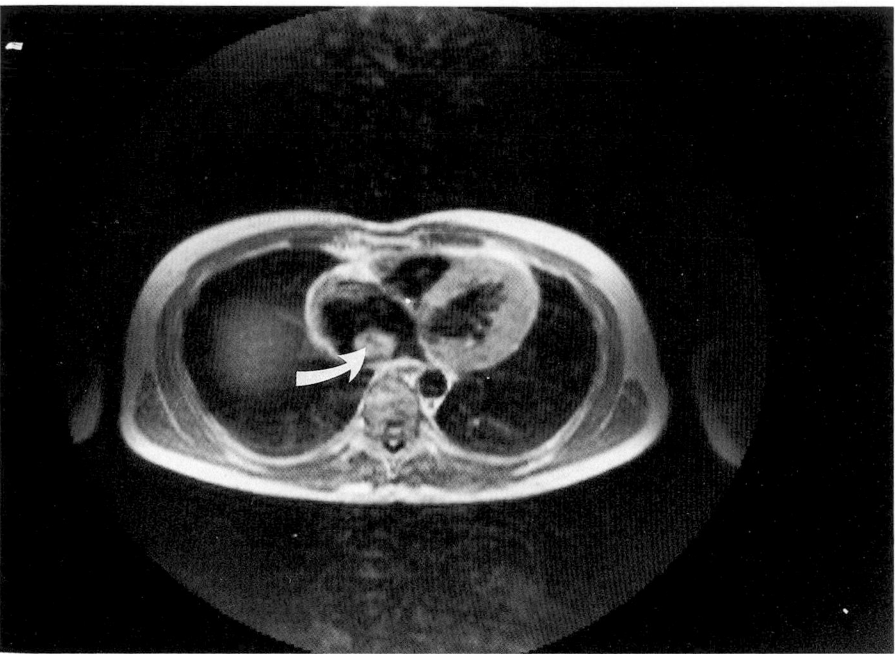

FIGURE 7. *Atrial myxoma. A right atrial myxoma is seen in this transaxial spin-echo image (arrow).*

and fibromata (low signal), it can be difficult to distinguish between different tumors. Thrombus is the most common intracavitary filling defect and is readily seen using a spin-echo sequence. Confusion between thrombus and slowly moving blood can be avoided by using a cine sequence, where blood gives high signal and the thrombus appears as a filling defect.

The Pericardium

The normal fibrous pericardium is best seen anteriorly and appears as a thin dark line around the heart using a short spin-echo sequence. The appearance of pericardial thickening and effusion depends upon the pathology. Thickened pericardium usually has a low signal, although it may have an intermediate or high signal if there is active inflammation.[15] In contrast to x-ray computed tomography, pericardial calcification is not demonstrated. Pericardial fluid usually has a high signal, although it may lose signal with motion. If it is difficult to distinguish pericardium from fluid, cine imaging is helpful because the motion of the heart within the pericardial sac is seen. The functional difference between constriction and restriction cannot be appreciated, but in the former, abnormal pericardium is invariably seen, and in the latter it is not.[16]

Ventricular Function

Cavity volumes can be measured by a number of techniques, but the most accurate is to sum cavity areas in multiple parallel contiguous slices. This is usually performed in the transverse plane and is accurate to at least 5%.[17] The technique makes few assumptions about chamber geometry and is therefore particularly useful for the right ventricle, the atria, and the infarcted left ventricle. By gating the acquisition to both end diastole and end systole the individual chamber stroke volumes and output may be calculated. A more rapid method for the left ventricle alone uses standard area-length calculations on oblique images containing the long axis.[18]

Valvular Regurgitation

In patients with regurgitation affecting a single valve, the multiple slice technique allows quantification of regurgitant volume and fraction by comparison of the ventricular stroke volumes that are equal in normal hearts.[19] In patients with regurgitation of one valve on both sides of the heart, this technique fails and comparison must then be made between the individual ventricular output and the actual forward flow in the pulmonary artery and aorta that is found using velocity mapping. Isolating the severity of combined regurgitant lesions on one side of the heart (eg, aortic and mitral regurgitation) is under investigation by quantifying the aortic regurgitant fraction alone from backflow measurements. Semiquantitative measurements of the severity of valvular regurgitation can be made from the area of signal loss in the proximal chamber associated with turbulence that causes signal loss in a manner similar to color flow Doppler echocardiography (Figure 8).

Ventricular Muscle

Ventricular mass may also be accurately measured using the multislice technique; this is useful for hypertension studies to demonstrate regression.[20] The distribution of ventricular muscle is also well demonstrated and MRI provides a better three-dimensional assessment of hypertrophic cardiomyopathy than does echocardiography.[21] Spectroscopic measurements of the relaxation parameter T_2 have shown higher values than normal in hypertrophied muscle.[22]

Muscle thinning is easily detected and previous infarction can be quantified by the presence and extent of thinning and wall-motion abnormality (Figure 9).[23] Wall motion is usually measured from diastolic and systolic images by superimposition of endocardial contours, but this assumes that the time of end systole is known and that it is the same for all parts of the ventricle. These assumptions are avoided by cine acquisition.

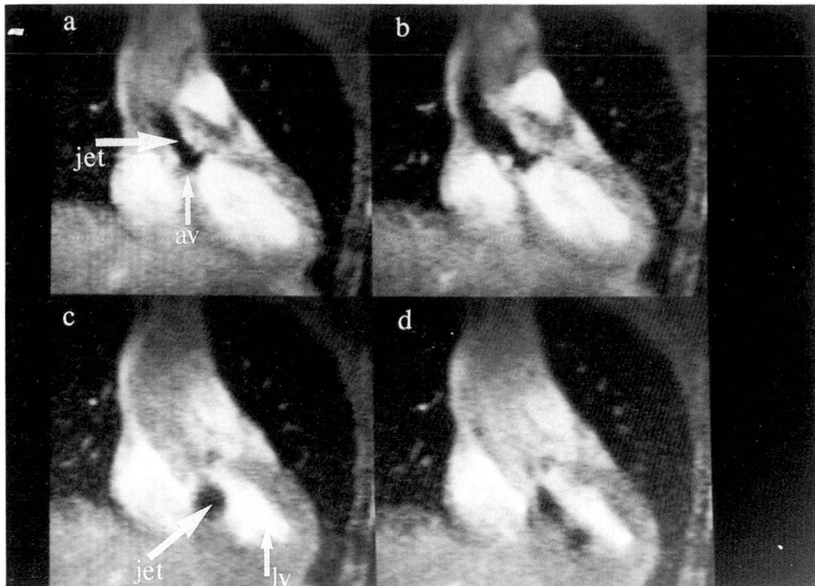

FIGURE 8. *Valvular regurgitation. Four frames from a cine gradient-echo acquisition in the coronal plane through the aortic valve. In systole (a and b), a turbulent jet (Jet) causing signal loss is seen in the aorta just distal to the aortic valve (AV). In diastole (c and d) a regurgitant jet (Jet) is seen below the aortic valve in the left ventricle (LV).*

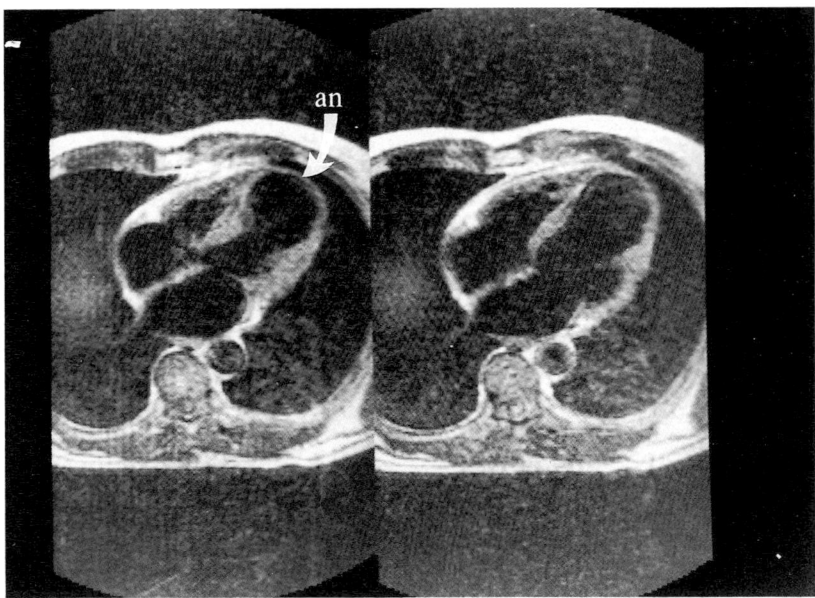

FIGURE 9. *Left ventricular aneurysm. Transaxial spin-echo images in systole (left) and diastole (right). The apex of the left ventricle is thinned with paradoxical wall motion typical of an aneurysm (An).*

Cine Imaging and Velocity Mapping

The spin-echo sequence cannot be repeated quickly in a single plane to acquire images as in a movie, but a modified gradient echo sequence can be repeated rapidly with a minimum temporal resolution of 6 msec, so that a multiframe cine acquisition can be made in the same time as a single spin-echo image (approximately 3 minutes). Moving blood does not lose signal, but instead it gives a very high signal and appears white. The only exception to this is where turbulent blood flow occurs, such as when blood flows across a stenotic or regurgitant valve.

Using cine imaging ventricular wall motion is more comprehensively defined than by end-diastolic and end-systolic frames alone. It is also helpful in the differentiation of thrombus and other filling defects from slowly moving blood. The loss of signal from turbulence can be used to detect and quantify valvular regurgitation and intracardiac shunts although more accurate measurements are made from chamber volumes as described above.

The combination of cine MRI with pharmacologic stress has permitted a comparison between wall motion and myocardial perfusion assessed by thallium emission tomography using dipyridamole and dobutamine (Figure 10).[24,25] The value of these techniques in the assessment of coronary artery disease requires further evaluation.

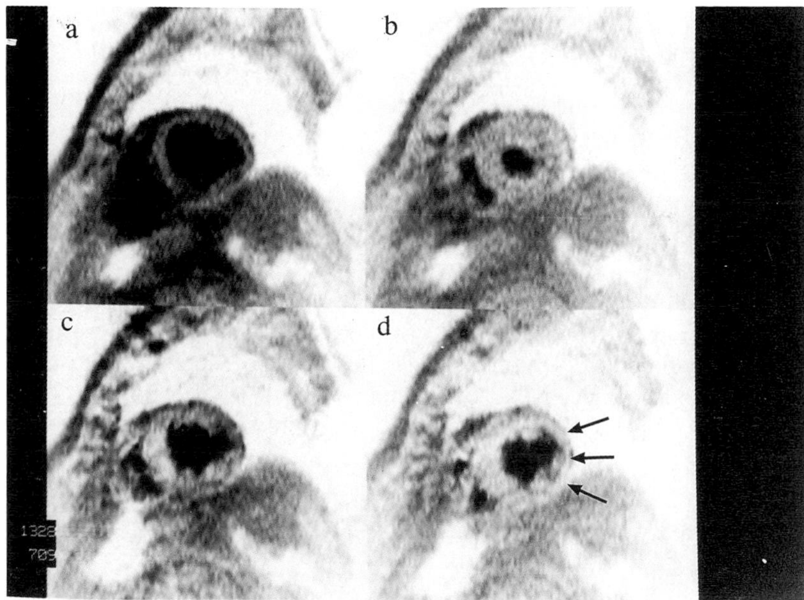

FIGURE 10. *Imaging of reversible ischemia during dobutamine stress. A patient with a proximal left circumflex lesion was stressed using dobutamine. Magnetic resonance imaging in a short-axis plane prior to stress shows normal wall motion and thickening from diastole* **(a)** *to systole* **(b).** *During dobutamine infusion, motion and thickening of the lateral wall become abnormal (***c** *and* **d,** *arrows). Reversible ischemia in this territory was confirmed by thallium myocardial perfusion tomography using dobutamine stress.*

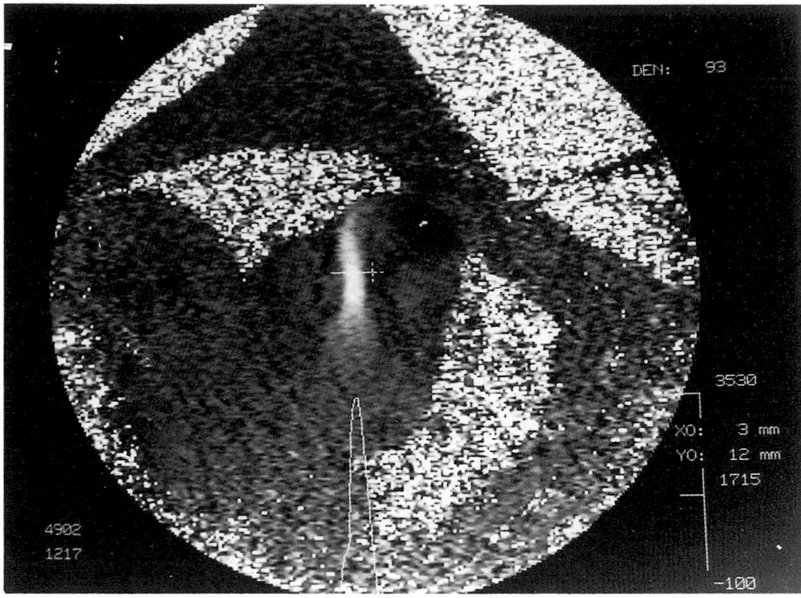

FIGURE 11. *Aortic stenosis pressure gradient. A midsystolic velocity map in a coronal plane that is rotated to align the jet with the direction of velocity encoding (bottom to top of image). The peak velocity was 3.53 m/s representing a gradient of 50 mm Hg.*

Cine velocity mapping provides accurate measurements of flow in the heart and vessels with an accuracy of approximately 5% in large vessels.[26] If the velocity information is color encoded and superimposed upon the gray scale anatomical image, then both anatomy and flow can be seen in a single display similar to that of color Doppler cine velocity mapping.[27] The technique has become an important part of the assessment of congenital heart disease with measurements of flow through shunts and conduits,[28] and the assessment of pressure gradients across stenoses from the peak velocity in the poststenotic jet (Figure 11).[26] The measurement of velocity and flow in coronary artery bypass grafts has also been achieved.[29]

Conclusion

Magnetic resonance imaging of the cardiovascular system has progressed across a broad front in recent years and it has now earned a place in the management of a variety of clinical problems. In those centers fortunate enough to have access to a machine, MRI contributes to patient management, and as scanners become tailored to the examination of the cardiovascular system, its use can only increase. The contribution of MRI to the assessment of coronary artery disease may become important if the combination of increased resolution with real-time imaging allows the coronary arteries to be imaged reliably.

References

1. Dooms GC, Higgins CB: The potential of magnetic resonance imaging for the evaluation of thoracic arterial disease. *J Thorac Cardiovasc Surg* 1986;92:1088–1095.
2. Goldman AP, Kotler MN, Scanlon MH, et al: Magnetic resonance imaging and two dimensional echocardiography. Alternative approach to aortography in diagnosis of aortic dissecting aneurysm. *Am J Med* 1986;80:1225–1229.
3. Goldman AP, Kotler MN, Scanlon MH, et al: The complementary role of magnetic resonance imaging, Doppler echocardiography, and computed tomography in the diagnosis of dissecting thoracic aneurysms. *Am Heart J* 1986;111:970–981.
4. Nienaber CA, Spielmann RP, van Kodolitsch Y, et al: Diagnosis of thoracic aortic dissection. Magnetic resonance imaging versus transoesophageal echocardiography. *Circulation* 1992;85:434–447.
5. Bogren HG, Underwood SR, Firmin DN, et al: Magnetic resonance velocity mapping in aortic dissection. *Br J Radiol* 1988;61:456–462.
6. Schaefer S, Peshock RM, Mallot CR, et al: Nuclear magnetic resonance imaging in Marfan's syndrome. *J Am Coll Cardiol* 1987;9:70–74.
7. Boxer RA, Singh S, LaCorte MA, et al: Cardiac magnetic resonance imaging in children with congenital heart disease. *J Pediatr* 1986;109:460–464.
8. Rees RSO, Somerville J, Underwood SR, et al: Magnetic resonance imaging of the pulmonary arteries and their systemic connections in pulmonary atresia: comparison with angiographic and surgical findings. *Br Heart J* 1987;58:621–626.
9. Didier D, Higgins CB: Identification and localisation of ventricular septal defect by gated magnetic resonance imaging. *Am J Cardiol* 1986;57:1358–1363.
10. Diethelm L, Déry R, Lipton MJ, Higgins CB: Atrial-level shunts: sensitivity and specificity of MR in diagnosis. *Radiology* 1987;162:181–186.
11. Fletcher BD, Jacobstein MD, Abramowsky CR, Anderson RH: Right atrioventricular valve atresia: anatomic evaluation with MR imaging. *Am J Radiol* 1987;148:671–674.
12. Sampson C, Martinez J, Rees S, et al: Evaluation of Fontan's operation by magnetic resonance imaging. *Am J Cardiol* 1990;65:819–821.
13. Rees RSO, Somerville J, Warnes CA, et al: Magnetic resonance imaging in the assessment of cardiac function and anatomy following Mustard's operation for transposition of the great vessels: a comparison with echocardiography and radionuclide angiography. *Am J Cardiol* 1988;61:1316–1322.
14. Barakos JA, Brown JJ, Higgins CB: MR imaging of secondary cardiac and paracardiac lesions. *AJR* 1989;153:47–50.
15. Sechtem U, Tscholakoff D, Higgins CB: MRI of the abnormal pericardium. *AJR* 1986;147:245–252.
16. Sechtem U, Higgins CB, Sommerhoff BA, et al: Magnetic resonance imaging of restrictive cardiomyopathy. *Am J Cardiol* 1987;59:480–482.
17. Longmore DB, Klipstein RH, Underwood SR, et al: Dimensional accuracy of magnetic resonance in studies of the heart. *Lancet* 1985;i:1360–1362.
18. Underwood SR, Gill CRW, Firmin DN, et al: Left ventricular volume measured rapidly by oblique magnetic resonance imaging. *Br Heart J* 1988;60:188–195.
19. Underwood SR, Klipstein RH, Firmin DN, et al: Magnetic resonance assessment of aortic and mitral regurgitation. *Br Heart J* 1986;56:455–462.
20. Eichstädt HW, Felix R, Langer M, et al: Use of nuclear magnetic resonance imaging to show regression of hypertrophy with ramipril treatment. *Am J Cardiol* 1987;59:98D–103D.
21. Berghöfer G, Köhler D, Schmutzler H, et al: Die magnetresonanztomo-graphische Darstellung bei hypertropher Kardiomyopathie im Vergleich zur Echokardiographie. *Herz/Kreisl* 1987;19:135–139.
22. Fried R, Boxt LM, Miller RH III, et al: Nuclear magnetic resonance spectroscopy of rat ventricles following supravalvar aortic banding. A model of left ventricular hypertrophy. *Invest Radiol* 1986;21:622–625.

23. Underwood SR, Rees RSO, Savage PE, et al: The assessment of regional left ventricular function by magnetic resonance. *Br Heart J* 1986;56:334–340.
24. Pennell DJ, Underwood SR, Ell PJ, et al: Dipyridamole magnetic resonance imaging: a comparison with thallium-201 emission tomography. *Br Heart J* 1990;64:362–369.
25. Pennell DJ, Underwood SR, Manzara CC, et al: Magnetic resonance imaging during dobutamine stress in patient with coronary artery disease. *Am J Cardiol* 1992;70:34–40.
26. Kilner PJ, Firmin DN, Rees RSO, et al: Valve and great vessel stenosis: assessment with magnetic resonance jet velocity mapping. *Radiology* 1991;178:229–235.
27. Klipstein RH, Firmin DN, Underwood SR, et al: Colour display of quantitative blood flow and cardiac anatomy in a single magnetic resonance cine loop. *Br J Radiol* 1987;60:105–111.
28. Rees RSO, Firmin DN, Mohiaddin RH, et al: Application of flow measurements by magnetic resonance velocity mapping to congenital heart disease. *Am J Cardiol* 1989;64:953–956.
29. Underwood SR, Firmin DN, Klipstein RH, et al: Magnetic resonance velocity mapping: clinical application of a new technique. *Br Heart J* 1987;57:404–412.

Chapter 2

Assessment of Pericardial Disease Using Nuclear Magnetic Resonance Imaging Techniques

Roxann Rokey, MD, G. Wesley Vick III, MD, PhD, and Richard E. Wendt III, PhD

Pericardial disease may result from a wide variety of etiologic factors. These factors include: bacterial, viral, and fungal infections; connective tissue and metabolic disorders; pericardiotomy; drug reactions; congestive heart failure; uremia; neoplasia; and radiation therapy. Congenital anomalies of the pericardium also occur and may cause symptoms. Because of this considerable diversity in causation, the signs and symptoms of pericardial disease are highly variable and often nonspecific. Indeed, when pericardial disease occurs secondary to another primary condition or in association with a more readily apparent affliction, clinical manifestations of the pericardial disorder are often confused with those of the primary or more evident malady. Thus, clinicians have come to rely heavily on imaging technology in their efforts to improve diagnostic delineation of pericardial disorders.

Echocardiography has been the mainstay of diagnosis of pericardial disease for almost 20 years. Echocardiography has a high sensitivity and specificity for detection of pericardial effusion, and is generally accurate in determining the relative size of pericardial effusions. However, echocardiography has substantial inherent limitations. In patients with poor echocardiographic windows due to body habitus, postoperative changes, or lung disease, suboptimal studies may be acquired that do not allow adequate definition of size and location of the pericardial process. Furthermore, there are a number of important parameters, such as pericardial thickening and pericardial fluid characteristics, that are difficult to reliably evaluate by echocardiography.

This chapter will focus on the utility of cardiac nuclear magnetic resonance (NMR) imaging in the assessment of acquired pericardial disease. Nuclear magnetic resonance imaging methods inherently have a wide field of view and are much less

---

Supported in part by: NIH Physician Scientist Award, #1K11-HL02009 (RR); American Heart Association, Texas Affiliate, #89G-205 (GWV); and Siemens Medical Systems (REW).
From Pohost GM (ed.), *Cardiovascular Applications of Magnetic Resonance*. Mount Kisco, NY, Futura Publishing Co., Inc., © 1993.

affected by individual variations in subject anatomy than are ultrasonic imaging techniques. Additionally, the relationships of the tomographic NMR imaging planes are precisely defined in relation to each other. These advantages, together with the potential of this technique in allowing characterization of tissues and fluids, makes NMR imaging a valuable tool for evaluation of pericardial disease.

Anatomy of the Pericardium

The pericardium is composed of two continuous layers, the visceral and parietal pericardium, which are separated by a potential space, the pericardial cavity (Figure 1).[1–3] The visceral pericardium is a serosal membrane composed of mesothelial cells containing microvilli. It is adjacent to the chambers of the heart and overlies any subepicardial fat that is present. The parietal pericardium provides the general shape and strength of the pericardium. It is composed of three distinct sublayers: the serosa, fibrosa, and epipericardium. The inner serosal sublayer of the parietal pericardium, like the visceral pericardium, contains mesothelial cells with numerous microvilli. It is continuous with the serosal visceral pericardium and the pericardial reflections indicate the junction of these two layers. The middle fibrosa sublayer contains collagen and elastic fibrils. It is this sublayer that provides much of the elasticity of the pericardium. The outer epipericardial sublayer contains collagen, elastic fibrils, nerves, lymphatic vessels, blood vessels, and adipose tissue. This sublayer forms the

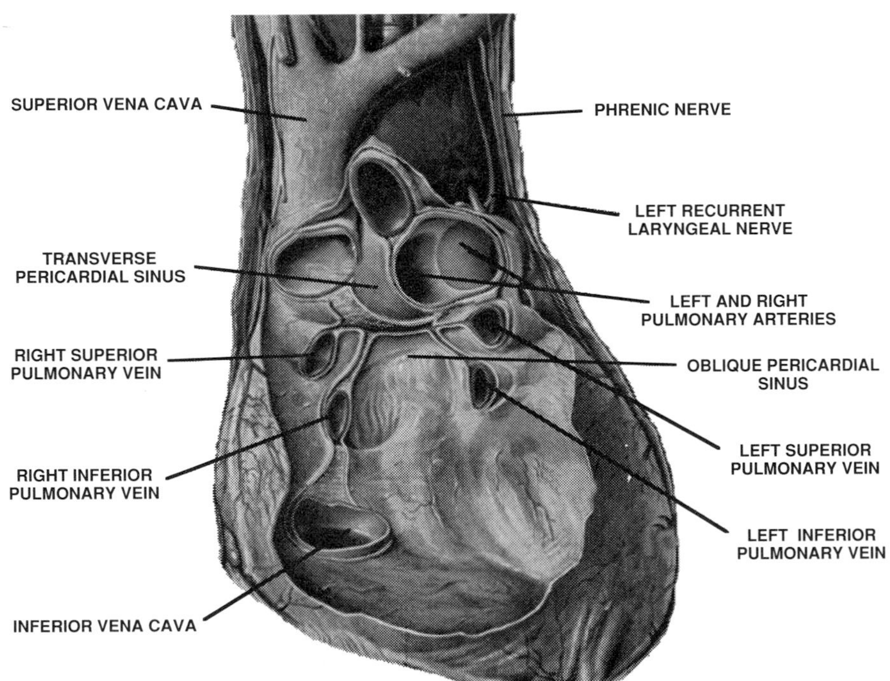

FIGURE 1. *View of the pericardium with the anterior aspect removed.*

anterior and posterior ligamentous attachments of the pericardium to the body. It is continuous with the parietal pleura laterally and with the adventitia of the great vessels at the pericardial reflections. The attachments of the pericardium to the manubrium, the xiphoid process, the vertebral column, and to the diaphragm by way of the superior pericardiosternal ligament, inferior pericardiosternal ligament, the pericardiovertebral ligament, and the phrenicopericardial ligament (central tendon of the diaphragm), respectively, in concert with its attachments to the great vessels, limit the amount of anterior-posterior motion of the heart.

The three sublayers of the parietal pericardium total approximately 0.8 to 1 mm in thickness.[4] However, its size varies and it is thickest at its insertions into the diaphragm, sternum, and great vessels. The visceral pericardium thickness is substantially less because it is composed of only a serosal membrane. The pericardial space normally contains between 10 and 50 cc of straw-colored fluid that is similar in composition to an ultrafiltrate of plasma and contains proteins in reduced concentration (1.74–3.5 g/dl) compared to plasma.[2] However, the ratio of albumin to protein concentration of this fluid is higher than that in the plasma. The pericardial fluid is thought to arise from the visceral pericardium, but may also arise from the overflow of myocardial interstitial fluid.[5,6] When pericardial fluid increases to an abnormal amount or is pathologic in nature, the fluid is termed an effusion. In pathologic myocardial and pericardial processes of the visceral or parietal pericardium, effusions may be detected in the subvisceral pericardium or between the visceral and parietal pericardium.

Nuclear Magnetic Resonance Imaging of the Pericardium

Cardiac NMR imaging of the pericardium to define the anatomy of the pericardium, its size, and the location and characterization of fluid requires synchronization of the imaging sequences to the cardiac cycle. The information desired from the NMR study will dictate the imaging protocol used.

Neither the visceral nor parietal pericardium is well visualized with NMR imaging techniques.[7,8] The presence of a pericardium is inferred because of a signal void observed between the myocardium and subepicardial fat, and the epipericardial fat and mediastinal fat.[8–10] The void is usually detected over the right ventricle and atrium because subepicardial fat is more prominent in these areas. The void detected in normal volunteers cannot represent pericardium alone, because reported NMR measurements are larger (1.4–2.6 mm) than those obtained anatomically.[8,11] The two pericardial layers, in addition to pericardial fluid, most likely contribute to the signal void, and in some instances, a chemical shift artifact may further augment the apparent abnormality.[12,13]

Nuclear Magnetic Resonance Imaging of Pericardial Fluid

Although echocardiography remains the noninvasive procedure of choice in the diagnosis of pericardial fluid and effusions, cardiac NMR imaging is an excellent adjunctive technique in specific cases and can provide information that the ultrasound technique cannot. The NMR technique is useful in: 1) detecting small pericardial effusions that are strongly suspected clinically, but remain undetected by the ultrasound technique; 2) demonstrating loculated pericardial effusions, particularly when the fluid is located posteriorly at the left ventricular apex, medial to the right atrium, or superiorly at the site of the aortic pericardial reflection; 3) distinguishing pericardial fluid/effusions from fat; 4) differentiating between pericardial and pleural effusions; 5) characterizing the nature of pericardial fluid; and 6) distinguishing fibrotic or calcified pericardium from pericardial fluid.

As little as 5 cc of pericardial fluid, which would produce a signal void of approximately 2 mm (range 0.1 to 3.2 mm), may be detected in an experimental preparation using NMR imaging techniques.[14] Although the exact delineation of distance measurements for normal versus abnormal amounts of fluid has not been established, experimental data indicate that measurements over 5 mm exceed 40 cc.[14] Clinical data also indicate that measurements >5 mm are abnormal.[7,15]

The etiology of pericardial effusions is diverse and the composition of the effusion is dependent upon the etiology.[16] In addition to the presence of pericardial fluid from the specific etiology, pericardial inflammation and/or thickening may also be present. Thus, when NMR imaging of pericardial effusions is performed, not only should the presence or absence of fluid be sought, but also the nature of the fluid and the possibility of pericardial inflammation or thickening should be evaluated.

The basis for characterization of the pericardium and pericardial effusions lies in the relaxation characteristics (T_1 and T_2) of the pericardium, pericardial fat, and fluid within the pericardium. Fluid with increased protein, cells, and/or lipid have relaxation characteristics that may allow for characterization of different effusion types. In general, information for anatomy and tissue characterization is obtained with data acquisition synchronized to the electrocardiogram (R wave). Multislice spin-echo sequences with variable TR times can be used to define anatomy and to help characterize effusions. Velocity compensated gradient-echo sequences are valuable in confirming the presence or absence of fluid within a suspected pericardial space.

Several clinical investigations have indicated the potential utility of NMR imaging in the detection and characterization of pericardial disease.[7,11,17,18] Measurements of pericardial fluid size in the NMR images correlate well with gross echocardiographic measurements and qualitatively with the volume of fluid within the pericardial space. Transudative pericardial effusions associated with congestive heart failure have been demonstrated to have a low signal intensity compared to myocardium on the first spin-echo image in comparison with exudative effusions secondary to uremic or tuberculous effusions.[11,18] Although the NMR findings in these clinical studies have agreed with the clinical diagnoses of suspected effusion type, adequate appraisal of the capabilities and limitations of the NMR imaging technique in evaluating pericardial effusions has been limited due to the lack of experimental data.

Recently, an experimental study using an animal model where pericardial effusions were created by introduction of fluid with known volume and composition into the pericardium has been reported.[14] In this study, the pericardium was instrumented, and a fluid of known composition was given either in incremental amounts or as a single fixed volume. The fluids were chosen to simulate pericardial effusions observed clinically. Effusions with different cell counts, protein concentration, and fat were chosen to resemble: 1) hemorrhagic/nonhemorrhagic; 2) transudative/exudative; and

3) chylous effusions, respectively. Fluid composition consisted of either: blood with 10% or 20% hematocrit, saline, plasma; or lipid (saturated and polyunsaturated triglycerides). Multislice, multispin-echo (TE of 34, 68, 102, or 136 msec) NMR images were obtained synchronized to the R wave of the electrocardiogram, and the effective TR time was varied by acquiring images either every heartbeat (400 msec), every other heartbeat (800 msec), or every sixth heartbeat (2,400 msec).

As little as 5 cc of fluid could be detected and a linear correlation was present between distance measurements and effusion size (Figures 2 and 3). On the basis of distance measurements, small effusions (≤40 cc; average of <5 mm in distance) could be separated from large effusions (≥120 cc). However, there was considerable overlap in measurements for moderately sized effusions (>40 cc and <120 cc).

The effects of cardiac motion influenced NMR imaging of experimental pericardial effusions. Adequate characterization of pericardial fluid composition was not possible in effusions with volumes containing <40 cc of fluid and loss of pericardial effusion signal intensity in vivo compared to postmortem studies was noted in images obtained with TE times >34 msec (Figures 4 and 5).

Pericardial effusions larger than 40 cc could be characterized when using the first spin-echo image (TE = 34 msec) on the basis of differential response to varying TR times (Figures 6 to 8). Effusions with fat had a high NMR signal intensity at a short TR time and an elevated signal intensity ratio of effusion to myocardium that declined as TR increased. The remaining effusions had a range of image brightness with respect to the myocardium but the signal intensity ratio uniformly increased with increasing TR time. Transudative, nonhemorrhagic effusions were darker (hypointense) than the myocardium at a TR time of 800 msec. In contrast, exudative nonhemorrhagic and hemorrhagic effusions were either the same intensity (isointense) or brighter (hyperintense) than the myocardium at a TR time of 800 msec. Only when the TR time was sufficiently short (400 msec) was differentiation of exudative from hemorrhagic effusions possible.

From the experimental study, several conclusions having clinical relevance can be drawn. First, because as little as 5 cc of fluid can be detected with NMR imaging techniques, detection of a signal void around the heart suggestive of pericardial fluid does not necessarily indicate a pathologic process. However, a distance measurement of 5 mm or greater implies fluid exceeding 40 cc in volume. Second, small nonloculated effusions (≤40 cc) will appear as a signal void regardless of effusion type because of cardiac motion. Thus, in order to determine if a signal void represents fluid or effusion versus pericardial fibrosis or calcification, imaging protocols that enhance the appearance of fluid in motion such as velocity compensated gradient-echo sequences should be used. The signal intensity of mobile pericardial fluid will change, whereas no substantial change in the signal void due to fibrosis or calcification will be noted. Third, characterization of pericardial effusions with more than 40 cc may be very difficult when using standard spin-echo imaging sequences with TE times of ≥68 msec because of the effects of cardiac motion. Thus, when attempting to characterize fluid, relatively short TE times (less than or equal to the 34 msec used in the experimental study) should be used. Fourth, characterization of fluid can be facilitated after the initial spin-echo images are obtained by increasing the effective TR time and measuring the changes in signal intensity and the pericardial to myocardial signal intensity ratio. Using the imaging protocol described in the experiment, transudative effusions

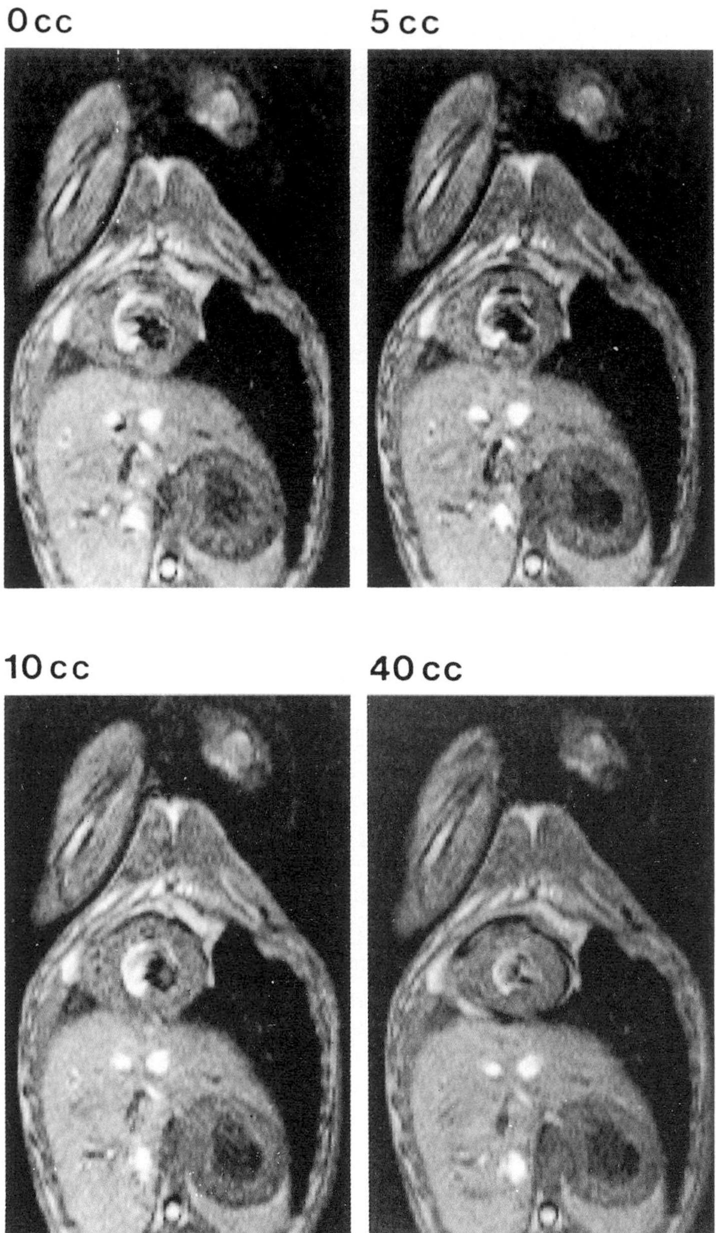

FIGURE 2. *Magnetic resonance images of the heart and pericardium in an experimental model of pericardial effusion obtained at baseline and with infusion of incremental amounts of fluid. With increasing volume, progressive separation of pericardial fat and the myocardium is noted. Regardless of fluid type, the signal void around the heart with ≤40 cc was very evident. Reprinted from Reference 14 with permission.*

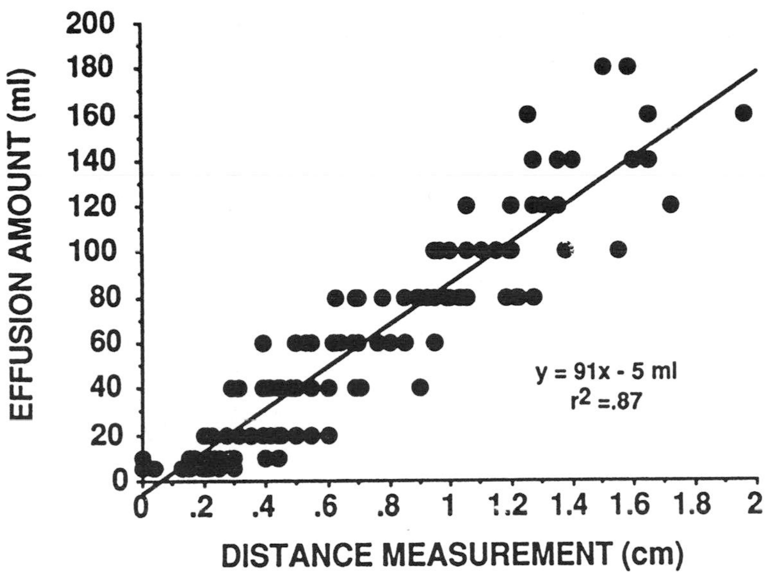

FIGURE 3. *Correlation of pericardial effusion volume versus distance measurements in the magnetic resonance images of experimental pericardial effusion. Reprinted from Reference 14 with permission.*

and those with a high lipid content can be differentiated from those that are exudative or hemorrhagic. However, given the relatively slower heart rates in patients compared to the experimental preparation, distinguishing between exudative or hemorrhagic effusions will be difficult using standard multislice spin-echo imaging sequences. Figure 9 is the flow diagram used at our institution for the assessment of pericardial processes.

Nuclear Magnetic Resonance Imaging of Pericarditis, Pericardial Thickening, and Constrictive Pericarditis

Pericarditis with subsequent pericardial thickening may involve the parietal or visceral pericardium and can result from a number of etiologies. When pericardial thickening compromises cardiac function, a diagnosis of constrictive pericarditis (effusive constrictive, constrictive [fibrotic or calcific], and occult constrictive) should be considered.[19–21] Recent studies indicate that flow and pressure changes can be accurately detected with MR imaging methods.[22,23] However, until further studies are validated in models of pericardial disease, MR imaging techniques should not be used to assess the hemodynamic changes associated with constrictive disease. Thus, in

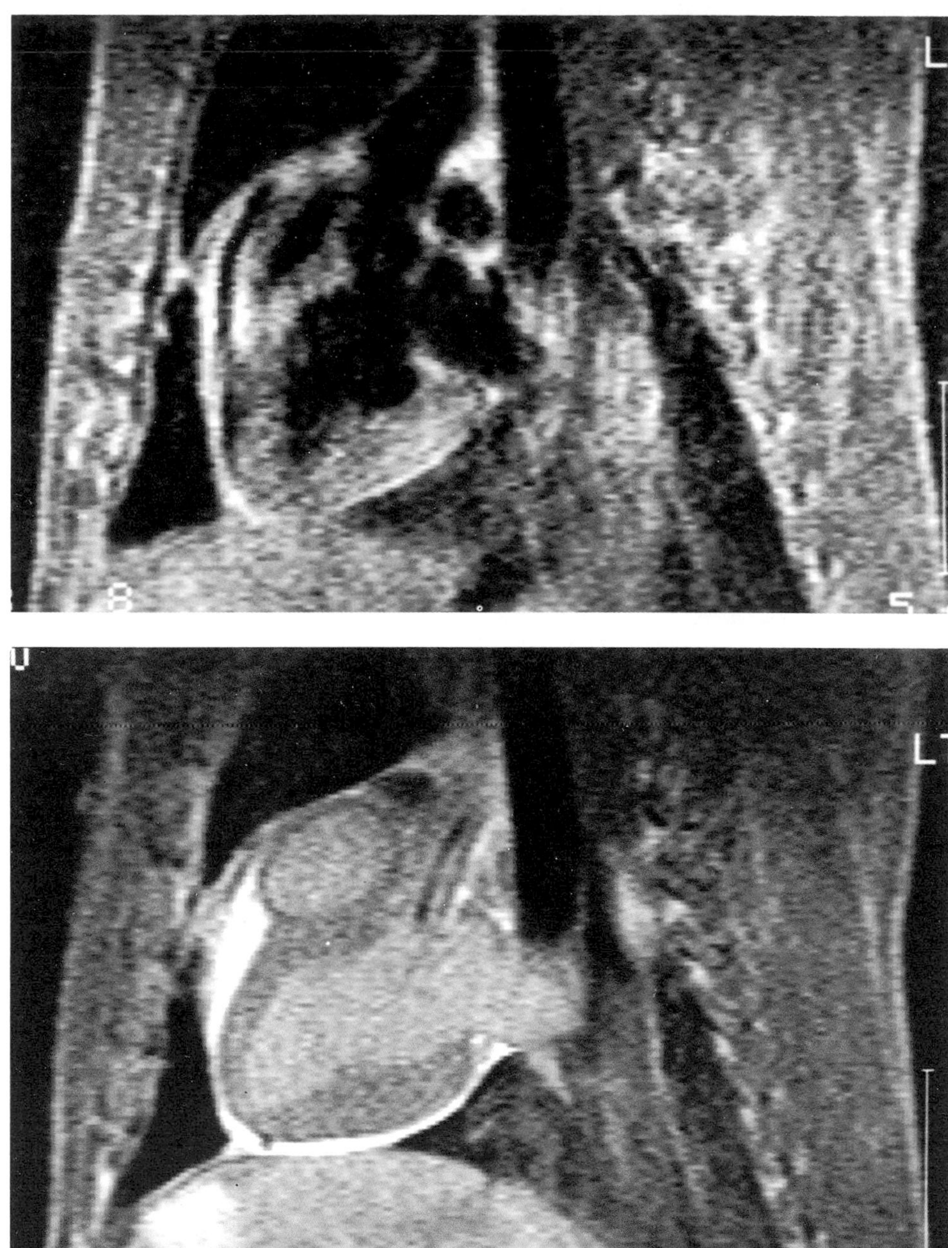

FIGURE 4. *In vivo* **(A)** *and postmortem* **(B)** *images of a small (40 cc) lipid pericardial effusion. Note the signal void adjacent to the heart in the in vivo image that is not present in the postmortem image.*

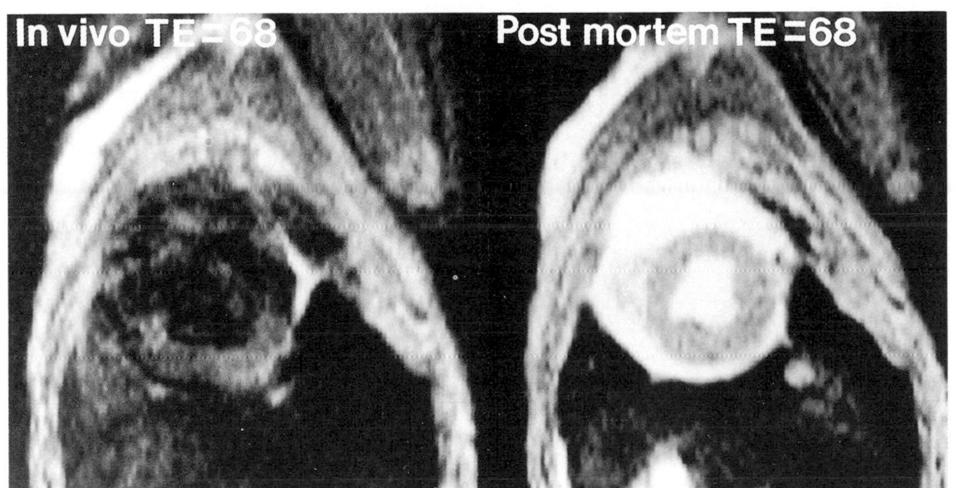

FIGURE 5. *In vivo and postmortem images of a plasma pericardial effusion using a TE of 68 msec and a TR of 2,400 msec. There is substantial loss of pericardial signal intensity compared to the postmortem image. The in vivo image obtained with a TE of 34 msec and same TR (not shown) was qualitatively similar in signal intensity to the postmortem image shown. Reprinted from Reference 14 with permission.*

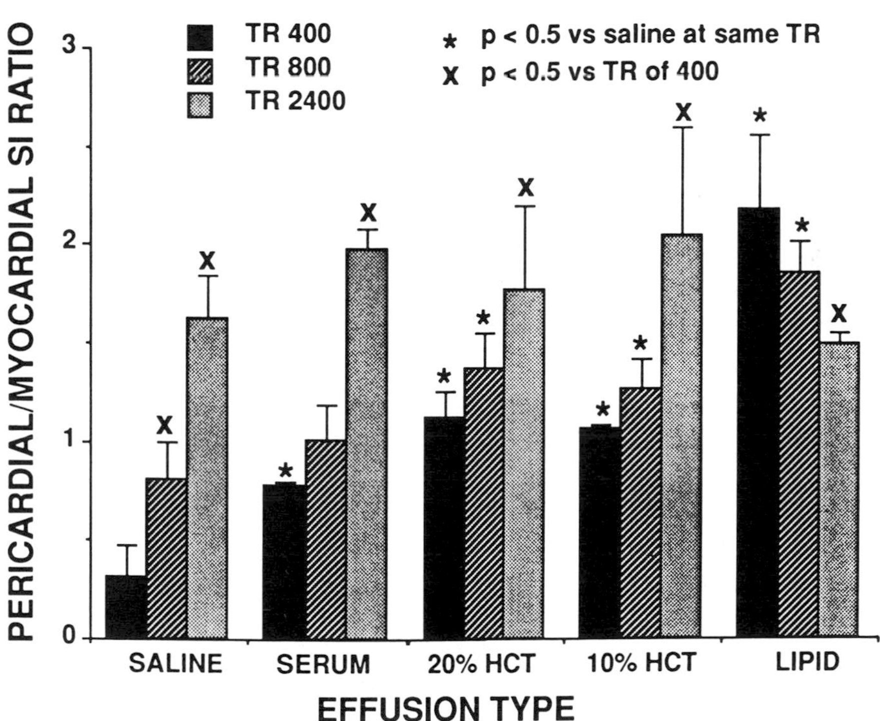

FIGURE 6. *Comparison of in vivo pericardial to myocardial signal intensity ratios at different TR times for different effusion types. Reprinted from Reference 14 with permission.*

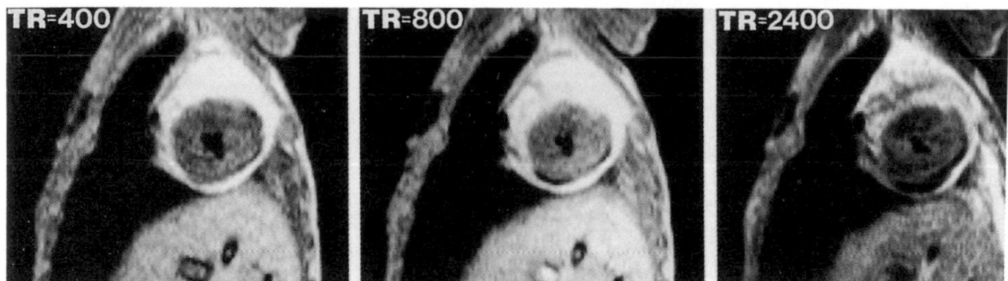

FIGURE 7. *Experimental lipid pericardial effusion at different TR times. The effusion is brighter (hyperintense) than myocardium at all imaging times. Reprinted from Reference 14 with permission.*

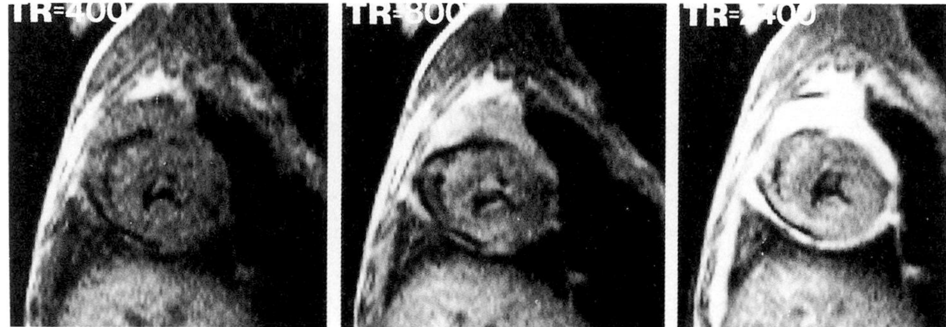

FIGURE 8. *Magnetic resonance images of experimental 20% hematocrit pericardial effusion at different TR times. The effusion is the same intensity (isointense) as the myocardium with TR times of 400 and 800 msec. At 2,400 msec, the effusion is brighter (hyperintense). Reprinted from Reference 14 with permission.*

suspected constrictive pericarditis, cardiac MR imaging techniques currently are best suited for the anatomical diagnosis of pericardial thickening.

The pathology of acquired pericardial disease represents a spectrum of processes, ranging from inflammation of either pericardial surface to the frankly calcified pericardium. Hence, the anatomical manifestations of acute pericarditis, pericardial thickening, and fibrosis/calcification as detected by the MR imaging technique are numerous. Inflammation of the pericardium may result in an increased protein concentration and/or cell count (prolonged T_2 relaxation time) adjacent to the pericardium and/or a subvisceral or subparietal effusion. In this case, the multislice first spin-echo images may show increased MR signal at the location of the visceral and parietal pericardium. The signal intensity of the pericardial effusion can be darker (hypointense), the same (isointense), or brighter (hyperintense) compared to myocardium, depending upon the size and composition of the effusion. Thickened pericardium that is not fibrotic can have a range of image brightness depending upon the composition and size of the fluid and the degree of organization. Thickened pericardium that is fibrotic has no MR-detectable signal and will appear darker than the myocardium. Calcified pericardium is not easily detected with the MR imaging techniques and appears as a signal void.

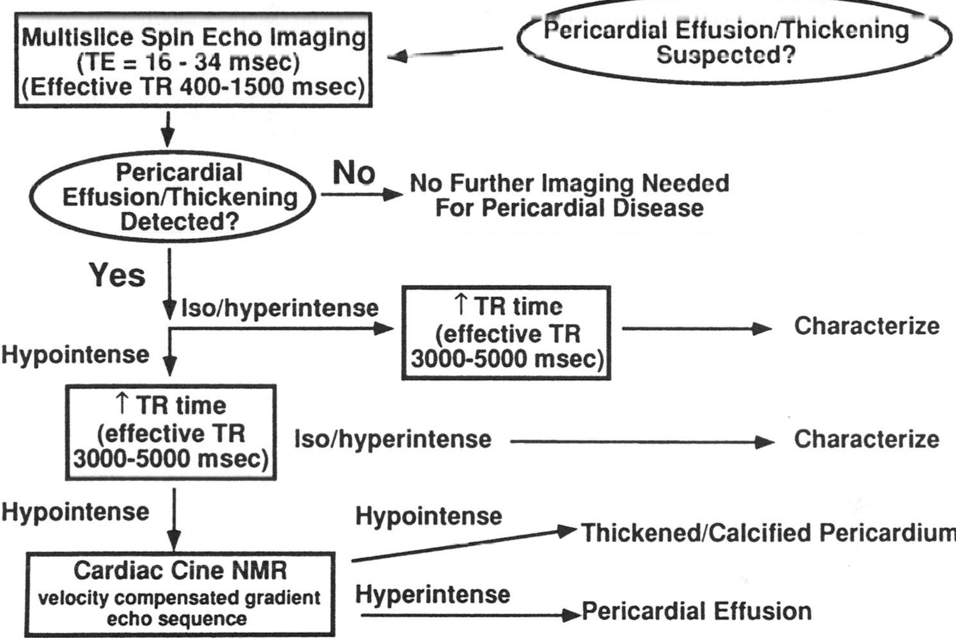

FIGURE 9. *Example of a nuclear magnetic resonance (NMR) imaging protocol for evaluation of pericardial disease.*

Thus, a thickened fibrotic pericardium, calcified pericardium, or a small pericardial effusion may all appear as a signal void when using a multislice, spin-echo MR imaging protocol. In these cases, velocity compensated gradient-echo sequences (cine MR) are valuable in confirming the presence or absence of fluid within a suspected pericardial space (Figure 10). These sequences demonstrate a "wash-in" effect of mobile fluid within the pericardial space. Therefore, a signal void within the pericardial space detected on spin-echo images that becomes hyperintense with cine MR sequences is consistent with pericardial fluid. In contrast, the signal void of fibrosed or calcified pericardium detected with spin-echo imaging would not substantially change in signal characteristics with the cine MR sequences.

Conclusion

The potential advantages of cardiac MR imaging in pericardial disease include the ability to detect very small pericardial effusions and loculated pericardial processes, to characterize the nature of suspected pericardial effusion, and to distinguish effusions from thickened or calcified pericardium. Although a few clinical reports have promoted this technique, recent experimental studies provide a more detailed appraisal of its limitations and capabilities. The influence of cardiac motion, despite the use of image acquisition synchronized to the electrocardiogram, degrades the image of the

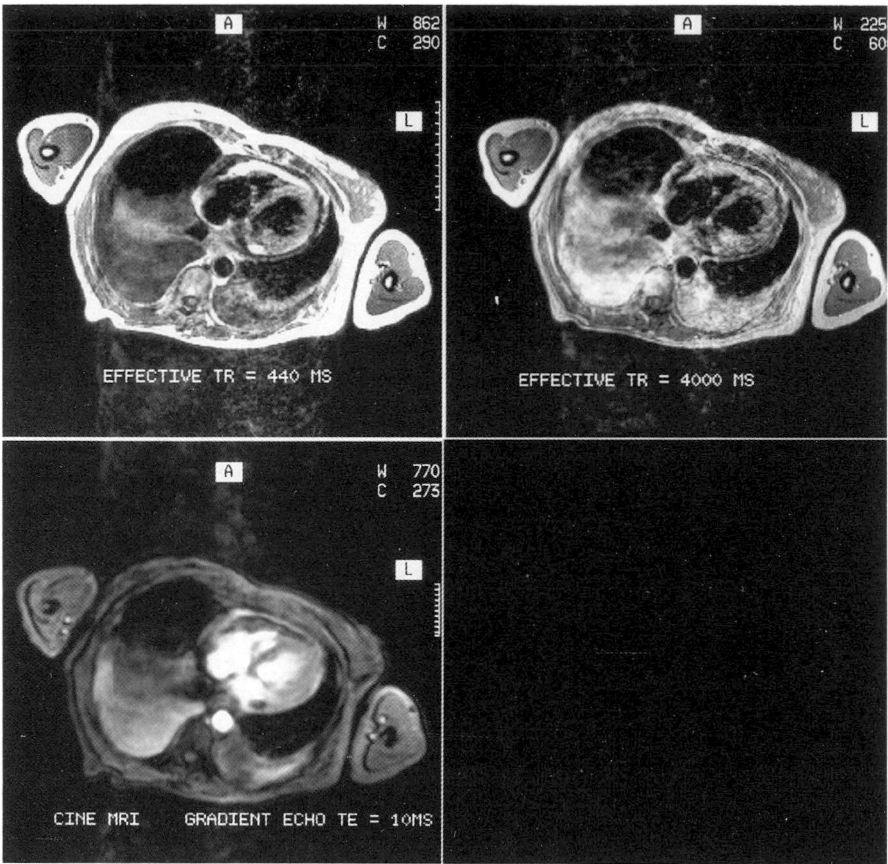

FIGURE 10. *Example of a signal void extrinsic to the myocardium noted in a standard spin-echo imaging protocol of the heart that might represent pericardial thickening, calcification, or fluid (upper two panels). A velocity compensated gradient-echo sequence demonstrates increased signal in this area and indicates that this most likely represents fluid (lower panel).*

pericardial process. Signal voids suggestive of pericardial effusion can represent either fluid, thickened fibrotic pericardium, or calcified pericardium, and techniques that emphasize the effects of flow should be used to differentiate the fluid from the abnormal pericardium. Distinguishing between fibrotic and calcified pericardium is not easy with this technique, and other imaging modalities that allow detection of a calcific process should be used when indicated. Small effusions cannot be reliably characterized because of the effect of cardiac motion. Similarly, larger effusions cannot be adequately characterized when using late spin-echo (long TE) imaging times. In addition, given heart rates of <150 beats per minute, characterization of exudative from hemorrhagic effusions is not reliable. However, MR imaging can be effectively used to detect effusions as small as 5 cc and to characterize specific types of fluid in larger effusions. These include differentiation of transudative, chylous, and exudative/hemorrhagic effusions.

References

1. Shabetai R: Function of the pericardium. In: Fowler NO, ed. *The Pericardium in Health and Disease*. Mount Kisco, NY: Futura Publishing Company, Inc.; 1985:19–20.
2. Holt JP: The normal pericardium. *Am J Cardiol* 1970;26:455–465.
3. Ishihara T, Ferrans VJ, Jones M, et al: Histologic and ultrastructural features of normal human parietal pericardium. *Am J Cardiol* 1980;46:744–753.
4. Ferrans VJ, Ishihara T, Roberts WC: Anatomy of the pericardium. In: Reddy PS, Leon DF, Schaver JA, eds. *Pericardial Disease*. New York: Raven Press; 1982:15–30.
5. Roberts WC, Spray TL: Pericardial heart disease: a study of its causes, consequences and morphologic features. In: Spodick D, ed. *Pericardial Diseases*. Philadelphia, PA; FA Davis Co; 1976:17.
6. Miller AJ: The lymphatics of the heart. *Arch Intern Med* 1964;112:501–511.
7. Stark DD, Higgins CB, Lanzer P, et al: Magnetic resonance imaging of the pericardium: normal and pathologic findings. *Radiology* 1984;150:469–474.
8. Sechtem U, Tscholakoff D, Higgins CB: MRI of the normal pericardium. *AJR* 1986;147:239–244.
9. Rokey R, Mulvagh SL, Cheirif J, et al: Lipomatous encasement and compression of the heart: antemortem diagnosis by cardiac nuclear magnetic resonance imaging and catheterization. *Am Heart J* 1989;117:952–953.
10. Roberts WC, Roberts JD: The floating heart or the heart too fat to sink: analysis of 55 necropsy patients. *Am J Cardiol* 1983;52:1286–1289.
11. Sechtem U, Tscholakoff D, Higgins CB: MRI of the abnormal pericardium. *AJR* 1986;147:245–252.
12. Brateman L: Chemical shift imaging: a review. *AJR* 1986;146:971–980.
13. Smith RC, Lange RC, McCarthy SM: Chemical shift artifact: dependence on shape and orientation of the lipid-water interface. *Radiology* 1991;181:225–229.
14. Rokey R, Vick GW, Bolli R, et al: Assessment of experimental pericardial effusion using nuclear magnetic resonance imaging techniques. *Am Heart J* 1991;121:1161–1169.
15. Stark DD, Higgins CB, Lanzer P, et al: Magnetic resonance imaging of the pericardium: normal and pathologic findings. *Radiology* 1984;150:469–474.
16. Agner RC, Gallis HA: Pericarditis-differential diagnostic considerations. *Arch Intern Med* 1979;139:407–412.
17. Soulen RL, Stark DD, Higgins CB: Magnetic resonance imaging of constrictive pericardial disease. *Am J Cardiol* 1985;55:480–484.
18. Mulvagh SL, Rokey R, Vick GW, et al: Usefulness of nuclear magnetic resonance imaging for evaluation of pericardial effusions, and comparison with two-dimensional echocardiography. *Am J Cardiol* 1989;64:1002–1009.
19. Hanock EW: On the rigid and elastic forms of constrictive pericarditis. *Am Heart J* 1980;100:917–923.
20. Wood P: Chronic constrictive pericarditis. *Am J Cardiol* 1961;7:48–61.
21. Hirschmann JV: Pericardial constriction. *Am Heart J* 1978;96:110–122.
22. Wendt RE, Rokey R, Wong Wai-Fan, et al: Nuclear magnetic resonance velocity measurements in small arteries: comparison with Doppler ultrasonic measurements in the aortas of normal rabbits (In Press).
23. Wendt RE, Wong Wai-Fan: Nuclear magnetic resonance velocity spectra of pulsatile flow in a rigid tube (In Press).

Chapter 3

Magnetic Resonance Imaging for the Evaluation of Intracardiac Masses and Thrombi

Udo Sechtem, MD, Peter Theissen, MD,
Hans-Josef Deutsch, MD,
and Markus Jungehülsing, MD

Cross-Sectional Imaging Techniques in the Diagnosis of Intracardiac Masses

The number and spectrum of intracardiac masses diagnosed in vivo has increased considerably since the introduction of modern noninvasive imaging techniques. Whereas in the past, the diagnosis had to be suspected clinically, transthoracic two-dimensional echocardiography (TTE) is now widely used in patients with nonspecific cardiac symptoms leading to identification of more and smaller tumors.

The challenge in patients with cardiac masses is to:

- identify or exclude a tumor
- demonstrate the exact localization, origin, size, extent, and hemodynamic implications of the tumor
- distinguish between malignant and benign tumors and between tumors and thrombi; differentiate primary from metastatic disease
- select the best therapeutic strategy.

Transthoracic two-dimensional echocardiography provides accurate assessment in the majority of patients with intracardiac masses.[1] Image quality, however, may be suboptimal and information about tissue composition is often not available. The

From Pohost GM (ed.), *Cardiovascular Applications of Magnetic Resonance*. Mount Kisco, NY, Futura Publishing Co., Inc., © 1993.

differentiation between myxoma and thrombus remains difficult. Moreover, depending on the acoustic properties of the tumor, even large masses located within the left atrium may not be apparent at TTE.[2] The limitations of TTE compared to transesophageal echocardiography (TEE) in detecting thrombi in the left atrial appendage, small and flat thrombi in the left atrium, thrombi and tumors in the superior vena cava, and masses attached to the right heart and the descending thoracic aorta have recently been described.[3] Computed tomography (CT) has also been used successfully to detect intracardiac masses.[4] However, CT requires the application of contrast material and the depiction of intracardiac structures is limited. Therefore, this technique has not gained widespread acceptance among cardiologists. Cine CT provides better delineation of the internal morphology of cardiac chambers, but the technique is not widely available and experience with cardiac tumors is limited.

Magnetic resonance imaging (MRI) is the latest imaging modality used in the diagnosis of cardiac masses. Its unique attributes, which include the large field of view, unlimited imaging planes, excellent soft tissue contrast, and intrinsic contrast between blood and myocardium, make MRI attractive for cardiac imaging. In this chapter, the use of MRI for the diagnosis of intracardiac tumors and thrombi will be reviewed and differential indications in comparison to other imaging techniques will be outlined.

Magnetic Resonance Imaging Protocol

With MRI, to achieve as much tissue differentiation as possible, dual spin-echo images (TE 30 and 60 msec) should be acquired. This will permit identification of lipomatous or angiomatous structures, whereas calcification is better diagnosed using gradient-echo MRI. However, CT is probably the most accurate technique for delineation of small calcifications.[5] In our experience, gradient-echo MRI is also superior for identifying small and mobile masses.

The choice of the imaging plane depends on the suspected localization of the mass, which in most instances has been previously diagnosed by echocardiography. Usually, the transverse plane provides the highest image quality and is well suited to demonstrate masses within the atria including the atrial appendages and paracardiac masses, which are most often located at the right, left, anterior, and posterior borders of the heart. Scans should be obtained from the level of the aortic arch down to the inferior wall of the ventricles. To optimize visualization of left ventricular thrombi, additional oblique sagittal and/or oblique transverse sections through the apex of the left ventricle should be obtained. Tumors in the right ventricular outflow tract or the great arteries should be imaged using additional straight sagittal and oblique sagittal planes, respectively. If tumorous structures lie parallel to the transverse plane, images should also be acquired in perpendicular planes, such as the sagittal or coronal plane. Depending on the number of scans necessary to answer the clinical question, examination time ranges from 30 to 90 minutes.

Intracardiac Tumors

Primary Intracardiac Tumors

Myxoma

Although most recent reports stress the limitations of TTE in the diagnosis of cardiac masses, this technique provides complete information in many patients with the most common cardiac tumor: atrial myxoma. In contrast to other cardiac tumors, Freedberg et al.[5] did not find any additional diagnostic benefit of MRI performed in four patients with a previous TTE diagnosis of atrial myxoma. This agrees with the findings of Mügge et al.[3] who reported a lack of additional information to TTE by TEE in 12 of their 15 myxoma patients. Tumor attachment to the interatrial septum was better delineated by TEE in the other 3 patients.

Administration of gadolinium-DTPA may help to distinguish between myxoma and thrombus. Schratter et al.[6] found that myxomas usually enhance after contrast application, whereas thrombi do not alter their signal intensity. However, it seems likely that similar enhancement could occur in old, vascularized left atrial thrombi.

In 12 patients with a left atrial myxoma, our own experience indicates that the presence of the mass, its size, and its attachments are clearly visualized on spin-echo magnetic resonance images in most patients. However, distinction of the mass from blood flow signal, which is sometimes present in the left atrium, especially when the myxoma causes some obstruction to left atrial outflow, may be difficult. In addition, volume averaging of flow signal and myxoma may result in spurious signal changes that are difficult to interpret. Gradient-echo images provide better delineation of the tumor and improve the visualization of calcifications that are easily distinguished due to their low signal intensity compared to the gray tumor and bright blood. In addition, gradient-echo images show tumor motion into the mitral valve plane (Figure 1) and depict valvular function as well as flow disturbances within the left atrium caused by tumor obstruction.

We compared the information provided by MRI with that provided by TTE in 12 patients. Eight patients also had TEE and 11 had angiocardiography. The diagnosis of myxoma could be made in all patients by TTE although image quality was very poor in 3. Magnetic resonance imaging provided superior images compared to TTE in 10 of 12 patients, which was helpful in identifying tumor composition and attachment. However, TEE image quality was considered superior to MRI in 5 of 8 patients, and was considered similar in the other 3 patients. The correct diagnosis was obtained in 10 of the 11 patients who underwent angiocardiography, although the diagnosis was clear before the procedure and the angiographer could tailor the procedure accordingly in all patients. This fact definitely contributed to the diagnostic success of angiocardiography because right ventricular or pulmonary injections with documentation of the levophase might have been omitted otherwise. In no patient was the tumor stalk visualized by angiocardiography. Due to the excellent images obtained at low cost, TEE must be considered the procedure of choice in patients with left atrial myxomas.

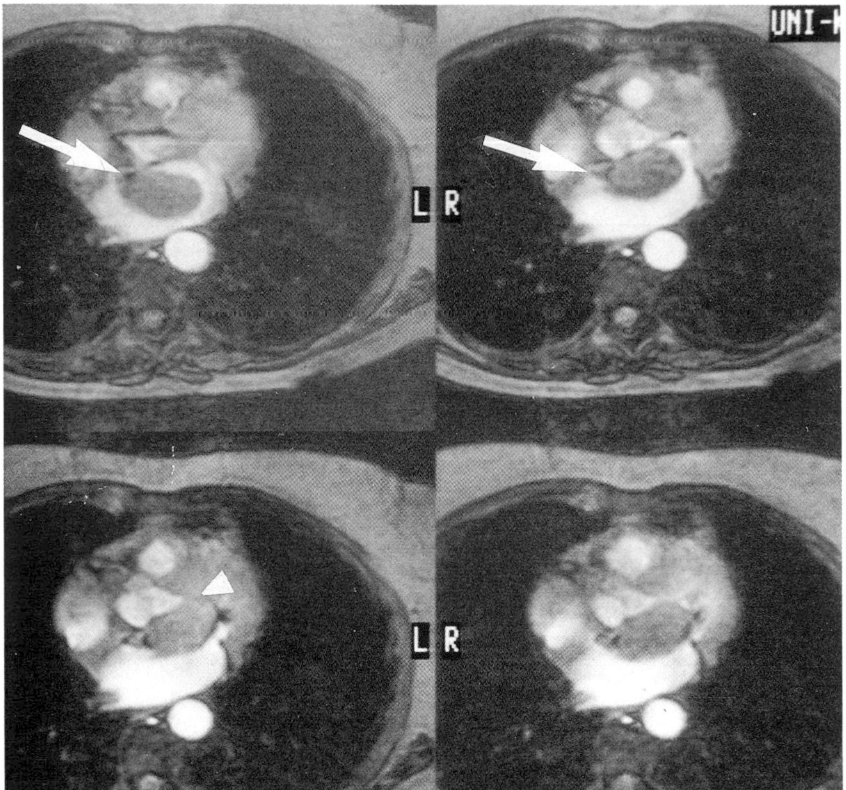

FIGURE 1. *Gradient-echo magnetic resonance images of a large left atrial myxoma.* **Upper left:** *End-diastolic image showing the tumor that has approximately the same signal intensity as the myocardium. The attachment to the interatrial septum is clearly seen (arrow). There is no connection to the anterior leaflet of the mitral valve.* **Upper right:** *Early diastole. Tumor moves into mitral valve plane.* **Lower left:** *Later in diastole. Tumor extends into the left ventricle and touches interventricular septum (arrowhead).* **Lower right:** *Mid-diastole.*

Other Primary Intracardiac Tumors

Primary tumors other than myxomas are exceedingly rare. Therefore, the experience with the MRI diagnosis of such masses is limited. Reports on the MRI diagnosis of angiosarcoma,[5,7,8] leiomyosarcoma,[9] lymphoma,[5,9] fibroma,[10,11] rhabdomyoma,[10] phaeochromocytoma,[12] lipoma,[13,14] and our own experience in eight patients with primary tumors indicate that MRI is highly accurate in achieving most of the diagnostic goals mentioned. In particular, MRI is well suited to localize the tumor and describe its relationship to normal intracardiac components and its extension to adjacent vascular and mediastinal structures.[5] This may be essential for determining surgical resectability of a tumor and planning of surgical intervention.[9]

Lipomatous intracardiac tumors (Figure 2) represent one condition where MRI can provide additional tissue diagnosis.[13] In lipomatous hypertrophy of the interatrial

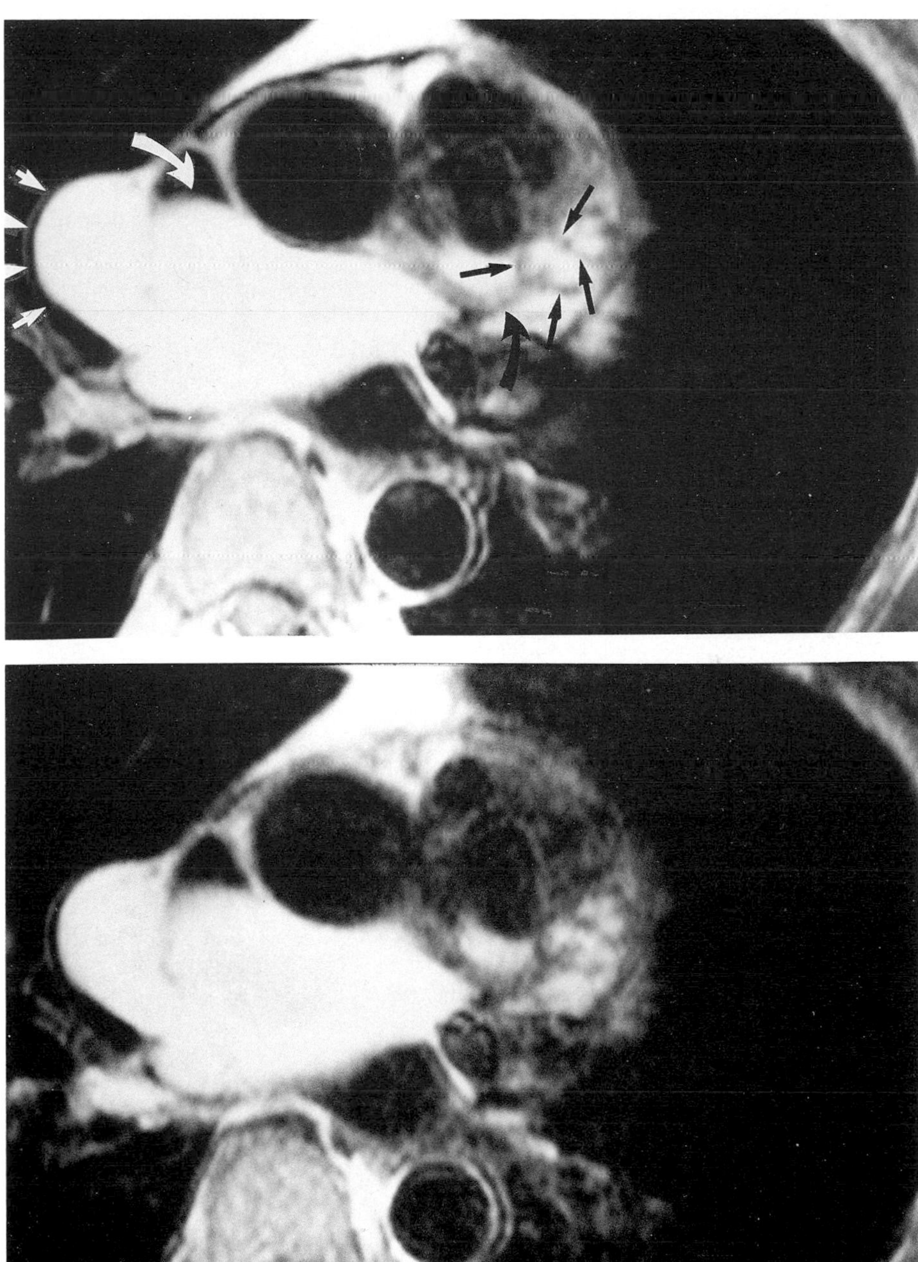

FIGURE 2. *Epicardial lipoma and coronary arteriovenous fistula between left anterior descending (LAD) and main pulmonary artery.* **Top:** *First spin-echo image (TE = 30 msec). The large, high signal intensity lipoma is clearly distinct from the pericardial space (small arrows). There is slight compression of the superior vena cava (curved arrow). Additional vascular structures (black arrows) arise from the left anterior descending artery (black curved arrow).* **Bottom:** *Second spin-echo image (TE = 60 msec). Unchanged signal intensity of tumor.*

septum, transverse magnetic resonance images typically show a thickened and bulging interatrial septum that has high signal intensity on both first and second echo images. Signal intensity is similar to pericardial and thoracic fat. Computed tomography can also identify fat as low-radiodensity lesions.[13,15] In contrast, fat cannot be routinely differentiated from myxoma or other tumors by ultrasound on the basis of the texture of reflected echoes. Only if the classic appearance of a bilobed mass sparing the fossa ovalis is present can TTE suggest the correct diagnosis. Magnetic resonance imaging may also be able to make the correct histologic diagnosis in angiomatous tumors because of the typical appearance of large, tortuous vascular structures (Figure 2).[9,10] Low signal intensity calcifications are easier to identify on gradient-echo magnetic resonance images than on spin-echo images because they can be better distinguished from high-intensity blood and myocardium (Figure 3). However, CT seems to be more sensitive in the identification of small calcifications.

True histologic diagnosis cannot be provided by MRI because different histologies may show similar magnetic resonance relaxation times resulting in identical signal intensities of tumors. Although signal enhancement of the tumor after gadolinium-DTPA (Figure 4) gives some clues to its vascularization, this sign is nonspecific and does not aid in the distinction between benign and malignant lesions. Therefore, benign lesions cannot be consistently distinguished from malignant ones on the basis

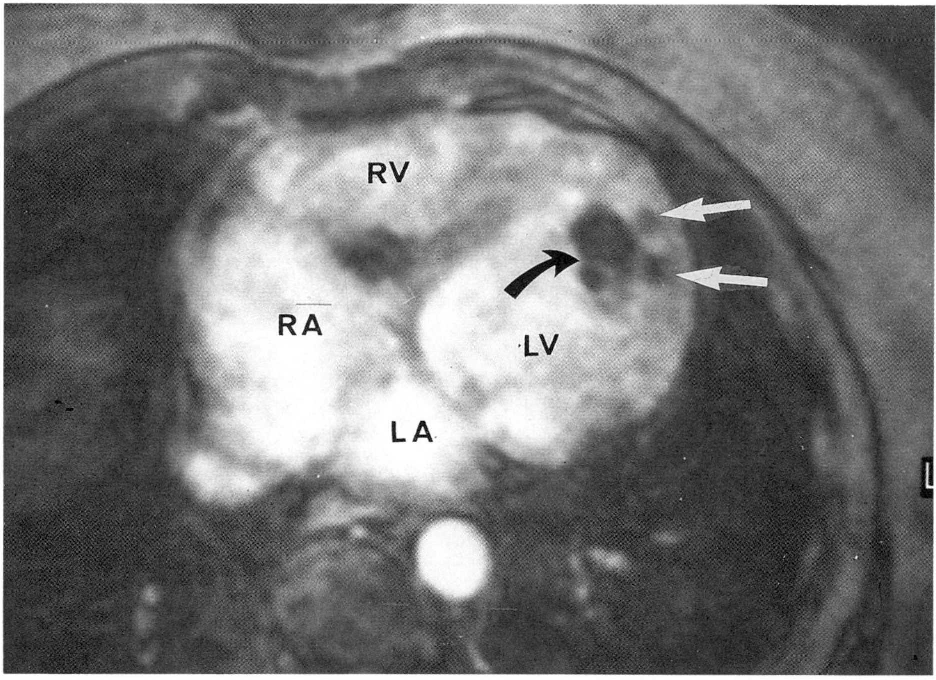

FIGURE 3. *Early systolic gradient-echo image in a patient with calcified endomyocardial fibrosis. Large calcifications are clearly seen as areas of low signal intensity within the left ventricular cavity (curved arrow). There is some infiltration of the myocardium by calcific deposits (white arrows). LA, left atrium; LV, left ventricle; RA, right atrium; RV, right ventricle.*

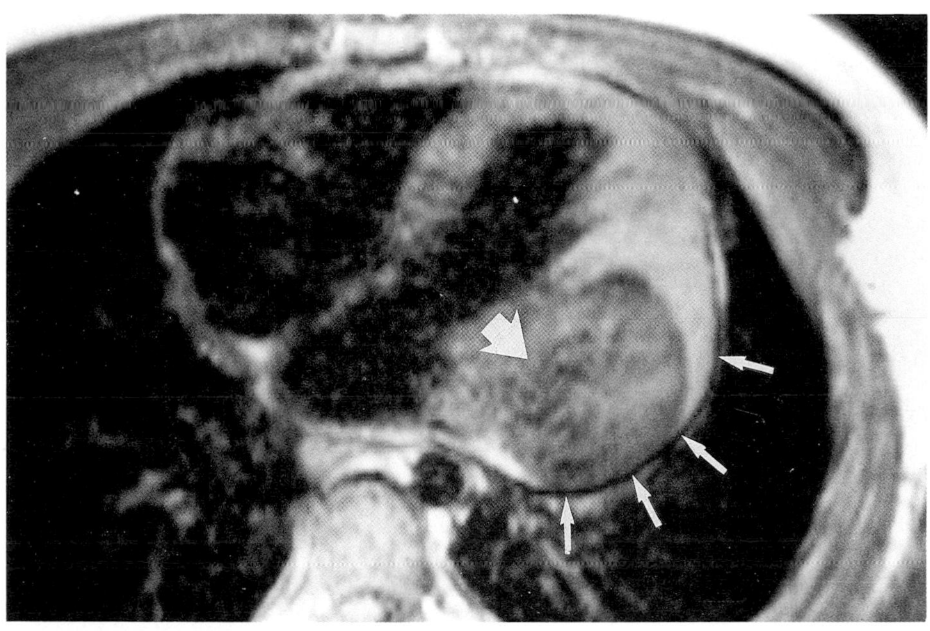

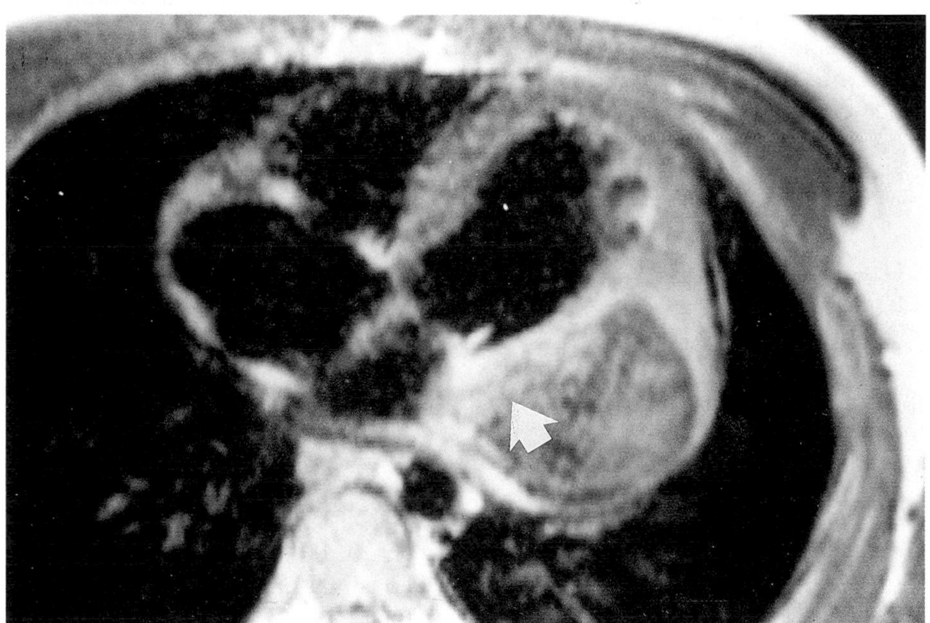

FIGURE 4. *Large fibroma located laterally to the left ventricle and left atrium.* **Top**: *First spin-echo image (TE=30 msec) before gadolinium-DTPA. The fibrous tumor tissue (large arrow) has lower signal intensity than myocardium. The tumor is clearly distinguished from the pericardium (small arrows) and abuts the left atrial wall, the mitral ring area, and parts of the left ventricular myocardium. At surgery, the potential large defect created by tumor removal made complete resection impossible.* **Bottom**: *After gadolinium-DTPA there is partial enhancement of parts of the tumor (arrow). This section is located a few millimeters lower than in the top panel.*

of tissue characteristics alone. Nevertheless, the combination of signal characteristics, morphology, and the clinical picture allows a correct diagnosis to be made in many instances.

The detection of intramural rhabdomyomas in children with tuberous sclerosis may be more difficult with MRI than with TTE.[10] In these patients, rhabdomyomas of <0.5-cm diameter bulging into the cardiac cavities may be missed by MRI, but diagnosed by TTE.[10] The reported echocardiographic findings were not independently verified.

Cardiac Metastases

Cardiac metastases are approximately 20 to 40 times more frequent than primary cardiac neoplasms. In some patients, early diagnosis may lead to the institution of specific therapy. Although TTE allows the diagnosis of metastatic disease in some patients,[16] many echocardiographers prefer TEE for more accurate depiction of these lesions.

Magnetic resonance imaging may have a complementary role in defining the extent of metastatic disease in patients with suspect echocardiographic findings. The field of view is considerably larger than that of TEE, which may be advantageous for the detection of bronchogenic carcinoma or additional metastases of melanoma, both of which cause the majority of cardiac metastases in males. In a patient with metastatic malignant fibrous histiocytoma, only MRI revealed the full extent of infiltration into the myocardium. This allowed preoperative planning of palliative surgery rather than finding the lesion unresectable at the time of surgery.[17] Magnetic resonance imaging is particularly useful to delineate the involvement of the pericardium by tumor and identify tumor extension into the pericardium in paracardiac neoplasms.

One of the strengths of MRI in metastatic cardiac masses is its ability to simultaneously depict tumor origin. This has been documented in renal cell carcinomas[5,18] that often extend to the right atrium after invasion of the renal vein. Because of its multiplanar capabilities, MRI can depict abdominal and thoracic tumor involvement in a single image. However, as with primary tumors, MRI cannot provide a histologic diagnosis of tumor composition.

Comparative Studies of MRI and TTE

Lund et al.[9] demonstrated that MRI provided additional diagnostic information affecting clinical management or surgical planning in 53 (87%) of 61 patients with suspected cardiac tumors or paracardiac masses; 51 patients had TTE previously. The primary contribution of MRI in these patients was not to obtain a tissue diagnosis, but rather to delineate the anatomical extent of the tumor and to aid in treatment planning. Freedberg et al.[5] emphasized that TTE remains the procedure of choice in the initial evaluation of cardiac tumors. Transthoracic two-dimensional echocardiography is widely available, can be performed at the bedside, is noninvasive and harmless, is not time consuming, and is not expensive. In this study, MRI expanded TTE findings in

10 of 14 patients, mainly in those patients with poor TTE studies and patients with extracardiac tumor extension.

In another smaller study, MRI provided information additional to TTE in only 2 of 8 patients with cardiac masses.[19] Magnetic resonance imaging did not improve on the diagnosis provided by TTE in any of the 6 patients with intracavitary lesions. On the contrary, TTE real-time imaging was superior to MRI in depicting tumor attachment and its interference with atrioventricular valves. In this study, however, only static spin-echo images were used.

In our clinical experience, pericardial involvement by tumor is better identified or excluded by MRI than by TTE or CT. This is due to more accurate and more complete visualization of the pericardium, as compared to TTE, and better soft tissue contrast compared to CT. There are several anatomical structures that can be misinterpreted as a tumor by echocardiography such as a prominent eustachian valve, abnormally located papillary muscles, or prominent epicardial fat. In these patients, MRI has been helpful in excluding intracardiac tumors. Information provided by MRI may also be useful in deciding against surgery if tumors can be unequivocally identified as either benign or too far advanced to be resectable. Magnetic resonance imaging is often of diagnostic value in patients with technically suboptimal TTE studies. However, to date it is unclear as to whether TEE would be able to provide similar information to MRI at a lower cost.

The limitations of MRI include difficulty in examining acutely ill patients and nondiagnostic image quality in some patients with cardiac arrhythmias or irregular breathing patterns. Examination times may become longer than 1 hour if additional multiplane gradient-echo images have to be obtained. Finally, MRI is more expensive than echocardiographic studies.

In the future, it can be expected that cardiologists will become aware of limitations of transthoracic echocardiography and TEE will become more widespread for better delineation of intracardiac masses. However, TEE still has a limited field of view and MRI (or CT) should be used as complementary techniques if extracardiac tumor extension or intramural growth is suspected. Magnetic resonance imaging has the unique advantage of being able to visualize both the heart and surrounding structures, whereas CT does not provide high-quality images of the internal cardiac morphology. Moreover, MRI is almost examiner-independent, which may be helpful in follow-up studies.

Cardiac Thrombi

Left Atrial Thrombi

Atrial thrombi are easily detected on spin-echo and gradient-echo magnetic resonance images.[6,7] However, there are no systematic comparative studies between TTE and MRI. It is conceivable that MRI will not be able to provide a higher diagnostic accuracy than TEE, which has become the technique of choice for the diagnosis of left atrial thrombi, especially those located in the left atrial appendage.[3]

Left Ventricular Thrombi

Transthoracic two-dimensional echocardiography has been the principal imaging modality for the diagnosis of left ventricular thrombi. However, the low specificity of TTE is a well-known problem[20] and the cardiac apex cannot be adequately examined. Transesophageal echocardiography does not improve the diagnostic capabilities of ultrasound because visualization of the apical area of the left ventricle is also not possible.

The sensitivity and specificity of imaging techniques that can be used for the diagnosis of left ventricular thrombi such as TTE, angiocardiography, CT, and spin-echo MRI was recently compared in patients with chronic anterior myocardial infarcts.[21] In all patients, the diagnosis was verified at left ventricular aneurysmectomy. In contrast to CT and MRI, one (4%) angiographic and six (24%) echocardiographic studies were technically inadequate for assessment. Sensitivity of all four techniques in patients with adequate studies was similar for all imaging techniques and ranged from 80% for CT to 93% for MRI. Specificity was 70% for angiography and TTE, 85% for MRI, and 100% for CT. If technically inadequate studies were included, the correct diagnosis was provided by TTE in only 15 of 25 (60%) patients. Hence, MRI or CT examinations should be considered in patients in whom thrombus is suspected and who cannot be adequately examined by TTE.

Interpretation of spin-echo magnetic resonance images is sometimes complicated by the presence of intraventricular flow signal due to stagnant blood within the aneurysm. Although slow flow usually increases in signal intensity from first to second spin-echo images and thrombus intensity decreases, this behavior is not sufficiently consistent to always distinguish both entities with certainty.[22] Moreover, the mobility of thrombi cannot be appreciated using spin-echo imaging.

The diagnostic capabilities of MRI are further enhanced by the introduction of gradient-echo MRI.[22] Contrast between bright blood and lower intensity thrombus is more consistent (Figure 5) and review of magnetic resonance images in a closed cine loop facilitates identification of hypokinetic or akinetic myocardium with adjacent thrombotic material and permits assessment of thrombus motion. Therefore, if MRI is only applied to detect thrombi at a prespecified site, gradient-echo MRI seems to be the technique of choice. However, spin-echo MRI provides a fast overview of cardiac anatomy, and may therefore be of additional use if the extent of the infarcted area is not yet known and time consuming gradient-echo imaging of the entire left ventricle would be necessary to obtain this information.

Small and highly mobile thrombi may be more difficult to visualize by gradient-echo MRI than by real-time TTE. Such thrombi move slightly differently from cardiac cycle to cardiac cycle, which may result in blurring on magnetic resonance images because they are collected from several cardiac cycles. However, MRI is undoubtedly superior to echocardiography for the detection of broad-based, laminar apical thrombi that are more common than pedunculated mobile ones.

Transthoracic two-dimensional echocardiography will remain the primary imaging technique to screen patients with left ventricular aneurysms because of its low cost and real-time imaging. However, in patients with low-quality echocardiograms, MRI represents a noninvasive, accurate second line technique; its diagnostic capabilities are further enhanced by the application of gradient-echo sequences in patients with suspected intraventricular thrombus.

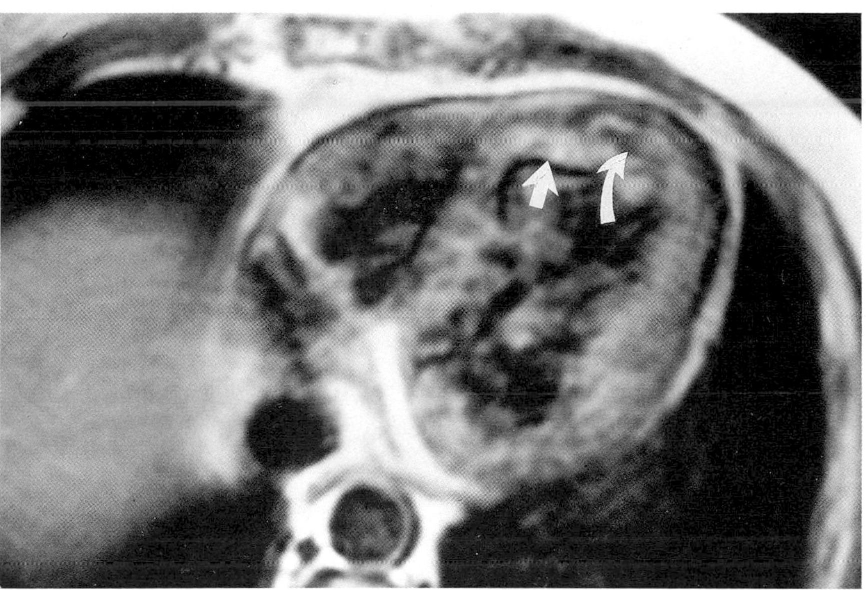

FIGURE 5A. *First spin-echo (TE = 30 msec) transverse image of a patient with left ventricular aneurysm and laminar thrombus. A part of the thrombus (curved arrow) has slightly lower signal intensity than myocardium and can be distinguished from slowly flowing blood (arrow) that has higher signal intensity. However, the remaining intraventricular, normally flowing blood appears slightly darker than thrombus. Reprinted from Reference 22 with permission.*

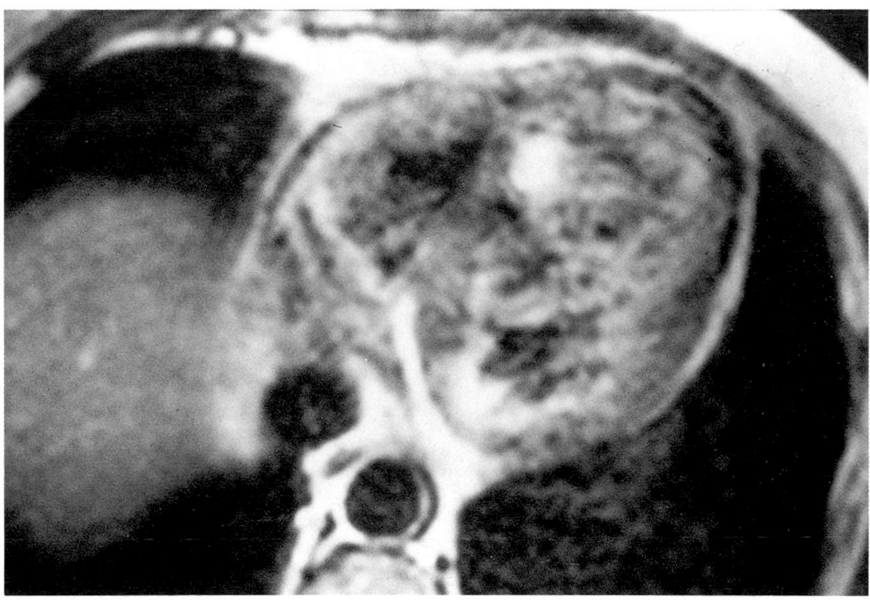

FIGURE 5B. *Second spin-echo (TE = 60 msec) transverse image in the same patient as in Figure 5A. In this image, identification of thrombus was not possible because of prominent flow artifacts. Reprinted from Reference 22 with permission.*

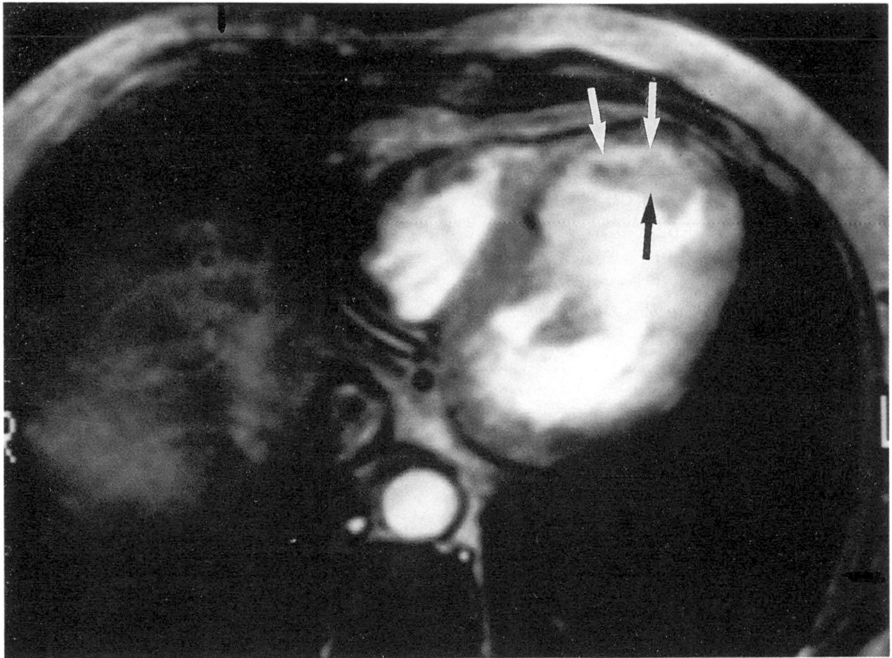

FIGURE 5C. *Transverse gradient-echo magnetic resonance image in the same patient as in Figure 5A; thrombus outlines are more clearly defined due to high contrast between blood and thrombus. Thrombus (black arrow) and myocardium, which have similar signal intensity on this image, can be differentiated because of a thin line of blood (small arrows) interposed between these two structures. Reprinted from Reference 22 with permission.*

References

1. Fyke FE, Seward JB, Edwards WD, et al: Primary cardiac tumors: experience with 30 consecutive patients since the introduction of two-dimensional echocardiography. *J Am Coll Cardiol* 1985;5:1465–1473.
2. Come PC, Riley MF, Markis JE, et al: Limitations of echocardiographic techniques in evaluation of left atrial masses. *Am J Cardiol* 1981;48:947–953.
3. Mügge A, Daniel WG, Haverich A, et al: Diagnosis of noninfective cardiac mass lesions by two-dimensional echocardiography. Comparison of the transthoracic and transesophageal approaches. *Circulation* 1991;83:70–78.
4. Gross BH, Glayer GM, Francis IR: CT of intracardiac and intrapericardial masses. *AJR* 1983;140:903–907.
5. Freedberg RS, Kronzon I, Rumanick WM, et al: The contribution of magnetic resonance imaging to the evaluation of intracardiac tumors diagnosed by echocardiography. *Circulation* 1988;77:96–103.
6. Schratter M, Mayr H, Tscholakoff D, et al: MRT mit Gd-DTPA in der Diagnostik tumoröser und pseudotumoröser intrakardialer Raumforderungen. *Fortschr Röntgenstr* 1990;152:16–22.
7. Gomes AS, Lois JF, Child JS, et al: Cardiac tumors and thrombus: evaluation with MR imaging. *AJR* 1987;149:895–899.

8. Dichek DA, Holmvang G, Fallon JT, et al: Angiosarcoma of the heart: three year survival and follow-up by nuclear magnetic resonance imaging. *Am Heart J* 1988;115:1323–1324.
9. Lund JT, Ehman RL, Julsrud PR, et al: Cardiac masses: assessment by MR imaging. *AJR* 1989;152:469–473.
10. Rienmüller R, Lloret JL, Tiling R, et al: MR imaging of pediatric cardiac tumors previously diagnosed by echocardiography. *J Comput Assist Tomogr* 1989;13:621–626.
11. Amparo EG, Higgins CB, Farmer D, et al: Gated MRI of cardiac and paracardiac masses: initial experience. *AJR* 1984;143:1151–1156.
12. Kawasuji M, Matsunaga Y, Iwa T: Cardiac phaeochromocytoma of the interatrial septum. *Eur J Cardiothorac Surg* 1989;3:175–177.
13. Kamiya H, Ohno M, Iwata H, et al: Cardiac lipoma in the interventricular septum: evaluation by computed tomography and magnetic resonance imaging. *Am Heart J* 1990;119:1215–1217.
14. Kaplan KR, Rifkin MD: MR diagnosis of lipomatous infiltration of the interatrial septum. *AJR* 1989;153:495–496.
15. Levine RA, Weyman AE, Dinsmore RE, et al: Noninvasive tissue characterization: diagnosis of lipomatous hypertrophy of the interatrial septum by nuclear magnetic resonance imaging. *J Am Coll Cardiol* 1986;7:688–692.
16. Lestuzzi C, Biasi S, Nicolosi GL, et al: Secondary neoplastic infiltration of the myocardium diagnosed by two-dimensional echocardiography in seven cases with anatomic confirmation. *J Am Coll Cardiol* 1987;9:439–445.
17. Lee R, Fisher MR: MR imaging of cardiac metastases from malignant fibrous histiocytoma. *J Comput Assist Tomogr* 1989;13:126–128.
18. Gindea AJ, Gentin B, Naidich DP, et al: Unusual cardiac metastasis in hypernephroma: the complemental role of echocardiography and magnetic resonance imaging. *Am Heart J* 1988;116:1359–1361.
19. Casolo F, Biasi S, Balzarini L, et al: MRI as an adjunct to echocardiography for the diagnostic imaging of cardiac masses. *Eur J Radiol* 1988;8:226–230.
20. Visser CA, Kan G, David GK, et al: Two dimensional echocardiography in the diagnosis of left ventricular thrombus. A prospective study of 67 patients with anatomic validation. *Chest* 1983;83:228–232.
21. Sechtem U, Theissen P, Heindel W, et al: Comparison of magnetic resonance imaging, computed tomography, echocardiography, and angiography in the diagnosis of left ventricular thrombi. *Am J Cardiol* 1989;64:1195–1199.
22. Jungehülsing M, Sechtem U, Theissen P, et al: Left ventricular thrombi: evaluation with spin-echo and gradient-echo MR imaging. *Radiology* 1992;182:225–230.

Chapter 4

Magnetic Resonance Imaging for the Evaluation of Myocardial Disease

Kerry M. Link, MD,
Steve P. Loehr, BA,
and Nadja M. Lesko, MD

Magnetic resonance imaging (MRI) has proved to be extremely useful for the evaluation of the entire spectrum of myocardial disease. It is an entirely noninvasive and nonionizing technique that does not depend on traditional contrast agents. Its multiplanar capabilities make MRI essentially a three-dimensional imaging technique. Perhaps its greatest strength is its ability to show the inherent contrast between the intracardiac cavities and the surrounding cardiovascular structures. This contrast results in sharp delineation between the cardiac chambers, the myocardium, the pericardium, and surrounding fat.

The technique was initially used for the depiction of anatomical abnormalities affecting the myocardium and pericardium. Through the use of various pulse sequences, gross qualitative tissue characterization was possible. With the advent of dynamic or cine MRI, assessment of normal physiology and pathophysiology of the myocardium is now routine. Truly quantitative measurements of contraction dynamics, infarction size, and volumetric data give MRI clear advantages over angiography and echocardiography.

This chapter will review the role of MRI in the evaluation of both anatomical and physiologic abnormalities of the myocardium.

Techniques

For anatomical assessment of the myocardium, ECG-gated multislice spin echo is routinely performed. Imaging planes will vary depending on the abnormality and its

From Pohost GM (ed.), *Cardiovascular Applications of Magnetic Resonance*. Mount Kisco, NY, Futura Publishing Co., Inc., © 1993.

location. Two important imaging planes are the long-and short-axis views of the heart. The long-axis view unfolds the spiral nature of the interventricular spectrum and overcomes the problem of foreshortening of the myocardium, which is associated with the transverse plane. Additionally, the long-axis view demonstrates the continuity of the aortic and mitral valves and their relationship to the left ventricular outflow tract (Figure 1). This view has proven very useful in assessing the anterior mitral valve leaflet in asymmetrical hypertrophic cardiomyopathies. The short-axis view is important in assessing systolic wall thickening (SWT) and the overall contraction dynamics of the myocardium (Figure 2). Because the myocardium advances toward the cardiac base during its clockwise corkscrew contraction cycle, the myocardium visualized at one portion of the cardiac cycle may not be in plane at other phases. This becomes

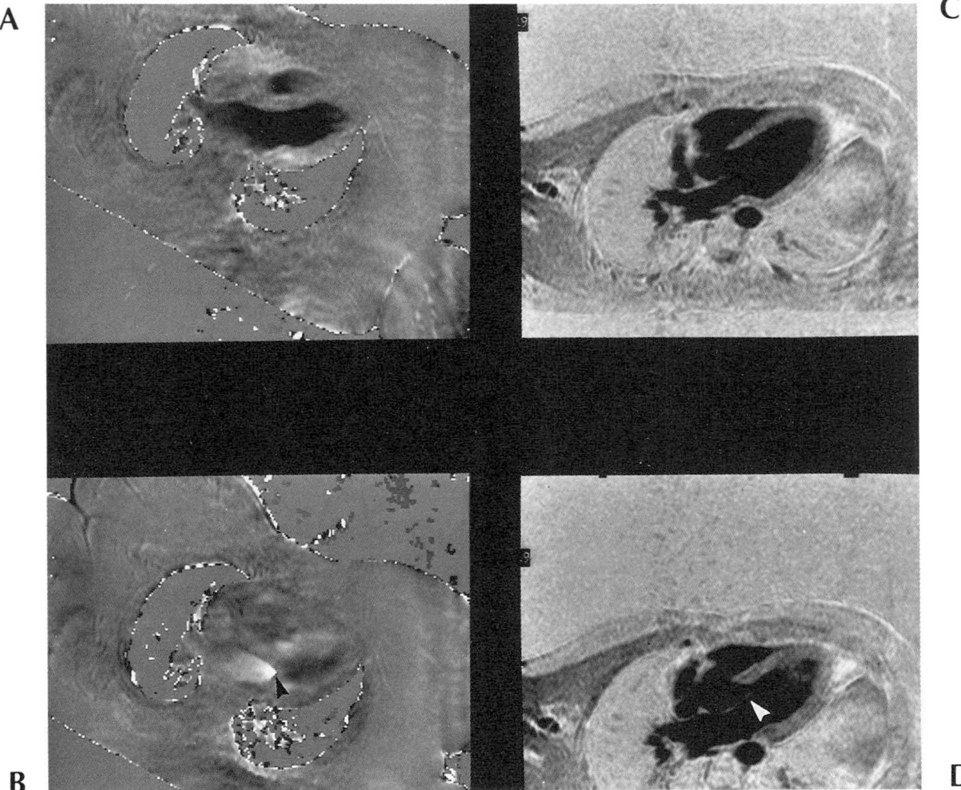

FIGURE 1. A *and* **B:** *Phase map through the midaspect of the heart performed in the long-axis plane during diastole (A) and systole (B). The black signal in the left atrium and left ventricle (A) demonstrates diastolic filling of the left ventricle. The white signal within the left atrium (B) represents mitral regurgitation (black arrow) in a patient with papillary infarction.* **C** *and* **D:** *"Black blood" cine MRI performed in long-axis view in late diastole (C) and early diastole (D) demonstrating the relationship of the anterior leaflet (white arrow) of the mitral valve to the left ventricular outflow tract.*

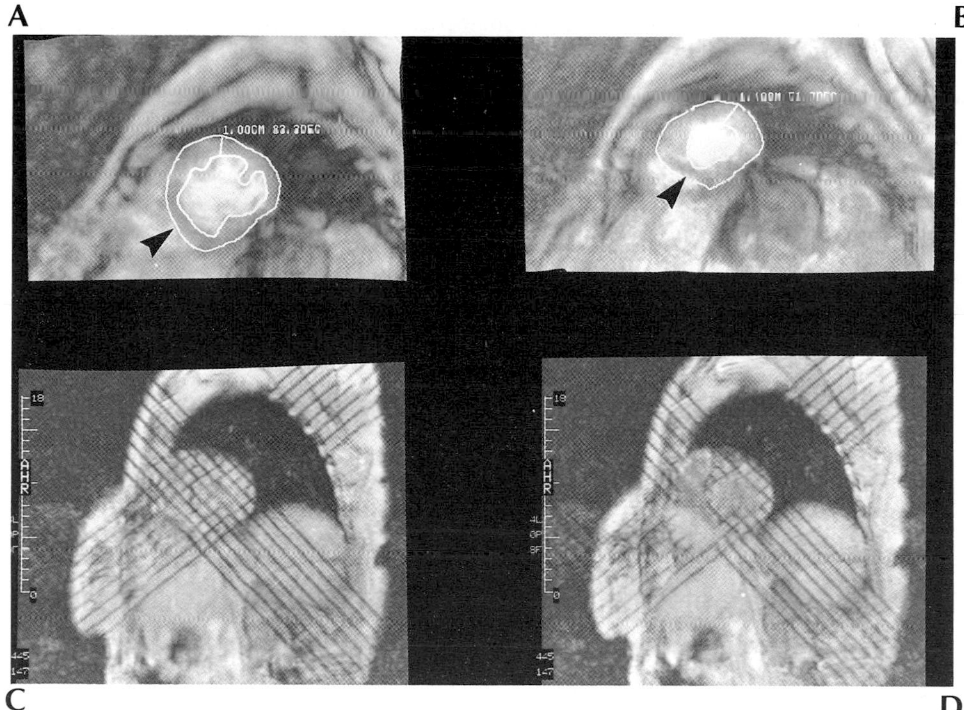

FIGURE 2. **A** *and* **B:** *ECG-referenced cine MRI obtained in the midaspect of the ventricles. Planimetry from end diastole (A) and end systole (B) are used to calculate volumes and to quantify SWT. There is thinning of the distal septum with abnormal thickening (arrow) in this patient with acute MI.* **C** *and* **D:** *Short-axis myocardial tagging study in diastole (C) and systole (D). The grid lines tagged to blood within both ventricles "disappear" as blood is ejected from the cavities.*

more of a problem with quantitative "tagging" techniques, but not with the qualitative assessment of overall contraction dynamics.

Dynamic MRI of the myocardium may be thought of as a continuum of techniques that range from qualitative to quantitative assessment. These techniques acquire images of the same slice at various phases of the cardiac cycle. Temporal resolution will vary depending upon the patient's R-R interval and the software capabilities of the various manufacturers. These techniques collectively are acquired in a more rapid fashion than spin-echo sequences.[1] They rely on short TE and TR and use short or narrow flip (or tip) angles on the order of 30°. Because the TR is shorter than the patient's R-R interval, it is not strictly ECG-gated. Data are acquired and then reordered according to a reference point in the cardiac cycle. They are, therefore, ECG-referenced techniques similar to dynamic nuclear cardiology examinations. On the whole, with these techniques the blood assumes a high signal and appears white. The blood can be made to appear black through the use of saturation slabs (Figure 1). Cine or gradient refocused echo MRI allows for the qualitative assessment of both blood flow and wall dynamics (eg, determination of hypokinesia, akinesia, and dyskinesia). Through planimetry, volumetric data and quantitative assessment of

SWT can be obtained (Figure 2). Phase mapping or velocity mapping MRI quantitatively assesses blood flow[2] and very recently has been used to quantitatively assess myocardial motion.[3] The information gathered during a magnetic resonance examination consists of an amplitude or magnitude component as well as a phase component. The former is used to form the anatomical (static or dynamic) images. The latter is actually a measurement of the motion of a hydrogen proton ($H+$) over time, and therefore, provides information regarding the velocity of blood or the motion of a piece of myocardium during the cardiac cycle (Figure 1). The last dynamic technique commonly used is that known as myocardial tagging.[4] Saturation stripes or grids are placed on the myocardium (and blood) in diastole (Figure 2). As the heart contracts, these strips or grids "stick" to the myocardium (or blood) it was originally "tagged" to and allows for assessment of the stress and torque that the myocardium undergoes. (Because blood exits the imaging planes very quickly these tags "disappear.")

Cardiomyopathy

The ability of MRI to directly visualize the endocardial and epicardial surfaces of the myocardium allows for accurate assessment of cardiomyopathic processes. This is especially true using the long-and short-axis views. Functional analysis, both qualitative and quantitative, is possible with the dynamic techniques. Tissue characterization can also play a role in assessing the infiltrative cardiomyopathies.

Hypertrophic Cardiomyopathy

Hypertrophic cardiomyopathy as described by Teare in 1958 is a disorder of unknown etiology resulting in varying degrees of myocardial hypertrophy and associated encroachment on ventricular cavity size. There is no ventricular dilatation; however, there is significant myocardial fiber disarray. There is a broad spectrum of the extent and severity of myocardial involvement. The most common form of hypertrophic cardiomyopathy is an asymmetrical variant that involves the hypertrophy of the left ventricular outflow portion of the interventricular septum (Figure 3). There may be asymmetrical involvement of the apex of the midseptal segment or free walls (Figure 3). There is a symmetrical type that involves the entire septum and free wall but does not involve the apex (Figure 3). An autosomal dominant or familial inheritance pattern has been suggested.[5] All forms result in decreased diastolic compliance and, therefore, restricted left ventricular filling. With or without subaortic outflow obstruction cardiac failure is the end result.

Magnetic resonance imaging is quite accurate in delineating the location and extent of the cardiomyopathic process, regardless of the type or severity.[6,7] The long-axis view is perhaps best suited to studying the various types of hypertrophic cardiomyopathies. No significant relaxation abnormalities are noted with hypertrophic cardiomyopathy using T_1 and T_2 relaxations parameters.[8] Therefore, hypertrophic cardiomyopathy is an anatomical diagnosis when using spin-echo MRI.

Compared to other imaging modalities used in the evaluation of hypertrophic

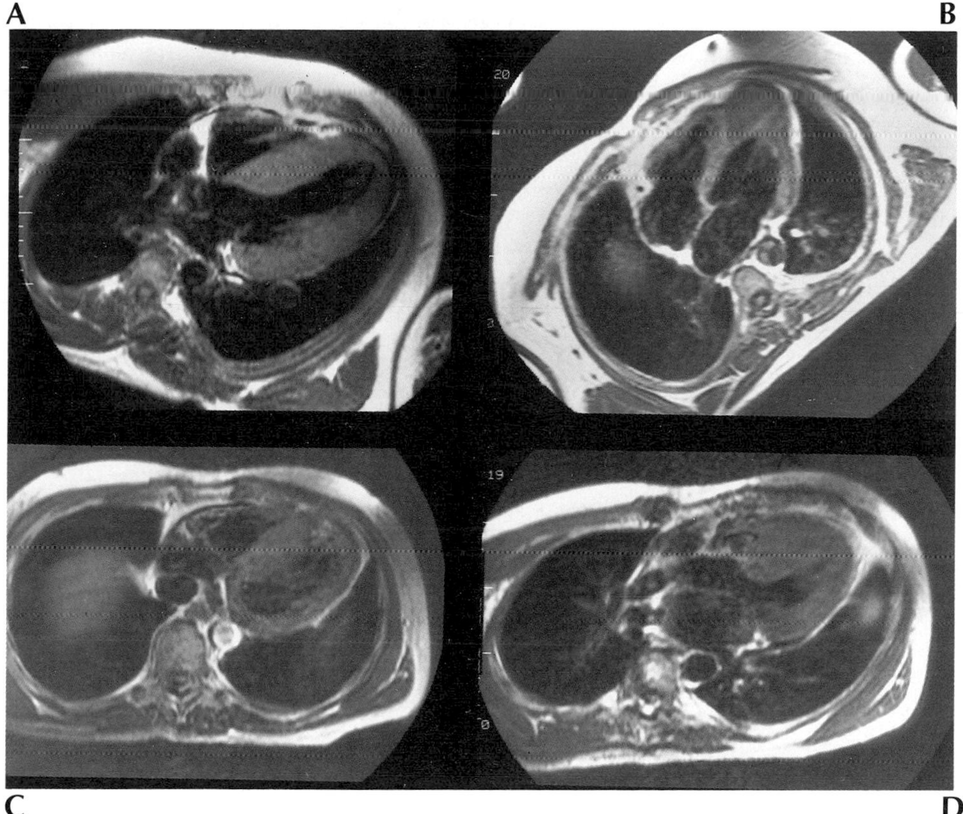

FIGURE 3. *Hypertrophic cardiomyopathy. Long-axis, ECG-gated spin-echo MRI of* (**A**) *symmetric,* (**B**) *apical,* (**C**)) *midseptal, and* (**D**) *subaortic hypertrophic cardiomyopathy. The images were obtained in mid- to end diastole.*

cardiomyopathy, MRI appears superior and maintains impressive advantages. These include: 1) no artifacts from calcium deposition (possible in hypertrophic cardiomyopathy) that may appear on radiographs or computed tomography (CT); 2) a high accuracy in calculating ventricular volumes despite large papillary muscles, which may hinder the ability to precisely assess the volume on ventriculography; and 3) a larger field-of-view than two-dimensional echocardiography.

Additionally, using dynamic techniques impaired SWT and global or regional or altered contraction dynamics can be assessed with MRI, a clear advantage over angiography and echocardiography.[9,10] With the newer velocity mapping techniques, pressure gradients across regions of midseptal or apical hypertrophic cardiomyopathy can be obtained using a modified Bernoulli's equation $\Delta P = 4v^2$ ($v = m/sec$). Associated mitral valve regurgitation can be identified by a signal void on cine MRI or by reversal of flow using phase mapping (Figure 1).[11]

Left ventricular hypertrophy is a concentric hypertrophy of the left ventricle (LV) due to an underlying systemic process such as hypertension or aortic valvular stenosis. There is not only concentric hypertrophy of the myocardium but also of the papillary muscles. Unlike the symmetrical form of hypertrophic cardiomyopathy the ventricular apex is also hypertrophied in left ventricular hypertrophy, as well as the trabecular conus cordis. Endocardial fibrous thickening may be present. Left ventricular volume is also decreased.[12]

With left ventricular hypertrophy both SWT and overall contract dynamics are essentially the same as in normal individuals. In hypertrophic cardiomyopathy, although absolute SWT is normal, the percent SWT is markedly decreased within the hypertrophic segment. This can easily be evaluated in either the long- or short-axis views using white or black blood cine MRI or myocardial tagging techniques.

Furthermore, advances have been made in the evaluation of tissue characterization methods using MRI. These methods involve the differentiation of the tissue qualities of hypertrophied versus normal tissue. On visual inspection, hypertrophic myocardial tissue reveals an inhomogeneous signal intensity pattern, with low signal intensity zones interspersed intramyocardially. Normal myocardial tissue displays a smooth increase in signal intensity from endocardium to midwall and then a decrease smoothly outward with no apparent area of interspersed low signal. It has been reported that this effect can be measured using tissue heterogeneous indexes derived from images processed with semiautomatic edge detection and a tissue characterization algorithm. It appears that as the degree of hypertrophy increased, there was a statistically significant rise in the tissue heterogeneous indexes.[13]

Magnetic resonance imaging can, therefore, identify the presence and extent of the various forms of hypertrophic cardiomyopathies as well as qualify and quantitate their associated pathophysiologic consequences. Differentiation of concentric hypertrophic cardiomyopathy from left ventricular hypertrophy is possible through evaluation of the apex SWT and tissue characterization.

Restrictive Cardiomyopathy

Both restrictive cardiomyopathy and constrictive pericarditis have similar clinical presentations and are difficult to differentiate. This is an important distinction as the latter can be improved or cured by a pericardiectomy.

With restrictive cardiomyopathy there is usually hypertrophy of both the right and left ventricles as well as marked dilatation of the right atrium (RA) and inferior vena cava (IVC). The pericardium is not thickened.

In constrictive pericarditis, the pericardium is thickened (>2 mm) and the ventricles are small and have a tubular shape. There is usually no evidence of hypertrophy. Due to the constriction of the ventricles, the RA and IVC may be dilated.

With its multiplanar format, MRI can readily display the associated anatomical abnormalities of either disease process on spin-echo images.[14]

Cine MRI can graphically display any associated atrioventricular regurgitation in either entity as well as the normal SWT. A delayed diastolic filling pattern is associated with restrictive cardiomyopathy. This is in contrast to constrictive pericarditis in which there is an abrupt termination of late diastolic filling.[15]

Dilated Cardiomyopathy

Magnetic resonance imaging has real advantages over both echocardiography and ventriculography in the evaluation of dilated cardiomyopathy. Due to the marked dilatation of the ventricular chamber it may be difficult to see the entire structure with echocardiography or to completely opacify it with contrast.

Spin-echo MRI nicely demonstrates the dilated LV as well as the thinning of the interventricular septum. Overall functional analysis including volumetric data and wall-motion analysis is easily accomplished with cine MRI. There have been no specific changes in T_1 and T_2 relaxation times to characterize dilated cardiomyopathy.[8] Using a short-axis view, end-systolic meridional wall stress of the LV can be determined and has been found to be significantly elevated in cases of dilated cardiomyopathy.[6]

Infiltrative Diseases

Unlike the other cardiomyopathies, tissue characterization plays a more important role in assessing infiltrative processes of the myocardium. Areas of edema secondary to viral myocarditis or sarcoidosis will result in focal regions of increased myocardial signal on T_2 images.[16] It must be remembered that artifactual signal increase may be induced by motion artifact and can result in false-positives. In addition to an increase in myocardial signal, Fabry's disease and amyloidosis are also associated with global ventricular hypertrophy.[17]

Myocardial Tumors

Spin-echo MRI is excellent in identifying the existence and extent of myocardial tumors. With cine MRI, the physiologic consequences of tumors, whether there is obstruction or interference with valve function, can be graphically assessed.[18]

Although MRI has not been proven useful in differentiating benign from malignant tumors based on T_1 and T_2 parameters, it has proved useful in assessing general tissue composition.[19] Lipomatous tumors have a high signal on T_1-weighted spin-echo images and a moderately high signal on T_2-weighted images. Calcium and dense fibrous tissue when present in large enough quantities will display a dark signal on T_1-and T_2-weighted images. Cystic tumors will have a low signal on T_1-weighted and a high signal on T_2-weighted images. Generally, most tumors have a relatively low signal on T_1-weighted and high signal on T_2-weighted images. Discerning tissue composition may be complicated by the presence of associated edema, hemorrhage, and necrosis. Gadolinium-DTPA has proven useful in increasing the sensitivity of tumor detection and extent.[20] Most tumors accumulate gadolinium-GTPA more than myocardium and allow for better quantitation of tumor volume.

Despite the versatility of MRI in assessing myocardial tumors both anatomically and functionally, echocardiography remains the screening modality of choice. Interestingly, MRI has proven most useful in assessing patients in whom echocardiography is ambiguous. Most often the suspected presence of a mass is excluded with MRI.[21]

The ability of MRI to identify paracardiac tumors and intracavitary tumors has been clearly established. Although fewer examples of purely myocardial tumors have been described, MRI has proven to be very useful in their evaluation. This is especially true when T_1-weighted studies are performed in conjunction with gadolinium-GTPA.[21] It is extremely important to delineate the entire extent of the tumor as well as its relationship to the ventricular cavity. If the tumor extends to the chamber, some type of patch graft will be required when the tumor is completely excised. Therefore, MRI plays an important role in the surgical work-up of myocardial masses.

Myocardial Infarction

Ischemic heart disease accounts for 80% to 90% of all heart disease related deaths in the United States. Recent strategies in MRI have investigated the efficacy of MRI to delineate areas of injury in the myocardial wall following myocardial infarction (MI). These strategies include examining the wall for thinning and abnormal wall motion, the determination of volumetric data, and the identification and quantification of the actual infarct. Recent work in the area of tissue characterization and paramagnetic contrast agents suggest that MRI may be able to predict myocardial viability.

With standard spin-echo techniques, the myocardial wall can be evaluated for the presence or absence of thinning. This is typically seen in patients with previous or chronic infarction. Although it may be subtle, relative wall thinning will be seen with an acute MI and is the most specific marker for acute MI.[22] Either true or false aneurysms may occur after MI and are easily identified with spin-echo MRI. The true aneurysms are associated with wall thinning and outward bulging. Cine MRI can demonstrate whether the aneurysm is akinetic or dyskinetic. False aneurysms have a narrow neck and are very thin "walled."[23] Associated thrombus is usually easily differentiated from slow flow. Thrombus appears as a low signal stationary mass on cine MRI or phase mapping studies and are invoked when doubt exists on spin-echo examinations. In acute MI, wall thinning may be difficult to recognize. In these cases, intracavitary stagnant blood by the affected wall segment may be used to localize the infarct.[24]

Analysis of contraction dynamics is not only a sensitive means of identifying acute and remote infarction, but also has prognostic value.[25] It is easy to outline the epicardial and endocardial surfaces at various phases of the cardiac cycle on either white or black blood cine MRI. Qualitative assessment of hypokinesia, akinesia, or dyskinesia is possible as well as quantitative evaluation of SWT. There is decreased SWT in areas of MI. The ability to directly visualize the myocardium and quantitate SWT allows for differentiation of truly hypokinetic segments from the passive motion of akinetic segments that are notoriously interpreted as being hypokinetic on left ventriculography.

Myocardial tagging techniques have proven to be even more accurate in wall-motion analysis in normal patients. The application of myocardial tagging techniques to ischemic disease awaits further investigation. It would appear, however, that this will be a more sensitive means of studying contraction dynamics and patient prognosis. In addition to qualitatively evaluating wall motion, cine MRI provides information regarding mitral regurgitation and, indirectly, the integrity of the papillary muscles. Although the muscles can be seen in the short-axis plane, it is difficult to assess their thickening because of their proximity to the LV wall.[26]

Multiphasic spin-echo, cine, or "black blood" cine MRI have all been used to calculate ejection fraction. Because of the excellent edge detection, planimetry of the endocardial surface can be performed in end diastole and end systole. These areas can be added together from multiple adjacent slices to calculate end-diastolic and end-systolic volumes. Alternatively, the length-area method can be used to generate volumes and ejection fraction.[27]

The actual size of infarction is an important prognostic indicator. It is also important to determine the infarction size and myocardium at risk after thrombolytic therapy in order to plan additional therapeutic intervention. The ability of MRI to quantitate infarction volume is undergoing continued investigation and is dependent upon its characterization from normal myocardium.[28]

Acute MI begins as a subendocardial process and spreads to the epicardial surface as a function of time. Endocardial necrosis begins within 20–40 minutes. Myocardial necrosis is complete within 3–6 hours. Reperfusion will limit infarction size if there are still viable myocytes. Within 8 hours, edema is noted in the interstitial space of the myocardium at risk and progresses for approximately 3 days. After this time, necrotic tissue is removed and replaced with granulation tissue beginning at the periphery of the infarct.[29]

As a result of this complex process, T_1 and T_2 relaxation parameters will vary depending on the time interval between infarction and scanning, and whether there has been reperfusion. In most clinical settings, there is little change in T_1 but an increase in T_2 relaxation time. Acute MI is, therefore, recognized by a high signal on T_2-weighted spin-echo images. The intensity will be at a maximum at approximately 3 days and slowly decreases after 20 days. It should be noted that increased signal has been seen in normal individuals and that signal patterns may be altered by the presence of hemorrhage, increased triglyceride content, and increased signal from poorly contracting myocardium.

Gadolinium-GTPA enhances the ability to detect acute MI on T_1-weighted spin-echo examinations. Image quality is markedly improved and there are fewer problems within motion-induced artifacts when compared with T_2-weighted sequences. In fact this protocol improves the detection and definition of acute MI. Although gadolinium-GTPA has been shown experimentally to be able to distinguish between reperfused and nonreperfused myocardium, it has not proven to be as useful in the clinical setting.[29]

When compared with studies of postmortem specimens, both T_2-weighted and T_1- weighted gadolinium-GTPA studies accurately localize the site of infarction but overestimate its volume. This implies that MRI is detecting not only infarction but also reversibly damaged myocardium. Using either of these techniques, planimetry

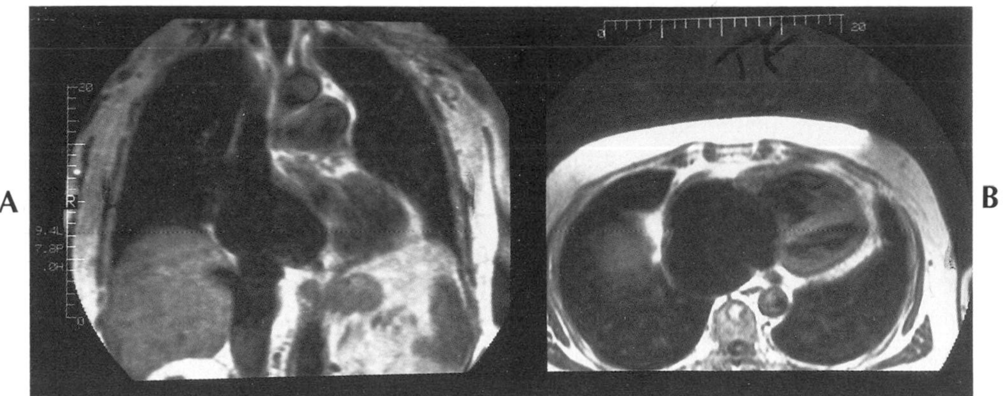

FIGURE 4. (A) *Coronal and* **(B)** *transaxial ECG-gated spin-echo MRI through the midaspect of the heart. The study demonstrates marked enlargement of the right atrium and inferior vena cava. There is mild hypertrophy of the right ventricular wall as well as some thickening of the pericardium along the free wall. The findings are consistent with constrictive pericarditis.*

can be performed to determine MI volume, knowing that injured myocardium is also being measured. Chronic infarction is identified by areas of decreased signal on T_2-weighted images, presumably due to the formation of fibrous tissue at the site of infarction. Additionally, no differential contrast enhancement after gadolinium-DTPA occurs.

The ability of MRI to determine myocardial viability is presently under investigation. To date, significant differences in T_1 and T_2 parameters have not proven useful in the clinical setting. Chemical shift MRI can detect areas of lipid deposition and may prove useful in detecting alterations in myocardial lipid content after acute MI. Hopefully, this will allow for better characterization of reversibly damaged myocardium.[18] There is some indication that gadolinium-DTPA may be of some use in determining viability using standard spin-echo sequences. Reversibly damaged myocardium may not enhance after infusion of gadolinium-DTPA (Figure 5).[30,31] However, reliable differentiation will probably require ultrafast imaging techniques that are not universally available at this time. At present, assessment of viability will depend on a combination of T_2 relaxation, gadolinium-DTPA, wall thickness, and motion analysis. Both infarction and reversibly injured myocardium display decreased end-systolic wall thickening. Viable myocardium has been described as having normal diastolic wall thickness. However, this finding may be difficult to assess. In addition, it may be impossible to determine the exact border between injured and infarcted myocardium. Despite these limitations experimental work would indicate that MRI will play a role in the clinical evaluation of myocardial viability.

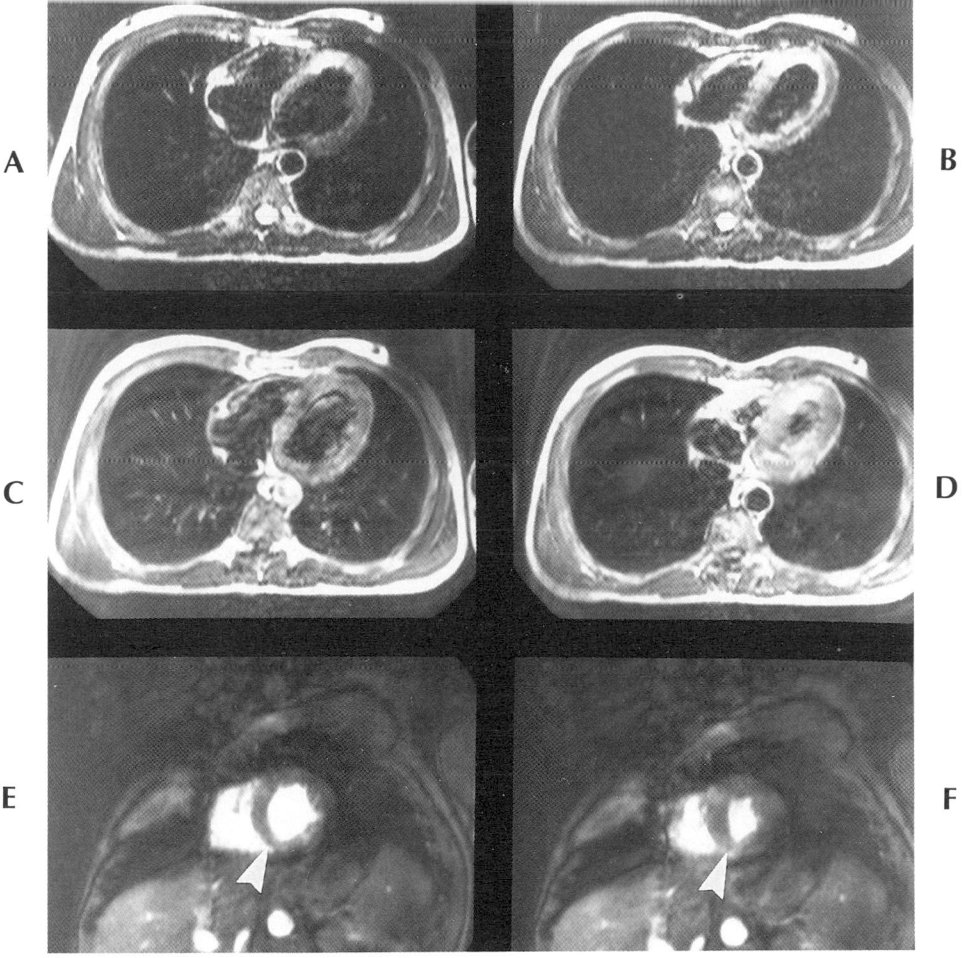

FIGURE 5. *Myocardial infarction.* **A** *and* **B:** *T_2-weighted spin-echo MRI images in transaxial plane demonstrating increased transmural signal in the distal septal and apical segments and subendocardial signal along the free wall in a patient with an acute MI.* **C** *and* **D:** *Gadolinium-DTPA enhanced T_1-weighted spin-echo MRI images corresponding to A and B. There is enhancement in the distal septal segment implying that the regions of increased signal on A and B that did not enhance are viable.* **E** *and* **F:** *Short-axis cine MRI in diastole and systole demonstrating wall thinning in distal septum (arrowhead in E) and abnormal thickening (arrowhead in F).*

References

1. Glover GH, Pelc NJ: A rapid gated cine MRI technique. In: Kressel HY, ed. *Magnetic Resonance Annual*. New York: Raven Press Publishers; 1988:299–333.
2. Bryant DJ, Payne JA, Firmin DN, Longmore DB: Measurement of flow with NMR imaging using a gradient pulse and phase difference technique. *J Comput Assist Tomogr* 1984;8:588.
3. Pelc NJ, Stanford CA, Herfkens RJ, et al: Three-dimensional motion analysis by means of phase-contrast cine MR imaging. *Radiology* 1991;181:281.
4. Zerhouni EA, Parish DM, Rogers WJ, et al: Human heart: tagging with MR imaging—a method for noninvasive assessment of myocardial motion. *Radiology* 1988;169:59.
5. Maron BJ, Bonow RO, Cannon RO, et al: Hypertrophic cardiomyopathy: interrelations of clinical manifestations, pathophysiology, and therapy. *N Engl J Med* 1987;316:844–852.
6. Higgins CB, Holt W, Pflugfelder P, et al: Functional evaluation of the heart with magnetic resonance imaging. *Magn Reson Med* 1988;6:121–139.
7. Johns JA, Leavitt MB, Newell JB, et al: Quantization of acute myocardial infarct size by nuclear magnetic resonance imaging. *J Am Coll Cardiol* 1990;15:143–149.
8. Caputo G, Fisher MR, McNamara MT, et al: Myocardial tissue characterization with the use of magnetic resonance imaging. *Circulation* 1986;72(suppl):III-23.
9. Higgins CB, Herfkens R, Lipton MJ, et al: Nuclear magnetic resonance imaging of acute myocardial infarction in dogs: alterations in magnetic relaxation times. *Am J Cardiol* 1983;52:184–188.
10. Roberts WC, Ferrans UJ: A survey of the causes and consequences of pericardial heart disease. In: Reddy PS, Leon DF, Shaver YA, eds. *Pericardial Disease*. New York: Raven Press Publishers; 1982:49–75.
11. White RD, Lenz GW, Silver MS, et al: Cine cardiovascular MRI: applications and attributes versus limitations of gating strategies. *Magn Res Imaging* 1989;7(suppl 1):94.
12. Saul S, Tomaszewski J: The heart. In: LiVolsi VA, et al: ed. *Pathology*. Media, PA: Harwal Publishing Co./John A. Wiley & Sons Inc.; 1984:45–60.
13. Sechtem U, Sommerhoff BA, Markewics W, et al: Regional left ventricular wall thickening by magnetic resonance imaging: evaluation in normal persons and patients with global and regional dysfunction. *Am J Cardiol* 1987;59:145–151.
14. Sechtem U, Higgins CG, Sommerhoff BA, et al: Magnetic resonance imaging of restrictive cardiomyopathy. *Am J Cardiol* 1989;59:480–482.
15. White RD, Zisch RJ: MRI of pericardial disease and paracardiac and intracardiac masses. In: Elliott LP, ed. *The Fundamentals of Cardiac Imaging in Children and Adults*. Philadelphia, PA: JB Lippincott, (in press).
16. Chandraratna PAN, Bradely WG, Kortman KE, et al: Detection of acute myocarditis using nuclear magnetic resonance imaging. *Am J Med* 1987;83:1144–1146.
17. Matsui S, Murakami E, Takekoshi N, et al: Myocardial tissue characterization by magnetic resonance imaging in Fabry's disease. *Am Heart J* 1989;117:472–474.
18. Bouchard A, Wilson R, Doyle M, et al: NMR lipid imaging: a new strategy for assessing the myocardial ischemic insult. *J Am Coll Cardiol* 1989;18:200A.
19. Brown JJ, Barakos JA, Higgins CB: Magnetic resonance imaging of cardiac and paracardiac masses. *J Thorac Imaging* 1989;4:58–64.
20. Niwa K, Tashima K, Terai M, et al: Contrast-enhanced magnetic resonance imaging of cardiac tumors in children. *Am Heart J* 1989;118:424–425.
21. Lund JT, Ehman RL, Julsrud PR, et al: Cardiac masses: assessment by MR imaging. *AJR* 1989;152:469–473.
22. Fisher MR, McNamara MT, Higgins CB: Acute myocardial infarction: MR evaluation in 29 patients. *AJR* 1987;148:247–251.
23. Ahmad M, Johnson RF, Fawcett HD, et al: Left ventricular aneurysm in short axis: a comparison of magnetic resonance, ultrasound and thallium-201 SPECT imaging. *Magn Reson Imaging* 1987;5:293–300.
24. Sechtem U, Theissen P, Heindel W, et al: Diagnosis of left ventricular thrombi by

magnetic resonance imaging and comparison with angiocardiography, computed tomography and echocardiography. *Am J Cardiol* 1989;64:1195–1200.

25. Filipchuk NG, Peshock RM, Malloy CT, et al: Detection and localization of recent myocardial infarction by magnetic resonance imaging. *Am J Cardiol* 1986;58:214–219.
26. Sechtem U, Pflugfelder PW, Gould RG, et al: Measurement of right and left ventricular volumes in healthy individuals with cine MR imaging. *Radiology* 1987;163:697.
27. Link KM: Cardiac imaging. In: Potchen ET, Gottschalk A, Haack EM, Siebert J, eds. *Magnetic Resonance Angiography: Concept and Applications*. St Louis, MO: CV Mosby Co.; 1991. (In press).
28. De Roos A, Matheijssen NAA, Doornbos J, et al: Myocardial infarct size after reperfusion therapy: assessment by gadolinium-DTPA-enhanced MR imaging. *Radiology* 1990;176:512–521.
29. Canby RC, Reeves RC, Evanochko WT, et al: Proton nuclear magnetic resonance relaxation times in severe myocardial ischemia. *J Am Coll Cardiol* 1987;10:412–420.
30. De Roos A, Van Rossum AC, Van der Wall EE, et al: Reperfused and nonreperfused myocardial infarction: potential of gadolinium-DTPA enhanced MR imaging. *Radiology* 1989;172:717–720.
31. McNamara MT, Tscholakoff D, Revel D, et al: Differentiation of reversible and irreversible myocardial injury by MR imaging with and without gadolinium-DTPA. *Radiology* 1986;158:765–769.

Chapter 5

Magnetic Resonance Imaging of Congenital Heart Disease

Richard D. White, MD

The use of magnetic resonance imaging (MRI) for the clinical evaluation of congenital heart disease (CHD) has become commonplace. In many medical centers, MRI is now regarded as a valuable adjunct to two-dimensional and Doppler echocardiography in the noninvasive assessment of CHD, including congenital abnormalities of the cardiac chambers, valves, great arteries and veins, and surrounding pericardium. It is now possible to derive much of the necessary qualitative and quantitative information regarding the various anatomical abnormalities (eg, presence versus absence, number, size, location and distribution, connections) and physiologic abnormalities (eg, intracardiac/vascular hemodynamics, systolic and diastolic chamber dynamics, passive motion or expansion) of the central cardiovascular structures associated with CHD using MRI. In fact, when used in combination with the anatomical and physiologic capabilities of Doppler echocardiography, the need for contrast cardioangiography, with its attendant risks (ie, risks related to vascular manipulation, contrast administration, and radiation exposure), can be greatly restricted. Accordingly, the role of catheterization procedures in the assessment of CHD can become more focused on pressure measurements.

In order to understand how MRI can be used to investigate such a wide range of clinically valuable parameters, it is necessary to appreciate the ever-expanding capabilities of this imaging modality and recognize the state of the art of cardiovascular MRI. Currently, several electrocardiographically gated two-dimensional MRI techniques are established enough to be used regularly to acquire clinically valuable information about CHD. They provide information in the form of either static or dynamic tomographic displays of the central cardiovascular system, with data acquired orthogonal to either the body axes (eg, transaxial) or the inherently oblique axes of the cardiovascular structures themselves (eg, cardiac short axis). These techniques include the following: 1) multilevel spin-echo MRI to produce a series of conventional static "dark-blood" images, each representing one of multiple adjacent anatomical levels (eg, 12 levels) at a point in the cardiac cycle that is uniformly delayed from the

From Pohost GM (ed.), *Cardiovascular Applications of Magnetic Resonance.* Mount Kisco, NY, Futura Publishing Co., Inc., © 1993.

previous level; 2) dynamic gradient-echo MRI to produce "bright-blood" magnitude images representing many evenly dispersed time segments of the cardiac cycle (eg, 16 segments) at a few select anatomical levels (eg, 3 levels) for display as "cine" image loops; and 3) dynamic gradient-echo phase velocity mapping (VMap) to record spatially, using a gray scale, the calibrated velocity-dependent phase shifts related to blood flow within the intracardiac/vascular spaces on a segment-to-segment basis thoughout the cardiac cycle; an image loop corresponding spatially and temporally with its magnitude cine counterpart is produced. These three techniques are described in greater detail elswhere.[1]

Overview

Anatomical Evaluation

The identification and delineation of abnormal cardiovascular structures has traditionally been, and presently remains, the foundation of MRI efforts in CHD. Accordingly, multilevel spin-echo MRI has continued to be the most commonly used technique for anatomical evaluation of CHD because of its well-recognized ability to provide accurate anatomical information about the cardiac chambers, valves, great arteries and veins, and pericardium with excellent tissue differentiation. As demonstrated in previous work dating back to the earlier years of clinical cardiovascular MRI, these qualities allow spin-echo MRI to acquire a wide range of valuable data regarding both abnormalites in segmental anatomy and structural malformations of the central cardiovascular system found in CHD.[2] At the same time, some shortcomings in the anatomical evaluation of CHD by spin-echo MRI have become apparent.[3] They are related to inherent limitations of the spin-echo technique, including both its static nature, which often hinders complete visualization of thin mobile structures (eg, fossa ovalis at the atrial level and the membranous septum at the ventricular level), and its display of all rapidly flowing blood as dark, which precludes differentiation between normal flow and abnormally complex flow. The clinical drawbacks of these limitations tend to be the false-positive diagnosis of some abnormalities (eg, secundum atrial septal defect [ASD] and membranous ventricular septal defect [VSD]) and the false-negative detection of either small communications with altered flow (eg, patent foramen ovale with left-to-right shunting) or abnormal courses of intrapulmonary vasculature (eg, anomalous pulmonary venous drainage). Nevertheless, because of the generally high success in providing useful information about both major categories of anatomical abnormalities, spin-echo MRI has become immensely helpful clinically for the definitive evaluation of several simpler forms (eg, pulmonary artery atresia, coarctation of the aorta, vascular ring, annuloaortic ectasia due to Marfan's syndrome) and many more complex and often interrelated forms (eg, situs ambiguus, univentricular heart conditions, double outlet ventricle) of CHD. In the future, newer techniques such as real-time echo planar scanning and three-dimensional magnetic resonance angiography should assist in the anatomical evaluation of CHD using MRI.

Segmental Anatomy

To date, several large series have clearly demonstrated the excellent capabilities of spin-echo MRI to provide accurate information regarding abnormalities in segmental anatomy associated with various forms of CHD.[4–10] With generally high sensitivity at high-specificity levels (Table 1), spin-echo MRI may be used to detect abnormalities of visceral-atrial situs, venous-atrial connection (Figure 1), atrial-ventricular connection (Figure 2), bulboventricular loop, ventricular-arterial connection, and great artery relationship.

Reduced sensitivity for detecting the return connections of the pulmonary veins by spin-echo MRI is probably related to the previously mentioned inherent limitations in this technique. In particular, diagnosis of abnormalities of pulmonary veins by spin-echo MRI may be difficult because closely neighboring anatomical structures (eg, lung parenchyma, bronchi, and pulmonary arteries) are also characterized by low signal intensity.

Structural Malformations

Several large series evaluating spin-echo MRI for the detection of various specific structural malformations in CHD have also been reported.[4,11–16] Although with somewhat greater variability in sensitivity than for the assessment of abnormal segmental anatomy (Table 2), spin echo may be used effectively to detect a number of congenital defects of the intracardiac septae at either the atrial or ventricular levels (Figure 3), abnormalities of the valves, and great artery abnormalities (Figure 4).

Problems with the exclusion of malformations involving thin mobile structures or the identification of small defects have been noted, most likely due to the limitations in the spin-echo technique. Although a good correlation between spin-echo measurements of the diameter of septal defects and surgical findings has been reported, accurate determination of the area of a septal defect with spin-echo MRI is inherently limited because consecutive images of adjacent anatomical levels do not accommodate for changes in position of the septae from both through-plane and in-plane motions during the cardiac cycle. While medium-sized and large septal defects, especially VSDs, are clearly demonstrated on spin-echo MRI, small septal defects at either level

TABLE 1. Detection of Abnormalities in Segmental Anatomy with S-E MRI

Anatomic Level	Sensitivity (%)	Specificity (%)
Visceral-Atrial Situs	100	100
Venous-Atrial Connection		
Systemic	98–100	NA
Pulmonary	66–95	98–100
Atrial-Ventricular Connection	100	NA
Bulboventricular Loop	100	NA
Ventricular-Arterial Connection	100	95
Great Artery Relationship	100	90–95

(text continues on p.66)

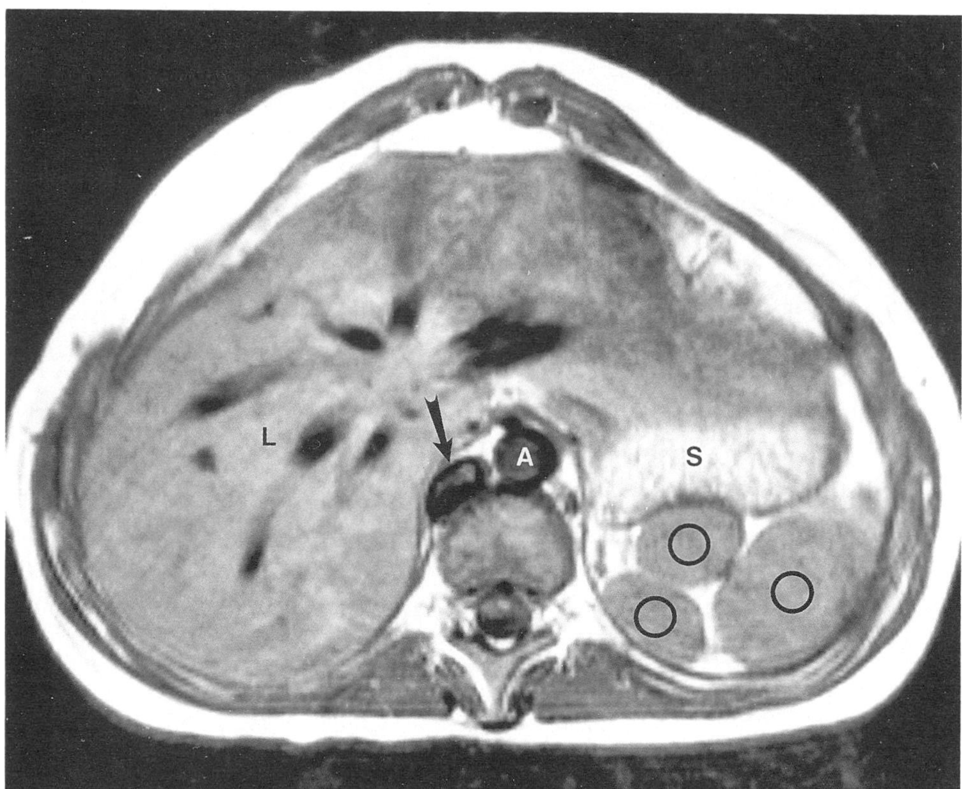

FIGURE 1. *Levo-isomerism with azygos continuation (spin echo; transaxial). Situs ambiguus with bilateral left-sidedness of the thoracic anatomy is accompanied by characteristics of polysplenia at the abdominal level. In addition to the multiple small spleens (circles), an enlarged retrocrural azygos vein (arrow) is identified. It provides venous drainage from the abdomen, because of the associated congenital interruption of the inferior vena cava below the liver. A, aorta; L, liver; s, stomach.*

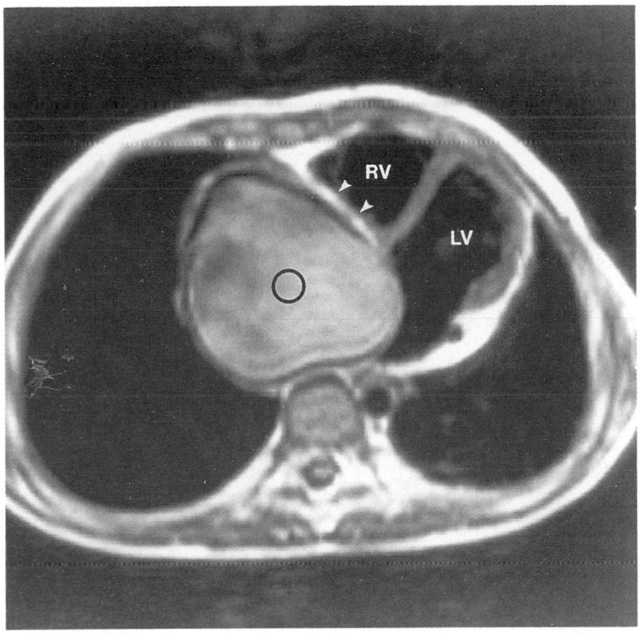

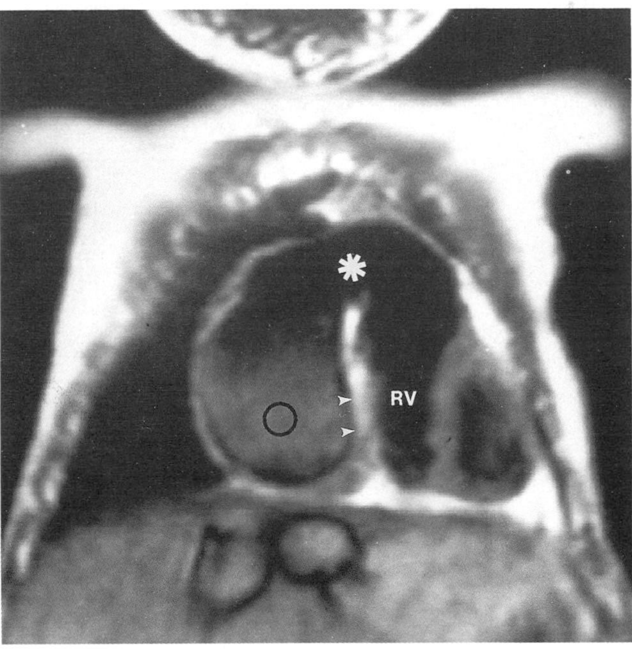

FIGURE 2. *Tricuspid atresia (spin echo; transaxial and coronal). Both the extension of the right atrioventricular groove (arrowheads), including its bright adipose tissue, to the level of the intracardiac septae* **(A)** *and the accompanying absence of the tricuspid valve leaflets is indicative of tricuspid atresia. The enlarged right atrium (circles) is filled with abnormal blood signal due to stagnation, despite a prior Fontan procedure with surgical communication (asterisk) established between the right atrial appendage and the proximal main pulmonary artery* **(B)**. *LV, left ventricle; RV, right ventricle.*

TABLE 2. Detection of Structural Malformations with Spin-Echo Magnetic Resonance Imaging

Structural Malformation	Sensitivity (%)	Specificity (%)
Septal Defects		
Atrial	35–98	90–95
Ventricular	84–100	90–95
Valvular Abnormalities		
Mitral	61–62	90–95
Tricuspid	75–76	90–95
Aortic	39–51	90–95
Pulmonic and Right Ventricular Outflow Tract	88–95	90–95
Great Artery Abnormalities		
Aorta	91–94	90–95
Pulmonary Artery	97–100	NA

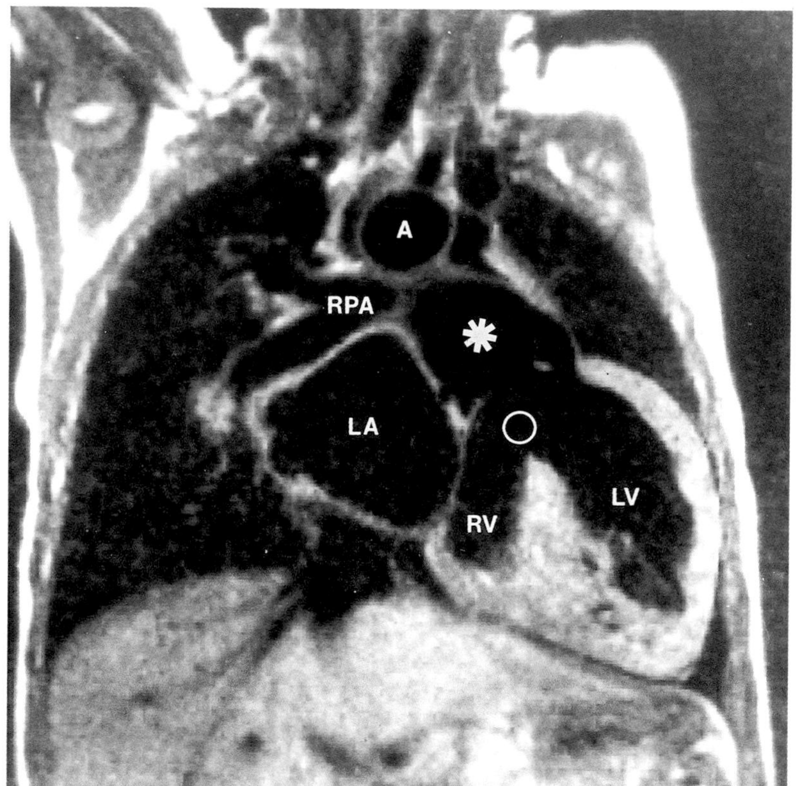

FIGURE 3. *Conotruncal VSD in truncus arteriosus (spin-echo; oblique coronal). Below the origin of the common great artery (asterisk), a large outflow defect of the interventricular septum (circle) is identified. A, aorta; LA, left atrium; LV, left ventricle; RPA, right pulmonary artery; RV, right ventricle.*

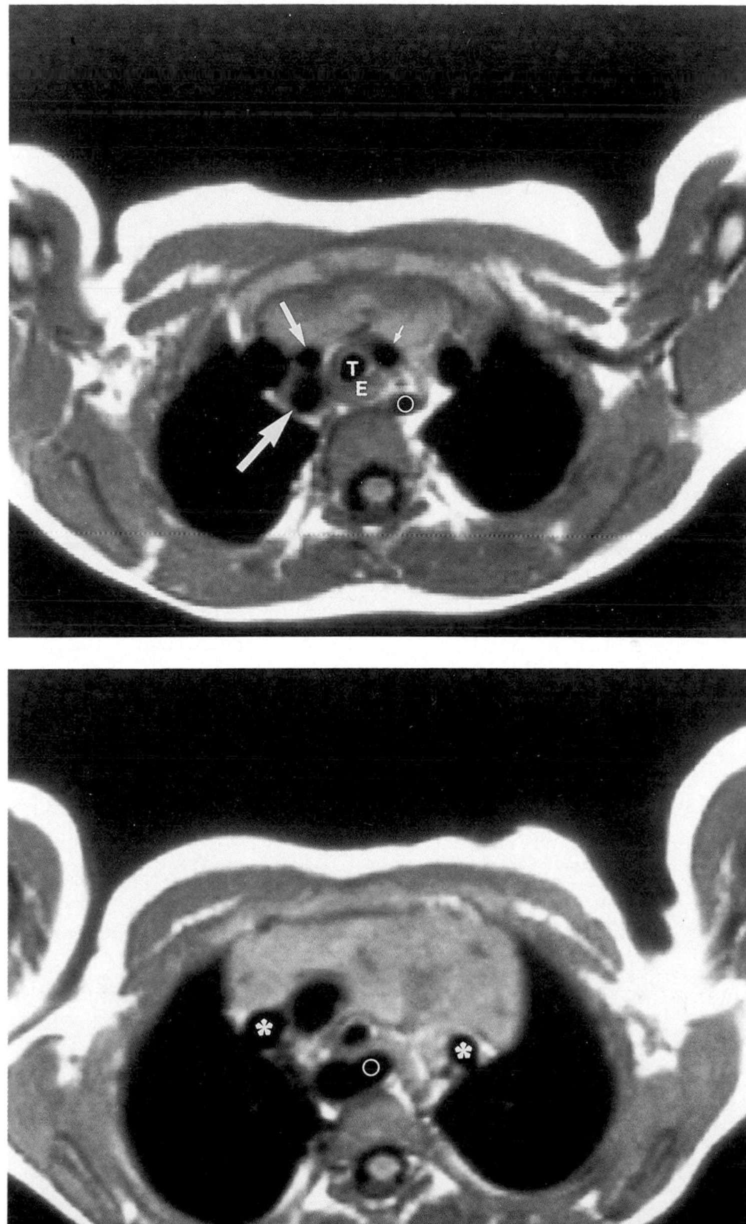

FIGURE 4. *Right-sided aortic arch with aberrant origin of the left subclavian artery (spin echo; transaxial). Just above the right-sided aortic arch, the origins of the left common carotid artery (small arrow), followed by that of the right common carotid artery (medium arrow), and then followed by that of the right subclavian artery (large arrow) are identifiable* **(A)**. *Last to arise, the aberrant left subclavian artery (circles) passes behind the trachea and esophagus* **(B)**. *Incidentally noted are noncommunicating bilateral superior venae cavae (asterisks). E, esophagus; T, trachea.*

may not be appreciated. Similar limitations reduce the ability of structural malformations of the valves to be diagnosed with spin-echo MRI.

Physiological Evaluation

While the value of static spin-echo MRI in detecting and defining anatomical abnormalities of the central cardiovascular system is well established, its value in assessing the associated physiologic abnormalites appears to be quite restricted largely because of its static nature. Use of multiphasic versions of spin-echo MRI help to overcome this restriction, but they remain limited by inadequate temporal resolution for the evaluation of contraction of the cardiac chambers, by a lack of ability to fully characterize blood flow patterns, and by the excessive length of scan time required.[1] Conversely, the various forms of dynamic gradient-echo MRI offer an alternative to invasive catheterization and to noninvasive two-dimensional echocardiography for evaluating the pathophysiology associated with various forms of CHD. Dynamic gradient-echo MRI techniques segment temporally the cardiac cycle into a sufficient number of images to provide adequate representation of the changes in the central cardiovascular structures and blood pools throughout the cardiac cycle. Hence, cardiac chamber dynamics and intracardiac/vascular hemodynamics can be assessed using dynamic gradient-echo MRI methods. In the process, the overall ability of MRI to detect and characterize anatomical abnormalites of CHD is greatly enhanced.

The signal from resonating protons recorded during MRI image data collection is a vector uniquely defined by magnitude (ie, intensity) and phase (ie, direction) components.[1] Just as the magnitude can be used to produce standard anatomy-based images, the phase component can be used to generate flow-based images that reflect the movement of protons spins during known time intervals within the pulse sequence. Both components have been used to develop the two previously mentioned versions of dynamic gradient-echo MRI. The standard "bright-blood" (ie, cine) version is the product of the magnitude component, and the flow mapping (ie, VMap) version the product of the phase component.

The cine version has grown in popularity for functional assessment of cardiovascular disease, including CHD, because of its ability to display dynamically the contracting cardiac chambers, moving valves, and the pulsatile central vasculature throughout the cardiac cycle with high temporal resolution.[1,17] When tomographic cine image loops are acquired at all anatomical levels encompassing the heart, MRI serves as a three-dimensional volume imaging technique. Because of variations in the signal of flowing blood in relation to cyclical blood flow patterns within the cardiac chambers and vasculature, intracardiac/vascular hemodynamics can also be appreciated.

With the VMap version, information regarding the direction and velocity of blood proton motion is displayed both spatially relative to the anatomy of the central cardiovascular structures and temporally relative to the time segments of the cardiac cycle.[1,3] Calibrated phase signal intensities on a gray scale reflect different blood flow velocities, and these intensities are displayed on a voxel-by-voxel basis to produce a velocity map corresponding spatially to a standard magnitude data image. By region-of-interest inspection, instantaneous mean velocity of blood flow can be determined over a defined area of multiple voxels. When the mean flow velocity for the complete cross-sectional intravascular area of a vessel is determined and multiplied by that area, instantaneous flow volume (cm^3/sec) can be assessed. Integration of the curve resulting from a plot of instantaneous volume flow per time segment of the cardiac cycle then provides a measure of net blood flow volume through that cross section of the vessel over the complete cardiac cycle (cm^3/cycle).

Together, both versions of dynamic gradient-echo MRI have certain advantages over two-dimensional and Doppler echocardiography for physiologic evaluation of CHD; they are generally less operator dependent, use a three-dimensional display, and more easily evaluate the vasculature in the mediastinum and lungs. However, only a few small series of CHD patients studied by these dynamic MRI methods have to date been reported. Newer techniques, such as myocardial tagging and ultrafast gradient-echo imaging with first-pass scanning of a circulating intravascular paramagnetic contrast agent, may also play important future roles in the physiological evaluation of CHD using MRI.

Qualitative Evaluation

Qualitative evaluation by visual inspection of the physiologic abnormalities associated with CHD is better accomplished with cine MRI than with VMap image loops because of the nature of the anatomy-based images provided by cine MRI.

Chamber Dynamics

Most of the work to date describing the use of cine MRI in the evaluation of cardiac chamber contraction and relaxation has applied to acquired cardiovascular diseases rather than to CHD.[1,17] For this purpose, cine MRI has been used primarily to assess segmental wall thickening of the left ventricle (LV) in normals and in cases of ischemic heart disease. Evaluation of wall thickness at end diastole and end systole in different LV regions at the equatorial level on transaxial image loops revealed heterogeneity of systolic wall thickening in both groups. In cases of ischemic disease, the degree of thickening within undamaged regions was within normal limits, but proportionately decreased in hypokinetic, akinetic, and dyskinetic ischemia damaged regions. Descriptions of regional LV dysfunction by cine MRI have correlated well with the results from two-dimensional Doppler echocardiography and ventriculography.

In a similar fashion, cine MRI could be used to evaluate qualitatively the contraction patterns of the ventricular walls in the setting of CHD; diastolic relaxation could also be assessed. Initial results indicate that cine MRI may be particularly useful in the qualitative, if not quantitative, evaluation of contraction abnormalities of the right ventricle (RV). Regions of impaired systolic wall thickening in the anterior wall of the infundibulum and body of the RV, indicating congenital dysplastic changes in the myocardium, have been identified by cine MRI with high sensitivity in cases of idiopathic RV outflow tract tachycardia; they are, in general, undetected by both two-dimensional Doppler echocardiography and RV ventriculography.[18] Right ventricular infundibular stenosis, as found in the setting of tetralogy of Fallot, is a dynamic entity that is better defined on cine image loops than on static spin-echo images. Muscular contraction and narrowing can be appreciated on cine MRI and the signal changes characterizing post-stenotic flow within the narrowed RV outflow tract are demonstrated.[19]

Hemodynamics

The principles governing tissue contrast and signal intensity of flowing blood on cine MRI have been described.[1] Basically, the blood pools within the central cardiovascular structures generate high signal intensity on cine MRI under normal physiologic conditions, but the intensity of blood varies somewhat over the cardiac cycle with the changing flow patterns. Nevertheless, the signal of the blood pools in the cardiac chambers and great arteries and veins normally remains greater than that of the surrounding myocardium and vessel walls. This signal enhancement of flowing blood on cine MRI facilitates the qualitative evaluation of the intracardiac/vascular spaces in CHD, thereby assisting in the differentiation between the walls of the cardiac chambers and vessels and the contained blood pools.

Abnormal blood flow is manifested by regional loss of signal within the blood pools.[1,17] The factors responsible for signal loss caused by abnormal flow patterns have been examined in phantoms; signal void on cine MRI is caused by the combined factors of flow through a narrow orifice, turbulence, and changing high flow velocities.[1,17] Accordingly, signal void jets of variable dimension and duration have been observed clinically in the setting of congenital valvular stenosis and insufficiency, a hemodynamically significant vascular narrowing, and a flow restricting septal defect or vascular communication.[1,17,19] It is important to recognize that the appearances of both normally and abnormally flowing blood on cine MRI is variably influenced by imaging parameters; for example, the amount of signal loss is reduced with decreasing TE.[1]

Using spin-echo MRI, false-positive diagnoses of intracardiac or intervascular shunt lesions may occur due to the previously mentioned difficulties with the differentiation between a situation of poor visualization of thin mobile structures and actual shunt lesions within these structures. Just as color flow Doppler echocardiography superimposes a display of intracardiac/vascular blood flow patterns on an image of the cardiovascular anatomy, cine MRI clearly demonstrates blood flow patterns relative to anatomy.[20] Therefore, the separation of the blood pools by an intact septum can be easily appreciated and differentiated from their communication through an ASD or VSD with (ie, restrictive) or without (ie, nonrestrictive) signs of associated complex flow. Because complex flow through a small restrictive shunt lesion may produce a jet of signal void, small defects are detected better on cine MRI than on spin-echo MRI (Figure 5).[1,17,20,21] Uncomplicated small septal defects with shunting at either the atrial or ventricular level have been demonstrated by jets of complex transseptal flow passing from left to right; the jet size depends on various factors related to the condition (eg, defect size, transseptal pressure gradient, and flow direction).[21] For similar reasons, it is possible to recognize the signal void caused by complex flow of blood shunted from right to left (eg, VSD of tetralogy of Fallot) or in either direction across a vascular communication (eg, patent ductus arteriosus).[22] Cine MRI allows three-dimensional reconstruction of septal defects because of temporally consistent demonstration of the missing portion of the septum at adjacent anatomical levels.[20] On properly oriented images, it has been also possible to determine the cross-sectional area of some defects on the basis of the diameter of the signal void jet of shunted blood at its origin.[21]

With spin-echo MRI, valve leaflets are only infrequently seen adequately enough to detect direct anatomical evidence of valve abnormalities, and the appreciation of the associated transvalvular flow disturbances is beyond the capabilites of this static technique. Thus, the diagnosis of valvular lesions by spin-echo MRI is largely predicated on the detection of secondary changes (eg, dilatation of the ascending aorta due to post-stenotic flow beyond a stenotic aortic valve). Both abnormal valve leaflet structure and motion (eg, doming) can be appreciated within the signal enhanced blood pools on cine MRI, and complex blood flow distal to a stenotic valve or proximal to an incompetent valve causes signal loss on cine MRI.[1,17] Valvular insufficiency is manifested on cine MRI as a signal void jet extending retrograde into the recipient chamber during the appropriate phase of the cardiac cycle. The sensitivity and specificity of cine MRI for the identification of acquired insufficiency involving the aortic and mitral valves have been shown to be approximately 95%.[1,17,20] Turbulent high-velocity blood flow beyond a stenotic valve leads to signal loss that can be observed emanating from the stenotic lesion.[1] However, unlike regurgitant flow, this signal loss from abnormal antegrade flow must be differentiated from normal signal decrease from physiologic forward flow through that valve. Presumably, the applications of cine MRI to the qualitative assessment of congenital valvular dysfunction are comparable to those reported for acquired dysfunction. Hence, cine MRI may be used to evaluate valvular insufficiency (eg, from a cleft anterior mitral valve leaflet in a partial atrioventricular canal), valvular stenosis (eg, from a bicuspid aortic valve), or subvalvular stenosis.

Compared to spin-echo MRI, improved evaluation of the number, size, distribution, and connections of the mediastinal and pulmonary vasculature can be performed with cine MRI because of the dynamic imaging format and the signal enhancement of intravascular flow.[19] Therefore, the location and severity of areas of congenital stenoses or aneurysmal dilatation of the central vasculature can be better assessed using cine MRI. As with the previously mentioned flow restricting lesions, cine MRI can be used to detect hemodynamically significant vascular stenoses of the great arteries. Cine MRI has been used in the evaluation of the relationship between flow disturbance and the vascular narrowing in cases of coarctation.[23] In cases of coarctation studied with cine MRI, the high signal intensity of blood within the aorta produces a striking similarity between cine MRI and angiographic images. Signal void jets due to complex flow caused by the narrowing are common and aid in the detection and characterization of the lesion. However, with high-grade obstruction, signal void may not be observed distal to the narrow segment if large collateral vessels exist.[20,23]

Cine MRI may also be useful in several respects in the evaluation of congenital conditions involving the pulmonary arteries (eg, tetralogy of Fallot).[19] On cine MRI, the pulmonary arteries can be distinguished from veins both by their pulsatile changes in signal intensity and their more prominent motion during the cardiac cycle. Stenoses of the main and central pulmonary arteries can be detected using cine MRI.[19] Compared to the pulmonary arteries, the pulmonary veins are relatively immobile and exhibit high signal intensity that remains relatively constant during the cardiac cycle. They are easily distinguished from the adjacent bronchial structures, which are

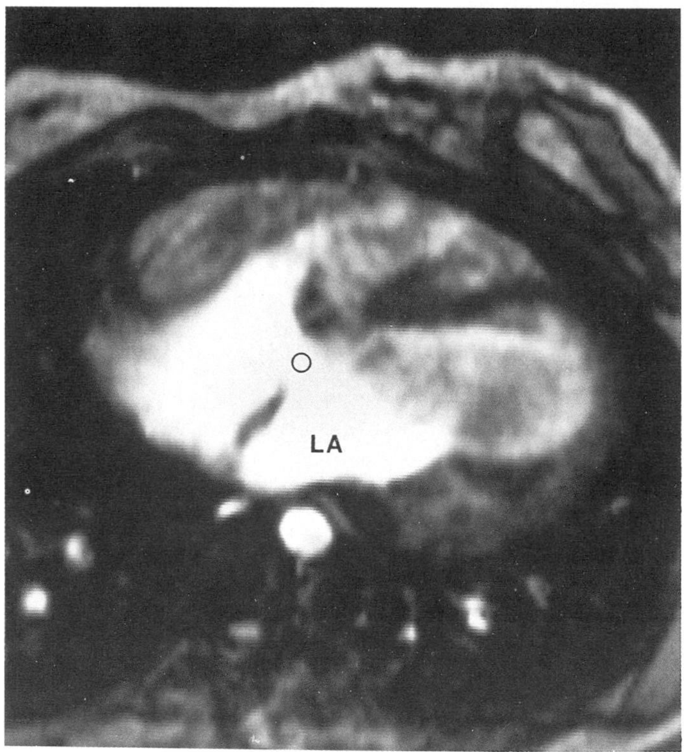

FIGURE 5. *Shunting and valvular insufficiency in a partial atrioventricular canal (cine; transaxial and oblique coronal). On the diastolic image* **(A)**, *a defect of the lower interatrial septum adjacent to the atrioventricular valves is revealed; it is consistent with a primum ASD (black circle). The corresponding midsystolic image* **(B)** *and the midsystolic frontal image* **(C)** *both demonstrate a large signal void jet (white circles) of complex shunted flow passing through the cleft anterior mitral valve leaflet (arrowheads), followed by the defective atrioventricular and lower interatrial septal regions, into the enlarged right atrium. A small jet of complex flow marks additional left-to-right shunting through a restrictive VSD (curved arrow). Two jets from mitral insufficiency, one more anterior (short arrow) and one more posterior (long arrow), are also identifiable. AA, ascending aorta; LA, left atrium; LV, left ventricle; MPA, main pulmonary artery; RV, right ventricle.*

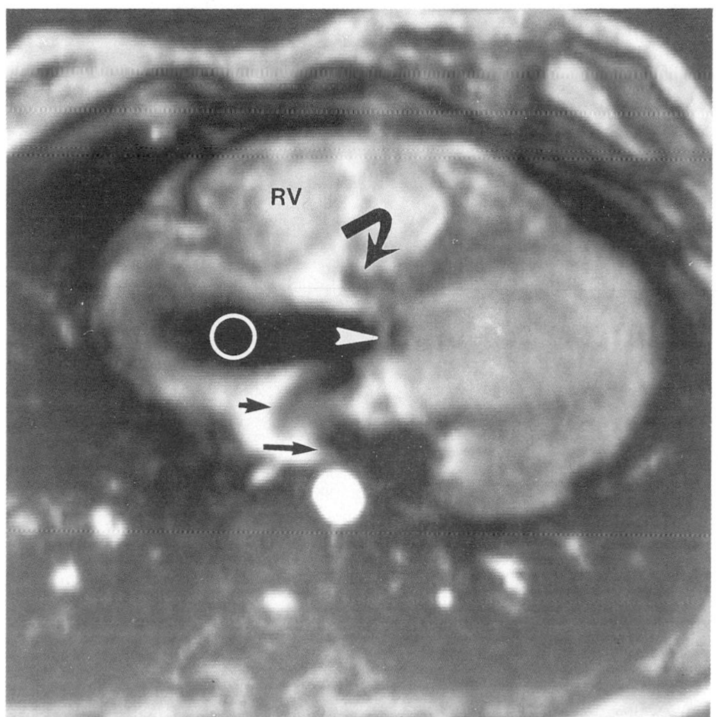

B

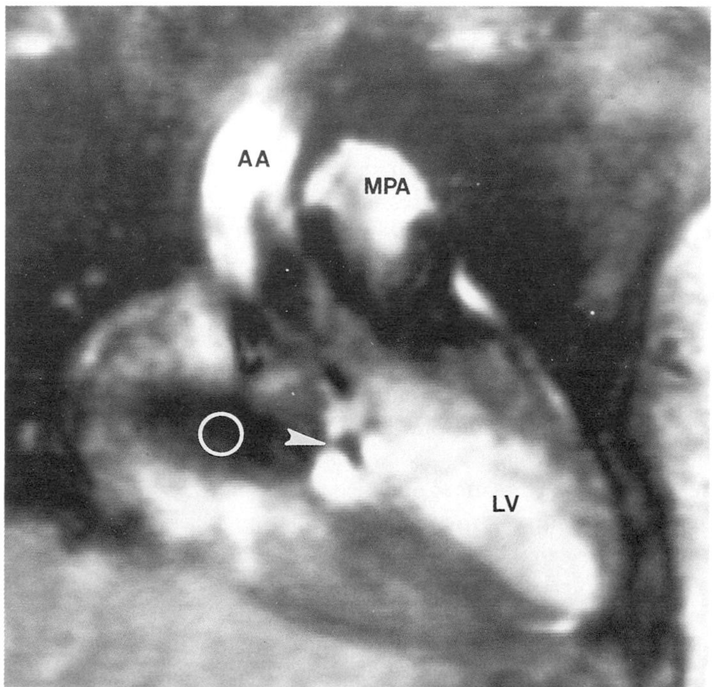

C

characterized by low signal intensity due to the contained air and susceptibility changes. Consequently, cine MRI is preferable to spin-echo MRI for the identification of anomalous pulmonary venous drainage, and it may aid in the diagnosis of congenital abnormalities of the systemic veins.[19,20,24] For both types of veins, however, the visualization of signal void jets from venous stenoses is less likely than with arterial stenoses because of the lower pressure gradients across such areas of narrowing.

Quantitative Evaluation

Chamber Volume Analysis

Ventricular volumes can be determined accurately directly from a series of cine MRI image loops encompassing the full extent of the two ventricles without the need for geometric assumptions.[1,17,25] For this purpose, the blood pool of each ventricle is outlined at end diastole and end systole from each dynamic tomogram and the volumes are calculated at that anatomical level based on both the number of voxels in the region outlined and the known volume of each voxel; the volumes calculated for each anatomical level representing the ventricular cavities are then summed to provide the total ventricular volumes by a modified Simpson's algorithm.[1,17,25] From the measured end-diastolic and end-systolic ventricular volumes, a stroke volume (SV) can be calculated each for the RV and the LV. Such values derived from cine MRI have shown good correlation with those derived from two-dimensional Doppler echocardiography and ventriculography.[1,17,25]

Complete cine MRI examination of the two ventricles provides the basis for three-dimensional determination of SV.[1,17,25] In the absence of a concurrent volume overloading condition affecting the ventricles (ie, additional shunt lesion or valvular insufficiency), several absolute and relative quantitative measures of cardiovascular physiology can be determined in the setting of CHD using cine MRI.[1,17,25] These SV measurements can provide the basis for determination of cardiac output or ejection fraction (EF) to assess impaired overall ventricular function, or regurgitant volume or regurgitant fraction to assess the severity of valvular insufficiency.

Direct quantitation of the amount of shunt flow as an indicator of the anatomical size of a defect related to prognosis is a useful parameter for planning corrective surgery.[25] For an ASD with left-to-right shunting, this can be accomplished with cine MRI in the absence of associated valvular insufficiency or additional shunts by evaluating the difference between the larger RV and smaller LV SV (Figure 6). This approach has been used to derive estimates of the shunt volume, shunt fraction, or Qp/Qs to indicate the hemodynamic importance of an uncomplicated ASD.[1,17,25] This method yields good correlations with shunt determinations obtained by catheterization.[24]

Similar to an ASD, shunt size in a VSD is an important clinical parameter. When SV of both ventricles is calculated from a three-dimensional cine MRI series, LV SV reflects both systemic and shunt volumes and should correspond to the augmented pulmonary blood flow, while RV SV should represent systemic blood flow alone.[1,17,21,25] Therefore, shunt volume for a VSD could theoretically be derived by subtraction of the smaller RV SV from the larger LV SV. However, it has been found that RV SV is also increased in such left-to-right shunts depending upon the location

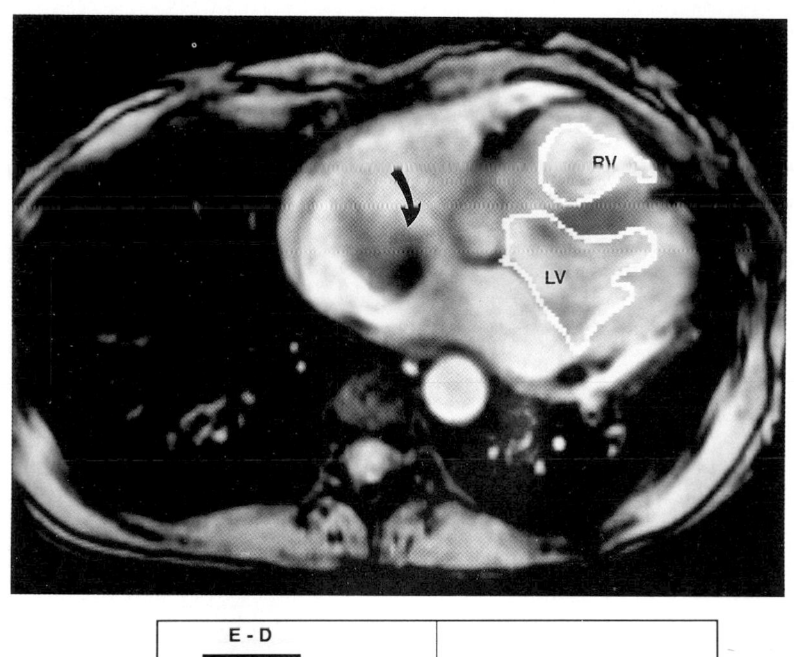

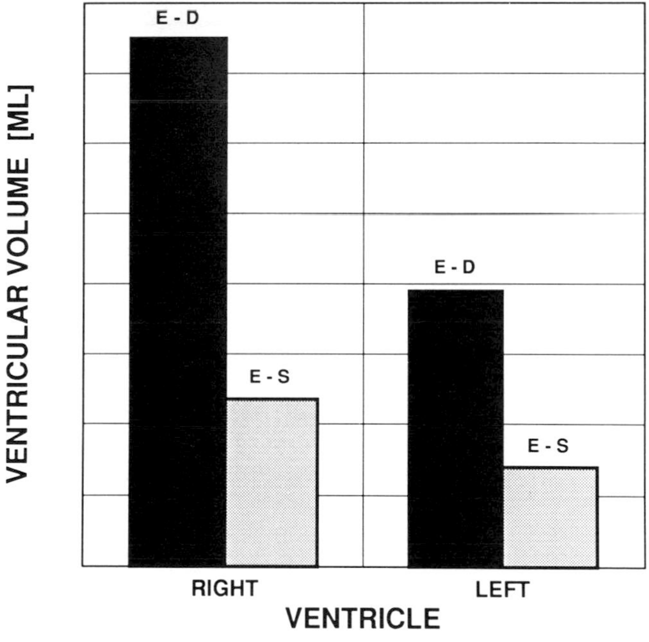

FIGURE 6. *Chamber volume analysis of an ASD with left-to-right shunting. On images from a cine MRI image loop at the midventricular level, endocardial borders of both the RV and LV can be easily recognized and delineated by region of interest methods to quantitate chamber volume changes over the cardiac cycle at that anatomical level* (top). *The observed signal void jet (curved arrow) is due to flow disturbance related to left-to-right shunting through a secundum ASD. Chamber volume analysis of a series of image loops covering the cardiac chambers permits accurate determinations of SV for both the RV and LV based on the difference between end-diastolic (E-D) and end-systolic (E-S) volumes* (bottom). *This approach allows assessment of overall function of each ventricle (eg, EF). In the absence of concurrent volume overloading conditions, it also permits quantitation of the amount of shunting by the evaluation of the difference between the larger SV of the RV (representing systemic SV plus shunt volume) and the smaller LV SV (representing only systemic SV). LV, left ventricle; RV, right ventricle.*

of the VSD.[21,25] Therefore, the ventricular volume method may not be as accurate in the setting of a VSD as an ASD.

Flow Volume Analysis

Some of the previously mentioned limitations of ventricular volume analysis for shunt quantitation may be overcome using flow volume analysis of great artery flow with the VMap version of dynamic gradient-echo MRI. With this approach, quantitation of shunt size can be accomplished by measurement of net blood flow volumes within the pulmonary artery and ascending aorta over a cardiac cycle. Normally, the integrated areas under the VMap curves for the main pulmonary artery and ascending aorta are equal. Conversely, shunts produce discrepant pulmonary and systemic arterial flows, with the former exceeding the latter in left-to-right shunts and the converse in right-to-left shunts (Figure 7).[1,26] This difference can be expressed either in absolute terms (eg, shunt volume) or in relative terms (eg, Qp/Qs). Values for shunting derived by flow volume analysis have correleted well with the results from cardiac catheterization or nuclear first-pass ventriculography.[26]

Flow Pattern Analysis

Quantitative analysis of the altered intracardiac/vascular flow patterns in CHD can be pursued using either the cine or VMap versions of dynamic gradient-echo MRI.

For cine MRI, at least semi-quantitative assessment of complex flow changes can be based on the size of the resulting signal void jet.[1,17] In addition to the previously described ventricular volume approach to quantitation of valvular insufficiency, the dimensions or volumes of the signal void within the recipient chamber itself may be exploited. The most useful expression of this approach is the measurement of the total volume of the signal void at its maximum on all tomographic image loops showing evidence of such flow disturbance; the total maximum volume has been found to be significantly different between grades of severity of valvular insufficiency.[1,17,20] The signal void jet size beyond a stenotic lesion has also been assessed as a measure of the severity of flow disturbance.[1] In coarctation, jet length on cine MRI correlates well with angiographic severity of coarctation.[23] Similarly, early experience indicates that valvular aortic stenosis can be graded, at least semiquantitatively, using cine MRI; there is significant correlation between the severity of the pressure gradient across the stenotic aortic valve and the length of the signal void jet.[1] In cases of patent ductus arteriosus, the size of the jet on cine MRI correlates with the degree of stenosis determined by either Doppler echocardiography or angiography.[22]

In general, the proton phase changes due to hemodynamic abnormalities with complex flows causing signal void on the cine version limits the measurement of velocity of regurgitant or post-stenotic flows on the VMap version, but technical advancements (eg, short TE gradient-echo sequences) should help overcome this limitation. Indeed, promising initial clinical results have been reported.[27] Conversely, the capabilities of the VMap method in slow flow conditions are not limited in this fashion. In cases of ASD, pulmonary artery flow has been measured using the VMap version, and marked differences between cases with and cases without secondary

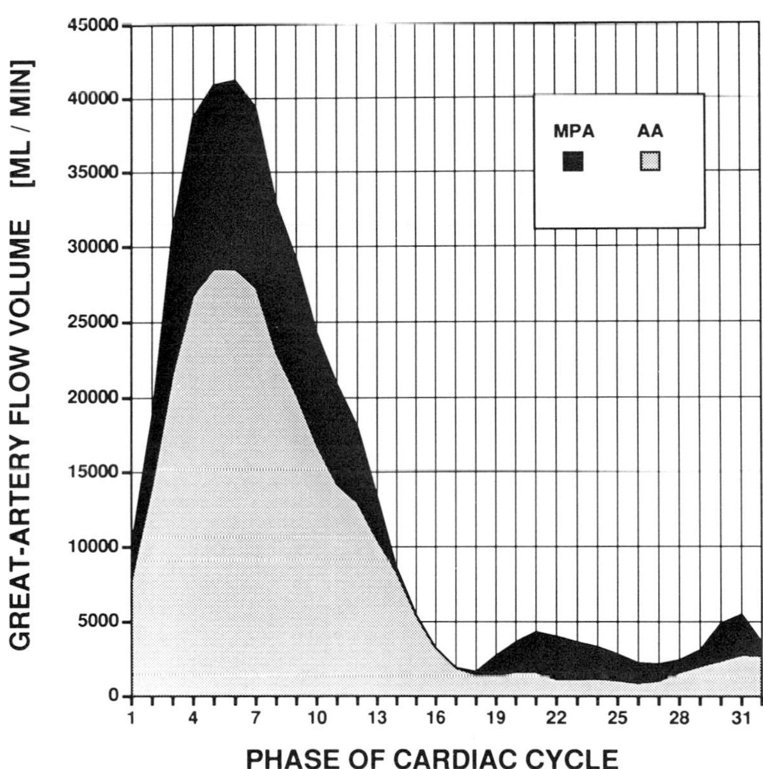

FIGURE 7. *Flow volume analysis of an ASD with left-to-right shunting. In the same case as in Figure 6, flow volume analysis using the VMap method permits direct measurement of the great artery flow volumes over the cardiac cycle after integration of the areas under the curves resulting from plotting of mean instantaneous volume flows passing through a cross section of each artery. The relative difference in flow volumes between the main pulmonary artery (MPA) (representing systemic SV plus shunt volume) and the ascending aorta (AA) (representing only systemic SV) may be used to derive a quantitative measure of left-to-right shunting (eg, Qp/Qs).*

pulmonary arterial hypertension have been observed; specifically, decreased antegrade and increased retrograde flows, along with early peaking of systolic flow velocity, have been observed in those with significantly elevated pulmonary arterial pressures.[28]

Postoperative Evaluation

As more patients with CHD undergo corrective surgery and survive longer, postoperative clinical evaluation becomes increasingly important. The combination of capabilities described earlier for the evaluation of anatomical and physiologic aspects makes MRI uniquely suited for the noninvasive evaluation following surgical repair of CHD. In contrast to Doppler echochocardiography, MRI is not restricted by limited acoustic windows or postoperative scarring.

Important postoperative anatomical features of various surgical procedures for CHD (eg, Fontan procedure for tricuspid atresia; aortic conduit placement for coarctation; systemic pulmonary artery shunts, including Blalock-Taussig, Glenn, Waterston shunts; Norwood procedure for hypoplastic left heart syndrome) have been successfully detected and delineated using spin-echo MRI.[29–32] Again, cine MRI has the advantage over spin-echo MRI of improved differentiation between blood vessels and air-filled structures, and this feature proves to be particularly valuable in the assessment of surgical shunts between the systemic and pulmonary arterial circulations placed for congenitally restricted pulmonary flow. However, the artifacts from metallic surgical materials are more prominent on gradient-echo MRI than on spin-echo MRI due to greater sensitivity of the former to local magnetic field inhomogeneities, and this may hinder adequate visualization of structures.

Cine MRI has also been used successfully for postoperative functional evaluation. Following intra-atrial baffle procedures for transposition of the great arteries, cine MRI has been used to derive accurate RV EF values, establish patency of the RV and LV outflow tracts, and differentiate patency from obstruction of the superior vena cava.[33] When compliance of the ascending aorta was measured with cine MRI following coarctation repair, derived values were found to be abnormally low, suggesting that poor compliance may be a factor in ongoing systolic arterial hypertension.[34] In addition, improved flow patterns on cine MRI have been noted after surgical repair of coarctation, but most signal void jets beyond the site of repair do not relate to a residual gradient, but rather to the luminal irregularity due to surgery.[34] Following pulmonary artery banding, cine MRI has demonstrated significant systolic and early diastolic signal void jets distal to the narrowing in all cases, indicating satisfactory banding.[19] Finally, using cine MRI, postoperative complications (eg, peripatch leak after VSD repair) have also been detected based on the presence of signal void jets.

Summary

With its multiple capabilities, MRI is able to provide a great deal of the fundamental information regarding the changes in anatomy and physiology of the central cardiovascular system characterizing the various forms of CHD. Especially when used in combination with Doppler echocardiography, most of the clinically important parameters that are necessary to accurately establish specific diagnoses of CHD, judge prognosis, and plan therapy can be addressed noninvasively. Hence, the need for catheterization can, in many instances, be restrictive to the acquisition of needed pressure measurements. Similar to this preoperative role, the potential role of MRI in the postoperative period of CHD is also great. With further technical advancements, these roles for MRI in the evaluation of CHD should continue to increase.

References

1. White RD, Paschal CB, Tkach JA, et al: Functional cardiovascular evaluation by magnetic resonance imaging. *Top Magn Reson Imag* 1990;2:31–48.

2. Fletcher BD, Jacobstein MD, Nelson AD, et al: Gated magnetic resonance imaging of congenital cardiac malformations. *Radiology* 1984;150:137–140.
3. Link KM, Lesko NM: Magnetic resonance imaging in the evaluation of congenital heart disease. *Magn Reson Q* 1991;7:173–190.
4. Kersting-Sommerhoff BA, Diethelm L, Teitel DF, et al: Magnetic resonance imaging of congenital heart disease: sensitivity and specificity using receiver operating characteristic curve analysis. *Am Heart J* 1989;118:155–161.
5. Fisher MR, Hricak H, Higgins CB: Magnetic resonance imaging of developmental venous anomalies. *AJR* 1985;145:705–709.
6. Fletcher BD, Jacobstein MD, Abramowsky CR, et al: Right atrioventricular valve atresia: anatomic evaluation with MR imaging. *AJR* 1987;148:671–674.
7. Kersting-Sommerhoff BA, Diethelm L, Stanger P, et al: Evaluation of complex congenital ventricular anomalies with magnetic resonance imaging. *Am Heart J* 1990;120:133–142.
8. Guit GL, Bluemm R, Rohmer J, et al: Levotransposition of the aorta: identification of segmental cardiac anatomy using MR imaging. *Radiology* 1986;161:673–679.
9. Parsons JM, Baker EJ, Anderson RH, et al: Double-outlet right ventricle: morphologic demonstration using nuclear magnetic resonance imaging. *J Am Coll Cardiol* 1991;18:168–178.
10. Formanek AG, Witcofski RL, D'Souza VJ, et al: MR imaging of the central pulmonary arterial tree in conotruncal malformation. *AJR* 1986;147:1127–1131.
11. Diethelm L, Dery R, Lipton MJ, et al: Atrial-level shunts: sensitivity and specificity of MR in diagnosis. *Radiology* 1987;162:181–186.
12. Lowell DG, Turner DA, Smith SM, et al: The detection of atrial and venticular septal defects with electrocardiographically synchronized magnetic resonance imaging. *Circulation* 1986;73:89–94.
13. Didier D, Higgins CB: Identification and localization of ventricular septal defect by gated magnetic resonance imaging. *Am J Cardiol* 1986;57:1363–1368.
14. Gomes AS, Lois JF, George B, et al: Congenital abnormalities of the aortic arch: MR imaging. *Radiology* 1987;165:691–695.
15. Soulen RL, Fishman EK, Pyeritz RE, et al: Marfan syndrome: evaluation with MR imaging versus CT. *Radiology* 1987;165:697–701.
16. Vick GW, Rokey R, Huhta JC, et al: Nuclear magnetic resonance imaging of the pulmonary arteries, subpulmonary region, and aorticopulmonary shunts: a comparative study with two-dimensional echocardiography and angiography. *Am Heart J* 1990;119:1103–1109.
17. Higgins CB, Holt W, Pflugfelder P, et al: Functional evaluation of the heart with magnetic resonance imaging. *Magn Reson Med* 1988;6:121–139.
18. Carlson MD, White RD, Trohman RG, et al: Cine magnetic resonance imaging scan detects previously unrecognized anatomical abnormalities in patients with right ventricular outflow tract ventricular tachycardia. (abstract) *Circulation* 1991;84(suppl II):II-646.
19. Chung KJ, Simpson IA, Newman R, et al: Cine magnetic resonance imaging for evaluation of congenital heart disease: role in pediatric cardiology compared with echocardiography and angiography. *J Pediatr* 1988;113:1028–1035.
20. Assessment of cardiac function with cine magnetic resonance imaging. In: Higgins CB, Silverman NH, Kersting-Sommerhoff BA, Schmidt KG. *Congenital Heart Disease: Echocardiography and Magnetic Resonance*. New York: Raven Press Publishers; 1990:335–343.
21. Sechtem U, Pflugfelder P, Cassidy MC, et al: Ventricular septal defect: visualization of shunt flow and determination of shunt size by cine MR imaging. *AJR* 1987;149:689–692.
22. Chien CT, Lin CS, Hsu YH, et al: Potential diagnosis of hemodynamic abnormalities in patent ductus arteriosus by cine magnetic resonance imaging. *Am Heart J* 1991;122:1065–1073.
23. Simpson IA, Chung KJ, Glass RF, et al: Cine magnetic resonance imaging for evaluation of anatomy and flow relations in infants and children with coarctation of the aorta. *Circulation* 1988;78:142–148.
24. Theissen P, Sechtem U, Linden A, et al: Noninvasive assessment of atrial septal defects

and anomalous connections of pulmonary veins by magnetic resonance imaging. (abstract) *Radiology* 1988;169(P):270.

25. Sechtem U, Theissen P: Evaluation of congenital heart disease with gradient echo (cine) magnetic resonance imaging. In: Higgins CB, Silverman NH, Kersting-Sommerhoff BA, Schmidt KG. *Congenital Heart Disease: Echocardiography and Magnetic Resonance*. New York: Raven Press Publishers; 1990:345–359.
26. Rees S, Firmin D, Mohiaddin R, et al: Application of flow measurements by magnetic resonance velocity mapping to congenital heart disease. *Am J Cardiol* 1989;64:953–956.
27. Kilner PJ, Firmin DN, Rees RS, et al: Valve and great vessel stenosis: assessment with MR jet velocity mapping. *Radiology* 1991;178:229–235.
28. Bogren HC, Klipstein RH, Mohiaddin RH, et al: Pulmonary artery distensibility and blood flow patterns: a magnetic resonance study of normal subjects and of patients with pulmonary arterial hypertension. *Am Heart J* 1989;118:990–999.
29. Sampson C, Martinez J, Rees S, et al: Evaluation of Fontan's operation by magnetic resonance imaging. *Am J Cardiol* 1990;65:819–821.
30. Pucillo AL, Schechter AG, Kay RH, et al: Magnetic resonance imaging of vascular conduits in coarctation of the aorta. *Am Heart J* 1989;117:482–485.
31. Jacobstein MD, Fletcher BD, Nelson AD, et al: Magnetic resonance imaging: evaluation of palliative systemic-pulmonary artery shunts. *Circulation* 1984;70:650–656.
32. Kondo C, Hardy C, Higgins SS, et al: Nuclear magnetic resonance imaging of the palliative operation for hypoplastic left heart syndrome. *J Am Coll Cardiol* 1991;18:817–823.
33. Chung KJ, Simpson IA, Glass RF, et al: Cine magnetic resonance imaging after surgical repair in patients with transposition of the great arteries. *Circulation* 1988;77:104–109.
34. Rees S, Somerville J, Ward C, et al: Coarctation of the aorta: MR imaging in late postoperative assessment. *Radiology* 1989;173:499–502.

Chapter 6

Left Ventricular Function: Pathophysiologic Considerations

Louis J. Dell'Italia, MD

The complete evaluation of left ventricular function includes an assessment of preload, afterload, and contractility. In addition to heart rate, these parameters play a major role in determining the oxygen demand (MVO_2) of the heart.[1,2] In response to any stress, whether it is the intermittent physical activity of the marathon runner or the continuous pressure overload of the patient with systemic hypertension, the heart must adapt to maintain stroke output in the face of increased systolic tension. This adaptation results in an increase in left ventricular mass and is mediated by an increase in myocyte size in the adult heart.[3,4] This hypertrophy process is also accompanied by a structural remodeling of chamber geometry and of the components of the myocardium, including its collagen matrix and capillaries, as well as the biochemical properties of the myocytes themselves.[5] This process is a physiologic response as long as oxygen supply exceeds oxygen demand at rest and especially during physical activity. However, when an imbalance in oxygen supply and demand results, the adaptive process is no longer physiologic, but instead is pathologic. This transition from a physiologic to a pathologic response is poorly understood and as yet is not clearly defined by any one or any combination of clinical or functional parameters.

Current evaluation of ventricular function includes a history and physical examination in addition to a functional assessment of the pump function of the heart by some imaging modality. However, by the time the left ventricular dysfunction becomes manifest by symptoms and a decreased ejection fraction, irreversible myocyte damage may have already occurred. However, a diagnostic approach that provides insight into how the adaptive process affects remodeling of the chamber (eg, left ventricular geometry and volume), afterload at the myocardial level (eg, wall stress and left ventricular mass), and myocardial oxygen supply and demand (eg, high-energy phosphate metabolism) might alert the clinician to early decompensation before irreversible myocyte damage. Cine magnetic resonance imaging (MRI) and phosphorus-31 nuclear magnetic resonance spectroscopy (^{31}P NMR) offer a window to follow morphologic and functional parameters as they relate to the bioenergetic profile of the heart.

From Pohost GM (ed.), *Cardiovascular Applications of Magnetic Resonance.* Mount Kisco, NY, Futura Publishing Co., Inc., © 1993.

Evaluation of Preload

Preload is defined in studies of isolated muscle as the resting stress (force/cross-sectional area) prior to electrical stimulation.[6] Extrapolation of this definition to the intact heart is difficult and has been substituted by an end-diastolic, atrial, or pulmonary capillary wedge pressure. However, there are a number of factors that can affect the diastolic pressure of the heart chamber, including: physical properties (eg, mass, composition of the wall); intrinsic dynamic factors (eg, myocardial relaxation); and extrinsic factors (eg, pericardium and ventricular interdependence).[7] A better insight into how these factors might affect cavitary pressure could be provided by the ratio of wall thickness to chamber radius, an estimate of overall mass, a diastolic time-volume curve, and an index of diastolic interference of one ventricle on the other as gleaned from the geometric configuration of the shared interventricular septum. Magnetic resonance imaging offers a detailed assessment of the heart that evaluates these qualitative and quantitative estimates and provides insight into the adaptive (or de-adaptive) responses to mechanical stress. This, in addition to an accurate estimate of volume, provides a comprehensive assessment of preload.

Studies have demonstrated that MRI of the heart yields accurate estimates of left ventricular mass[8,9] and cardiac chamber dimensions.[10] Cardiac MRI produces distinct visualization of endocardial borders and inherently three-dimensional information for the measurement of ventricular volumes. These features offer significant advantages for calculation of accurate ventricular volumes because there are no assumptions of geometry. In vitro cast studies of the left and right ventricles in both human[11] and canine[12] hearts demonstrate a high correlation (0.99) of water displacement volumes with MRI-derived volumes over a wide range of ventricular volumes. Markiewicz and co-workers[13] validated in vivo left ventricular volume estimates by demonstrating equal right and left ventricular stroke volumes calculated from the MRI-derived volumes. However, the MRI-derived stroke volumes underestimated those determined by thermodilution measurements of cardiac output. The spin-echo imaging technique used in that study had a low frame acquisition rate (100 msec between frames) that could not provide the temporal resolution to accurately identify end systole. The gradient-echo technique circumvents this problem by providing a better sampling frequency of 30 msec. Using this technique, we validated a serial short-axis method for obtaining absolute right and left ventricular volumes in our laboratory by using intact postmortem canine ventricles cast with silicone rubber.[14,15] Subsequent water displacement volumes of the right and left ventricular casts correlated with cine MRI derived volumes with high correlation coefficients and small standard errors ($r=0.99$, SE = 0.96 ml; and $r=0.99$, SE = 1.06, respectively).

In addition to the previously mentioned changes in chamber dimensions, wall thickness, and volume, there are adaptive changes in chamber geometry that can now be evaluated with the three-dimensional capabilities of MRI. Singleton[16] has recently developed automatic edge detection software in our laboratory that provides three-dimensional images of the left ventricle. Figure 1 demonstrates a three-dimensional reconstruction of the left ventricle at end diastole in a normal subject demonstrating the normal truncated elliptical configuration. Future work evaluating three-dimensional displays of the right and left ventricular chambers and interventricular

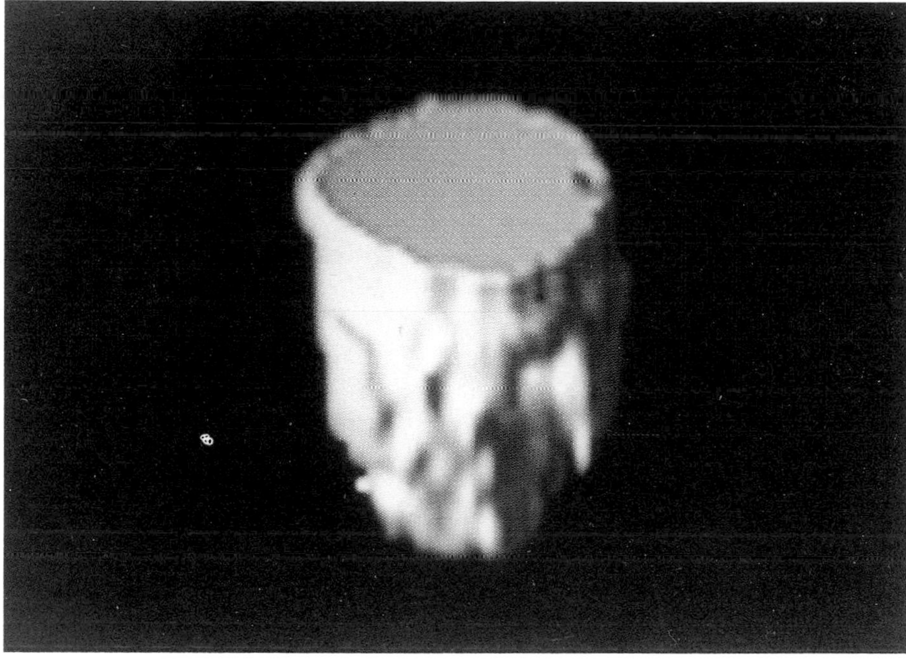

FIGURE 1. *Three-dimensional image of the left ventricle at end diastole in a normal human subject.*

septum will provide insight into how each ventricle adapts to its respective load during diastole and systole.[17]

Evaluation of Afterload

The force opposing the shortening of muscle fibers, or afterload, is a major determinant of myocardial performance in isolated muscle preparations and intact heart. Arterial blood pressure and systemic vascular resistance are the most commonly used clinical measures of afterload. However, these indexes are only a small part of the load faced by the ejecting ventricle. Aortic input impedance is better than pressure for characterizing afterload because it incorporates the complex relationship between pulsatile pressure and flow that is mainly determined by the viscoelasticity of the aortic wall, diameter of the vessels, and physical properties of the blood.[18] This dynamic relationship between pressure and flow provides estimates of vessel compliance and possible importance of wave reflection imparted by stiffened arterial vessels. However, acute or chronic changes in impedance do not reflect the interrelationship between ventricular wall thickness, chamber dimensions, and chamber pressure, all of which directly affect the response to afterload at the myocardial level. Therefore, in the left ventricular chamber, afterload is best approximated by application of the Laplace relation (pressure × radius/wall thickness).

In the ventricle subjected to a chronic pressure overload, the myocardial cell undergoes hypertrophy by the addition of new sarcomeres in parallel so that the chamber wall stress estimate and, presumably, the systolic force/myocardial cell relationship remain unchanged.[19] This adaptation produces concentric hypertrophy such that the wall thickness : chamber radius ratio is substantially increased. In contrast, the volume overloaded ventricle undergoes eccentric hypertrophy whereby wall thickness increases sufficiently to counterbalance the increase in chamber radius. These changes represent an important adaptive process in maintaining stable oxygen demand. Weber and Janicki[20,21] have demonstrated a close relationship between the integral of systolic force and MVO_2 for conditions of a constant contractile state and heart rate in both the ejecting and isovolumetrically beating heart. Therefore, serial estimates of chamber wall stress can provide an index of the appropriateness of the hypertrophy process in patients with chronic pressure or volume overload.[22,23]

Toward the goal of combining accurate MRI-derived dimensions and wall thickness with pressures to calculate estimates of wall stress, we have developed a catheter tip manometer to record high-fidelity pressures without distorting magnetic resonance images in an intact dog.[24] Furthermore, this catheter is inserted percutaneously so that the pericardium and thorax are never disturbed by a surgical procedure. Using this approach we obtained wall stress throughout the cardiac cycle during increases in afterload in six anesthetized dogs having depressed contractility produced by halothane anesthesia and intravenous propranolol. An assessment of wall stress versus time during left ventricular ejection demonstrated a linear slope that we have called time-varying wall stress.[14] In the mildly to moderately depressed ventricle, time-varying wall stress decreased as pressure was increased modestly with intravenous infusion of angiotensin. We applied a mathematical model that partitions each of the parameters of the wall stress calculation and demonstrated that the rising pressure component in the latter half of systole was the sole determinant of the decrease in slope of the wall stress-time relationship during ejection (Figure 2). We postulated that increased wave reflection in the arterial circulation is a plausible underlying mechanism of action. Evaluation of time-varying wall stress in patients with congestive heart failure before and after treatment with vasodilators may provide new insight into how these agents improve cardiac output without appreciably altering systemic arterial pressure.[25,26] These data can be obtained in patients because we and others have demonstrated that wall stress can be calculated throughout systolic ejection using time-matched MRI-derived dimensions and wall thickness and a noninvasive pressure recording.[27,28]

The previous discussion has referred to global wall stress calculations in a ventricle without wall motion abnormalities due to ischemia or previous myocardial infarction. However, left ventricular enlargement, or remodeling, frequently occurs after myocardial infarction involving a large amount of myocardium. There is now increasing evidence that geometric rearrangement of the wall and chamber provokes a substantial increase in stress of the noninfarcted wall segment.[29] This should provide a mechanical stimulus for myocyte growth, thereby maintaining a normal regional stress.[30] However, this adaptive process does not occur in a predictable manner nor can it be easily followed without an assessment of regional wall stress that requires a direct measurement of local geometry. The application of the three-dimensional capabilities of MRI can alert the clinician to subtle changes in geometry of the noninfarcted wall segment early after a myocardial

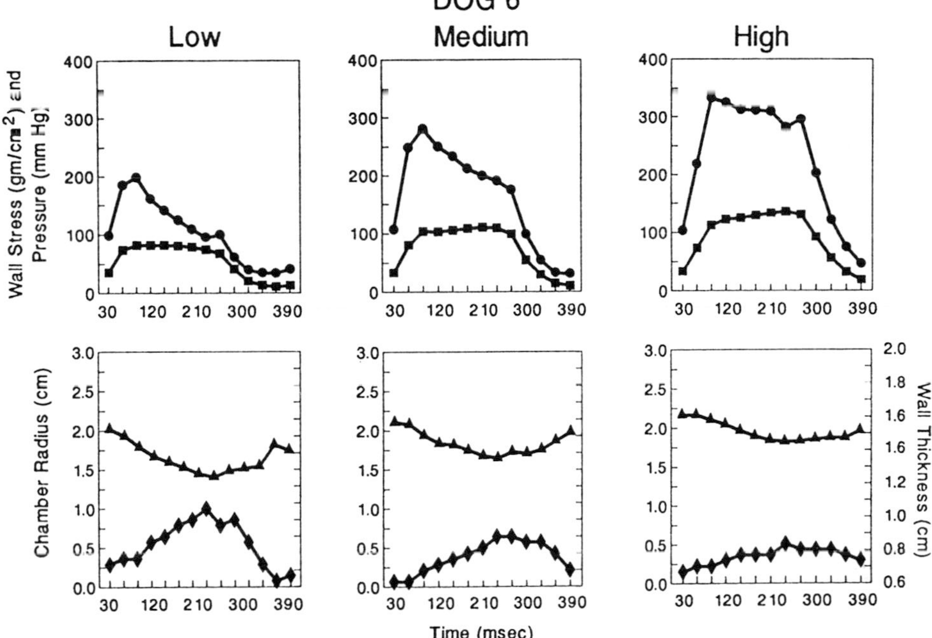

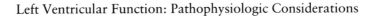

FIGURE 2. *Comparison of changes in left ventricular pressure (■ ■), circumferential wall stress (● ●), chamber radius (▲ ▲), and wall thickness (◆ ◆) throughout the cardiac cycle for control and angiotensin infusions at low, medium, and high loading conditions in a representative canine. With increasing load there is a decrease in the slope of the wall stress–time relationship during ejection (time-varying wall stress). Reproduced from the* American Journal of Physiology *with permission.*

infarction that, if not compensated for by an appropriate hypertrophy process, will lead to subsequent ventricular enlargement and heart failure.

Evaluation of Contractility

Ideally, the clinical evaluation of contractility of the heart should provide an index of the contractile performance of each myocardial cell. However, commonly used ejection phase indexes of pump performance such as ejection fraction and percent fractional shortening are affected by changes in loading condition independent of changes of muscle function. For example, in mitral regurgitation a normal ejection fraction can occur in the presence of muscle dysfunction because of the beneficial effects of an increase in preload due to the regurgitant lesion and a decrease in afterload due to ejection into the low-pressure left atrium. In contrast, extremes of cardiac loading conditions can produce failure of the heart as a pump, even when myocardial contractility is not depressed. Other hemodynamic indexes of pump performance including the ventricular function curve, dP/dt_{max}, or velocity of circumferential shortening are load-dependent measures of contractility.

The linear relation between end-systolic pressure and volume has been used as an index of contractility in studies of the isolated, in vivo animal, and human heart.[31,32] A limitation of the end-systolic pressure-volume relationship is that wall stress rather than pressure is a better index of afterload because it takes into account both left ventricular size and wall thickness. Accordingly, the determination of the relation between mean wall stress during ejection and mean velocity of circumferential shortening (force-velocity relation) has provided a reliable index for identifying depression of contractility.[31] However, use of these constructs of left ventricular performance require at least three loading conditions produced by infusion of a vasoconstrictor. This time-consuming and potentially hazardous maneuver has led to the use of a simple pressure-volume ratio as an index of contractility. Because a single point ratio assumes a zero intercept, it does not truly represent the end-systolic pressure-volume slope and, therefore, has resulted in variable success clinically. However, Carabello and co-workers[23] have successfully used the end-systolic stress–end-systolic volume index ratio to predict postoperative clinical status in patients undergoing mitral valve replacement for severe mitral regurgitation (Figure 3). The use of a wall stress calculation incorporates the adaptive compensation of the hypertrophy process as it relates to the volume at end systole. Although this study provided promising data for identifying contractile dysfunction in the difficult problem of mitral regurgition, further studies have not tested its usefulness in a large number of patients. Nevertheless, the concept of how chamber radius and wall thickness relate to the peak

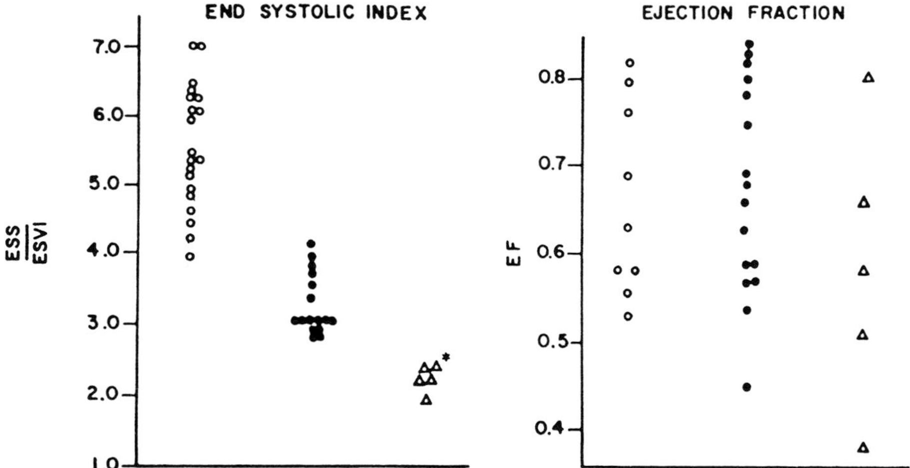

FIGURE 3. Left panel: *The end-systolic stress/end-systolic volume index ratio (ESS/ESVI) in normal subjects (open circles), in patients with severe mitral regurgitation who improved clinically after valve replacement (closed circles), and in patients who died or did not improve after mitral valve replacement (open triangles).* **Right panel:** *Use of the ESS/ESVI ratio allowed for separation of groups, whereas left ventricular ejection did not. Reproduced from the American Heart Association with permission.*

or end-systolic pressure is an important adjunct to the ejection fraction value when one is trying to determine whether irreversible muscle damage is present.

Evaluation of Bioenergetics

Because of the complexity in defining contractility of the heart, it should not be surprising that there is no single index that can be used and compared in all patients. However, as stated previously, the ventricle undergoes hypertrophy in response to a mechanical stress in order to maintain a stable myocardial tension and oxygen demand both at rest and during physical exertion. If this adaptive process could be monitored as it relates to the supply of oxygen or energy substrates for contraction, the onset of de-adaptation could be identified by an imbalance of myocardial oxygen supply and demand or by an imbalance between the adaptive process of the heart and its own energy supply.

Oxidative phosphorylation generates most of the energy for cardiac contraction through the production of adenosine triphosphate (ATP). One of the means by which ATP production increases in response to increased work is through the creatine kinase reaction that catalyzes the transfer of high-energy phosphate groups between phosphocreatine (PCr) and ATP:

$$H + Mg \cdot ADP + PCr\ 7\ Mg \cdot ATP + Creatine$$

The application of ^{31}P NMR to biological tissue studying both steady-state levels of high-energy phosphate compounds and creatine kinase kinetics has provided evidence that mitochondrial creatine kinase plays an important role in linking oxidative phosphorylation and cardiac contraction in normal and diseased hearts.[34,35] Because oxidative phosphorylation generates most of the ATP for cardiac work, MVO_2 correlates closely with cardiac energy utilization. In vivo studies in canines have related changes in high-energy phosphate metabolites to direct measurements of MVO_2 during alterations in loading conditions.[36] While PCr and inorganic phosphorus levels reflected changes in MVO_2, heart rate–systolic pressure product was similar in response to increases in afterload and contractility despite a marked disparity in MVO_2 during each load. This result is in accord with previous studies because rate pressure product does not account for changes in ventricular volume, geometric influences, and the contractile state of the myocardium.[1] As discussed previously, an accurate assessment of contractility is difficult. However, the integral of the wall stress-time relationship correlates with directly measured MVO_2.[20,21] Therefore, an analysis of wall stress in combination with high-energy phosphate metabolism could provide an estimate of energy demand as it relates to the functional adequacy of oxygen delivery in the absence of a direct measurement of MVO_2.

Using combined MRI, ^{31}P NMR, and our nonferrous high-fidelity catheter, we evaluated the relationship between high-energy phosphate metabolites and cardiac work as determined by wall stress estimates and dP/dt_{max} during angiotensin and dobutamine infusions in an intact canine model.[37] In spite of a marked increase in afterload and contractility, there was no significant change in the PCr/ATP ratio.

Hemodynamic and MRI evaluation of baseline left ventricular function demonstrated myocardial depression most likely due to the effects of halothane anesthesia. The significant increase in heart rate and dP/dt_{max} during dobutamine was balanced by the significant decrease in total systolic stress integral (area under the wall stress-time relationship curve) (Figure 4). In contrast, there was a tendency for the PCr/ATP ratio to decrease during angiotensin (Figure 5). This may be related to the twofold increase in the total systolic stress integral (Figure 4). The effects of acute alterations in workload on left ventricular MVO_2 and PCr/ATP are complex and are determined not only by changes in afterload, inotropy, and heart rate, but also by the baseline contractile state of the heart. In the absence of a direct measurement of MVO_2, wall stress should provide a better estimate of oxygen demand because its calculation incorporates both pressure and ventricular size. This was a study of the effects of acute alterations in load and contractility. However, the inclusion of ventricular dimensions and wall thickness becomes even more important in evaluating the ventricle subjected to a chronic pressure or volume overload because it provides information regarding the adequacy of the hypertrophy process in maintaining stable oxygen demands.

In the absence of a direct measurement of MVO_2 and coronary blood flow, the PCr/ATP ratio provides an estimate of the functional adequacy of coronary blood flow

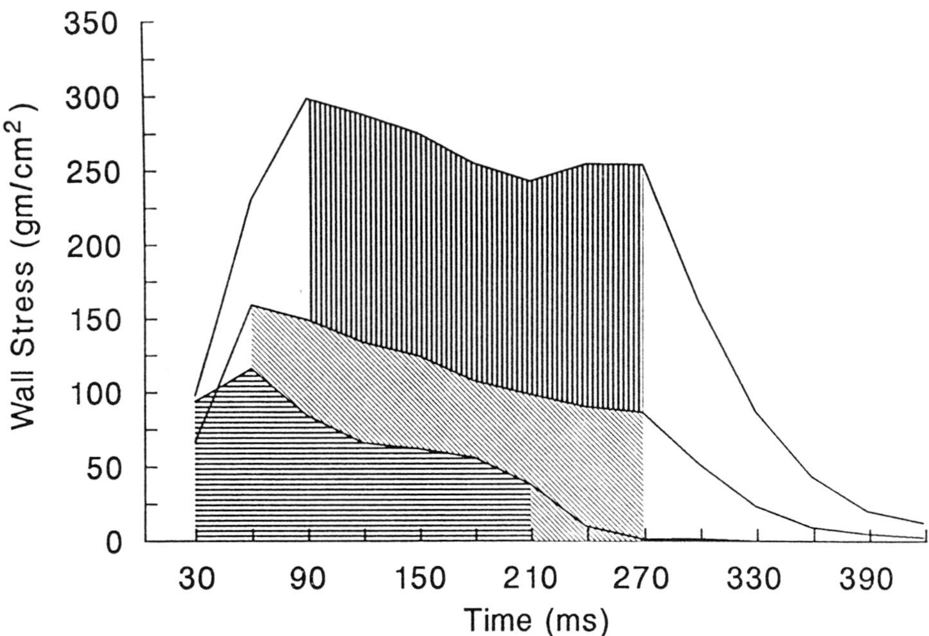

FIGURE 4. *Total systolic stress integral for control (diagonal cross-hatched lines), dobutamine (horizontal cross-hatched lines), and angiotensin (vertical cross-hatched lines) in a representative canine. The onset of the systolic stress integral was taken at the time when the ventricle demonstrated evidence of shortening in the cine magnetic resonance frames obtained at 30-msec intervals. The end-systolic stress was identified at the cine magnetic resonance frame closest to, but not occurring after,* $-dP/dt_{max}$.

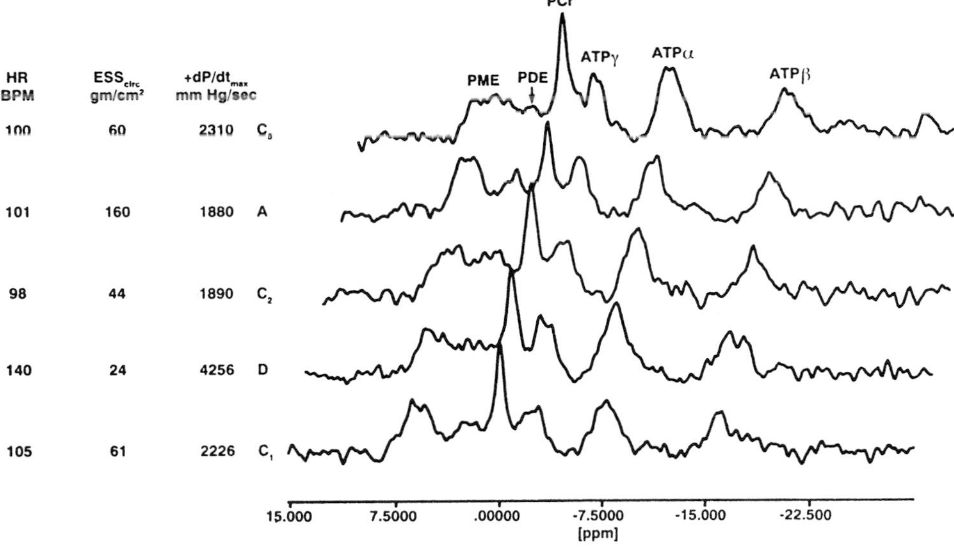

FIGURE 5. *Stacked plots of ^{31}P NMR spectra obtained at control 1 (C_1), dobutamine (D), control 2 (C_2), angiotensin infusion (A), and control 3 (C_3) in a representative animal. Corresponding heart rate (HR), end-systolic circumferential wall stress (ESS_{circ}), and peak $+dP/dt_{max}$ are listed to the left of each ^{31}P NMR spectra. PME, phosphomonoester; PDE, phosphodiester; PCr, phosphocreatine.*

(oxygen delivery) to the myocardium during acute alterations in load. There are other chronic cardiac conditions, however, that have been reported to decrease the PCr/ATP ratio by mechanisms other than a decrease in coronary blood flow. A low PCr/ATP ratio has been reported in patients with left ventricular hypertrophy secondary to aortic valvular disease,[38] and in animal models of heart failure resulting from chronic pressure overload.[34,40] In chronic left ventricular hypertrophy, the decreased PCr/ATP ratio has been associated with a decrease in creatine kinase activity and a fall in the total creatine content of muscle.[34,39,40]

Conclusions

The goal of the current discussion is to introduce an approach to the assessment of pump function of the heart that focuses on adaptive changes to mechanical stress as they relate to energy supply. Accordingly, changes in volume and geometry (preload), mass and wall stress (myocardial afterload), and the end-systolic stress/end-systolic volume index ratio (ESS/ESVI) (contractility) are related to energy supply (PCr/ATP ratio), thereby monitoring the balance of adaptation and oxygen requirements. It is hypothesized that the onset of de-adaptation is heralded by an imbalance of energy supply and demand and, if not checked, will result in irreversible myocyte damage. The capabilities of combined MRI and spectroscopy provide the possibility for such a comprehensive evaluation of mechanical and metabolic functions of the heart.

References

1. Baller D, Bretschneider HJ, Hellige G: A critical look at currently used indirect indexes of myocardial oxygen consumption. *Basic Res Cardiol* 1981;76:163–181.
2. Sonnenblick EH, Ross J, Braunwald E: Oxygen consumption of the heart: newer concepts of its multifactorial determination. *Am J Cardiol* 1968;22:328–336.
3. Weber KT, Clark WA, Janicki JS, Shroff SG: Physiologic versus pathologic hypertrophy and the pressure-overloaded myocardium. *J Cardiovasc Pharmacol* 1987;10:S37-S49.
4. Meerson FZ: A mechanism of hypertrophy and wear of the myocardium. *Am J Cardiol* 1965;15:755–760.
5. Swynghedauw B: Remodelling of the heart in response to chronic mechanical overload. *Eur Heart J* 1989;10:935–943.
6. Parmley WW, Talbot L: Heart as a pump. In: Berne RM (ed). *Handbook of Physiology—The Cardiovascular System (Section 2)*. Bethesda, MD: American Physiological Society; 1979:429-457.
7. Glantz SA, Parmley WW: Factors which affect the diastolic pressure-volume curve. *Circ Res* 1978;42:171–180.
8. Florentine MS, Grosskreutz CL, Chang W, et al: Measurement of left ventricular mass in in vivo gated nuclear magnetic resonance imaging. *J Am Coll Cardiol* 1986;8:107–112.
9. Maddahi J, Crues J, Berman DS, et al: Noninvasive quantification of left ventricular myocardial mass by gated proton nuclear magnetic resonance imaging. *J Am Coll Cardiol* 1987;10:682–692.
10. Dinsmore RE: Quantitation of cardiac dimensions from ECG-synchronized MRI studies. *Cardiovasc Intervent Radiol* 1987;10:356–364.
11. Rehr RB, Malloy CR, Filipchuk NG, Peshock RM: Left ventricular volumes measured by MR imaging. *Radiology* 1985;156:717–719.
12. Sechtem U, Pflugfelder PW, Gould RG, et al: Measurement of right and left ventricular volumes in healthy individuals with cine MR imaging. *Radiology* 1987;163:697–702.
13. Markiewicz W, Sechtem U, Kirby R, et al: Measurement of ventricular volumes in the dog by nuclear magnetic resonance imaging. *J Am Coll Cardiol* 1987;10:170–177.
14. Dell'Italia LJ, Blackwell GG, Thorn BT, et al: Time-varying wall stress: an index of ventricular vascular coupling. *Am J Physiol* 1992;32:H599-H605.
15. Pearce DJ, Dell'Italia LJ, Blackwell GG, et al: Simultaneous evaluation of the right and left ventricular pressure-volume relationship in an intact canine model (abstract). In: Proceedings of the Society of Magnetic Resonance in Medicine. 1990:1153.
16. Singleton HR: Automatic image segmentation using edge detection by tissue classification in local neighborhoods. *Proc IEEE, Southeastcon* 1992; 286–290.
17. Pearce DJ, Dell'Italia LJ, Blackwell GG, et al: Three-dimensional in-vivo analysis of the left ventricle following acute right ventricular hypertension. *Circulation* 1991; II-57.
18. O'Rourke MF: Vascular impedance in studies of arterial and cardiac function. *Physiol Rev* 1982;62:570–623.
19. Grossman W: Cardiac hypertrophy: useful adaptation or pathologic process? *Am J Med* 1980;69:576–584.
20. Weber KT, Janicki JS: Myocardial oxygen consumption: the role of wall force and shortening. *Am J Physiol* 1977;233:H421-H430.
21. Weber KT, Janicki JS: The metabolic demand and oxygen supply of the heart: physiologic and clinical considerations. *Am J Cardiol* 1979;44:722–729.
22. Carabello BA, Spann JF: The uses and limitations of end-systolic indexes of left ventricular function. *Circulation* 1984;69:1058–1064.
23. Carabello BA, Nolan SP, McGuire LB: Assessment of preoperative left ventricular function in patients with mitral regurgitation: value of the end-systolic wall stress-end-systolic volume ratio. *Circulation* 1981;64:1212–1217.
24. Dell'Italia LJ, Carter B, Millar H, Pohost GM: The development of a micro-tip catheter to record high-fidelity pressures during cine-gated NMR without significant image distortion. *Magn Reson Med* 1991;17:119–125.

25. Pepine CJ, Nichols WW, Curry RC Jr, Conti CR: Aortic input impedance during nitroprusside infusion. *J Clin Invest* 1979;64:643–654.
26. Pepine CJ, Nichols WW, Conti CR: Aortic input impedance in heart failure. *Circulation* 1978;58:460–465.
27. Baucum RW, Blackwell GG, Dell'Italia LJ, Pohost GM: Noninvasive determination of wall stress in humans using applanation tonometry and CINE MR (abstract). In: Proceedings of the Society of Magnetic Resonance in Medicine 1991:1001.
28. Auffermann W, Wagner S, Holt WW, et al: Noninvasive determination of left ventricular output and wall stress in volume overload and in myocardial disease by cine magnetic resonance imaging. *Am Heart J* 1991;121:1750–1758.
29. Capasso JM, Li P, Zhang P, Anversa P: Heterogeneity of ventricular remodeling after acute myocardial infarction in rats. *Am J Physiol* 1992;31:H486-H495.
30. Katz AM: Angiotensin II: hemodynamic regulator or growth factor? *J Mol Cell Cardiol* 1990;22:739–747.
31. Suga H, Sagawa K: Instantaneous pressure-volume relationships and their ratio in the excised, supported canine left ventricle. *Circ Res* 1974;35:117–126.
32. Sagawa K: The end-systolic pressure-volume relation of the ventricle: definition, modification, and clinical use. *Circulation* 1981;63:1223–1227.
33. Colan SD, Borow KM, Neumann A: Left ventricular end-systolic wall stress-velocity of fiber shortening relation: a load-independent index of myocardial contractility. *J Am Coll Cardiol* 1984;4:715–724.
34. Ingwall JS: The hypertrophied myocardium accumulates the MB-creatine kinase isozyme. *Eur Heart J* 1984;5:129–139.
35. Bittl JA, Ingwall JS: The energetics of myocardial stretch: creatine kinase flux and oxygen consumption in the noncontracting rat heart. *Circ Res* 1986;58:378–383.
36. Katz LA, Swain JA, Portman MA, Balaban RS: Relation between phosphate metabolites and oxygen consumption of heart in vivo. *Am J Physiol* 1989;256:H265-H274.
37. Dell'Italia LJ, Evanochko WT, Blackwell GG, et al: Relationship between shortening load, contractility, and myocardial energetics in an intact dog. *Am J Physiol* (in press).
38. Conway MA, Allis J, Ouwerkerk R, et al: Detection of low phosphocreatine to ATP ratio in failing hypertrophied human myocardium by ^{31}P magnetic resonance spectroscopy. *Lancet* 1991;338:973–976.
39. Ingwall JS, Kramer MF, Fifer MA, et al: The creatine kinase system in normal and diseased human myocardium. *N Engl J Med* 1985;313:1050–1054.
40. Bittl JA, Ingwall JS: Intracellular high-energy phosphate transfer in normal and hypertrophied myocardium. *Circulation* 1987;75(suppl I):I96-I101.

Chapter 7

Magnetic Resonance Imaging of Valvular Heart Disease

Charles B. Higgins, MD and
Gary R. Caputo, MD

Noninvasive imaging techniques have been used so increasingly during the past decade for the evaluation and monitoring of patients with valvular heart disease that currently the techniques have almost completely replaced angiocardiography for the diagnosis and assessment of the severity of valvular heart disease.[1–4] Cardiac catheterization and coronary angiography are still used in older patients prior to surgery in order to assess the status of the coronary arteries and also in circumstances of discrepancies between noninvasive studies and estimates of severity from clinical findings. Although echocardiography has been the primary technique used for the evaluation and monitoring of valvular heart disease, studies at several centers around the world during the past few years have demonstrated the considerable effectiveness of magnetic resonance imaging (MRI) for this purpose.[5–10] Magnetic resonance imaging, like echocardiography, is a completely noninvasive technique and consequently is an attractive technique for sequential monitoring of patients with valvular heart disease. An additional advantage of MRI is that it provides a three-dimensional data set that facilitates quantification of both valvular and ventricular function. The acquisition of a three-dimensional data set also eliminates uncertainties regarding reproducibility of the imaging data from one study to the next. Moreover, unlike echocardiographic and angiocardiographic measurements, it involves no geometric models for ventricular measurements that introduce potential errors in dilated and misshaped ventricles.

For the imaging technique to provide complete information in valvular heart disease, it is necessary to accurately detect the presence of a lesion, to quantify the severity of the valvular lesion, and to quantify ventricular dimensions, function, and pathological loading conditions. This chapter will discuss the capability of MRI for: 1) the detection and quantification of valvular regurgitation; 2) the detection and quantification of valvular stenosis; 3) the quantification of left ventricular dimensions, function, and loading conditions; and 4) monitoring of valvular and ventricular function.

From Pohost GM (ed.), *Cardiovascular Applications of Magnetic Resonance*. Mount Kisco, NY, Futura Publishing Co., Inc., © 1993.

Techniques

The evaluation of valvular and ventricular function requires the acquisition of images at multiple time frames during the cardiac cycle. While images at multiple time frames during the cardiac cycle can be accomplished using the spin-echo technique, it is generally advantageous to use the cine magnetic resonance technique. Fast gradient-echo techniques such as turbo gradient-echo imaging have been recently introduced and may have a role in the assessment of valvular heart disease in the future. Likewise, the instant imaging technique, referred to as echoplanar MRI, which obtains images in approximately 50 msec, will also likely have an important role in the assessment of valvular and ventricular function. However, the cine magnetic resonance technique has been the one applied in most studies for the evaluation of valvular heart disease up to the present.

Techniques Used in Assessing Valvular Heart Disease

Cine Magnetic Resonance Imaging

Cine magnetic resonance imaging acquires imaging data during short intervals during the cardiac cycle. The imaging data are acquired during a short TR interval. The length of the TR interval defines the time frame for each of the images. The TR is generally 20 to 30 msec and the TE is usually 5 to 10 msec. Usually some type of flow compensation technique is used as well in order to minimize signal loss caused by first-order motion effects. In general, the shortest TE available is used because artifacts caused by motion and the magnetic susceptibility effects are minimized with a short TE. The use of a flow compensation pulse has the unwanted effect of lengthening the TE. However, the use of a flow compensation technique along with a slightly higher TE value may be as efficacious as the use of the shortest TE available. As will be discussed later, the duration of the TE is important in the occurrence of a signal void used to recognize the presence of valvular regurgitation on cine magnetic resonance images.

Cine magnetic resonance images can be acquired at any field strength. The technique used in our laboratory uses a 1.5-T superconducting magnet. A gradient recalled acquisition by a steady-state technique utiiizes low flip angles of 30° and gradient refocused echoes with a TE of 5–10 msec and a TR of 20–30 msec. The acquisition matrix is usually 128×256 and uses a field of view of 32 cm, which is interpolated to 256×256 for display.

With the cine MRI technique used in our laboratory the TR is independent of the ECG signal. This independence of the pulse repetition from the ECG signal provides evenly spaced images throughout the cardiac cycle. The ECG is recorded, along with the imaging data, in order to accomplish retrospective sorting and reconstruction of the images in order to provide images at each time frame throughout the cardiac cycle. As indicated previously, the length of the time frame is equal to the TR interval. To generate the series of cine magnetic resonance images the data from 256 cardiac cycles is obtained.

Images can be acquired at a single tomographic level or at multiple tomographic levels during the same acquisition. The total number of images that can be acquired is equal to the R-R interval of the ECG divided by the TR interval. For instance, at a heart rate of 60 beats per minute the TR interval is 1,000 msec. If the TR is 20 msec, then 50 images can be acquired from one R wave to the next R wave. These 50 images can be acquired at a single tomographic level or they might be acquired at two or four tomographic levels, producing 25 and 12 images at each level, respectively. In our laboratory, 16 or more time frames are usually acquired at each tomographic level.

For the evaluation of valvular heart disease, images may be acquired in a variety of views (Figures 1 and 2). For the assessment of aortic regurgitation, images in the transverse and coronal views are generally acquired (Figure 1). For the evaluation of mitral regurgitation, transverse or horizontal long-axis (four-chamber) views are generally acquired. For tricuspid regurgitation, images in the transaxial or horizontal long-axis views are acquired. For the evaluation of ventricular function, images in the transverse or cardiac short-axis views are generally acquired. For the assessment of ventricular dimensions and function, occasionally a set of images in the cardiac long-axis and short-axis views are done in order to provide measurements based upon a biplane geometrical model similar to that used for angiographic measurements.[11,12]

For the evaluation of ventricular function, it is ideal to acquire images at each of the tomographic levels encompassing the entire ventricle. Images are done in either the transverse or cardiac short-axis views starting below the apex of the heart and extending to above the base of the left ventricle. Two or three tomographic levels are usually scanned at the same time, with a slice thickness of 10 mm and the interslice gap at 10 mm. The 10-mm gaps are acquired in subsequent imaging sequences. It usually requires 10–12 tomographic images to encompass the entire left ventricle. The short-axis images (perpendicular to the long axis of the left ventricle) are obtained by a double angulation of the slice selective gradient. Initially, a set of transverse images is acquired and from these transverse images a plane passing from the middle of the mitral valve to the cardiac apex is defined. Images acquired in this plane constitute the cardiac long-axis images. From a cardiac long-axis image positioned in the middle of the left ventricle, the short-axis plane is prescribed, perpendicular to a line passing between the mitral valve and the cardiac apex on the long-axis image. Short-axis and long-axis views of the valves may be acquired in order to assess flow across the valves using a flow encoded cine magnetic resonance technique (Figure 1).

Turbo Gradient-Echo Imaging

The short acquisition times available with the turbo gradient-echo technique offers the advantage of acquiring images within a single breath-hold. However, the total acquisition time of these images without the use of gating is usually 200 msec or more but can be as low as 125 msec using small acquisition matrices.[13,14] A new version of the turbo gradient-echo technique called segmented turbo gradient-echo has reduced the total acquisition time to approximately 50 msec.[15] However, it should be noted that the turbo gradient-echo, and even the segmented turbo gradient-echo sequences, do not acquire images at a sufficiently rapid frequency to isolate images corresponding to end diastole and end systole. The temporal frequency of these techniques for evaluating cardiac function is inferior to that provided by cine magnetic resonance.

(Text continues on p. 96)

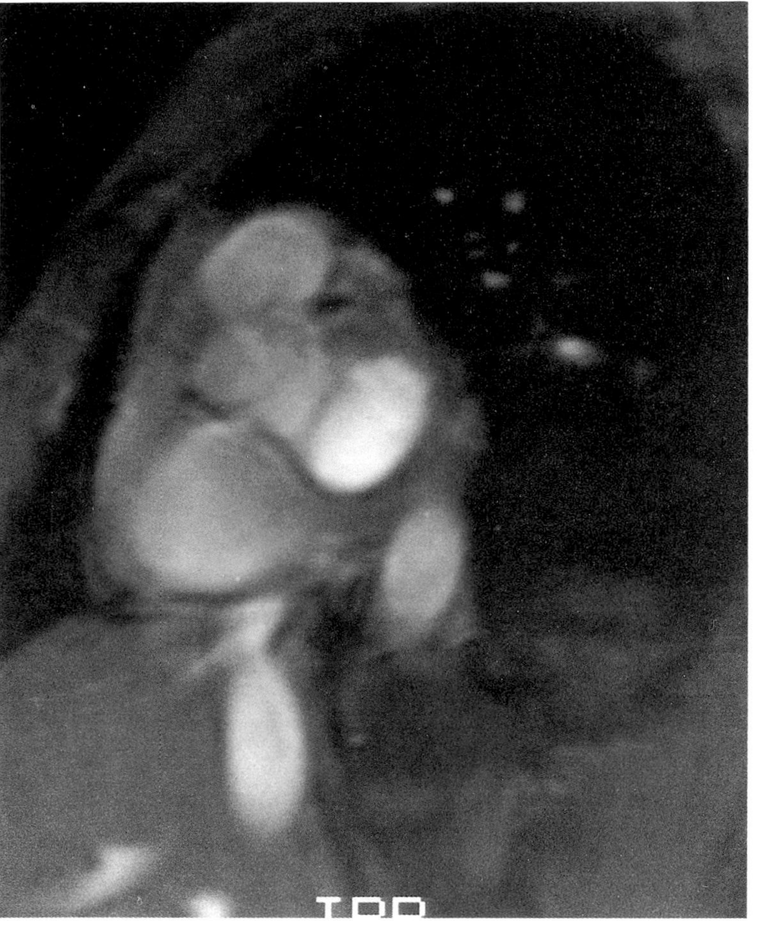

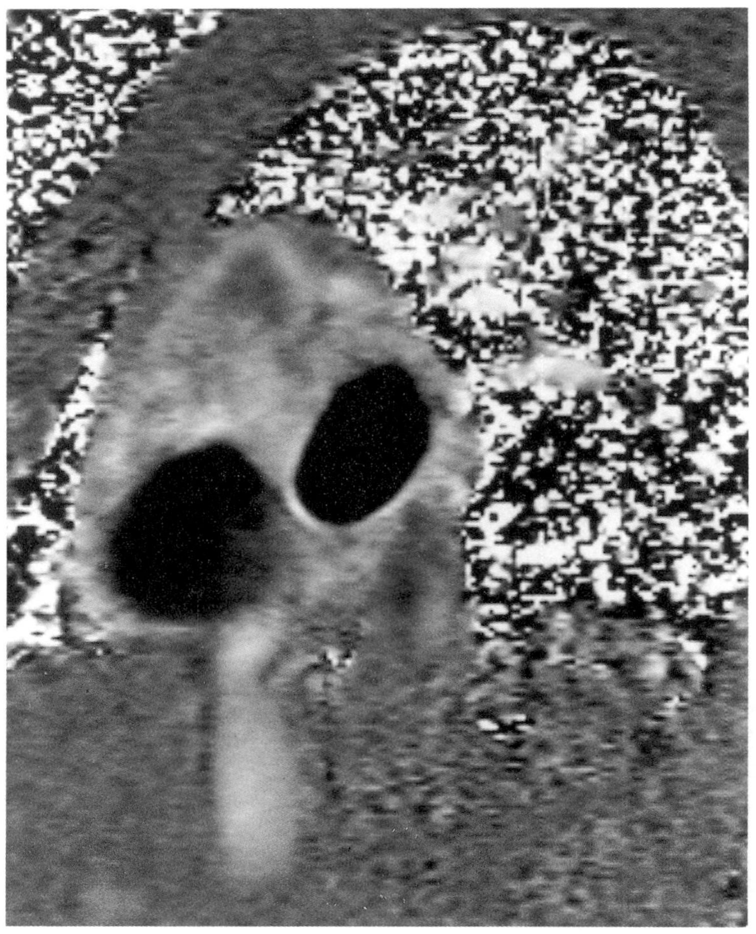

FIGURE 1. *Horizontal long-axis magnitude* **(left)** *and phase* **(right)** *images through the mitral (closed arrow) and tricuspid valves (open arrow). These images are acquired perpendicular to the atrioventricular valve annuli. The phase images can be used to measure blood flow across the valves.*

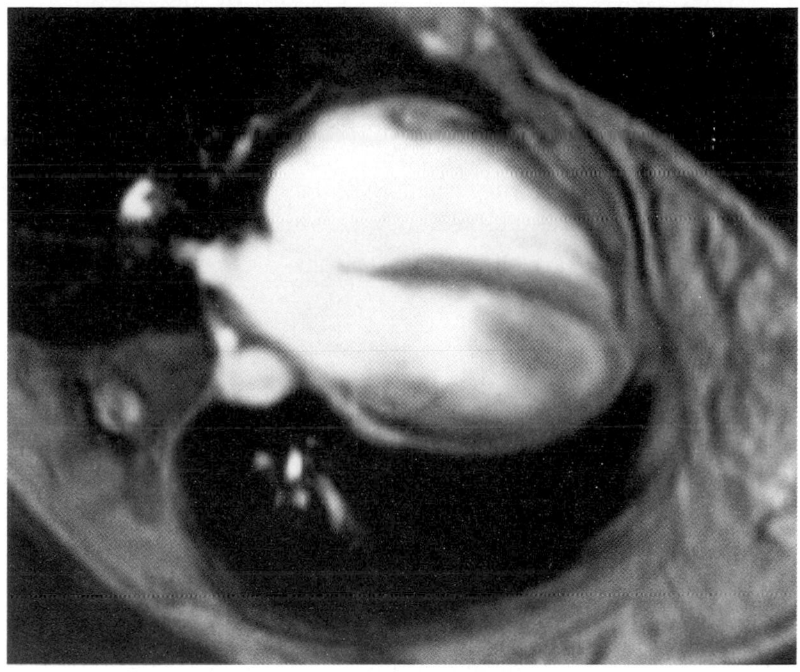

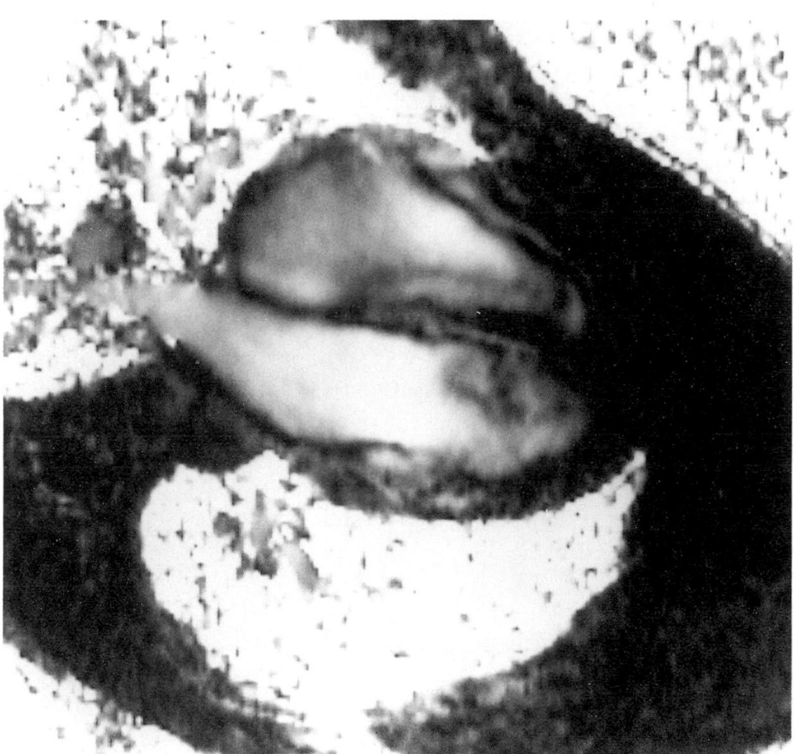

FIGURE 2. *Short-axis magnitude* **(top)** *and phase images* **(bottom)** *at the level of the mitral annulus (closed arrow) and the tricuspid annulus. These images are acquired perpendicular to the atrioventricular valve annuli. Each voxel on the phase image can be interrogated in order to derive a value for instantaneous velocity across the mitral or tricuspid valve.*

The turbo gradient-echo technique uses a TR of approximately 6–7 msec and a TE of 3–4 msec. For the evaluation of valvular heart disease these sequences are usually not adequate because they do not provide images at multiple phases of the cardiac cycle, permitting isolation of the end-diastolic and end-systolic phases, which is necessary for measurements of ventricular volumes and ejection fraction. In addition, these techniques generally result in images with low signal and in many cases, nonoptimal contrast.

Biphasic Spin-Echo Technique

The major advantages of the biphasic spin-echo technique are shorter acquisition times for imaging the entire volume of the heart and greater precision with the acquisition of images corresponding to end diastole and end systole.[16] In the use of the ECG-gated biphasic spin-echo technique, the interval from the peak of the R wave (end diastole) to the downslope of the T wave (end systole) is measured in milliseconds and entered as the duration of systole at the time of imaging. Images of the 16 sectional locations at both end diastole and end systole can be acquired in a total of approximately 1,000 heartbeats. The biphasic sequence consists of four rapid spin-echo sequences using a TE of about 14 msec. In each sequence the data for four sectional locations are acquired at end diastole and the data for four sectional locations are also acquired at end systole. Four separate acquisitions (16 sectional locations) are acquired sequentially during the complete biphasic acquisitions. Thus, a cluster of four images at four different anatomical locations are acquired during a 77-msec interval centered on the R wave of the ECG (end diastole) and another set of four images are acquired during a 77-msec interval occurring near the final slope of the T wave (end systole) of the ECG. These 77-msec intervals correspond approximately to the end-diastolic and end-systolic periods.

In general, the left ventricular volume and mass calculated from biphasic spin-echo images are comparable to those measured from stacks of cine magnetic resonance images.[16] However, the cine magnetic resonance defined end-systolic volume was significantly larger and ejection fraction was significantly smaller compared to measurements obtained by the biphasic acquisition technique, probably because of uncertainty in the isolation of end diastole from the series of cine magnetic resonance images. A major advantage of the biphasic spin-echo technique for measurement of ventricular volumes and ejection fraction is that the acquisition time of the entire study is less than half of that required for the acquisition of the stack of cine magnetic resonance images encompassing the entire heart.

Velocity Encoded Cine Magnetic Resonance Imaging

Velocity encoded cine magnetic resonance imaging (VEC) can be used to measure blood flow velocity (Figures 1 and 2). The VEC method used in our laboratory has been described in detail.[17] Briefly, VEC is performed by using a bipolar gradient pulse to modulate the phase of proton spins. To eliminate the phase shifts introduced by field nonuniformities and the chemical shift phenomenon, each acquisition consisted of two interleaved cine sequences. The two sequences were performed with different flow encoded gradients along the same direction. Velocity encoding could be selected either in the slice-select, phase encoded, or frequency encoded directions by the operator. Subtraction of phase data of one sequence from that of the other resulted in cancellation of all phase shifts except those resulting from flow along a velocity encoded direction. Velocity encoding can be done in a single direction, ie, in the flow direction, or can be done in all three dimensions. The phase difference between the two sequences is proportional to flow in the velocity encoded direction according to the formula:

$$\Delta \text{ phase} = g \times \text{velocity} \times T \times Ag$$

where g is a gyromagnetic ratio, T is the interval between gradient pulses, and Ag is the area of each lobe of the gradient pulse. When the gradients of the two sequences are chosen so as to keep the phase shift $<180°$ to avoid aliasing, the velocity component along the velocity encoded direction can be determined from the phase difference (Δ phase).

Identification of Valvular Stenosis and Regurgitation

Blood flow produces a very bright signal on gradient-echo images. The signal intensity of blood flow is influenced by the nature and magnitude of the flow during the time of acquisition of the cine magnetic resonance images. The physical principles determining the bright signal intensity of blood flow on cine magnetic resonance images and the relationship of the signal intensity to the velocity of blood flow have been described previously.[18,19]

Blood flow within the heart and great arteries produces bright signal during nearly all phases of the cardiac cycle. In the normal heart, transient signal loss is recognized at short periods during the cardiac cycle, especially consonant with the opening of the atrioventricular valves and occasionally with the opening of the semilunar valves.[20] There may also be transient signal loss immediately upon closure of the atrioventricular valves. In contrast to the bright signal of blood flow in the normal heart, abnormal flow patterns cause severe dephasing of spins in a voxel and result in loss of signal (signal void). This signal void in the blood pool is caused by high-velocity turbulent flow.[18] It is seen in association with valvular stenosis and regurgitation.[5,6,20] With cine magnetic resonance images, mitral regurgitation is identified by a circumscript area of signal loss emanation from the insufficient mitral valve into the left atrium during ventricular systole. This area of signal void can be clearly identified and separated from the high signal intensity of the blood pool. Aortic regurgitation is identified by an area of signal loss extending from the incompetent aortic valve into the left ventricle during ventricular diastole (Figure 3A and 3B). Likewise, tricuspid and pulmonic regurgitation can be identified as signal void associated with the respective valves occurring at the appropriate phase of the cardiac cycle. The ability to recognize the signal void and the apparent size of the signal void is influenced by the TE value used in the acquisition and the tomographic thickness and the volume of the acquisition voxels.[21] The signal void is more readily identified and larger in size, with a longer TE interval.

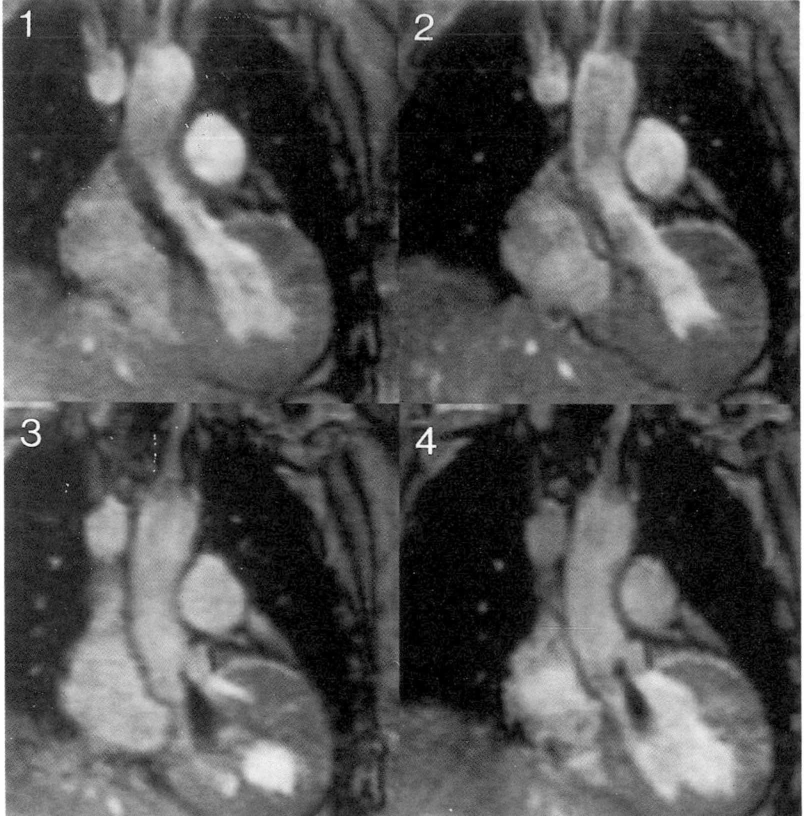

FIGURE 3A. *A series of coronal images in systole (above) and diastole (below) in a patient with aortic regurgitation. The signal void (arrow) emanating from the aortic valve in diastole is indicative of aortic regurgitation. Reprinted from Reference 20 with permission.*

High-velocity turbulent flow across valvular stenosis causes a signal void, which is projected into the downstream chamber of a great artery.[5,6,22] With the use of a short TE value, the central and peripheral components of a flow jet across valvular stenosis may be recognized (Figure 4).[22] The central component (vena contracta) produces a bright signal flow region and the central component, consisting of eddies, produces signal void.

The flow pattern on cine magnetic resonance images can be used to identify the precise site of stenosis or multiple sites of stenosis. For instance, these sequences have been used to identify the site of membranous subaortic stenosis and stenosis produced by a supravalvular mitral ring (Figure 5A and 5B).

The diagnostic accuracy of cine magnetic resonance for identifying aortic and mitral regurgitation was assessed in a study from our laboratory.[23] Sixty-two cine magnetic resonance studies of patients with regurgitation were blindly reviewed by three independent observers. In these patients regurgitation was documented by using Doppler and color flow echocardiography and/or angiography. Studies of 20 normal subjects were used to determine the specificity of the technique. Retrospective analysis

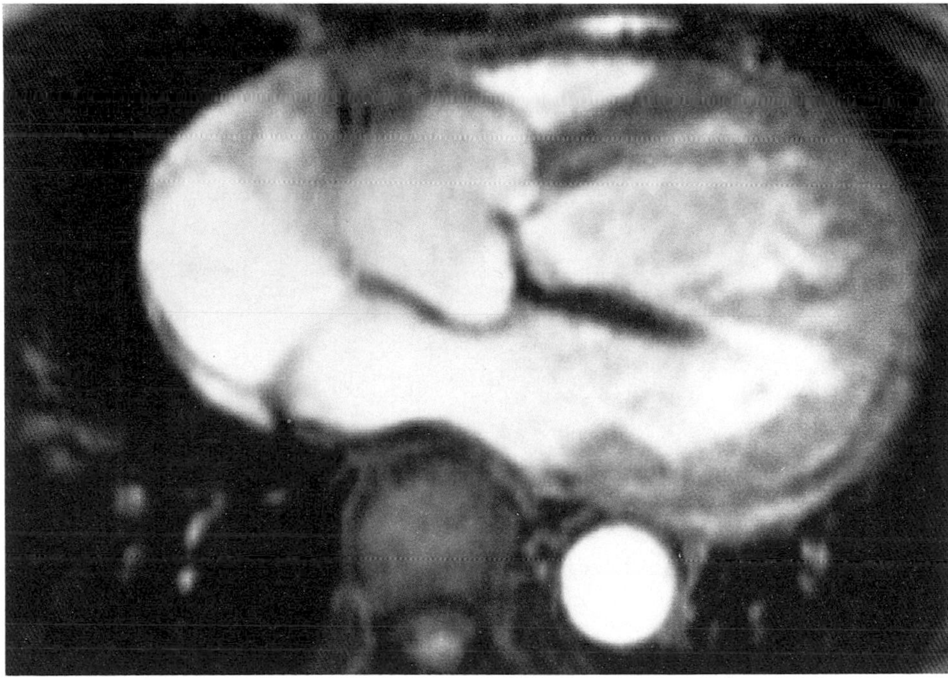

FIGURE 3B. *Transaxial image acquired beneath the aortic valve in diastole demonstrates a signal void originating from the aortic valve and projecting into the left ventricular outflow region.*

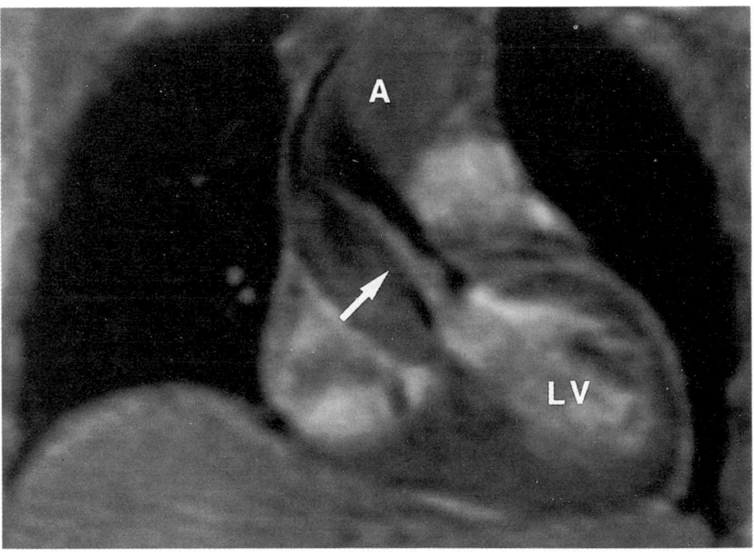

FIGURE 4. *Cine magnetic resonance image in systole demonstrates the eccentric flow jet across the aortic valve caused by aortic stenosis. The central region of the jet is the vena contracta, which has laminar flow patterns. The signal void at the margin of the jet (arrow) is caused by eddies. A, aorta; LV, left ventricle.*

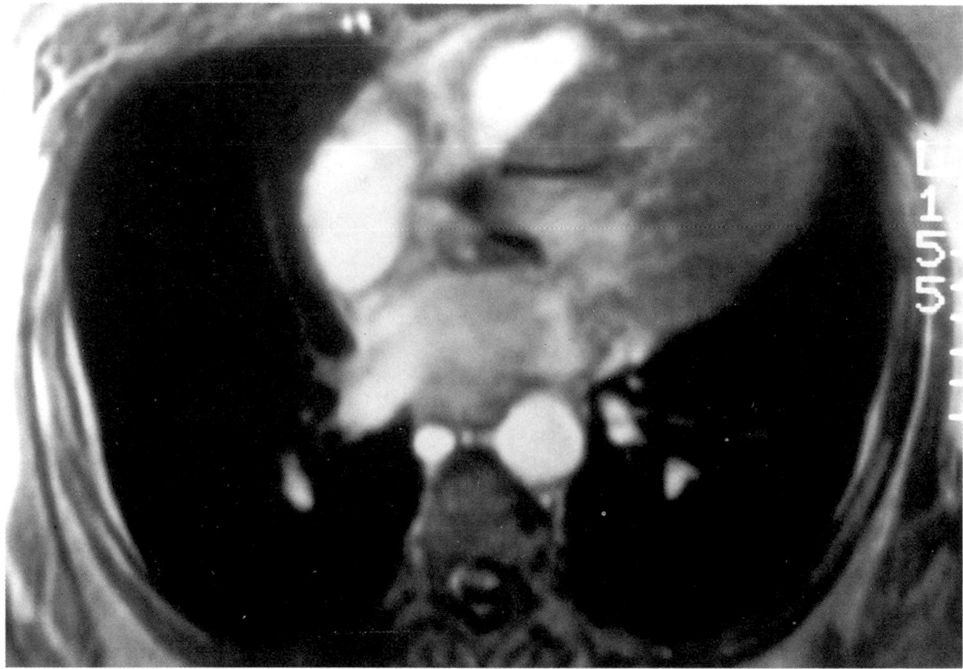

FIGURE 5A. *Cine magnetic resonance images acquired beneath the aortic valve in systole shows a signal void (arrows) arising beneath the valve, indicating membranous subaortic stenosis.*

for detection of mitral and aortic regurgitation by visualization of a signal void on cine magnetic resonance images showed a high specificity (>0.93), sensitivity (>0.89), and diagnostic accuracy (>0.92) for those lesions for the least experienced reviewer. The most experienced reviewer demonstrated a diagnostic accuracy of 0.96 for identifying mitral regurgitation and 0.94 for identifying aortic regurgitation. All lesions considered as moderate and severe were identified by all three observers. One instance of mild mitral regurgitation and four instances of mild aortic regurgitation were not identified by at least one of the observers (false-negative studies). There was one case in which all three reviewers detected aortic regurgitation on cine magnetic resonance, but echocardiography did not show the regurgitation (false-positive).

Quantification of Valvular Regurgitation

There are several methods by which valvular regurgitation can be estimated or precisely quantified using MRI. These methods are: 1) ventricular volumetric measurements;[9,10,24] 2) volumetric measurements of the signal void of regurgitation;[7,23,25] 3) direct measurement of retrograde blood flow using VEC;[26] and 4) area of the proximal acceleration flow signal void in aortic regurgitation.[27]

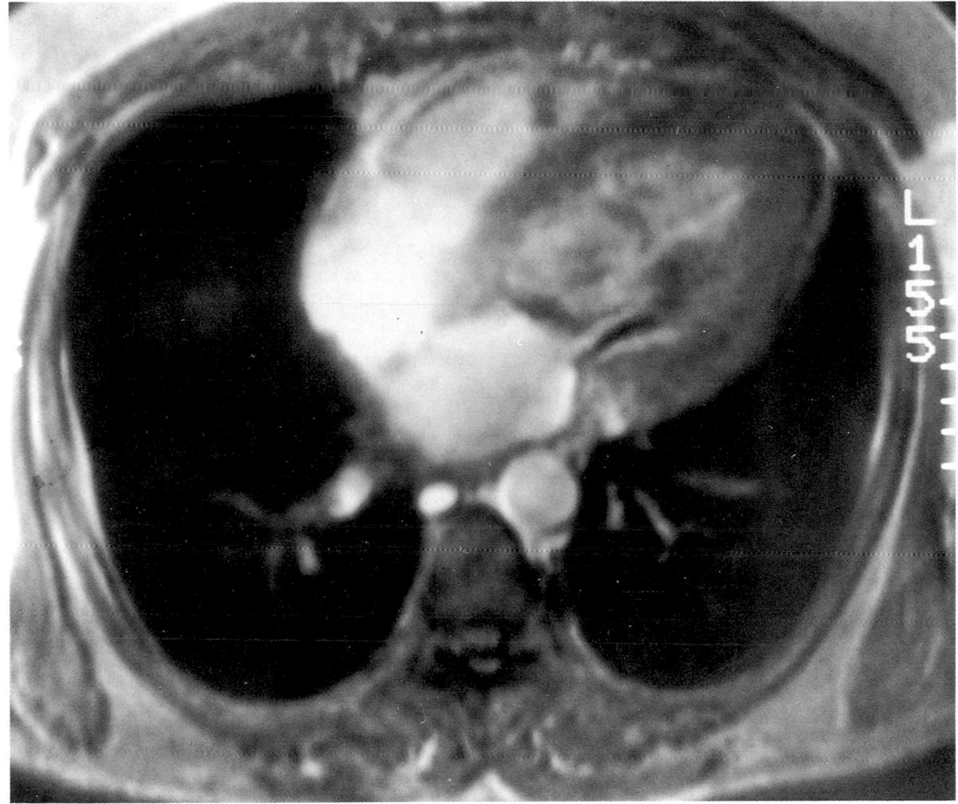

FIGURE 5B. *Cine magnetic resonance image at the level of the mitral valve shows a signal void (arrow) originating on the left atrial side of the mitral valve. This was caused by a supravalvular mitral ring.*

Quantification of Regurgitation by Ventricular Volumetrics

Several reports have verified that ventricular volumes are accurately measured from cine magnetic resonance images.[10–12,24,28–31] The difference between end- diastolic and end-systolic volumes for a ventricle with regurgitant valve includes both the forward stroke volume and regurgitant volume. The right and left ventricular stroke volumes are equal in normal hearts, while the differences in stroke volumes between a regurgitant ventricle (eg, left ventricle with aortic and mitral regurgitation) and a normal ventricle (eg, right ventricle) is regurgitant volume. The sum of the forward stroke volume and regurgitant volumes is called the total stroke volume of the regurgitant ventricle. Ventricular volumetric measurements by MRI in patients with aortic or mitral regurgitation have shown that the stroke volume in the left ventricle exceeds that of the right ventricle by a value equivalent to the stroke volume.[9,10,24] The regurgitant fraction can be calculated as regurgitant volume divided by the stroke volume of the regurgitant ventricle. The stroke volume ratio can also be calculated from the stroke volumes of the two ventricles. These measurements derived from cine magnetic resonance images have distinguished patients with mild, moderate, and severe left-sided regurgitation, as shown by independent imaging techniques (Figure 6).[9,10,24]

A limitation for using the stroke volume difference for quantification of regurgitation is in the presence of multivalvular disease. If both aortic and mitral regurgitation are present, the calculation will determine only the total volume of regurgitation. If regurgitation coexists on both sides of the heart, this calculation will not be meaningful. Another limitation of this approach may be low specificity in the presence of mild regurgitation.

Quantification of Regurgitation by Signal Void Volumetrics

The signal void emanating from the regurgitant valve can be demarcated on each image encompassing the chamber that receives the regurgitant flow.[7,23,25] For instance, the signal void can be outlined on each of the tomographic images encompassing the left ventricle from the level of the aortic valve to the cardiac apex in order to measure the volume of the signal void associated with aortic regurgitation. This measurement is done at the phase of diastole at which the signal void is maximum. The

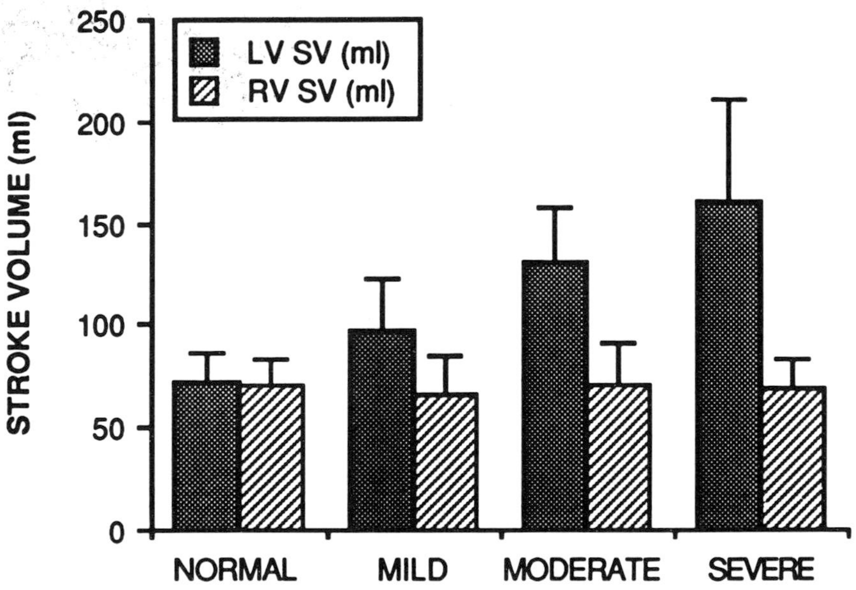

FIGURE 6. *Left and right ventricular stroke volumes are shown in normal subjects and in patients with mild, moderate, and severe regurgitation. Right ventricular stroke volume is similar among the groups, while there is a progressive increase in left ventricular stroke volume with increasing severity of regurgitation. Reprinted with permission from Auffermann W, Wagner S, Holt W, et al: Evaluation of valvular regurgitation by Cine magnetic Resonance. Am J Cardiac Imaging 1989;3:27–33.*

area of the signal void on each image is measured by planimetry and these areas for each of the tomographic images are summed to provide an estimate of the volume of the signal void. A study in our laboratory[23] has compared the volume of the signal void among groups of patients with mild, moderate, and severe aortic and mitral regurgitation. Measurements of the volume of the signal void were significantly ($p > 0.01$) different among mild, moderate, and severe lesions in both aortic and mitral regurgitation and correlated with the echocardiographic and/or angiographic gradings (Figure 7). The reproducibility of the measurements was good, as reflected by an interobserver correlation of 0.98 and an interobserver correlation of 0.94. In 23 studies of patients with isolated mitral regurgitation and 21 studies of patients with isolated aortic regurgitation, the regurgitant volume was determined by both the difference of left and right ventricular stroke volume and the volume of the signal void. Correlation for the two measurements in mitral regurgitation was 0.84 and in aortic regurgitation was also 0.84.

It should be noted that this method has several shortcomings. This technique suffers from some of the same limitations as encountered with color flow mapping for estimating the volume of regurgitation. A major factor is that the size of the signal void is influenced by the velocity of flow across the small regurgitant opening in the valve. Since this velocity is influenced by the pressure differential between the aorta and left ventricle or between the left ventricle and left atrium, the signal void will vary depending upon the level of aortic or ventricular pressure. Another practical limitation is the presence of disturbed flow emanating from two valves during the same phase of the cardiac cycle. The separation of the signal void resulting from aortic regurgitation and that resulting from mitral stenosis becomes problematic or impossible in some circumstances. Finally, it should be noted that the volume of the signal void from a regurgitant valve is importantly altered by changes in imaging parameters. Shortening of the echo delay time can cause reduction in the volume of the regurgitant signal void.[21] Consequently, comparison of regurgitant volume between studies in the same subject or among laboratories must be done with constant imaging parameters. The apparent size of the signal void can also be altered depending upon image display factors.

Quantitation of Regurgitation by Velocity-Encoded Cine MRI

This technique can distinguish between antegrade and retrograde flow, so that retrograde flow in diastole can be measured to directly quantify aortic regurgitation.[26] Figures 8A and 8B display magnitude and phase images for a normal individual in systole and diastole. The ascending aorta demonstrates white coloration of the voxels in systole, indicating forward flow in the ascending aorta. In diastole the intensity of the voxels in the region of the ascending aorta is similar to background intensity during diastole in the normal individual, indicating little or no flow. In aortic regurgitation, the coloration of the voxels of the ascending aorta during diastole is black, indicating retrograde blood flow in the ascending aorta at this stage of the cardiac cycle. Figures 9A and 9B show a plot of flow in the ascending aorta versus time during the cardiac cycle in a normal individual and in a patient with severe aortic regurgitation. Each point on this graph represents the flow measured for one of the VEC images acquired during the cardiac cycle. In the normal individual there is essentially no flow during diastole. In contrast, there is considerable negative flow (retrograde flow) in the ascending aorta

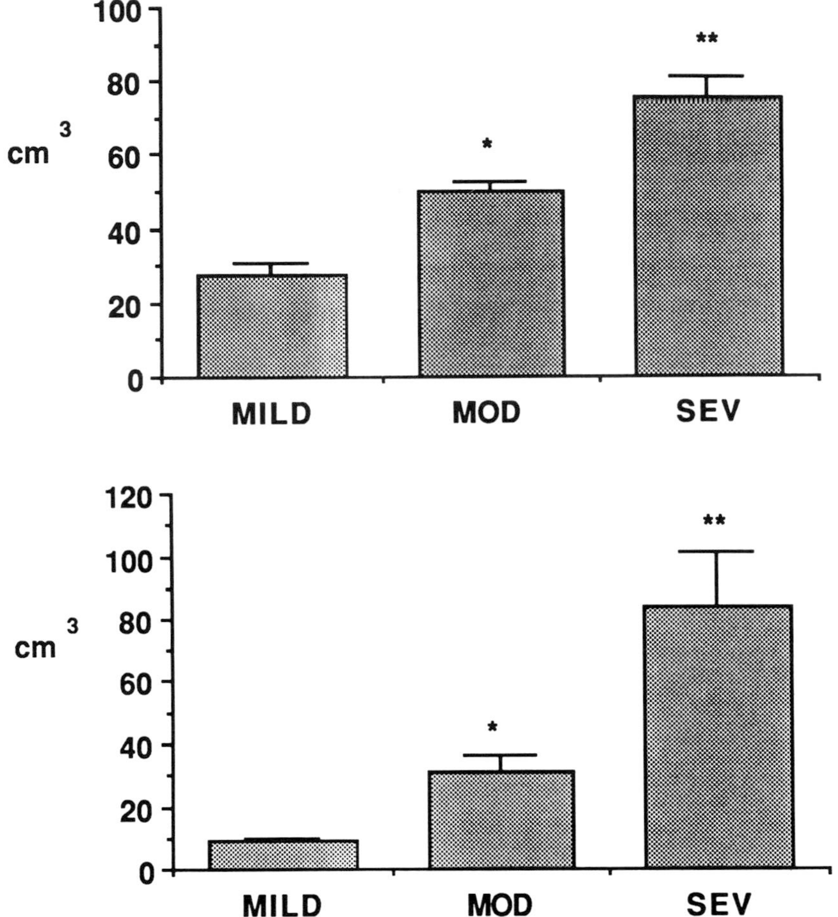

FIGURE 7. *Comparison of the volume of the flow void in aortic* (top panel) *and mitral* (bottom panel) *regurgitation in patients with mild, moderate, and severe regurgitation as defined by independent imaging studies. There are significant differences in the volume of the flow voids between mild and moderate (*) and moderate and severe (**) regurgitation. Reprinted from Reference 23 with permission.*

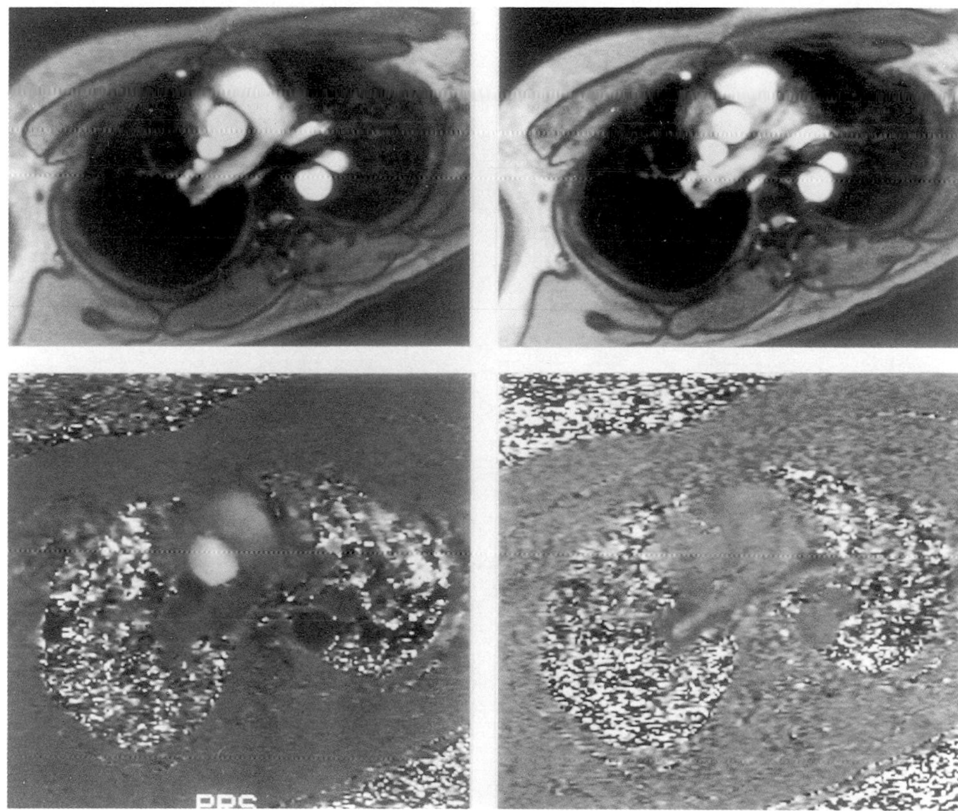

FIGURE 8A. *Magnitude (above) and phase (below) images acquired during systole (left) and diastole (right) in a normal subject. The phase image shows bright voxels in the ascending aorta in systole, indicating antegrade flow, while the intensity of the ascending aorta is similar to background during diastole, indicating little or no flow.*

during diastole. If the region under the diastolic retrograde flow curve is planimetered, this measurement represents the volume of aortic regurgitation.

A recent study in our laboratory[26] demonstrated that the preferred site for measurement of retrograde flow in the ascending aorta in order to estimate aortic regurgitation was in the pre-arch region. The measurement performed at the base of the ascending aorta is sometimes complicated by the swirling of blood in this region in patients with aortic regurgitation. A close correlation was demonstrated between the VEC method for measuring retrograde blood flow in the ascending aorta and ventricular volumetric measurements of the difference in stroke volume between the two ventricles in patients with pure aortic regurgitation.[26]

Recent experiments have evaluated the interstudy reproducibility of measurements of aortic regurgitation using the VEC technique.[33] Figure 10 demonstrates the measurements done on two separate occasions in 10 patients with aortic regurgitation. For the most part these measurements were done 1 to 2 weeks apart in patients with

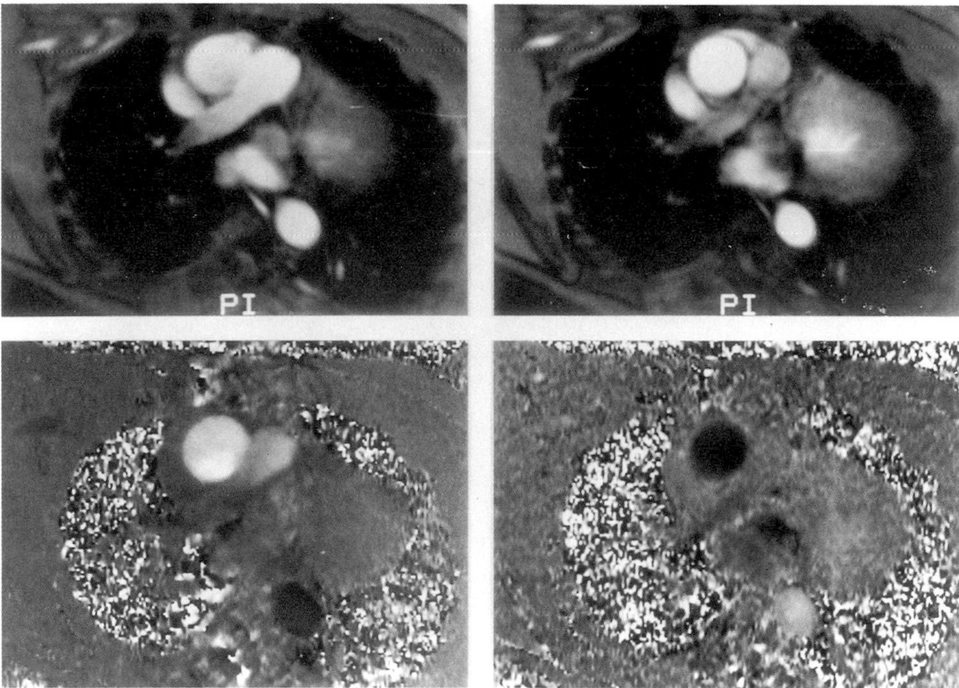

FIGURE 8B. *Magnitude (above) and phase (below) images in systole (left) and diastole (right) in a patient with aortic regurgitation. The voxels in the ascending aorta are bright in systole, indicating antegrade flow, while the voxels are dark in diastole, indicating retrograde flow caused by aortic regurgitation.*

pure aortic regurgitation in whom treatment had remained constant and aortic pressure and heart rates were nearly equivalent between the two studies. The correlation coefficient for the measurements between the two studies was 0.98, with a standard of the estimate of approximately 3%. This study demonstrates that the VEC technique might be useful in monitoring patients over time with aortic regurgitation and would be effective for assessing changes in the severity of regurgitation in response to therapy.

Quantification of Multivalvular Regurgitation

The combination of ventricular volumetrics and the VEC technique for measuring diastolic retrograde blood flow in the aorta can be used for the quantification of multivalvular regurgitation. In the presence of both aortic and mitral regurgitation, the total regurgitation on the left side of the heart can be calculated using ventricular volumetric measurements. The total regurgitant volume is equal to the difference between the left ventricular stroke volume and the right ventricular stroke volume. This relationship holds as long as there is no significant regurgitation within the right

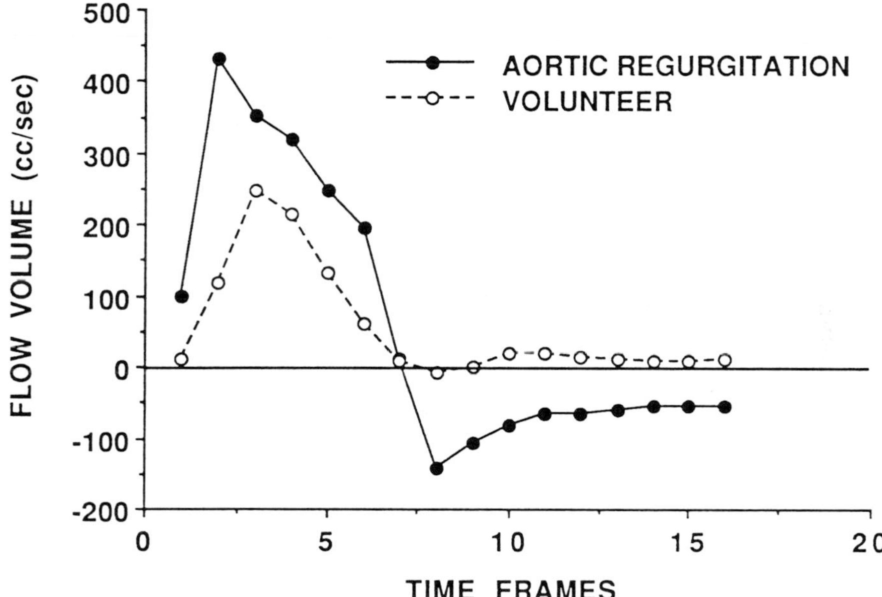

FIGURE 9. *Flow volume versus time curve for a normal subject* **(solid circles)** *and a patient with aortic regurgitation* **(open circles)**. *Each point on the curve represents the flow measured on the phase image acquired at each specific point in the cardiac cycle. There is nearly no flow in the ascending aorta in diastole in normal subjects. There is considerable negative (retrograde) flow in the aorta in diastole in the patient with aortic regurgitation. The area under the retrograde flow curve in diastole is a direct measure of the volume of aortic regurgitation. Reprinted with permission from Mostbeck GH, Caputo GR, Higgins CB: MR measurement of blood flow in the cardiovascular system. AJR 1992;159:453–462.*

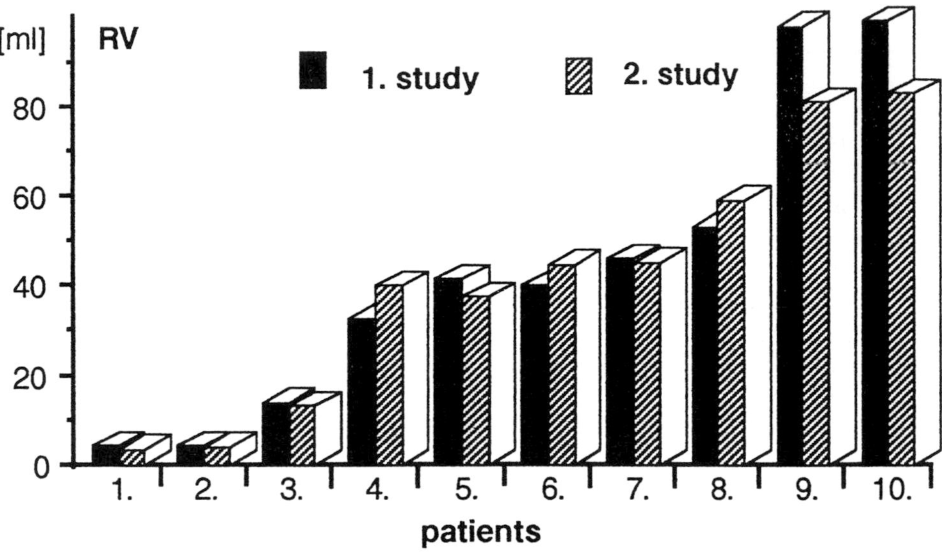

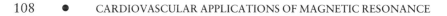

FIGURE 10. *Block diagram shows the regurgitant fraction measured by velocity encoded cine magnetic resonance (VEC) in 10 patients studied on two separate occasions. The values are nearly identical between the two VEC studies. Reprinted from Reference 33 with permission.*

side of the heart. Aortic regurgitation can be directly measured as the retrograde diastolic blood flow from VEC images. Mitral regurgitation, then, is calculated as the difference between the volumetric total regurgitant volume and the aortic regurgitation as measured by the retrograde diastolic blood flow. In this manner, both mitral regurgitation and aortic regurgitation can be quantified in the presence of left-sided multivalvular regurgitation.

Quantification of Aortic Regurgitation by Volume of Proximal Acceleration Flow Area

It is known from echocardiographic studies that flow accelerates proximal to a regurgitant orifice. This has been called the proximal acceleration flow area or proximal convergence zone; it is a laminar flow area located immediately upstream from the regurgitant valve. It produces a semicircular signal void in diastole at the base of the aorta contiguous with the aortic valve in aortic regurgitation. Yoshida et al.[27] showed that the area of the acceleration flow signal void measured on the long-axis image of the left ventricle correlated well with the angiographic grade of aortic regurgitation. This seems to constitute another semiquantitative estimate of aortic regurgitation. Its value for regurgitation of other valves has not yet been tested.

Quantification of Valvular Stenosis

Doppler echocardiographic studies have used the modified Bernoulli equation for estimating the gradient across stenotic valves by measuring the peak velocity across the site of stenosis. This measurement is based upon the measurement of peak flow velocity that is used in the following equation:

$$\Delta P \text{ peak} = 4V^2 \text{ peak}$$

where P is the peak pressure and V is the peak velocity across the stenosis. This relationship holds when the pressure distal to the stenosis is inconsequential in comparison to the pressure proximal to the stenosis. The same formula has now been used with VEC MRI techniques for the measurement of velocity and estimation of the pressure gradient across valvular and vascular stenoses. A phase image at the level of the aortic valve can be used to measure peak velocity and flow across the opened aortic valve (Figure 11). At the present time, only a small experience has been accumulated with the use of velocity encoded cine MRI techniques for the assessment of jet velocity mapping. Kilner et al.[22] have reported reasonable correspondence between measurements of peak velocity and estimates of pressure gradients across stenotic valves in comparison to Doppler ultrasonography and/or catheterization.

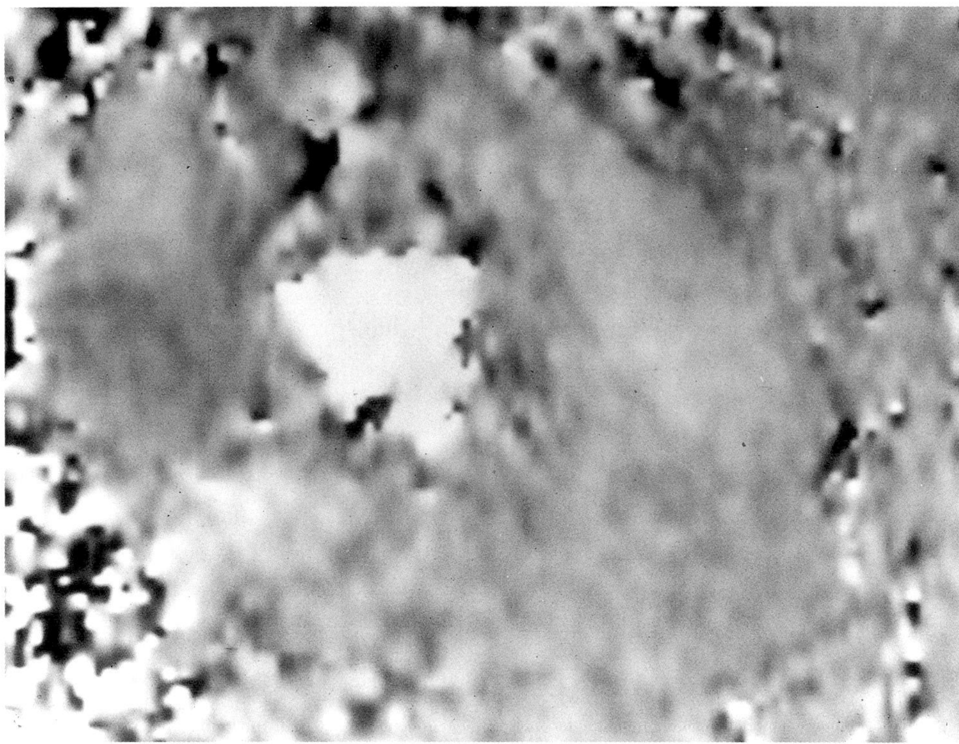

FIGURE 11. *Phase image at the level of the aortic valve. Velocity can be measured for each voxel contained within the opened aortic valve.*

Because of severe signal loss on cine magnetic resonance images at very high velocities associated with valvular stenoses, it has been proposed that it may be impossible to measure peak velocity of blood flow using standard magnetic gradients and standard TE values. The report by Kilner et al.[22] suggests that TE values must be <4 msec using a 0.5-T imager in order to measure velocities of blood flow up to 6 m/s. Our own experiments using a constant flow phantom demonstrated that velocities up to 6 m/s could be measured using a TE value of 6–7 msec with a 1.5-T imager. Regardless of the exact value of TE that is necessary for measuring high velocity, it seems axiomatic that the shortest value should be used. The maximum value that can be measured with a specific imaging system is related to a number of factors including slice thickness, TE value, and probably field strength.

Quantification and Monitoring of Ventricular Function and Loading Factors

The three-dimensional data set provided by a stack of images encompassing the entire heart at multiple phases throughout the cardiac cycle makes MRI a highly reproducible three-dimensional imaging technique. A number of studies have demonstrated accuracy and reproducibility of the technique for measuring left ventricular end-diastolic volume, end-systolic volume, stroke volume, ejection fraction, and left ventricular mass.[11,12,28–31] Likewise, several studies have suggested that similar accuracy and reproducibility of volumetric measurements can be achieved for the right ventricle as well,[29,34,35] which constitutes an advantage of MRI in comparison to echocardiography. Measurements of left ventricular mass are extremely important for estimating the severity and influence of valvular lesions on the left ventricle, especially aortic stenosis. Several studies now suggest that tomographic imaging techniques such as MRI and ultrafast computed tomography may be the most accurate techniques for measurements of left ventricular mass.[36–39] A recent study from our laboratory also suggests that MRI may be an accurate and reproducible method for quantifying right ventricular mass.[35] The values for right ventricular mass provided by MRI in a group of normal volunteers were similar to the previously established values for right ventricular mass in studies of right ventricular mass defined at postmortem examination in patients who died without evidence of heart disease.

The interstudy reproducibility of MRI for measurements of left ventricular volumes and functional parameters is also excellent. Recent studies comparing interstudy variability of the magnetic resonance measurements of left ventricular volume and mass and end-systolic wall stress demonstrated that the percent variability between studies for ventricular volumes and ejection fraction in normal ventricles and dilated ventricles was approximately 5%. The interstudy variability for left ventricular mass was <5%.[40,41] The interstudy variability for measurement of wall stress was on the order of 10% to 15%.

Estimation of Left Ventricular Wall Stress With Cine Magnetic Resonance Imaging

Acquisition of digital blood pressure recordings and carotid pulse tracing recordings in proximity to the cine magnetic resonance imaging study has permitted the estimation of left ventricular peak and end-systolic wall stress. Wall stress can be estimated using the following formula:

$$WS_{es} = \frac{1.35 \times P_{es} \times D_{es}}{4h\,(1 + h/D_{es})}$$

where h is wall thickness at end systole, D_{es} = left ventricular diameter at end systole, and P_{es} = pressure at end systole. The end-systolic pressure is estimated by relating the peak systolic pressure measured by the digital cuff technique and the position of the dicrotic notch on the carotid pulse tracing. The wall thickness and internal diameter of the left ventricle are measured from the cine magnetic resonance image corresponding to end systole. The end-systolic image is chosen as the image with the smallest luminal area.

A study from our laboratory in normal subjects and in patients with varying degrees of valvular regurgitation demonstrated that left ventricular wall stress was similar in patients with mild and moderate regurgitation compared to the normal subjects (Figure 12).[42,43] In valvular regurgitation of a severe degree, left ventricular wall stress was significantly increased. In patients with dilated cardiomyopathy with associated mild mitral regurgitation the left ventricular wall stress was considerably and significantly increased above the normal values. This finding suggests that noninvasive estimation of left ventricular wall stress by cine magnetic resonance might be used to identify the presence of myocardial disease in patients with valvular regurgitation and failure of the ventricle to compensate for the volume load.

Magnetic resonance imaging has also been used to provide a three-dimensional

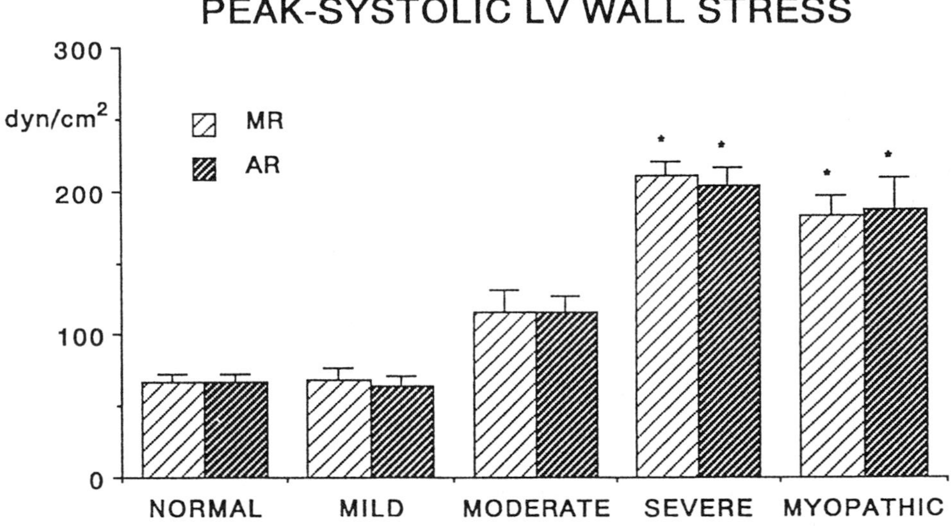

FIGURE 12. *Block diagram shows the peak left ventricular (LV) wall stress measured from cine magnetic resonance data in normal subjects and patients with varying degrees of severity of aortic (AR) and mitral (MR) regurgitation and patients with cardiomyopathy with mild regurgitation (myopathic).*

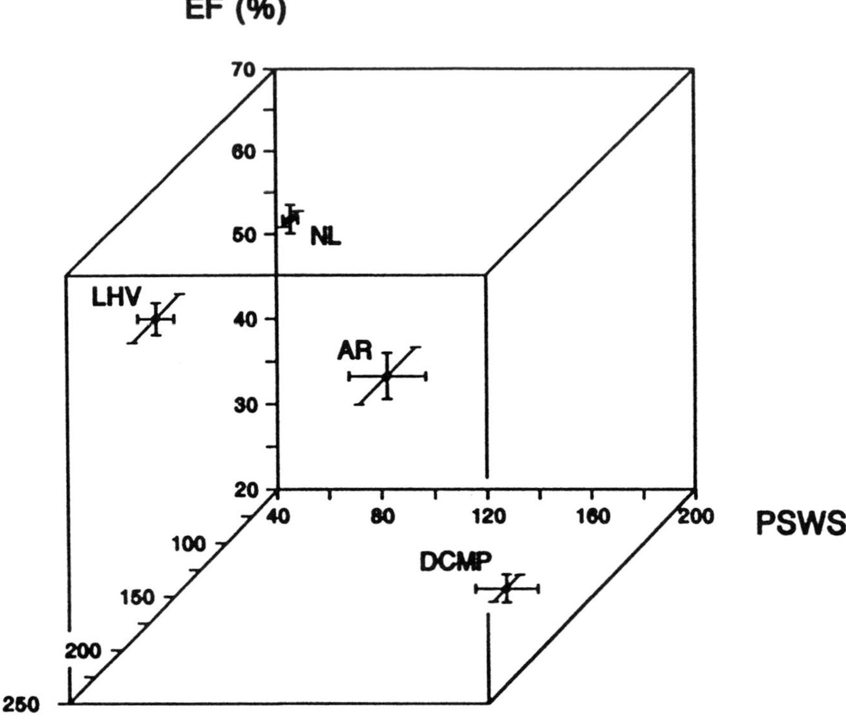

FIGURE 13. *Three coordinate plots of left ventricular (LV) ejection fraction, LV mass, and LV peak systolic wall stress (PSWS) in normal subjects and patients with left ventricular hypertrophy (LVH), severe aortic regurgitation (AR), and dilated cardiomyopathy (DCMP).*

description of the left ventricle in various cardiac disease states.[42] A plot of left ventricular mass versus wall stress in normal subjects, patients with severe aortic regurgitation, patients with concentric left ventricular hypertrophy, and patients with primary myocardial disease were substantially different (Figure 13). In comparison to normal subjects, patients with severe aortic regurgitation had a substantially increased left ventricular mass and increase in left ventricular wall stress. Coversely, in patients with primary myocardial disease and dilated cardiomyopathy, left ventricular mass was increased to a lesser degree and there was a substantially greater increase in end-systolic wall stress.

Monitoring Valvular and Ventricular Function

Magnetic resonance imaging has also been used to monitor the alterations in left ventricular function in response to therapy. In patients with dilated cardiomyopathy treated for 3 months with the new angiotensin converting enzyme inhibitor, sequential gradient-echo studies demonstrated progressive decreases in left ventricular end-systolic wall stress, end-systolic volume, left ventricular mass, and increase of ejection fraction.[44] As discussed previously, VEC gradient-echo can be used to monitor the severity of aortic regurgitation sequentially because the interstudy reproducibility of the measurement of regurgitant volume is excellent. Thus the combination of velocity encoded measurements of aortic regurgitation and cine magnetic resonance measurements of ventricular function and loading factors may provide an effective method for evaluating the response of patients with valvular heart disease to various therapeutic interventions.

Cine magnetic resonance may prove to be the most effective technique for the noninvasive assessment of the severity of valvular heart disease, and in addition, for the monitoring of patients with valvular heart disease. Concerns regarding the expense of MRI currently exist, but comparative costs of imaging studies suggest that such concerns may be exaggerated. A recent survey indicated that in the United States the cost of an MRI study was <1.5 times the cost of combined two-dimensional and Doppler echocardiography, and approximately one third the cost of left heart catheterization and angiography.[45] Moreover, these other studies do not provide a three-dimensional data set and consequently may not be able to quantify cardiac dimensions and function as precisely and reproducibly as a three-dimensional imaging technique.

References

1. Richards KL: Assessment of aortic and pulmonic stenosis by echocardiography. *Circulation* 1991;84(3)(suppl I):182–187.
2. Pearlman AS: Role of echocardiography in the diagnosis and evaluation of severity of mitral and tricuspid stenosis. *Circulation* 1991;84(suppl):193–197.
3. Cheitlin MD: Valvular heart disease; management and intervention, clinical overview and discussion. *Circulation* 1991;84(suppl):259–264.
4. Simpson IA, Sahn DJ: Quantification of valvular regurgitation by Doppler echocardiography. *Circulation* 1991;84(suppl):188–192.
5. Higgins CB, Wagner S, Kondo C, et al: Evaluation of valvular heart disease with cine gradient echo magnetic resonance imaging. *Circulation* 1991;84(suppl):198–206.
6. Cranney GB, Lotan CS, Pohost GM: Nuclear magnetic resonance imaging for assessment and follow-up of patients with valve disease. *Circulation* 1991;84(suppl):216–227.
7. Schiebler M, Axel L, Reichek N, et al: Correlation of cine MR imaging with two-dimensional pulsed Doppler echocardiography in valvular insufficiency. *J Comput Assist Tomogr* 1987;11:627–632.
8. Utz JA, Herfkens RJ, Heinsmimer JA, et al: Valvular regurgitation: dynamic MR imaging. *Radiology* 1988;168:91–94.
9. Underwood SR, Klipstein RH, Firmin DN, et al: Magnetic resonance assessment of aortic and mitral regurgitation. *Br Heart J* 1986;56:455–462.
10. Sechtem U, Pflugfelder PW, Cassidy MM, et al: Mitral and aortic regurgitation: quantification of regurgitant volumes with cine MR imaging. *Radiology* 1988;167:425–430.
11. Cranney GB, Lotan CS, Dean L, et al: Left ventricular volume measurement using cardiac axis NMR imaging—validation by calibrated ventricular angiography. *Circulation* 1990;82:154–163.
12. Underwood SR, Gill CRW, Klipstein RH, et al: Left ventricular volume measured rapidly by oblique magnetic resonance imaging. *Br Heart J* 1988;60:188–195.
13. Atkinson DJ, Burstein D, Edelman RR: First-pass cardiac perfusion: evaluation with ultrafast MR imaging. *Radiology* 1990;174:757–762.
14. Frahm J, Merboldt KD, Bruhn H, et al: 0.3-Second FLASH MRI of the human heart. *Magn Reson Med* 1990;13:150–157.

15. Atkinson DJ, Edelman RR: Cineangiography of the heart in a single breath hold with a segmented turborFLASH sequence. *Radiology* 1991;178:357–360.
16. Caputo GR, Suzuki J-I, Kondo C, et al: Determination of left ventricular volume and mass with use of biphasic spin-echo MR imaging: comparison with cine MR. *Radiology* 1990;177:773–777.
17. Kondo C, Caputo G, Semelka R, et al: Right and left ventricular stroke volume measurements with velocity encoded cine NMR imaging: in vitro and in vivo validation. *AJR* 1991;157:9–16.
18. Evans AJ, Blinder RA, Herfkens RJ, et al: Effects of turbulence on signal intensity in gradient echo images. *Invest Radiol* 1988;23:512–518.
19. Evans AJ, Hedlund LW, Herfkens RJ, et al: Evaluation of steady and pulsatile flow with dynamic MRI using limited flip angles and gradient refocused echoes. *Magn Reson Imaging* 1987;5:475–482.
20. Sechtem U, Pflugfelder PW, White RD, et al: Cine MR imaging: potential for the evaluation of cardiovascular function. *AJR* 1987;148:239–246.
21. Suzuki J-I, Caputo GR, Kondo C, et al: Cine MR imaging of valvular heart disease: display and imaging parameters affect the size of the signal void caused by valvular regurgitation. *AJR* 1990;155:723–727.
22. Kilner PJ, Firmin DN, Rees RSO, et al: Valve and great vessel stenosis: assessment with MR jet velocity mapping. *Radiology* 1991;178:229–235.
23. Wagner S, Auffermann W, Buser P, et al: Diagnostic accuracy and estimation of the severity of valvular regurgitation from signal void on cine MRI. *Am Heart J* 1989;118:760–767.
24. Pflugfelder PW, Landsberg JS, Cassidy MM, et al: Comparison of cine magnetic resonance imaging with Doppler echocardiography for the evaluation of aortic regurgitation. *AJR* 1989;153:729–735.
25. Pflugfelder P, Sechtem UP, White RD, et al: Noninvasive evaluation of mitral regurgitation by analysis of left atrial signal loss in cine magnetic resonance. *Am Heart J* 1989;117:1113–1119.
26. Caputo GR, Steinman D, Funari M, et al: Quantification of aortic regurgitation by velocity encoded cine MR. *Circulation* 1991;84(suppl II):II-203.
27. Yoshida K, Yoshikawa J, Hozumi T, et al: Assessment of aortic regurgitation by the acceleration flow signal void proximal to the leaking orifice in cinemagnetic resonance imaging. *Circulation* 1991;83:1951–1955.
28. Longmore DB, Underwood SR, Bland C, et al: Dimensional accuracy of magnetic resonance in studies of the heart. *Lancet* 1985;1:1360–1362.
29. Sechtem U, Pflugfelder PW, Gould RG, et al: Measurement of right and left ventricular volumes in healthy individuals with cine MR imaging. *Radiology* 1987;163:697–702.
30. Utz JA, Herfkens RJ, Heinsimer JA, et al: Cine NMR determination of left ventricular ejection fraction. *AJR* 1987;148:839–843.
31. Valk J, Roos JP: Evaluation of magnetic resonance imaging for determination of left ventricular ejection fraction and comparison with angiography. *Am J Cardiol* 1988;62:628–633.
32. Underwood SR, Firmin DN, Klipstein RH, et al: Magnetic resonance velocity mapping: clinical application of a new technique. *Br Heart J* 1987;57:404–412.
33. Dulce M, Mostbeck G, Cheitlin M, et al: Severity of aortic regurgitation: interstudy reproducibility of measurements with velocity encoded cine MR imaging. *Radiology* 1992;185:235–240.
34. Markiewicz W, Sechtem U, Kerby R, et al: Measurement of ventricular volumes in the dog by magnetic resonance imaging. *J Am Coll Cardiol* 1987;10:170–177.
35. Doherty NE, Fujita N, Caputo GR, et al: Measurement of right ventricular mass in normal and dilated cardiomyopathic ventricles using cine MRI. *Am J Cardiol* 1991;69:1223–1228.
36. Mogelvang J, Thomson C, Horn T, et al: Determination of left ventricular volume (mass) by magnetic resonance imaging. *Am J Noninvas Cardiol* 1987;1:231–236.

37. Caputo GR, Tscholakoff DT, Sechtem U, et al: Measurement of canine left ventricular mass by using MR imaging. *AJR* 1987;148:33–38.
38. Shapiro EP, Rogers WJ, Beyer R, et al: Determination of left ventricular mass by magnetic resonance imaging in hearts deformed by acute infarction. *Circulation* 1989;79:706–711.
39. Ostrzega E, Maddahi J, Honma H, et al: Quantification of left ventricular myocardial mass in humans by nuclear magnetic resonance imaging. *Am Heart J* 1989;117:444–452.
40. Semelka RC, Tomci E, Wagner S, et al: Normal left ventricular dimensions and function: interstudy reproducibility of measurements with cine MR imaging. *Radiology* 1990;174:763–768.
41. Semelka RC, Tomei E, Wagner S, et al: Interstudy reproducibility of dimensional and functional measurements between cine magnetic resonance studies in the morphologically abnormal left ventricle. *Am Heart J* 1990;119:1367–1373.
42. Wagner S, Auffermann W, Buser P, et al: Functional description of the left ventricle in patients with volume overload, pressure overload and myocardial disease using cine nuclear magnetic resonance imaging (NMRI). *Am J Cardiac Imaging* 1991;5:87–97.
43. Auffermann W, Wagner S, Holt WW, et al: Noninvasive determination of left ventricular output and wall stress in volume overload and myocardial disease by cine MRI. *Am Heart J* 1992;121:1750–1758.
44. Doherty NE, Seelos KC, Suzuki J-I, et al: Application of cine NMR imaging for sequential evaluation of response to angiotensin converting enzyme inhibitor therapy in dilated cardiomyopathy. *J Am Coll Cardiol* 1992 19(6):1294–1302.
45. O'Rourke RA: Relative patient costs: comparison of available techniques. In: Pohost GM, O'Rourke RA, eds. *Principles and Practice of Cardiovascular Imaging*. Boston, MA: Little, Brown & Co; 1991:857–858.

Part 2

Evolving Methods

Chapter 8

Fast Imaging:
Echo-Planar Imaging

Barry L.W. Chapman, PhD,
and Robert Turner, PhD

Since its beginnings in the early 1970s,[1] one fundamental problem of magnetic resonance imaging (MRI) has been resolution. Resolution is usually perceived as a purely spatial problem, but this is true only for structures that are free of motion. Indeed, MRI becomes more susceptible to motion artifacts as the pixel size becomes smaller, because spatial and temporal resolution are intrinsically coupled.

A partial solution to this problem has been to use gating procedures to remove the effect of periodic motions associated with cardiac function and breathing. In addition to lengthening the imaging time, gating also relies on perfect registration of the structures under investigation throughout the entire acquisition. Nevertheless, a band of signal intensity in the phase encode direction, known as phase encode ghosting, is almost always visible when faster moving organs or blood are included within a gradient-echo or spin-echo image. With the introduction of more rapid (10–25 msec) techniques,[2] imaging within a single breath-hold is possible. While this removes one motion it requires the active cooperation of the subject and is, of course, useless for other involuntary motions.

It was in response to the problems caused by long image acquisition times that echo-planar imaging was developed in 1977 at the University of Nottingham, by a group of physicists led by Peter Mansfield.[3] The first human images were limited by available gradient coil current to 6-mm in-plane resolution and had low (4:1) signal-to-noise ratio, due to the low field of 0.1 T.[4] In response to the growing demands of MRI, major improvements have been made in magnet and power supply technology. Main magnetic fields are now 4 T and higher, and gradient fields of up to 40 mT/m can be switched in under 0.5 msec. The echo-planar imaging technique, providing impetus for some of these developments, has improved to the point of clinical usefulness, and is now available at perhaps a dozen sites worldwide. Meanwhile, the technique has evolved, so that it is now usually used in the form of the variant modulus blipped echo-planar single-pulse technique (MBEST).[5] The resultant images enable

From Pohost GM (ed.), *Cardiovascular Applications of Magnetic Resonance*. Mount Kisco, NY, Futura Publishing Co., Inc., © 1993.

TABLE 1.

	EPI	TurboFLASH
Minimum imaging time (128 × 128)	40 msec	500 msec
Implementation	hard	easy
Contrast separation	flexible	limited
Radiofrequency power deposition	minimal	moderate
Motion artifact	none	little

echo-planar imaging to be used in a variety of clinical applications, in particular in the heart where complete cardiac movies have been obtained in a single cardiac cycle.[6] The methods and applications of echo-planar imaging have recently been reviewed in detail by Cohen and Weisskoff[7] and Stehling et al.[8]

For the imaging of fast moving structures echo-planar imaging is unrivaled. The fastest alternative, TurboFLASH, is capable of imaging an entire plane with a 128 × 128 pixel matrix in 500 msec. Typically, most of the information content in an image comes from the central 20% of k-space. Although the images produced are apparently free from phase encode artifact, this is still insufficient to capture the motion during systole, where imaging in <50 msec is required. As resolution is improved, even shorter acquisition periods are needed to ensure that the apparent gain in resolution is not negated by motional blurring.

Further major differences between echo-planar imaging and TurboFLASH are listed in Table 1. To summarize the content of this table, TurboFLASH is easier to implement, but echo-planar imaging offers better signal-to-noise ratio, greater flexibility in terms of MRI contrast and adaptability, and unparalleled temporal resolution, of particular value in cardiac studies.

Method

Echo-planar imaging and its variants are characterized by the ability to obtain the data for a complete image plane from a single radiofrequency excitation. In contrast, until the recent widespread implementation of the rapid spin-echo technique, standard MRI techniques obtained one line of data in sample space, or k-space, from each excitation. K-space is simply the name for the multidimensional (in this case two-dimensional) space in which MRI data is sampled, Fourier transformation of which yields the image.

To understand echo-planar imaging, it is sufficient to consider the principles of gradient-echo two-dimensional Fourier transform (2DFT) technique. In 2DFT, a slice-selective radiofrequency and gradient combination is used to excite the spins in a single slice through the subject (Figure 1, top). Subsequent phase encoded and read dephase gradients serve to initialize the point at which sampling in k-space is to begin (Figure 2, top). A single line of data is acquired for each increment of the phase encode

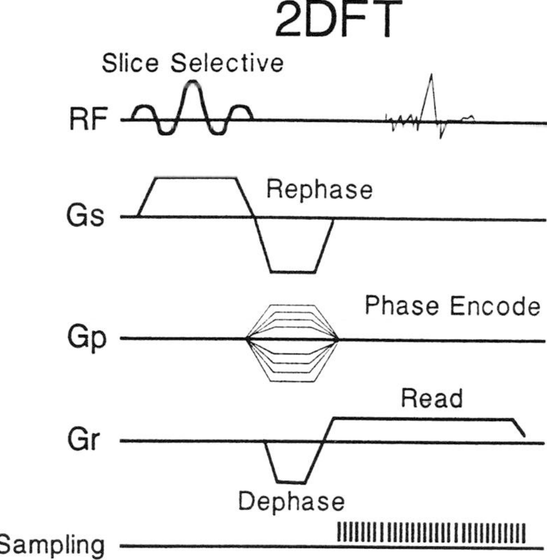

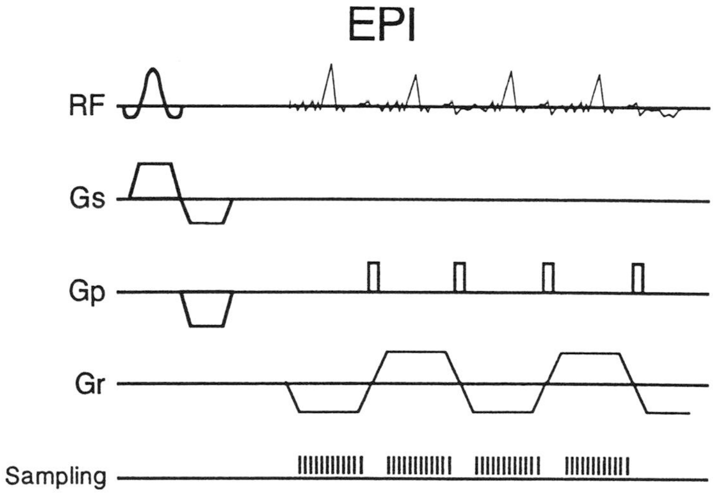

FIGURE 1. Top: *The gradient-echo two-dimensional Fourier transform (2DFT) gradient-echo pulse sequence. Following each slice selective radiofrequency (RF) excitation, phase encode gradients (Gp) of different strengths are used to obtain different k-space (sample) lines. These lines are subsequently sampled during the application of a read gradient (Gr) to provide discrimination in the second dimension.* **Bottom**: *The corresponding echo-planar imaging (EPI) pulse sequence. In echo-planar imaging following a single radiofrequency excitation a series of incremental phase encode gradients (Gp) is used to obtain the different k-space lines. Each line is again sampled during the application of a read gradient (Gr) that is repeatedly reversed to recall the necessary gradient echoes.*

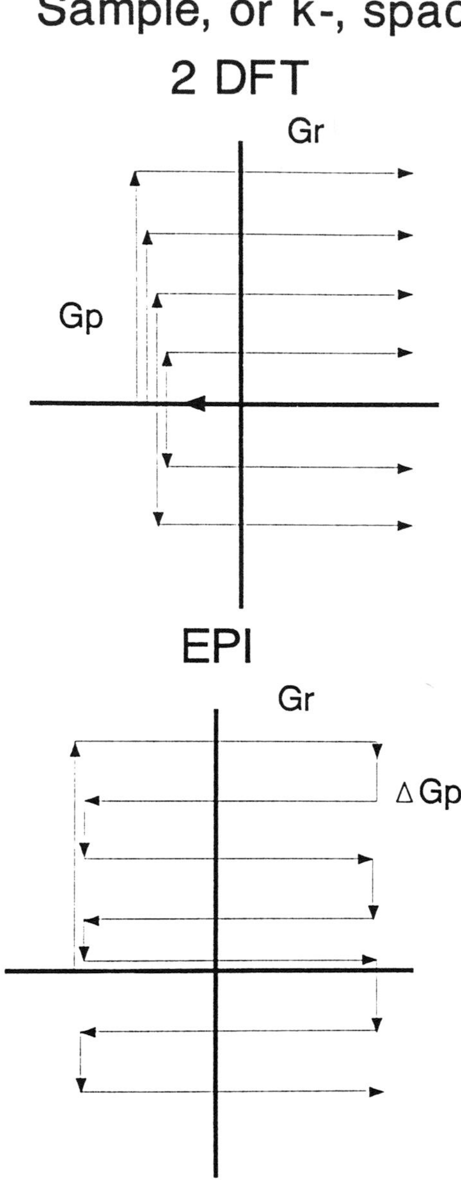

FIGURE 2. Top: *Data obtained by the 2DFT technique. The phase encode gradient (Gp) establishes the initial sampling point at the start of each line. Sampling then proceeds under the action of the orthogonal read gradient.* **Bottom:** *Data sampling in the MBEST variant of echo-planar imaging. Here the data from an entire sample plane are obtained following a single radiofrequency excitation by traversing the lattice by using a series of phase encode blips (Gp) and a repeatedly reversing read gradient (Gr).*

gradient. Successive lines are obtained simply by altering the amount of phase encoding to position the initial sample point appropriately.

In the echo-planar imaging variant MBEST, the slice selection is performed in the same manner as 2DFT (Figure 1, bottom.) Subsequently, the furthest point in k-space is selected as the initial sample point by use of the two remaining orthogonal gradients in exactly the same way as in 2DFT. The first line of k-space is then again obtained by sampling during the application of a readout gradient.

The difference between echo-planar imaging and 2DFT lies in the manner in which the second and subsequent k-space lines are obtained. In echo-planar imaging, a small phase encode difference is produced by the application of a short gradient pulse or blip. During this time the read gradient is reversed. The adjacent line in k-space is then sampled while this reversed read gradient is applied (Figure 2, bottom). Successive lines are obtained in a similar manner by the application of the phase encode gradient blip and read gradient reversal to repetitively recall a series of gradient echoes with differing amounts of phase encoding.

In this way the entire set of data required for a complete image is obtained following the application of a single radiofrequency excitation. Before Fourier transformation it is necessary to time-reverse alternate lines of data. If the gradient echoes are imperfectly centered in each data line, a conspicuous ghost image is introduced halfway across the field of view from the correct image. Elimination of this ghost is a major concern in the successful implementation of echo-planar imaging.

Hardware Requirements

In addition to being the fastest MRI technique, echo-planar imaging is also the most technologically demanding. The relatively prolonged sampling period (up to 128 msec) allows field inhomogeneities to have a severe effect on the phase coherence of the spins in the slice, and hence, extremely good static field uniformity is required. If this sampling time is shortened, the homogeneity requirement is reduced, but to achieve this entails higher switched read gradients. This introduces the most serious technical challenge: gradients. The spatial labeling of nuclear spins, fundamental to MRI, is achieved by applying a magnetic field gradient across the sample. The gradient G is related to the resolution Δl and the sampling time T by the simple formula:

$$G = \frac{2\pi}{\gamma \Delta l T}$$

where γ is the gyromagnetic ratio of the resonant nuclei. Consequently, for constant resolution, the shorter the spin evolution time, the greater the required gradient.

In practice, the in-plane resolution dictates the amount of spin evolution and hence the gradient strength per unit time required. In order to meet the requirements of echo-planar imaging for speed and to ensure that T_2^* dephasing of the signal throughout the data acquisition is minimal, echo-planar imaging requires short read times, which in turn entail high gradients. For the same reasons, the time for switching of these gradients must be kept to a minimum. Large gradients require large currents. Even if the inductance is kept to a minimum,[9] short rise times require power supplies capable of producing a large voltage. Consequently, the requirements of echo-planar imaging for both high gradients and rapid switching place great demands on the gradient power supply. Gradients adequate for echo-planar imaging have been achieved by the use of multiple amplifiers (connected in series and/or in parallel) coupled to one or more gradient coil sets,[6] the development of resonant gradient coil systems,[10] and more recently the development of hybrid inverter systems.[11,12]

Induced eddy currents in surrounding metal structures are associated with the rapid switching of magnetic fields. These eddy currents have their own spatial and temporal characteristics that introduce errors into the magnetic field, dependent on time and gradient strength, which can produce serious image artifacts. The greater gradient demands of echo-planar imaging coupled with the requirement for better homogeneity make it particularly sensitive to these field perturbations. The traditional method of gradient overdrive, or eddy current compensation to compensate for the temporal, though not the spatial dependencies of the eddy currents, has given way to the introduction of screened or shielded gradient coils.[13] Indeed, self-shielded gradient coils were originally developed for use with echo-planar imaging.

Systems comprising earlier types of gradient power supply and inadequate coils can still benefit from the introduction of hybrid echo-planar imaging and gradient-echo 2DFT, in which several successive lines in k-space are acquired on each radiofrequency excitation with an additional phase encode gradient used to move the initial sample point to the appropriate line.[14] In this way fewer cardiac cycles can be used, for example, to reduce the uncertainty in the registration of the structures throughout the imaging procedure.

Clinical Applications

Imagine an MRI system in which the patient is placed in the magnet and examination proceeds by observing magnetic resonance images updated twice a second. Echo-planar imaging provides just such a facility for real-time patient positioning and selection of appropriate contrast by interactive control of sequence parameters. This in turn has resulted in a great reduction in the necessity for subsequent time-consuming MRI studies. Additionally, while echo-planar imaging provides the fastest means of obtaining a set of images of static structures, its greatest advantages lie in the realm of functional rather than simply anatomical studies.

For example, nonreproducible motions may be captured, including peristalsis in the abdomen,[15] cerebrospinal fluid flow in the brain,[16] fetal and fetal heart motion in vivo,[17] and cardiac arrhythmias. For cardiac imaging, echo-planar imaging provides the only means of accurately capturing motion during systole, particularly in infants and fetuses in whom heart rates range from 120 to 180 beats per minute. The earliest clinical use of echo-planar imaging (1983) was in the diagnosis of congenital heart and major vessel abnormalities in infants.[18,19] With the rapidity of the entire procedure it was unnecessary to sedate the infants, most of whom were under 2 years of age. Despite the low resolution, originally 6 mm in-plane, and the low field (0.1 T), clinically useful images were obtained.

Subsequent improvements in MRI technology have enabled echo-planar imaging, with increased spatial and temporal resolution to be used in adults. A wide variety of pathologic conditions have been studied, including heart studies, though large-scale clinical trials have yet to be conducted. Bright (Figure 3) or black blood images, freezing the motion not only of the heart wall, but also of the blood itself, are routinely acquired. As a consequence, echo-planar imaging has been useful in the diagnosis of mitral and aortic valve regurgitation (Figure 4), in whom movie sequences have clearly demonstrated regurgitant jets. Echo-planar imaging of the heart has also demonstrated significant beat-to-beat variations even in healthy hearts. This explains the difficulty encountered by conventional slow MRI techniques, no matter how carefully gated, in depicting such narrow and rapidly moving structures as the coronary vessels. Developments in pediatric imaging have continued, culminating in

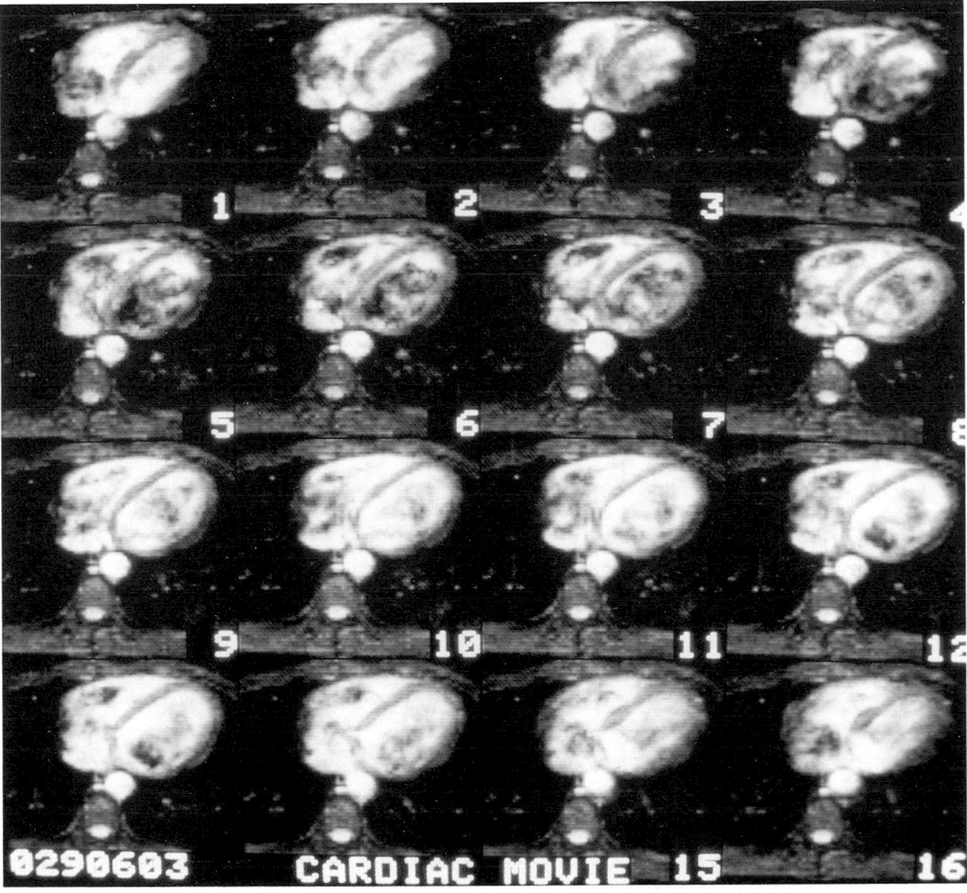

FIGURE 3. *Stills from a 16-frame cardiac movie, normal heart. Each image was acquired at 0.5 T using a gradient-echo echo-planar imaging sequence in 64 msec, with an in-plane resolution of 3 mm × 3 mm. The signal loss due to turbulent blood flow can easily be seen in images acquired near systole. The images were obtained from 16 consecutive cardiac cycles, the gated acquisition being delayed from the RR wave by successive time increments. (Figure courtesy of P. Mansfield, Department of Physics, University of Nottingham, England.)*

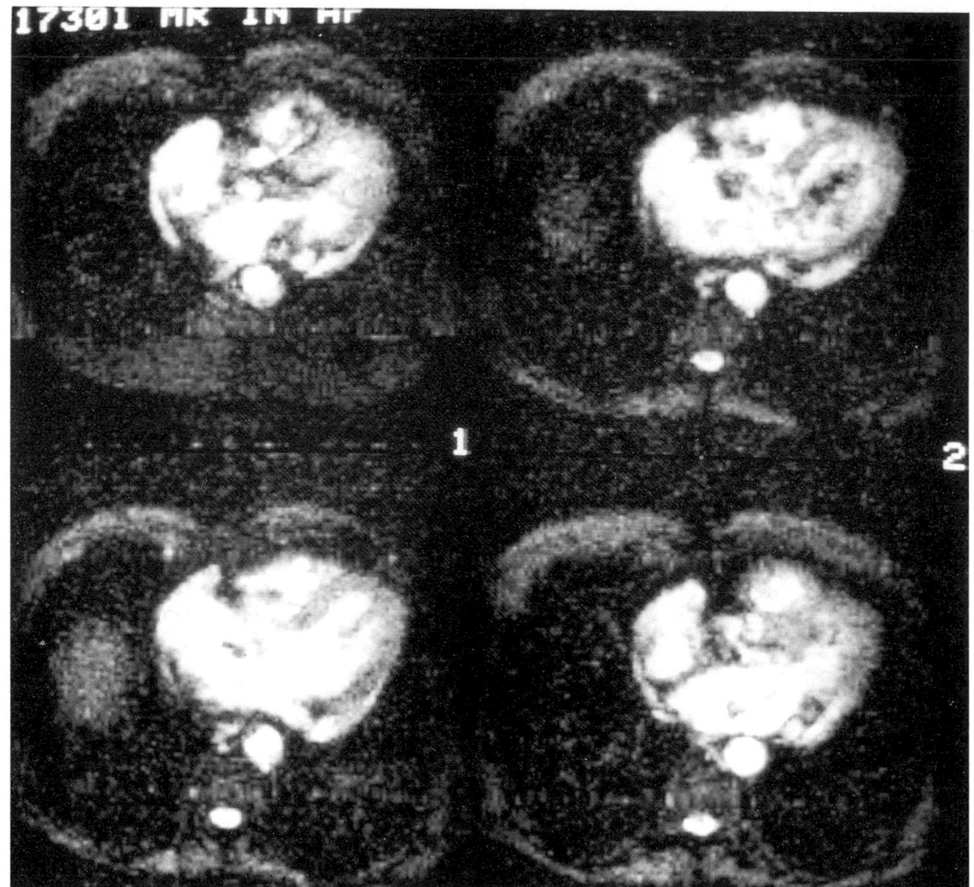

FIGURE 4. *Mitral valve regurgitation. The turbulent regurgitant jet is visible in frame 2 of these 128 × 128 pixel matrix echo-planar imaging images, taken from a set of 16 obtained at 0.5 T using a similar gradient-echo echo-planar imaging sequence as in Figure 3. (Figure courtesy of P. Mansfield and M.K. Stehling, Department of Physics, University of Nottingham, England.)*

remarkable images of the fetus in utero (Figure 5) that show the rapidly pulsating fetal heart at multiple phases of the cardiac cycle.

A significant advantage of echo-planar imaging over other fast-imaging methods lies in its ability to obtain multiple slices rapidly. Up to 15 slices, each with the full achievable signal-to-noise ratio, can be obtained in 1 second. This means that a set of complete volume maps of the heart, at 16 points in the cardiac cycle, could be made in 30 seconds or less. If procedures for patient handling were streamlined, this could mean a total examination time of perhaps 5 minutes, which is not unreasonable for an emergency case.

A further development of this approach has been made by Cohen and Weisskoff[7]

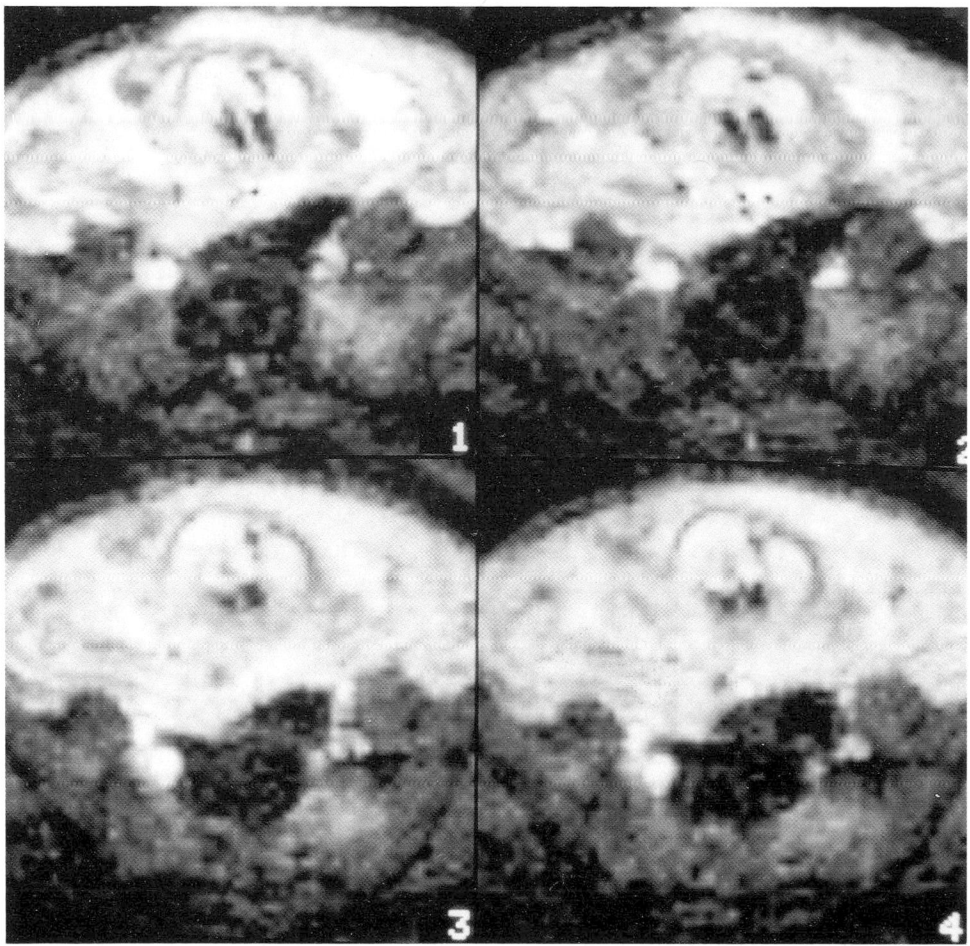

FIGURE 5. *Echo-planar images of the fetal heart in utero, showing the same slice at four phases of the cardiac cycle, in a 26-week gestation fetus. Matrix size was 128 × 128 pixels. The uninflated, liquid lungs appear bright, while the blood in left and right ventricles is generally dark in these spin-echo images. (Figure courtesy of P. Mansfield, Department of Physics, University of Nottingham, England.)*

using a direct volume acquisition. A thick slice is selected, and a series of gated acquisitions, each with a different phase encode gradient applied in the slice-select direction, allows the extraction of thin slices (Figure 6). Any residual motion artifact caused by beat-to-beat variations appears in the direction normal to the slice, where it does not significantly compromise image quality.

Finally, it should be mentioned that with adequate gradient supplies on each axis, slices of any orientation may be obtained, as in conventional gradient-echo 2DFT imaging. Long- and short-axis cardiac movies (Figure 7) have thus been obtained by the group at Massachusetts General Hospital.

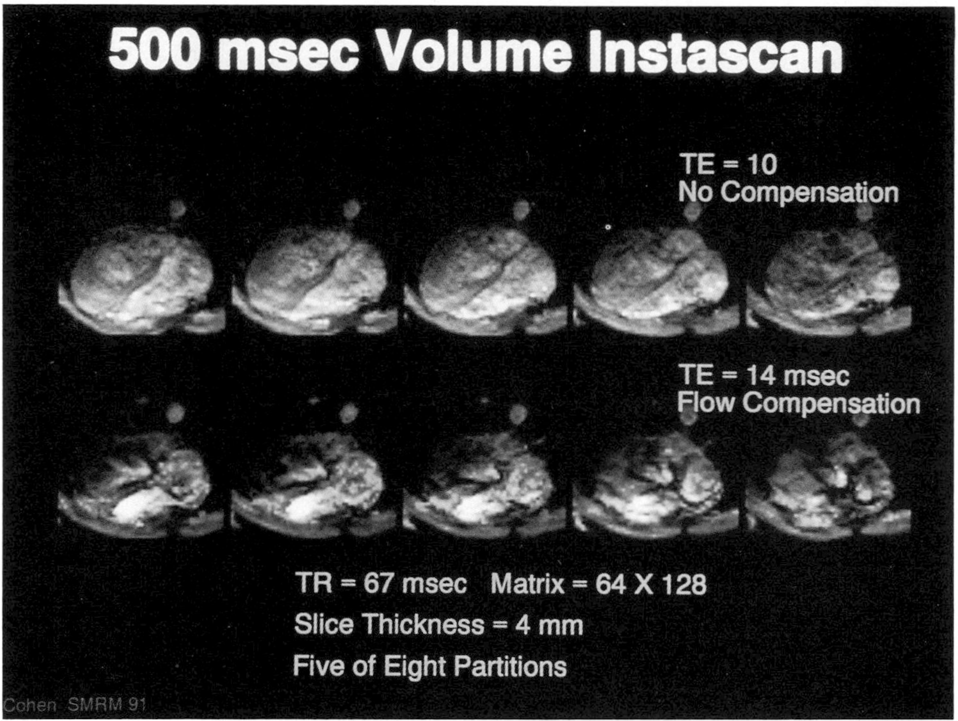

FIGURE 6. *Volume echo-planar images, normal heart. These images were obtained by selecting a thick slice, and making eight echo-planar imaging acquisitions while phase encode gradients are stepped in the slice-select direction. The resulting data set undergoes a further Fourier transformation to provide eight thin slices of the heart, with no visible motion artifact. The upper five images show five slices at a single phase of the cardiac cycle, with no motion compensation, while the lower five have motion-compensating gradient applied, with a slightly longer TE, as shown. The pixel matrix was 64 × 128. (Figure courtesy of M.S. Cohen, MRI, Massachusetts General Hospital, Boston, Massachusetts.)*

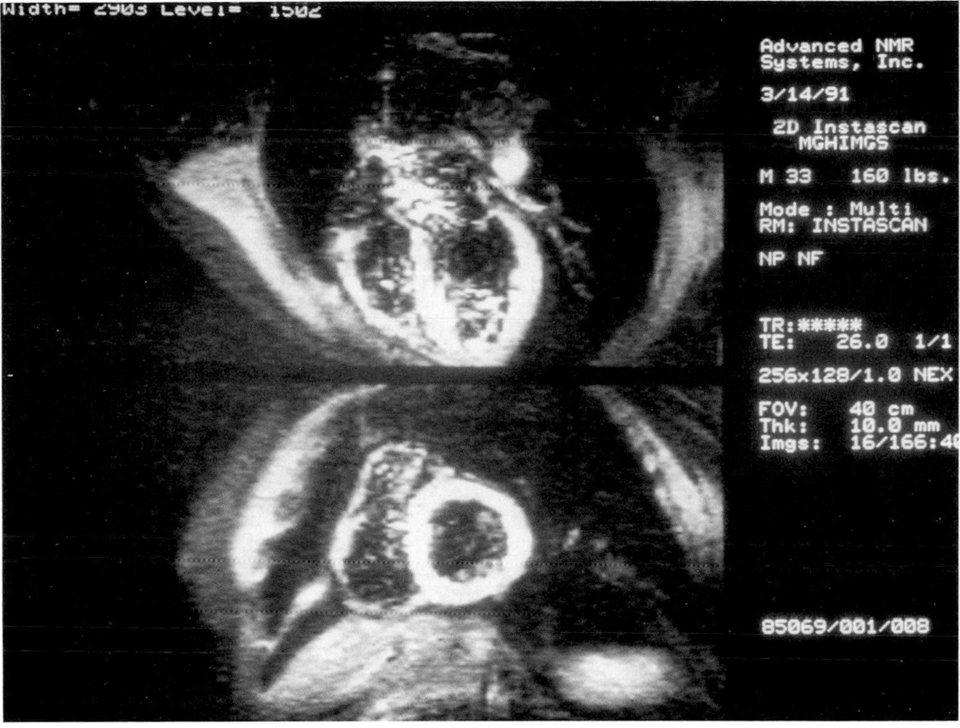

FIGURE 7. *Long- and short-axis views of normal heart acquired with oblique echo-planar imaging during diastole, extracted from a movie loop consisting of 26 frames within the cardiac cycle, obtained on successive cycles by appropriate gating. A spin-echo acquisition was used, causing the blood to appear dark, although turbulent flow causes small bright areas. The pixel matrix was 128 × 256, field of view was 40 cm, and the TE was 26 msec. (Figure courtesy of R.M. Weisskoff, MRI, Massachusetts General Hospital, Boston, Massachusetts.)*

Safety

Safety considerations in MRI fall into three main categories: those associated with the main field, the gradient field, and the applied rf. The normal concerns regarding patient exposure to the main field[20] apply equally to both standard MRI and echo-planar imaging and will not be discussed further in this chapter. Echo-planar imaging requires significantly higher gradients than other techniques and greater gradient switching rates. Slight stimulation of the peripheral nerves has been noted[21,22] using higher gradients than normal for echo-planar imaging. While no deleterious effects due to echo-planar imaging studies have been reported, this feature may ultimately limit the speed of acquisition and resolution of echo-planar imaging. Current data suggest that 1.5 mm × 1.5 mm resolution can be achieved over a matrix size of 256 × 256 pixels in an imaging time of 60 msec without any neural stimulation.

The major safety concern in MRI, generally speaking, is the amount of radiofrequency heating induced, particularly at higher fields in which the radiofrequency power requirements are greater. In this regard echo-planar imaging has an advantage in that it requires less radiofrequency power than any other MRI technique; the data for an entire image can be obtained from a single radiofrequency excitation.

Even at cine frame rates of >16 frames per single cardiac cycle, the low radiofrequency flip angles then used and the efficiency of the data acquisition process results in the total radiofrequency power absorption remaining low.

Discussion

Echo-planar imaging has been an established technique for 15 years. The relatively slow rate at which it has been introduced has been due partly to its technological demands and partly to the relative ignorance of its existence by the medical community at large.

Many of the technological problems have now been solved. The introduction of increasingly powerful superconducting magnets has resulted in far better signal-to-noise ratios. Improved gradient coil design[23] and the introduction of screened gradients[13] have lead to improved gradient fields and the elimination of transient eddy currents due to the rapid switching of large gradients proximal to surrounding metallic structures, respectively, both of which were originally devised for use in echo-planar imaging systems. The improvements in power supplies and the invention of resonant gradient systems[24] have reduced the gradient switching times and increased gradient strength, again in response to the requirements of echo-planar imaging. The continuing improvements in computer technology permit the higher data digitization rates and shorter reconstruction times necessary for the real-time acquisition and display of results.

Additionally, continuing innovations have continued to improve the quality and expand the range of capabilities of echo-planar imaging. In particular, the close similarity between echo-planar imaging and gradient-echo 2DFT enables all the prepulse sequences that can be used in conjunction with the former to be immediately applied to the latter. These include: spin-echo imaging, by introducing a 180° pulse; fat or water imaging by, eg, the Dixon method[25]; three-dimensional volume imaging by selecting a thick slice and incorporating a phase encode in the slice-select direction in exactly the same way that gradient-echo 2DFT does for its second dimension; and inversion recovery by introducing a 180° before the sequence. Echo-planar imaging has also been used to perform full three-dimensional imaging, flow imaging, and chemical shift imaging in a variety of applications ranging from clinical studies to the oil industry.

The potential benefits of echo-planar imaging to the clinician, and particularly to cardiologists, cannot be adequately stressed. Those who have been fortunate enough to have direct clinical experience with echo-planar imaging are uniformly enthusiastic about its usefulness. The technological demands of echo-planar imaging should not be minimized, but MRI researchers will continue to respond to these challenges.

References

1. Lauterbur PC: Image formation by induced local interactions: examples employing nuclear magnetic resonance. *Nature* 1973;242:190.
2. Haase A, Frahm J, Matthaei D, et al: FLASH imaging: rapid NMR imaging using low flip-angle pulses. *J Magn Reson* 1986;67:258–266.
3. Mansfield P, Maudsley AA: Planar spin imaging by NMR. *J Phys C* 1977;10:155.
4. Rzedzian R, Chapman B, Mansfield P, et al: Real-time nuclear magnetic resonance clinical imaging in paediatrics. *Lancet* 1983;2(8362):1281–1282.
5. Turner R, Chapman B, Howseman AM, et al: Snap-shot magnetic resonance imaging at 0.1T using double-screened gradients. *J Magn Reson* 1988;80:248–258.
6. Chapman B, Turner R, Ordidge RJ, et al: Real-time movie imaging from a single cardiac cycle by NMR. *Magn Reson Med* 1987;5:246–254.
7. Cohen MS, Weisskoff RM: Ultra-fast imaging. *Magn Reson Imaging* 1991;9:1–37.
8. Stehling MK, Turner R, Mansfield P: Echo-planar imaging: magnetic resonance imaging in a fraction of a second. *Science* 1991;254:43–50.
9. Turner R: Minimum inductance coils. *J Phys E: Sci Instrum* 1988;21:948–952.
10. Rzedian R, Pykett IL: Instant images of the human heart using a new, whole-body MR imaging system. *AJR* 1987;149:245.
11. Coxon RJ, Mansfield P: A method for the rapid switching of large gradients. (abstract) In: Proceedings of the 3rd Congress of the European Society of Magnetic Resonance in Medicine and Biology. 1986:45–46.
12. Mueller OM, Roemer PB, Park JN, Souza SP: A general purpose non-resonant gradient power system (abstract). In: Proceedings of the 10th Meeting of the Society of Magnetic Resonance in Medicine. 1991;1:130.
13. Mansfield P, Chapman BLW, Turner R, Bowley R: Magnetic field screens. UK Patent 861 1 1777, 1986; US Patent 4,978,920, 1990.
14. Haacke EM, Bearden FH, Clayton JR, Linga NR: Reduction of MR time by the hybrid fast-scan technique. *Radiology* 1986;158:521–529.
15. Stehling MK, Evans DF, Lamont G, et al: Gastrointestinal tract: dynamic MR studies with echo-planar imaging. *Radiology* 1989;171:41–46.
16. Mansfield P, Chapman B, Doyle M, et al: Observation of CSF and ventricular motion in the brain by real-time echo-planar imaging. (abstract) In: Proceedings of the Society of Magnetic Resonance in Medicine. 1986;3:699–700.
17. Mansfield P, Stehling MK, Ordidge RJ, et al: Echo planar imaging of the human fetus in utero at 0.5T. *Br J Radiol* 1990;63:833–841.
18. Small P, Chrispin A, Rutter N, et al: Echo-planar imaging (EPI) in evaluating septation at ventricular and bulbar in the normal infant heart and cyanotic congenital heart disease. In: Proceedings of the Society of Magnetic Resonance in Medicine. 1985;1:673.
19. Chrispin A, Small P, Rutter N, et al: Echo planar imaging of normal and abnormal connections of the heart and great arteries. *Pediatr Radiol* 1986;16:289–292.
20. Shellock FG, Kanal E: Policies, guidelines, and recommendations for MR imaging safety and patient management. *J Magn Reson Imaging* 1991;1:97–101.
21. Budinger TF, Fischer H, Hentschel D, et al: Neural stimulation dB/dt thresholds for frequency and number of oscillations using sinusoidal magnetic gradient fields. (abstract) In: Proceedings of the 9th Meeting of the Society of Magnetic Resonance in Medicine. 1990:276.
22. Bourland JD, Nyenhuis JA, Mouchawar GA, et al: Human peripheral nerve stimulation from z-gradients. (abstract) Proceedings of the 9th Meeting of the Society of Magnetic Resonance in Medicine. 1990:1157.
23. Turner R: A target field approach to optimal coil design. *J Phys D: Appl Phys* 1986;19:L147-L151.
24. Rzedzian RR, Pykett I: Ultra-fast MRI: the technical and clinical realization (plenary lecture). Proceedings of the 7th Annual Meeting of the Society of Magnetic Resonance in Medicine. 1988.
25. Dixon T: Simple spectroscopic imaging. *Radiology* 1984;153:189–194.

Chapter 9

Breath-Hold Cines Using Phase Encode Grouping

Moriel NessAiver, PhD

Motion leads to a variety of artifacts in magnetic resonance images. Cyclic motion due to the beating heart can be managed by gating, but noncyclic motion due to respiration or peristalsis is best managed by rapid image acquisition. We have developed a technique called phase encode grouping (PEG) for cardiac gated imaging of thoracic and abdominal structures in a single breath-hold (10–20 seconds) without the need for special hardware. This is achieved by trading temporal resolution for shorter total scan time. By doing breath-hold scans, respiratory artifacts are completely eliminated, significantly improving image quality. By setting up multiple contiguous acquisitions, it is possible, in <8 minutes, to obtain 10 good-quality cines covering the whole heart. By acquiring the images in a double oblique, short-axis orientation, both left and right ventricular volumes can be accurately measured throughout the cardiac cycle again in <8 minutes. Phase encode grouping can be used with myocardial tagging[1] to obtain breath-hold cines depicting myocardial motion. By acquiring a motion-compensated cine in one breath-hold and a motion-sensitized cine in a second breath-hold, we obtain up to 16 quantitative flow images, with 50 msec temporal resolution, in a total elapsed time of <1 minute.

Methods

Technical

Sequences were developed on a Picker International, Inc., 1.5-T HPQ system (Picker International, Inc., Highland Heights, OH). High temporal resolution field-echo sequences (TE ranges from 3.7 to 5.2; TR ranges from 8.7 to 14.6) can be used to acquire up to 64 views or lines of data per heartbeat. A diagram of a typical high temporal resolution sequence is illustrated in Figure 1. The usual approach is to apply a single phase encode step per heartbeat, resulting in a 64-frame cine that requires from 64 to 256

From Pohost GM (ed.), *Cardiovascular Applications of Magnetic Resonance*. Mount Kisco, NY, Futura Publishing Co., Inc., © 1993.

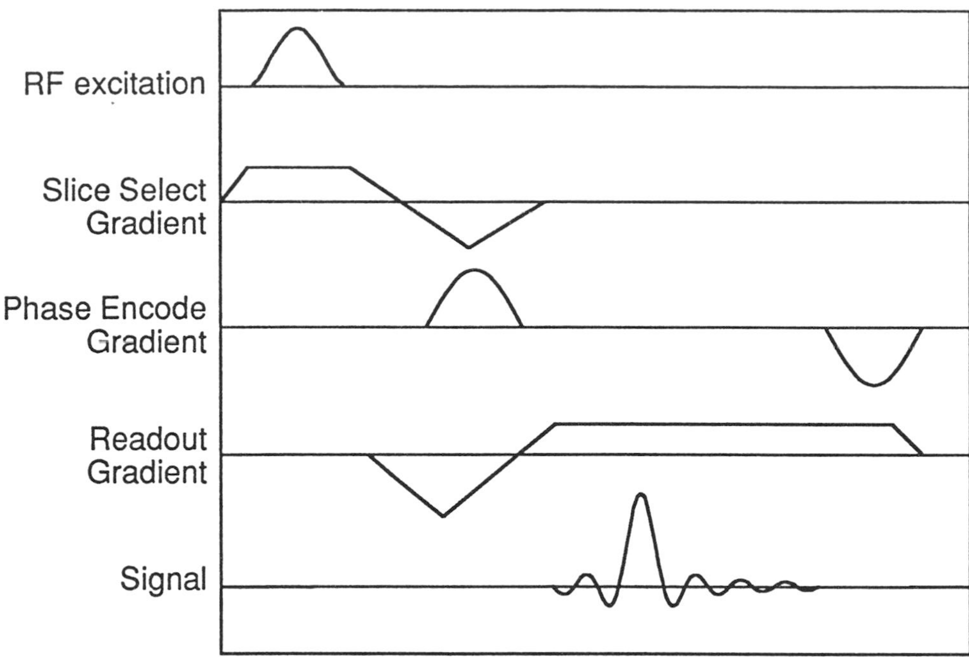

FIGURE 1. *Typical field-echo imaging sequence.*

heartbeats total acquisition time depending on the image matrix and number of averages. The temporal resolution of the cine is the time between data collections within a heartbeat, which in turn is determined by the TR of the field-echo sequence being used.

Another approach is to use PEG and divide the same 64 views into phase encode groups, ie, 32 groups of 2, 16 groups of 4, 8 groups of 8, etc. Each view within a group uses a different phase encode step. This results in a 2-to 64-fold decrease in total acquisition time at the expense of temporal resolution, which is now defined as the time between central views of phase encode groups. Depending upon the group size and acquisition matrix, a 16-frame cine could be acquired in as little as 16 heartbeats.

The key to good image quality using PEG is the order in which the phase encode steps are applied. Three different phase encode ordering schemes are shown in Figures 2 and 3 for a group size of 4. The first two schemes were reported by Atkinson et al.[1,2] The first moves sequentially through the phase encode views or k-space as shown in Figure 2. Since the central n views with the majority of the signal power (where n is the size of the group) are all acquired at n different points in the cardiac cycle, the images tend to suffer from significant blurring and ghosting artifacts. Atkinson et al.[2] dealt with this problem by switching to what they termed a "segmented k-space" approach to the phase encode ordering. As shown on the left side of Figure 3, they divided k-space into n segments and then took one line from each segment per heartbeat. The firing order within a group moves simply from segment A to segment D. We will refer to this method as a simple segmentation of k-space or SSOKS.

The SSOKS approach provides a significant improvement in image quality over the sequential ordering, but still has the disadvantage that the central $2n$ portion of

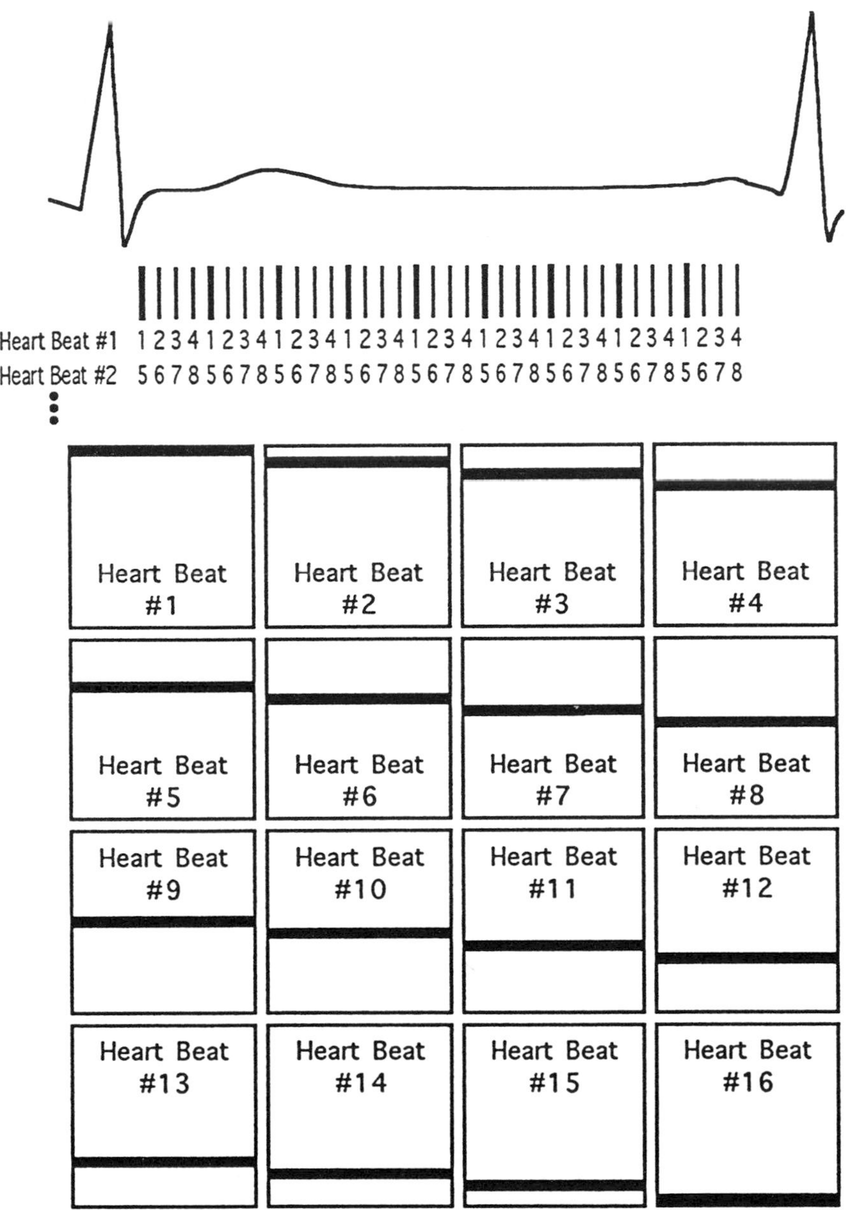

FIGURE 2. *Maps of k-space. When using a 64×256 matrix and a group size of 4, all k-space can be acquired in 16 heartbeats. Four adjacent lines of k-space are acquired in each heartbeat, moving sequentially through all k-space.*

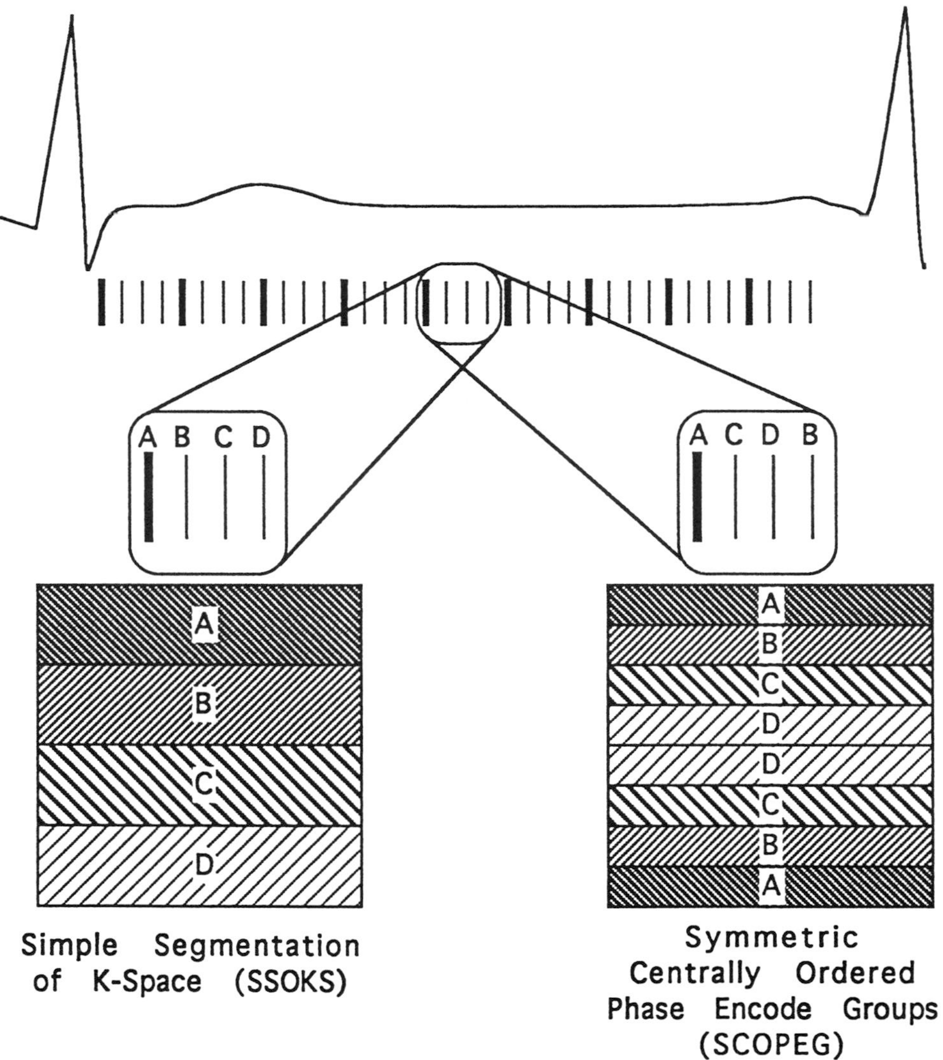

FIGURE 3. *Two different phase encode ordering schemes. The map of the k-space on the left shows a simple division into four segments. One line from each segment is used for each heartbeat. The firing order moves simply from top to bottom. The map of k-space on the right treats positive and negative k-space separately, resulting in a symmetric pattern. The firing within a group is centrally ordered to minimize the temporal distance of the lower-frequency views from the central view.*

k-space is acquired at two different points in the cardiac cycle. Another potential problem arises from the pattern of the phase encode gradient lobes within as well as between groups. Figure 1 shows a typical field-echo sequence. Note that the phase encode gradient has both an initial encoding lobe and a de-encoding or rewind lobe. The top panel of Figure 4 shows an example of the phase encode gradient pattern for two groups of four. Note that two lobes of the same sign and similar amplitude occur at the transition from positive-to-negative k-space within a group and from negative-to-positive k-space between two groups. This could be a potential source of artifact if eddy currents are present in the system.

Our method, as shown on the right side of Figure 3, uses a symmetric, centrally ordered phase encode grouping (SCOPEG) scheme.[3] In the first half of the acquisition all of the positive phase encode lines are acquired, while the negative lines are acquired in the second half. This ordering scheme has several advantages:

1) The central n portion of k-space is acquired at a single point in the cardiac cycle (the portion labeled D).
2) The remaining segments are ordered such that the lower-frequency portions are acquired temporally close to the central portion.
3) The phase encode gradients follow a very smooth transition during a single heartbeat as shown on the bottom panel of Figure 4. This tends to cancel out any eddy current effects.

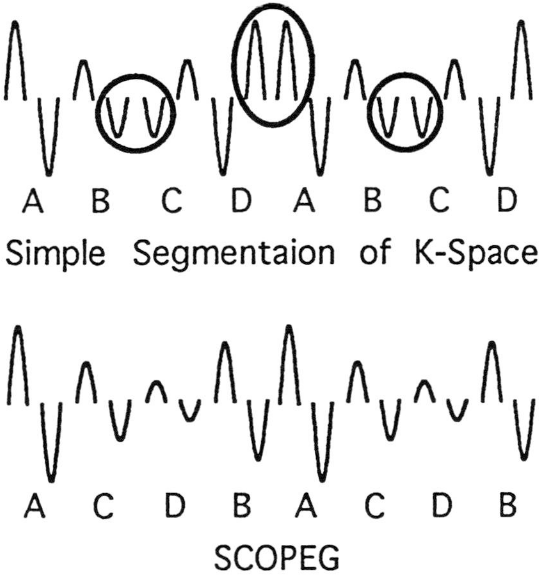

FIGURE 4. *A comparison of the phase encode gradient pattern for SSOKS and SCOPEG. The SSOKS method results in back-to-back positive and back-to-back negative phase encode lobes. The SCOPEG method moves smoothly through large-to-small-to large lobes, always alternating the sign.*

Comparisons of the different PEG schemes were obtained in both phantoms and volunteers at six different flip angles: 10°–60°.

Clinical

Cardiac gated, single breath-hold studies were obtained in 10 volunteers and two patients. Two of the volunteers had known bicuspid aortic valves. One patient had mitral regurgitation and the other had dilated cardiomyopathy and was scheduled for a transplant. Typically, square pixels of 2.7 to 3.1 mm on each side were used, with square field of views and 5–10-mm thick slices, although 1.7 mm × 3.4 mm pixels were also possible with good signal-to-noise ratios when using rectangular field of views and surface coils. Multiple cines were acquired in transverse, long-axis, and short-axis orientations. With the two volunteers with bicuspid aortas, several cines were acquired, both perpendicular and parallel to the outflow tract. Quantitative flow images were obtained in the aorta, the main pulmonary artery, and across the mitral valve.

Results

Technical

The sequential ordering of phase encode groups resulted in significant ghosting in both phantoms and volunteers and loss of edge definition in volunteers. The SSOKS method has been shown by Atkinson et al.[2] to decrease ghosting and improve edge definition at low flip angles (10°–15°) but still showed artifacts (spurious echoes) above 20°. Although we obtained the same improvement at low flip angles, we saw the same general improvement at higher flip angles and we were not able to reproduce the spurious echoes. This was most likely due to differences in the details of the sequences and hardware used.

In the phantom studies there was very little difference between SSOKS and SCOPEG in all but the first image of every cine. The first few views immediately after the R wave trigger have abnormally high signal due to the extra time for relaxation while waiting for the trigger. With SSOKS, this causes a significant asymmetry between the positive and negative views in k-space resulting in smearing in the final image. Because portions of k-space are acquired in a symmetrically interleaved fashion with SCOPEG, the same extra high signal results in a coherent ghosting. In volunteers, the smearing in the first case and ghosting in the second is present, but to a much smaller degree due to the significantly longer T_1 values in vivo. This smearing/ghosting can be virtually eliminated by processing the raw data prior to reconstruction.

As stated above, we did not experience any of the spurious echo artifacts reported by Atkinson et al.[2] at high flip angles, up to and including 60°. We used sequences with TE values ranging from 3.7 to 6.85 and TR values ranging from 8.3 to 13.5. The best signal-to-noise ratio and edge definition were obtained with a TE of 5 and a TR of 12.5, which used a 6.144-msec sampling window. Contrast between blood and myocardium was best with flip angles between 30° and 40°, depending on the slice orientation. The differences in the image quality using SSOKS or SCOPEG are subtle. The consensus of five observers was that SCOPEG gave slightly better edge definition on the average.

Clinical

Breath-hold cine imaging has proven to be very useful. Good-quality cine images can be acquired in <15 seconds. Figure 5 shows a typical 12-frame axial cine acquired in 14 seconds. Note that there is none of the respiratory-induced ghosting that is commonly present with cardiac imaging. Ten such cines covering the whole heart can be acquired in a total elapsed time of <8 minutes. These images can then be used as pilots for oblique studies. Figure 6 shows how one axial image of the main pulmonary artery was used to set up scans of the left and right pulmonary arteries.

One method of cardiac function analysis requires obtaining multiple short-axis views at end diastole and end systole. Prior to breath-hold cine imaging, this could take as much as 45 to 60 minutes. Figures 7A and 7B show good quality short-axis images at end diastole and end systole. A total of 10 short-axis cines were acquired in 7.5 minutes.

Breath-hold imaging presents no problem in normal volunteers but what about patients with serious cardiac problems? Figures 8A and 8B show long-axis and short-axis cines of a patient scheduled for a heart transplant due to dilated cardiomyopathy. Note how little the ventricle contracts and the swirling pattern of the blood. The patient reported no difficulty holding his breath for the 14 seconds necessary to acquire each cine.

We have encountered a number of cases in which the breath-hold cines were far superior to the standard 4- to 8-minute cines. One patient had a very consistent arrhythmia that made it virtually impossible to acquire normal cine images, yet the arrhythmia disappeared during a breath-hold. We were able to obtain quantitative flow images of this patient clearly demonstrating mitral regurgitation (Figure 9). Another patient would periodically cough during a normal cine scan, but had no difficulty holding his breath for 15 seconds without coughing.

Another application of breath-hold imaging is the quick identification of valvular abnormalities. Figures 10A and 10B show two 20-year-old males with bicuspid aortic valves; Figure 10C shows a normal tricuspid aortic valve. Ten different cines at a variety of orientations clearly show the extent of the turbulent jet and an increase in the size of the ascending aorta, but no evidence of regurgitation. Total study time was 15 minutes. The mother of one of the volunteers also has a bicuspid valve that demonstrated a small amount of regurgitation.

By using a flow-compensated sequence in one breath-hold and a flow-sensitized sequence in a second breath-hold, we were able to obtain up to 16 frames of quantitative flow information. The top two images in Figure 11 are part of a 64-frame high temporal resolution quantitative flow study showing flow in the aorta 125 msec after the detection of the R wave. Total acquisition time was 4 minutes. The bottom two images are part of a 16-frame quantitative flow study from the same volunteer, also acquired at 125 msec after the R wave, that required only two breath-holds; total time was 1 minute. The average flow in both studies was 1.05 m/s. Figure 11 shows an application of this technique in a patient with mitral regurgitation.

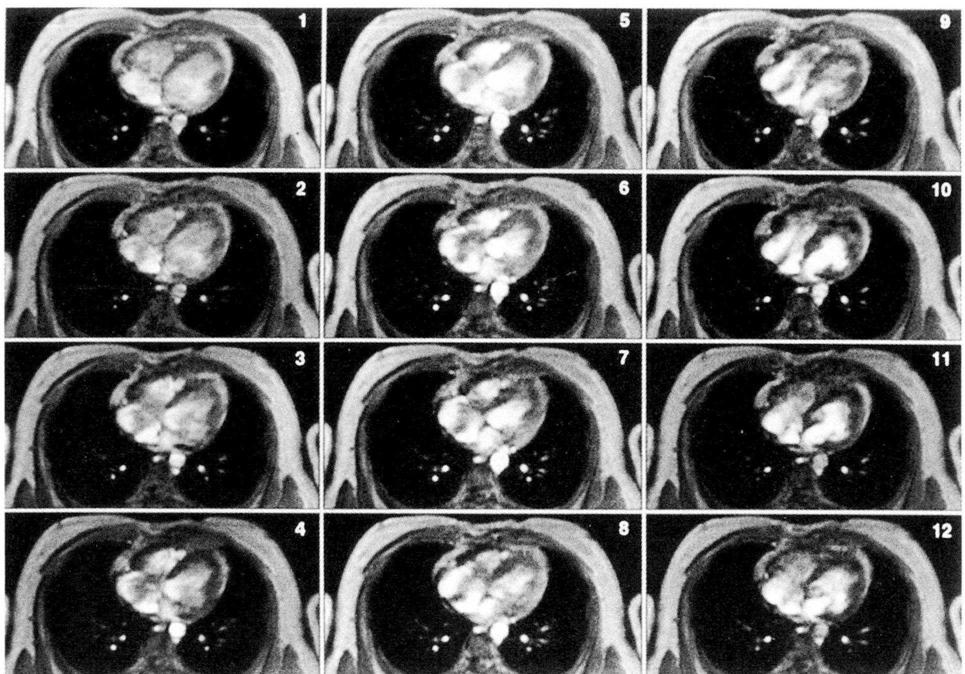

FIGURE 5. *A typical 12-frame axial breath-hold cine acquired in 14.2 seconds, one signal averaged 64 × 128 matrix, 20 × 40 cm field of view, 10-mm slice thickness.*

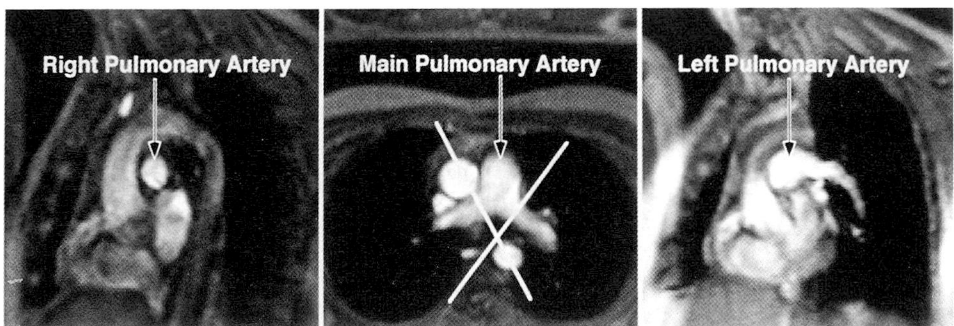

FIGURE 6. *The central image was one of 14 frames acquired as one of a batch of 10 cine acquisitions covering the whole heart. Each acquisition required <16 seconds. This image was then used to set up two oblique scans of the left and right pulmonary arteries.*

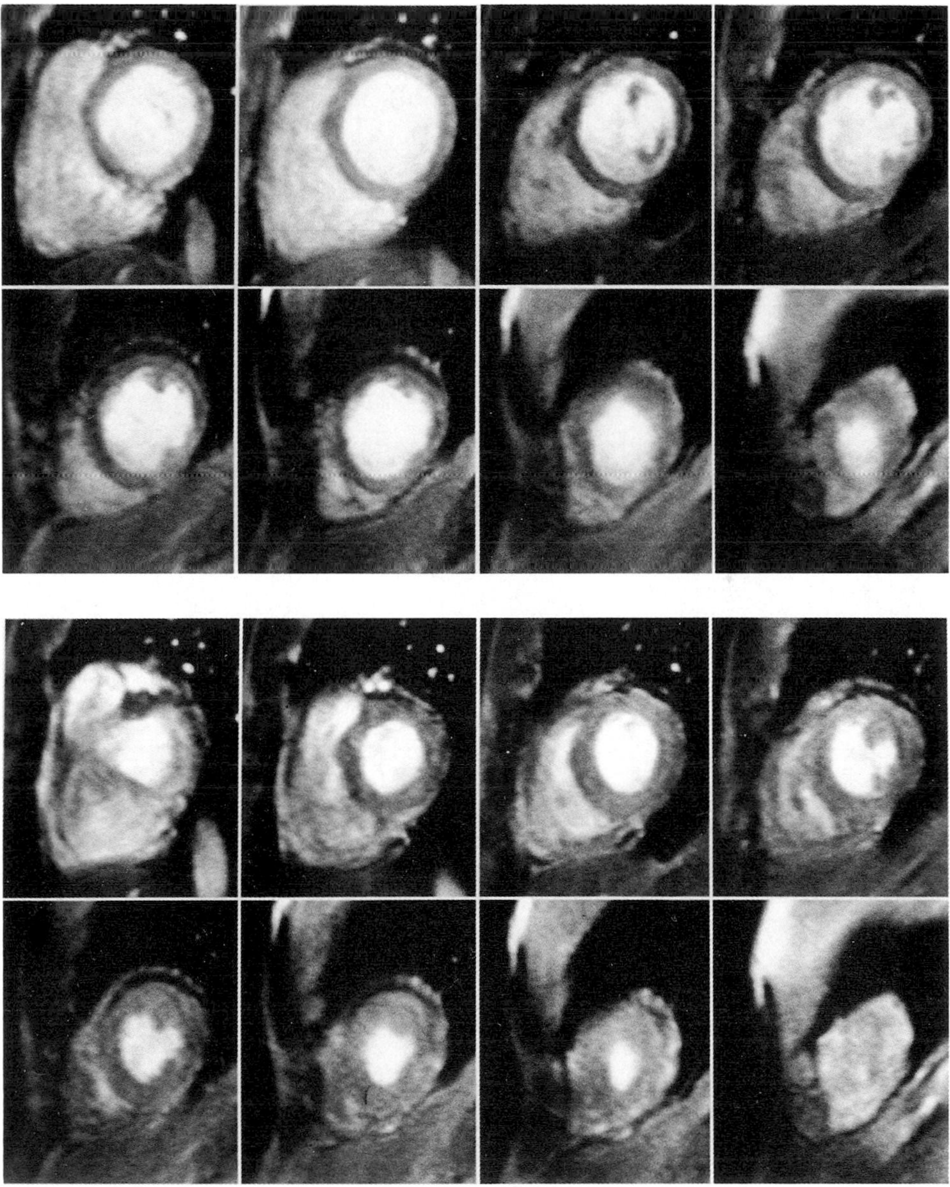

FIGURE 7. *Ten short-axis breath-hold cines acquired by moving from the base of the heart to the apex.* **(A):** *The first frame (end diastole) at eight anatomical positions from which both left and right ventricular volumes could be estimated.* **(B):** *The same anatomical positions at end systole.*

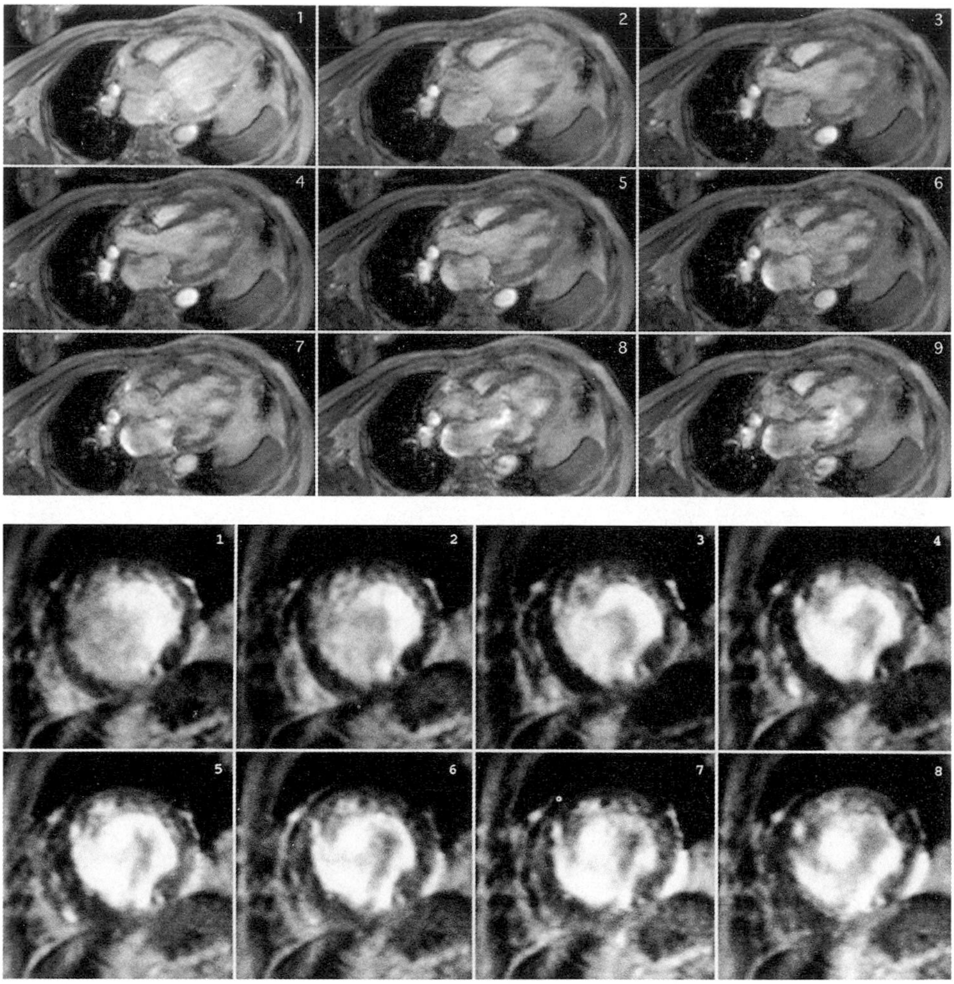

FIGURE 8. *Patient with dilated cardiomyopathy. Each acquisition was done in <15 seconds.* **(Top):** *Long-axis view: flow 3. Phase encode group size of 5, temporal resolution of 72 msec.* **(Bottom):** *Short-axis view. A slightly faster sequence was used, phase encode group size of 6, temporal resolution of 75 msec.*

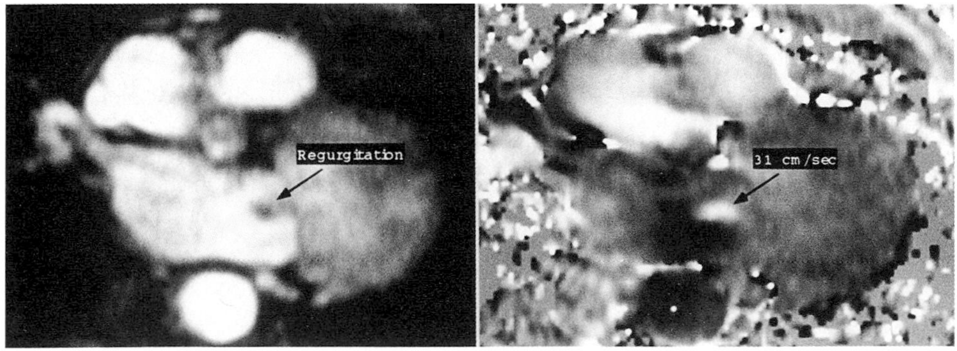

FIGURE 9. *Magnitude and quantitative flow image showing a 31 cm/s mitral regurgi-*

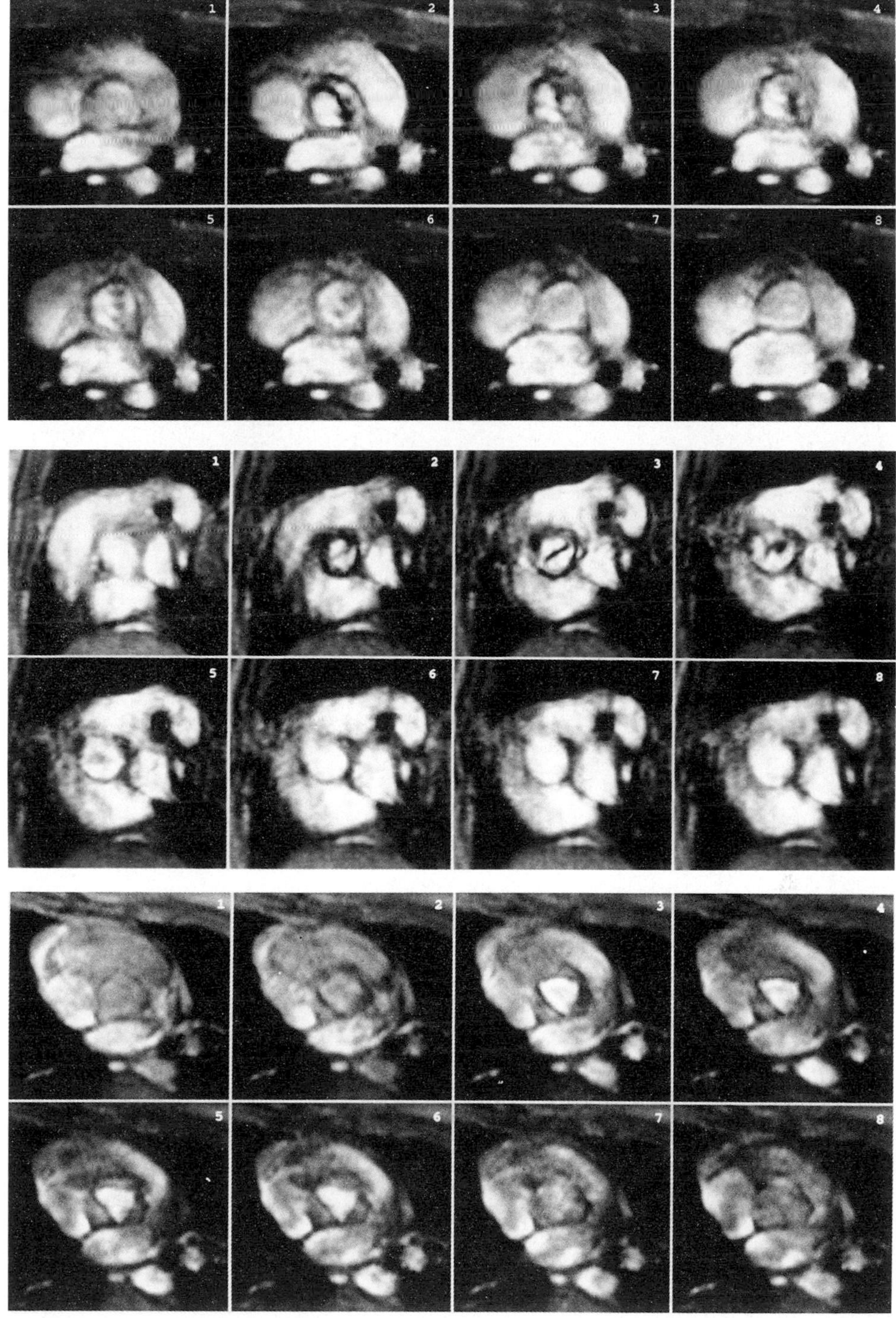

FIGURE 10. *Breath-hold cines perpendicular to the aortic outflow tract immediately above the aortic valve. Each is eight of 12 frames.* **(A-B):** *Two 20-year-old volunteers with bicuspid aortic valves. B is rotated 90° from A.* **(C):** *A normal tricuspid aortic valve.*

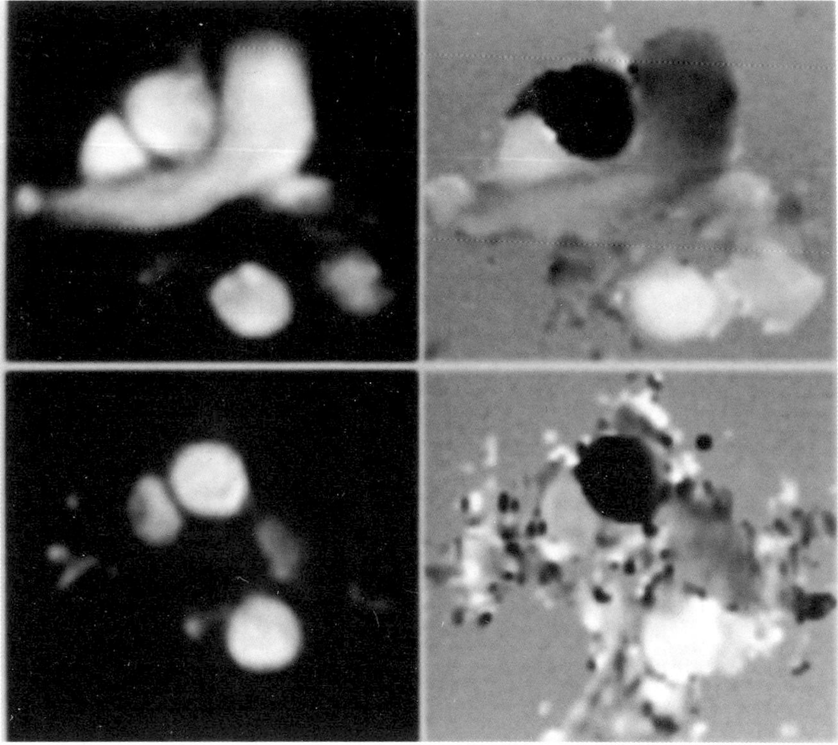

FIGURE 11. *Quantitative flow images 125 msec after the R wave. The top two are the magnitude and velocity images from a 64-frame study. The bottom two are from a 16-frame study in which the reference images were acquired in one breath-hold and the sensitized images in a second breath-hold. Both velocity maps show an average flow of 1.05 m/s.*

Discussion

Breath-hold cine imaging using PEG has a number of advantages over standard cine imaging techniques:

1) Elimination of respiratory ghosting.
2) Elimination of blurring due to respiratory motion.
3) Significant reduction in total study time.
4) Improved slice positioning by using gated pilot studies.
5) A larger number of scan orientations can be achieved in less time.
6) Cardiac function analysis with multiple short-axis cines is now practical.
7) Sufficient time to allow for error.

This last item is a little unusual, but in reality is very important. In a typical magnetic resonance imaging center, cardiac imaging plays a minor role. As a result, the technologists do not have a lot of experience with it. Because cardiac anatomy varies so greatly from individual to individual, it is not always easy to pinpoint the anatomy of interest. Since such scans take only a few seconds to perform, there is very little time lost if the slice positioning or scan parameters were not set right. Accordingly, PEG cine imaging could make cardiac magnetic resonance scanning a viable modality.

Acknowledgments

The author would like to thank Dr. Ron Peshock of the University of Texas Southwestern Medical Center and Dr. Kerry Link of the Bowman Gray School of Medicine for supplying clinical images for this chapter.

References

1. Atkinson DJ, Edelman RR, Chien D: High resolution, breath-hold cine MRI. (abstract) In: Proceedings of the 9th Annual Meeting of the Society of Magnetic Resonance in Medicine. 1990:397.
2. Atkinson DJ, Edelman RR: Cineangiography of the heart in a single breath-hold with a segmented turboFLASH sequence. *Radiology* 1991;178(2):357–360.
3. NessAiver MS, Erdman WA, Clarke G, et al: Breath hold cine MRI for the assessment of blood flow using symmetric, centrally ordered phase encode groups (SCOPEG): technical description and initial clinical evaluation. (abstract) In: Proceedings of the 10th Annual Meeting of the Society of Magnetic Resonance in Medicine. 1991:1159.

Chapter 10

Flow Quantitation

Peter G. Walker, PhD, Markus B. Scheidegger, PhD, Gregory B. Cranney, MBBS, Gerald M. Pohost, MD, and Ajit P. Yoganathan, PhD

This chapter outlines some of the current applications of nuclear magnetic resonance (NMR) to the quantitation of blood flow in the human cardiovascular system. We begin by mentioning some of the reasons for quantifying blood flow and discuss the pros and cons of the currently available techniques. We then focus on magnetic resonance imaging (MRI) methods showing some clinically obtained results of unidirectional velocity measurements in arteries and veins. Additionally, some of the limitations of the method such as turbulent signal loss are mentioned, as well as current research topics such as short TE imaging. Finally, some results showing bidirectional in-plane velocity fields within the human heart are shown and the possibilities of three-dimensional computer reconstruction are explored.

Why Blood Flow Quantitation?

Before looking into the different methods of blood velocity quantitation, it is worthwhile to consider the motivation behind such measurements. Table 1 shows a list of areas in which blood velocity measurement is or will be important.

The first category deals with the assessment of performance. For example, the cardiac output of the heart is a useful indication of its health and may be used in judging the need for a range of heart operations and as an indication of postoperative recovery or, in the case of shunts, in the evaluation of surgical and/or medical treatments. The second category deals with the quantitation and identification of cardiac valvular regurgitation. The decision to proceed with an operation to replace or repair a defective heart valve is obviously a very important one. This decision is made more reliably and more easily through the use of velocity measurements to quantify the exact regurgitant flow rate and through velocity visualization of the flow to indicate

The work described was partially supported by NIH grants R01-HL 42075; R01-HL 4548502.
From Pohost G (ed.), *Cardiovascular Applications of Magnetic Resonance.* Mount Kisco, NY, Futura Publishing Co., Inc., © 1993.

TABLE 1. Applications of Blood Flow Quantitation

Performance
- Cardiac output
- Shunt flow rate

Valvular regurgitation
- Identify location of leakage
- Quantify the severity of leakage

Stenosis: Valvular or vascular
- Aortic, mitral, coronary, femoral, iliac, etc.
- Identify location and structure, quantify the hemodynamic severity of stenosis

Basic research into blood flow-structure interaction
- Three-dimensional ventricular and atrial flow fields
- Three-dimensional flow in large vessels (eg, aorta, pulmonary artery)
- Flow fields in the vascular system, especially at bifurcations prone to atherosclerosis

the position of the leakage. Similarly, the location and hemodynamic severity of stenoses can also be assessed from velocity measurements through flow rate quantitation and flow field visualization. The final category differs from the preceding ones in that it involves the use of velocity measurements for investigating the relationship between blood flow and the function of the human body rather than as a diagnostic tool. As such it will of course not be used as often, but this is nonetheless a very important fundamental application to understanding disease processes. Examples of possible areas of research are the relationship between the pattern of blood flow through the carotid bifurcation and areas of plaque formation and the importance of ventricular flow on the initiation of systolic anterior motion of the mitral valve and mitral valve prolapse.

Current Flow Quantitation Methods

The previous section discussed of the reasons for the need to quantify flow. In this section some of the currently used techniques are considered and compared with NMR.

Table 2 is a list of five methods for blood flow quantitation (qualitative and quantitative). Each method has a number of advantages and disadvantages, some of which are listed.[1–5]

The various blood flow quantitation techniques shown in Table 2 can be divided into two groups. The first group, cine angiography, catheterization, and thermodilution, are all methods that measure flow indirectly. As a result they are at best semiquantitative and all have the disadvantage of being invasive. In addition, cine angiography involves ionizing radiation. These drawbacks increase the risk factor of the procedure and therefore limit the number of times that it can be applied. On the positive side, cine angiography has the advantage of being interactive and having good resolution. This results in a clear interpretation of the anatomy and flow, and catheterization can be used intraoperatively to provide an immediate assessment of valve performance through direct pressure drop measurement.

TABLE 2. Comparison Among Current Methods of Blood Flow Quantitation

Method	Advantages	Disadvantages
Cine angiography	Real time High resolution	Invasive Ionizing radiation Qualitative
Catheterization	Intraoperative Direct pressure measurement	Invasive
Thermodilution	Volume flow	Invasive Estimation
Doppler ultrasound	Relatively cheap Intraoperative Quick and easy to use Noninvasive Safe	Single velocity component Needs acoustic window No digital data at present Nyquist limit Turbulence
NMR	Full three-dimensional velocity information Large velocity range Inherently digital data Safe (?) Volume flow information Jet visualization	Can be slow for large studies Turbulent signal loss Well known MRI problems: motion artifacts, no ferrous metal, claustrophobia, etc.

The second group of techniques consists of Doppler ultrasound and NMR. Both are relatively new techniques and are the future as far as noninvasive velocity measurement techniques are concerned. They have major advantages over the first group because they measure velocity directly, are noninvasive, and are believed to be safe. Therefore, they can be applied repeatedly without putting the patient at any additional risk. Doppler ultrasound has the advantage of being relatively quick and inexpensive and involves small, portable machinery that can be used in the operating room. Its disadvantages are: 1) It measures only a single velocity component, the maximum value of which is limited in the pulsed Doppler mode; 2) It is unable to penetrate bone. This makes it difficult to obtain a suitable acoustic window. This is a particular problem when viewing the heart through the chest wall as the ribs tend to block the ultrasound beam; 3) The data are currently provided in video or print format only, making it difficult to do any in-depth computer analyses; and 4) Turbulent flows are too complicated to provide detailed reliable velocity field measurements. NMR has the advantage that it is theoretically possible to measure the full three-dimensional time-dependent velocity field anywhere in the body without any hindrance from obstructive bone and that this data is inherently available on computer. Unlike ultrasound, NMR does not require a window into the body in order to create an image. It is in fact possible to orientate the image slice in any direction, making it possible to image the desired area, such as the heart or head, from any angle, thus allowing the user the best possible view. By the very nature of NMR the acquired data are stored on a computer. Thus, the data cannot only be displayed to obtain a view of the structure or flow, but can also be used for immediate calculations such as stroke volume and flow rate. One of the disadvantages of NMR is that it can be slow for very large studies, although not for small ones. For instance, the time required to measure a single component of the blood velocity through the imaging plane may be only 10 minutes, which is acceptable for most patient studies. Contrast this with a more complicated study that involves measuring two or three velocity components in a number of image planes. The time required in this case may be on the order of hours, making it only feasible on healthy volunteers. Further drawbacks of NMR are that it currently cannot measure velocity if the flow is turbulent because this causes signal loss; image artifacts such as motion from breathing can create distortions of the image and velocity data; and it cannot be used for claustrophobic or critically ill patients or for those with some ferrous metal implants. Also, phase encoding techniques, although eddy in principle, require good hardware because of the need to rapidly switch gradients and to keep eddy currents low.

Magnetic Resonance Flow Techniques

The two main methods used to measure velocity by NMR are time of flight and phase velocity encoding.

Time-of-Flight Method

The time-of-flight method does not measure velocity directly, but relies on signal intensity variations to indicate areas of motion. Depending upon the type of imaging sequence used, moving fluid in the angiographic image will appear either brighter or darker than the surrounding stationary fluid or tissue. This can be used to visualize blood motion or, through methods such as bolus tracking, to quantify the blood velocity. Earlier approaches to velocity quantitation using NMR tried to use these effects, but were very difficult to perform in practice due to the need to calibrate the system or to perform a repeated number of measurements. These drawbacks, along with the advent of phase velocity encoding techniques, which will be demonstrated, are far easier to apply and much more reliable and accurate, have led to the decline in the application of this technique for flow quantification. Despite this, time-of-flight effects are still an important part of magnetic resonance angiography as they provide an excellent visual image of blood motion and can therefore provide a quick visual qualitative picture.

Another effect that deserves attention is turbulent signal loss. This is most obvious in regions of stenoses and intracardiac jets associated with cardiac valvular regurgitation. The increase in the velocity of these types of flow cause the flow to become turbulent. The rapid spatial and temporal changes in velocity associated with turbulence creates a reduction of the NMR signal intensity due to phase dispersion. Therefore, areas of high turbulence show up on the image as dark areas and contrast highly with the surrounding fluid or tissue. The extent of the signal loss is a reasonable qualitative/semiquantitative indicator of valvular regurgitation.

Phase Velocity Encoding

In simplified terms, phase velocity encoding works as follows. As the magnetic resonance signal can be thought of as a processing vector, it is possible to measure not only the magnitude of the signal but also the degree of rotation or phase. This phase will depend upon the speed of precession, and, therefore, the local field strength. Use can be made of this phenomenon by applying a bipolar gradient in the direction of the required velocity. Under the influence of such a gradient, a stationary proton will precede a given amount in one direction due to the first half of the gradient and an equal amount in the other direction due to the equal but oppositely applied second gradient. The proton will therefore have no net rotation due to this gradient sequence. If, however, the proton is moving, then it will experience a different gradient strength in each half of the sequence and will therefore end up with a net rotation or phase. For a proton moving with a constant velocity this phase shift will be directly proportional to the velocity and can, therefore, be used to quantify the velocity of blood motion.

The most common application of this technique is to make use of the fact that because much of the blood flow in the body's arteries and veins is oriented along the direction of the vessel axis, the flow field can therefore be very well described by measuring only one component of velocity. This can be achieved by astutely orienting the image slice so that it cuts perpendicularly to the vessel and then measuring the velocity through the imaging plane.

An example of this type of measurement is shown in Figure 1. The velocity perpendicular to the imaging plane is shown as a surface plot with the height representing velocity and the other two directions representing position. This type of plot is relatively easy to obtain using modern workstations and is even available on some MRI consoles. Software allows the free rotation of the plot or for an animation to be made from a number of images obtained at different times in the cardiac cycle. In this way a very clear visual image of the blood flow is obtained in either static or dynamic representation.

The plots shown in Figure 1 are from an in vitro study in which an aortic pericardium valve was altered to make it mildly stenotic. The flow field downstream of the valve was then imaged under steady flow conditions.[6] The image clearly shows the funneling of the flow due to the stenosis and the region of flow separation (ie, reversed flow) downstream of the stenosed section of the valve.

Although the ability to visualize blood flow through the production of images like those in Figure 1 is very useful in understanding the nature of the flow field, a far greater use for this type of velocity information lies in its ability to provide a quantitation of volumetric blood flow rate. This can be obtained by integrating the velocity of the blood over the lumen of the imaged vessel. In practice this involves no more than adding together the relevant velocity values and is therefore very quick and easy to perform. Figure 2 shows such an integration performed across the ascending aorta.[7] In this particular case the systolic outflow curve is normal but the negative flow rate present during diastole may indicate aortic regurgitation. If aortic regurgitation were present, then by integrating the area under the flow rate curve during diastole the regurgitant volume could be calculated and used to assess the regurgitant severity. Other researchers have also used this method to study other in vivo flow fields. Klipstein et al.[8] are among those who have obtained good images of flow in the ascending and descending aortas. Mohiaddin et al.[9] investigated disorders of the right side of the heart by studying flow in the superior and inferior vena cava. By comparing flow fields from normal subjects with those from patients with right side defects, such as tricuspid regurgitation, pulmonary hypertension, and right ventricular dysplasia,

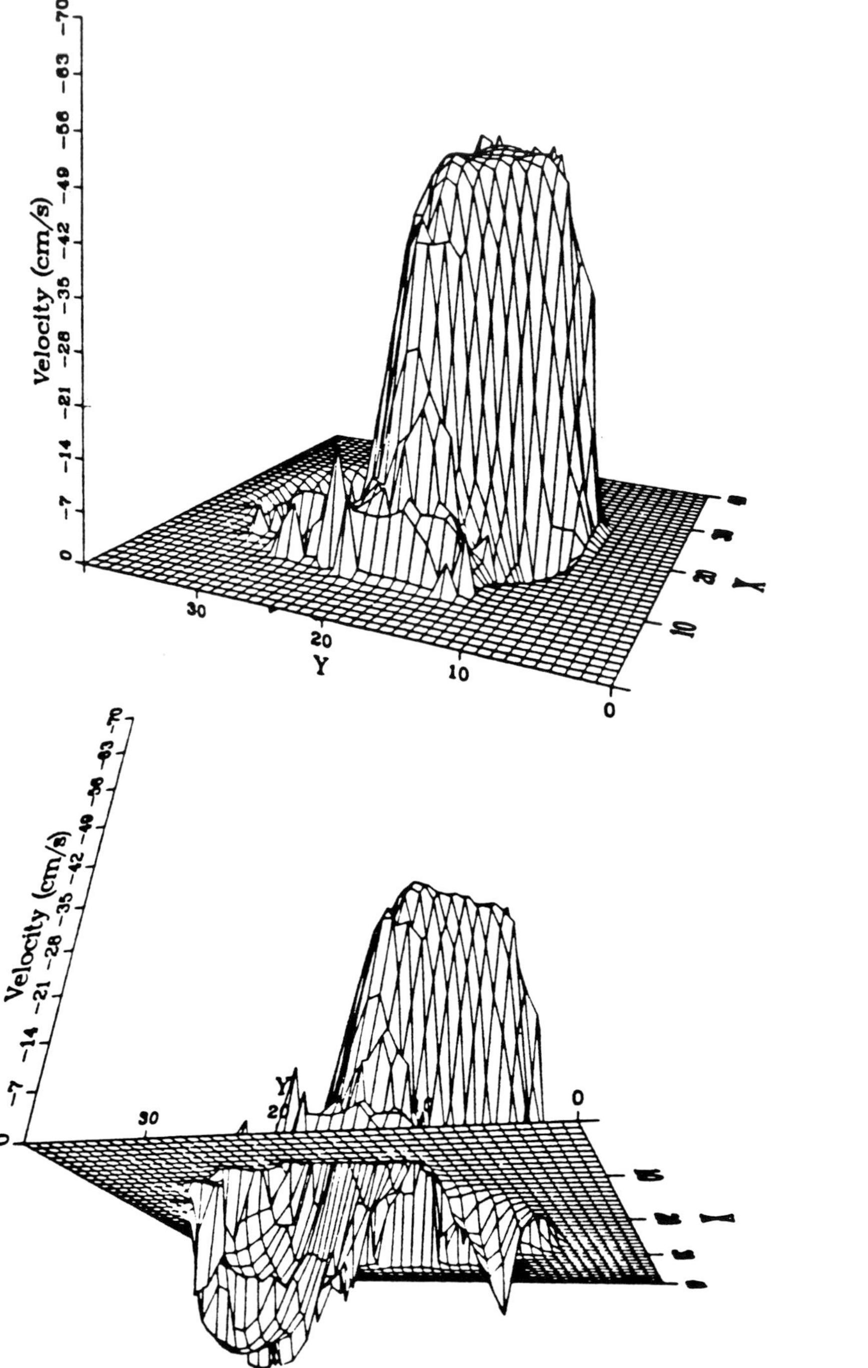

FIGURE 1. *Two views of the steady flow velocity profile through a stenotic pericardial valve measured in vitro by NMR phase velocity encoding.*

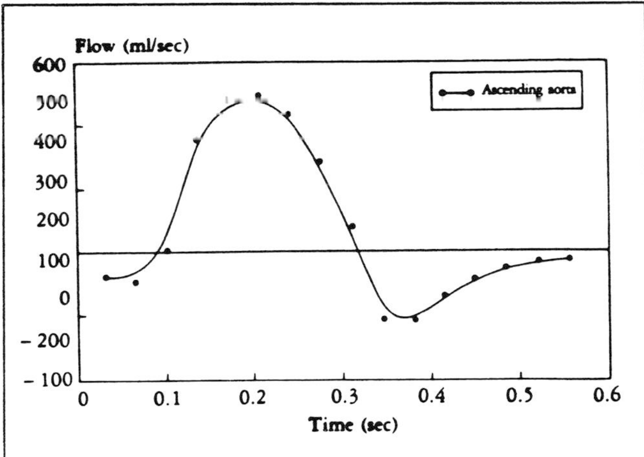

FIGURE 2. *An aortic flow curve from a patient with possible aortic regurgitation. The curve was obtained by integrating the NMR-obtained velocity across the area of the aorta. Reprinted from Reference 3 with permission.*

they were able in some cases to identify flow factors indicative of that defect. Martin et al.[10] determined shunt patency by quantifying cerebrospinal fluid shunt flow rates and Cranney et al.[11] have reviewed some phase velocity applications for assessment of valvular heart disease.

The quality of the velocity data will of course dictate how it can be applied. For this reason a number of investigations have been performed in order to assess the accuracy of phase velocity encoding measurements. Figure 3 shows an in vitro study in which the steady flow rate through a straight tube has been calculated from magnetic resonance measurements and compared with the known values.[6] As can be seen, there is an excellent agreement between the true and calculated flow rates at the lower flow rate end of the graph. The discrepancy at higher flow rates will be discussed shortly. This shows that under ideal laboratory conditions magnetic resonance phase velocity encoding is very accurate. In the clinical setting, however, there are a number of factors that decrease the accuracy of the measurement. These include motion artifacts due to the beating action of the heart and motion of the chest from respiration; effects due to the pulsatile nature of the blood flow that induces errors due to acceleration and jerk; turbulence that causes intravoxel dephasing; and variations in heart rate and beat-to-beat variations in the flow field itself. It is difficult to verify the effects these parameters have on the accuracy of in vivo results because the actual velocities are not known. A number of researchers have, however, compared in vivo magnetic resonance-measured velocities with Doppler ultrasound measurements. For example, Meier et al.[12] measured the flow in the human abdominal aorta and compared the results with Doppler ultrasound measusements and found good quantitative agreement. A different validation approach was used by Firmin et al.,[13] who compared the ventricular stroke volume obtained from planimetry with that derived from velocity maps in the ascending aorta. They found a good correlation and concluded that the magnetic resonance measurements have implications for the detection of atheroma in

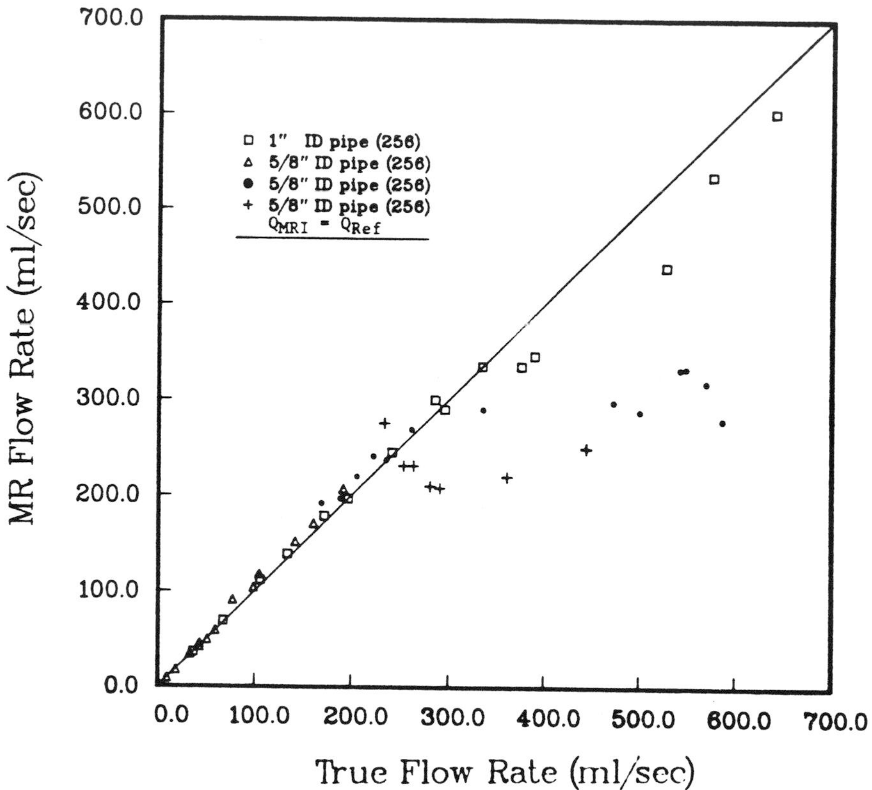

FIGURE 3. *Comparison between the NMR-measured flow rate and the true flow rate for the flow in a straight pipe over a range of different pipe diameters.*

arteries. Unfortunately, these factors hinder the use of magnetic resonance velocity measurements in certain cases, such as in the evaluation of the severity of valvular regurgitation. This is one of the areas in which an accurate flow rate measurement is very desirous and therefore deserves special attention. The high velocities and high degree of turbulence associated with regurgitant jets lead to signal loss and prevent a velocity measurement from being obtained. This is illustrated in Figure 3, where the signal loss at the higher flow rates leads to a large discrepancy in the measured flow rate. The problem is caused by changes in the flow field between the excitation pulse and signal sampling and between pulse excitations. This last effect will also be present in nonturbulent flow if the flow field is nonstationary. These problems should be reduced, if not fully overcome, in the near future with the development of faster, higher-quality gradients and new imaging schemes that eliminate many of the above factors through the use of very short TE and shorter scan times. Shorter TE is beneficial because it does not allow the fluid to fluctuate during the imaging slice time. This results in a narrower spread in velocities and a more coherent signal. Scheidegger et al.[14] have developed an imaging sequence that reduces the TE to between 3 and 4.5 msec. They achieve this by sampling the left and right k-space separately. With this method, motion-induced artifacts in the frequency encoding direction are also minimized.

All of the work discussed so far has been concerned with the flow in the vascular system, in which the velocity is largely one dimensional. For these flows it is often enough to measure one velocity component in order to obtain a good understanding of the flow. This approach is, however, not ideal when considering the flow in the heart because the size and shape of the atria and ventricles and the pulsatile nature of the system create a strongly three-dimensional flow field. In order to fully understand this flow field it is therefore necessary to measure at least two, if not all three, of the velocity components. Our group at the Georgia Institute of Technology, in collaboration with Dr. Pohost's group at the University of Alabama at Birmingham, have performed a number of measurements on the left side of the human heart. Figures 4A through 4E show a left ventricular outflow tract view of the heart of a healthy young male. The velocity has been measured in the plane of the image and is represented in vectorial form overlaid on top of the normal angiographic image.

Figure 4A has been labeled to show the major vessels visible in the image. On the left is the left ventricle, identifiable by its thick wall with the apex at the top right. The bright chamber in the lower center is the left atrium, and directly above this is the outflow tract leading to the aorta. The aortic valve and mitral valves are also labeled. The descending aorta is located at the bottom center of the image. On both images, the time of the image after the beginning of the R wave is shown in milliseconds at the lower left-hand corner. This first image is at the start of systole very shortly after the opening of the aortic valve. The flow in the outflow tract is visible and the ventricle is distended with very little flow inside.

Figure 4B is very close to peak ejection. The flow in the outflow tract is visible with velocities on the order of 1 m/s. The left ventricle is distended with very little flow inside. Flow is also visible in the descending aorta.

Figure 4C is at the very start of diastole. The left atrium is dilated and there is some motion of blood from the atrium toward the left ventricle. There is little motion within the ventricle and a small residual flow in the aorta due to the recent closure of the aortic valve.

Figure 4D shows the flow shortly after the mitral valve has opened. The anterior leaflet of the mitral valve is the dark horizontal line across the center of the image. The flow exiting the left atrium and flowing into the ventricle can be seen. There is very little flow in the region of the aortic valve as this is sheltered by the mitral valve leaflet.

Figure 4E is toward the end of diastole and shows the closure of the mitral valve. This motion of the valve creates a large eddy inside the left ventricle; later images have shown that this eddy remains after the full closure of the mitral valve.

These five images have been used to demonstrate the possibilities of this technique. They show that through the projection of the velocity field onto the modulus magnetic resonance image it is possible to obtain an insight into the function of the heart chambers and valve action. Through animation of a series of such images (Figures 4A through 4E show five images from a set of 20, spaced 40 msec apart throughout the heart cycle), it is possible to obtain a dynamic view of the ventricular function. In particular, the interaction of the blood flow with the valves is very well shown and could therefore be used to study blood flow patterns in the heart under normal and diseased conditions.

Currently we are expanding this work in order to visualize the full three-dimensional nature of blood flow inside the human heart. This is obtained by

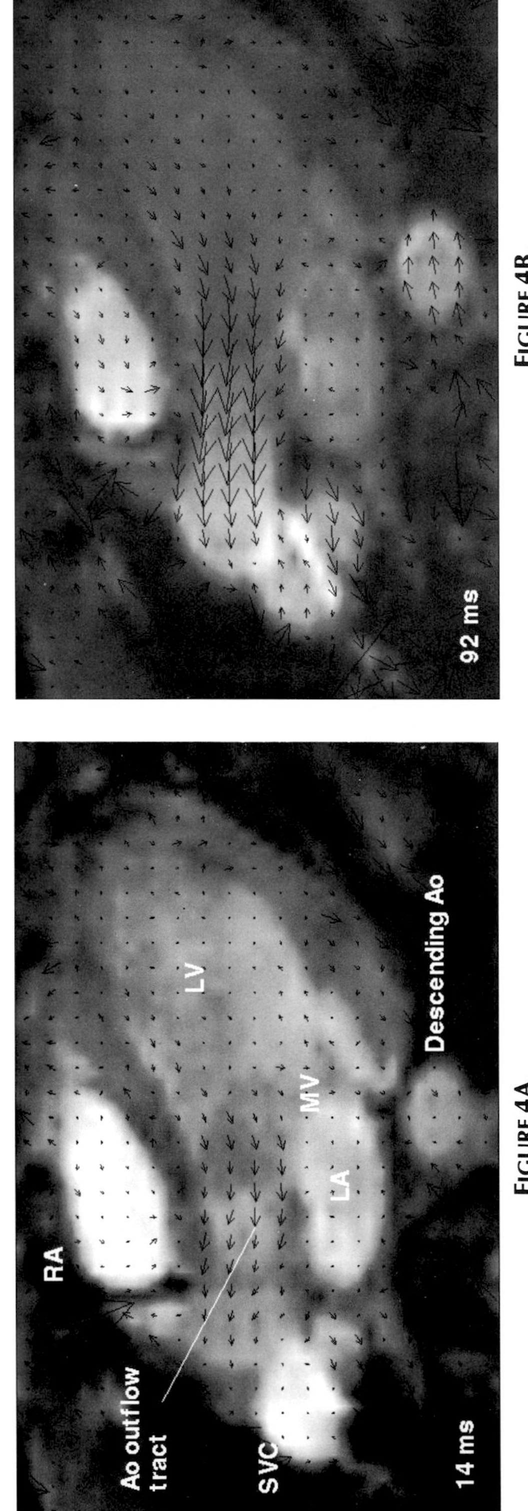

FIGURE 4B.

FIGURE 4A.

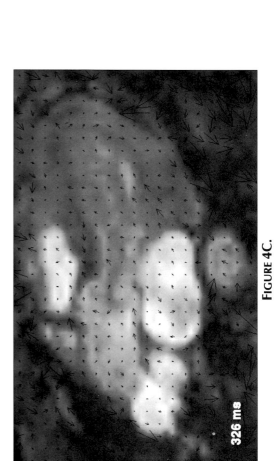

FIGURE 4C.

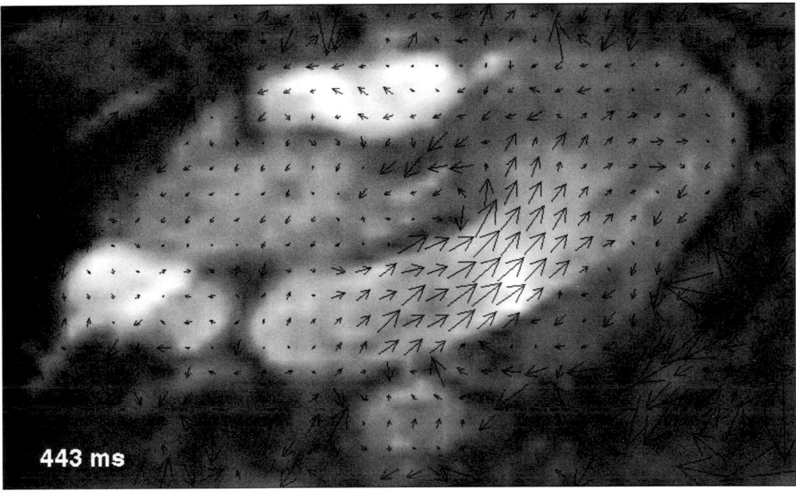

FIGURE 4D.

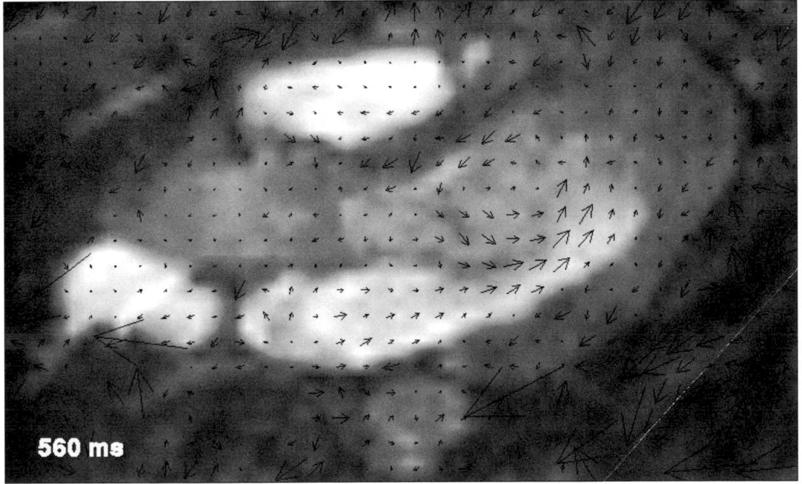

FIGURE 4E.

FIGURE 4. *The NMR-obtained velocities in the heart of a healthy male. Vectors representing the magnitude and direction of the velocities are plotted on top of the normal NMR angiographic image. The plane is a left ventricular outflow tract view with the time of the image after the R wave shown in the bottom left-hand corner.*

measuring all three components of velocity over a number of adjacent image planes. The velocity measurements from the different planes are then combined using a workstation in order to form a final three-dimensional image of the heart through which the passage of blood can be visualized.

Conclusions

Hopefully, this chapter has demonstrated that magnetic resonance phase velocity encoding is an excellent technique for the quantitation of blood flow. It has been shown that useful qualitative and quantitative images of flow through the vascular system can be easily obtained and that the more complicated flow through the heart can also be measured. Although problems are presently created by artifactual effects and signal loss in pathophysiologic cases, it is thought that these can be overcome in the near future by the development of techniques incorporating shorter TE and better pulse sequences.

References

1. Miller SW: Cardiac angiography. In: Pohost GM, O'Rourke RA (eds) *Principles and Practice of Cardiovascular Imaging*. Boston, MA: Little, Brown & Co; 1991:383–421.
2. Nanda NC, ed: *Textbook of Color Doppler Echocardiography*. Philadelphia, PA: Lea & Febiger; 1989.
3. Cranney GB, Doyle M: Magnetic resonance methods for cardiovascular studies. In: Pohost GM, O'Rourke RA (eds) *Principles and Practice of Cardiovascular Imaging*. Boston, MA: Little, Brown & Co; 1991:485–501.
4. Grossman W: *Cardiac Catheterization and Angiography*. 3rd ed. Philadelphia, PA: Lea & Febiger; 1986.
5. Weisel RD, Berger RL, Hechtman HB: Measurement of cardiac output by thermodilution. *N Engl J Med* 1975;292:682.
6. Poiseau E: Magnetic resonance imaging of flow using phase velocity encoding: an in vitro study. Thesis dissertation. Georgia Institute of Technology, 1989.
7. Cranney GB, Lotan CS, Pohost GM: Evaluation of aortic regurgitation by magnetic resonance imaging. *Curr Prob Cardiol* 1990;15:87–114.
8. Klipstein RH, Firmin DN, Underwood SR, et al: Blood flow patterns in the human aorta studied by magnetic resonance. *Br Heart J* 1987;58:316–323.
9. Mohiaddin RH, Wann SL, Underwood R, et al: Vena caval flow: assessment with cine MR velocity mapping. *Radiology* 1990;177:537–541.
10. Martin AJ, Drake JM, Lemaire C, Henkelman RM: Cerebrospinal fluid shunts: flow measurements with MR imaging. *Radiology* 1989;173:243–247.
11. Cranney GB, Lotan CS, Pohost GM: NMR for assessment and follow up of patients with valve disease. *Circulation* 1991;84:216–227.
12. Meier D, Maier S, Boesiger P: Quantitative flow measurements on phantoms and on blood vessels with MR. *Magn Reson Med* 1988;8:25–34.
13. Firmin DN, Nayler GL, Klipstein RH, et al: In vivo validation of MR velocity imaging. *J Comput Assist Tomogr* 1987;11:751–756.
14. Scheidegger MB, Maier SE, Boesiger P: FID-acquired-echos (FAcE). A short echo time imaging method for flow artifact suppression. *Magn Reson Imaging* 1991;9:517–524.

Chapter 11

Myocardial Tissue Characterization

Gerald Wisenberg, MD, Frank S. Prato, PhD, Ting Y. Lee, PhD, and Chun Y. Tong, MSc

Since its introduction as a major noninvasive modality in the early 1980s, MRI has often been described as the technique capable of unique tissue characterization. As applied to the heart, this ability may be defined as the identification of abnormalities in the composition or physical state of myocardium. This characterization is achieved through measurable changes in signal intensity on magnetic resonance images, or more accurately by alterations in myocardial relaxivity (the reciprocal of the nuclear magnetic resonance [NMR] relaxation parameters, T_1 and T_2). These changes are dependent on one or more of the following: 1) regional or global changes in proton density (water content), such as may occur in myocardial infarction or heart transplant rejection, respectively; 2) regional or global flow-dependent changes in relaxivity following injection of paramagnetic tracers; 3) regional or global changes in vascular permeability to injected paramagnetic tracers, at equilibrium, as may occur following myocardial infarction and reperfusion leading to changes in relaxivity; or 4) altered tissue concentration of relaxivity changing substances in disease, eg, iron deposition disorders.

Characterization of Myocardial Tissue

The characterization of myocardial tissue can be performed either qualitatively or quantitatively. Most readily, images can be examined subjectively or measured objectively for regional or global abnormalities in myocardial signal intensity. On spin-echo images, signal intensity is influenced not only by T_1 and T_2, but also by pulse TR. This is particularly important with regard to so-called T_1 effects on images. Put simply, everything else being equal, an increase in T_1 will tend to produce a decrease in myocardial signal, prolongation of T_2 leads to an increase in myocardial signal. Shortening TR will tend to increase T_1 weighting in images, ie, make more obvious

---

Supported in part by grant B1777 of the Heart and Stroke Foundation of Ontario and grant MA 9467 of the Medical Research Council of Canada.
From Pohost GM (ed.), *Cardiovascular Applications of Magnetic Resonance.* Mount Kisco, NY, Futura Publishing Co., Inc., © 1993.

the lower signal in regions of increased T_1, whereas lengthening TR will tend to increase the T_2 weighting of images, making regions of increased T_2 stand out (Figure 1).

Most changes in myocardial tissue composition will produce similar directional changes in T_1 and T_2, although not necessarily to the same degree. At rapid heart rates (>100 beats per minute) that determine TR on MRI, depending on the specific changes in T_1 and T_2, the T_1 and T_2 effects on images may largely cancel each other out, and no change in regional or global signal intensity will be detected. Therefore, dependence on signal intensity changes alone, as they are greatly influenced by heart rate, is not ideal for tissue characterization. Another more objective method is to compare myocardial signal to skeletal muscle signal, but this is still imprecise, subject to the vagaries of heart rate influence. Most appropriately, T_1 and T_2 should be measured from in vivo images, although myocardial motion and blood flow effects will interfere with precise quantitation. However, it is clear that measurement of these parameters offers the best method to enhance the sensitivity and specificity of MRI for detection of pathology.

T_1 values can be measured by determining signal intensity values from two separate spin-echo images with constant TE but with different TR values, eg, one and two RR intervals, and solving for T_1 in the following equation:

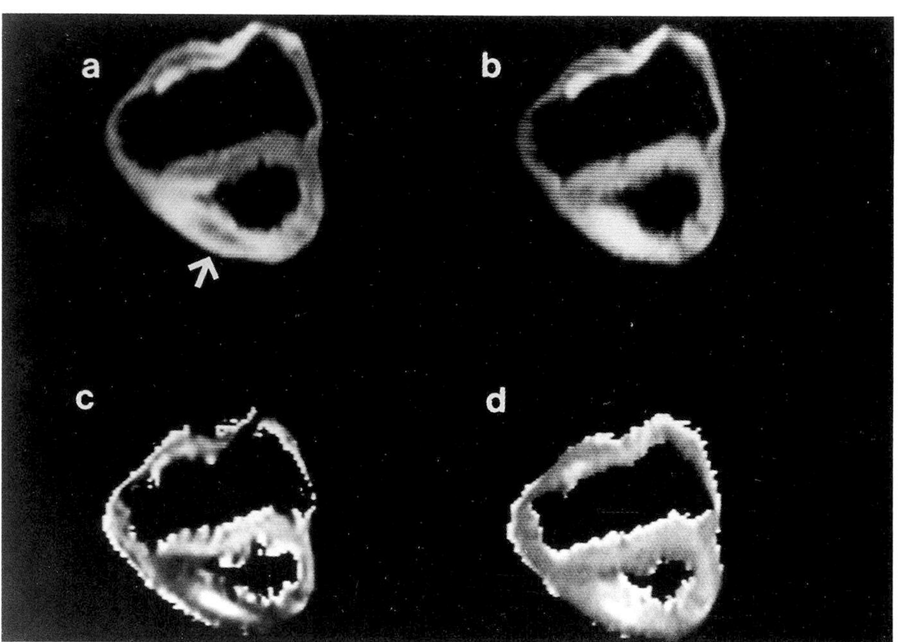

FIGURE 1. *Comparison of T_1- and T_2-weighted images acquired in a canine that had suffered an acute anterior myocardial infarction 1 week earlier. These images were obtained following gadolinium-DTPA administration in excised hearts imaged after sacrifice.* **a:** *TR/TE 150/35 msec (T_1 weighted);* **b:** *TR/TE 645/80 msec (T_2 weighted);* **c:** *T_1 map;* **d:** *T_2 map. On the T_1-weighted image, there is a central zone in the infarct of relatively increased T_1 that demonstrates reduced signal. On the T_2-weighted image, the entire zone of infarction demonstrates increased signal.*

$$S = \frac{C \exp(-TE/T_2 \sin(\alpha)\{1 - \exp[-(TR - TE)/T_1]\}}{1 + \cos(\alpha)\exp(-TR/T_1)}$$

where α = the tip angle obtained experimentally, and
where C = a constant determined experimentally for each instrument by imaging solutions of known T_1 and T_2 values.
where S = signal intensity

Similarly, T_2 can be determined from signal intensity values obtained from two spin-echo images with different TE, but constant TR values, either from a multi-echo sequence or separate spin-echo images.[1]

Regarding T_1, considerable inaccuracies (~30%) may occur when both TR values exceed the T_1 of tissue under examination.[2] With conventional spin-echo imaging, extra pulse trains may need to be interposed between successive R wave triggers without signal data being incorporated into images to effectively lower the TR of these images for more accurate T_1 measurement. Short T_1 values may occur in myocardium following paramagnetic tracer administration.

The methods noted above can be tedious and time consuming (~30 minutes), be affected by the slice selectively of radiofrequency application in multi-slice techniques, and be very hardware dependent.

Recently, so-called "turbo FLASH" sequences have been proposed for rapid image acquisition and T_1 measurement. Effectively limited to high-field systems, a proposed inversion recovery sequence by Larsson et al.[3] uses TE values of 2–3 msec, TR values of 5 msec, small flip angles (6°), and T_I of 200 msec. Such a technique has been used to measure myocardial and aortic blood T_1 values sequentially following a bolus injection of the paramagnetic tracer gadolinium-DTPA for absolute measurement of regional myocardial blood flow.[3] Our laboratory is currently developing a similar sequence for obtaining regional T_1 maps similar to Figure 1 toward the similar goal of flow quantitation.

Regional or Global Changes in Proton Density

Myocardial Ischemia

During brief periods of reversible ischemia, no significant changes in regional water content occur, and in the absence of paramagnetic flow tracers are not detectable by standard proton imaging. However, with a sufficiently long period of ischemia, endothelial and cellular membrane injury leading to enhanced permeability occurs. Higgins et al.[4] were among the first investigators to demonstrate an increase in regional T_1 and T_2 values in infarcted myocardium, measured by in vitro imaging performed 24 hours after coronary occlusion. Total water content increased from a mean of 76% in noninfarcted normal myocardium to 78.6% in infarcted myocardium. Subsequently, in vivo imaging was able to demonstrate changes in regional signal intensity within 4 hours after coronary occlusion (Figure 2).[5] Additionally, in our laboratory we have documented the changes that occur in myocardial T_1 and T_2 values over the weeks following myocardial infarction, with and without myocardial reperfusion (Table 1).[6] In essence, in nonreperfused infarcts, regional T_1 and T_2

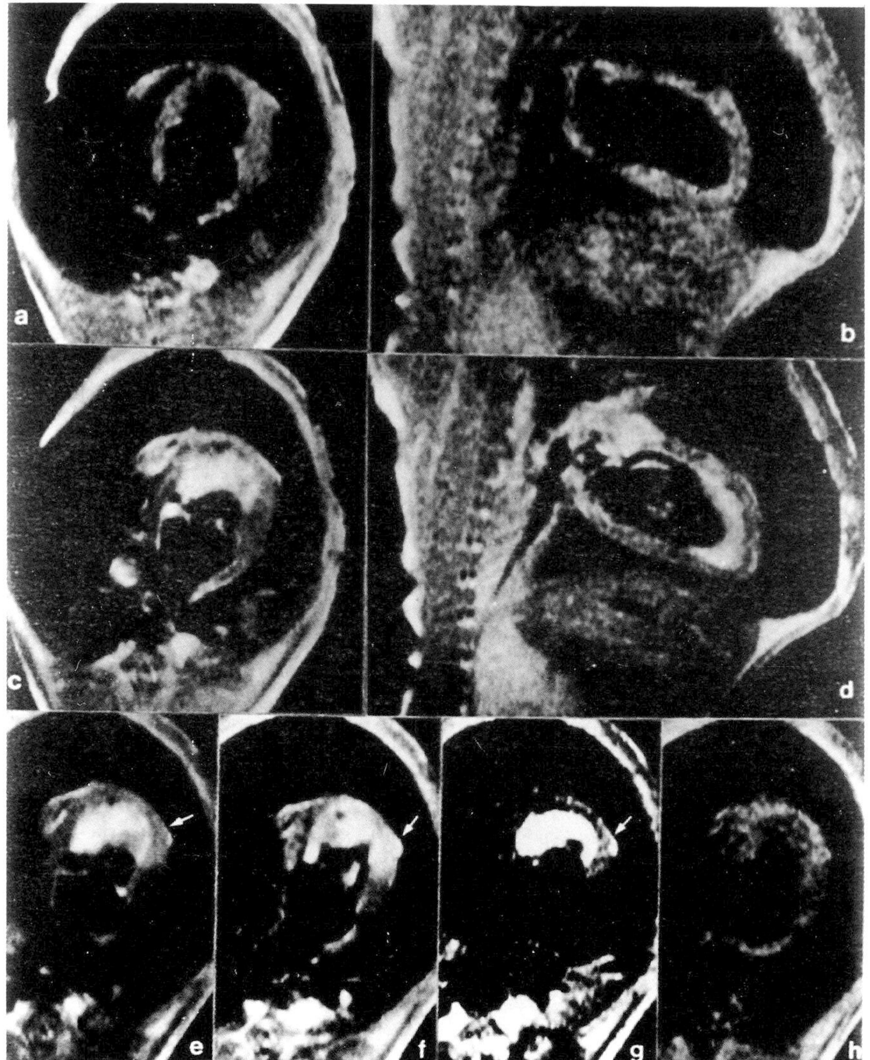

FIGURE 2. *Transverse* **(a)** *and sagittal* **(b)** *TE 30-msec images obtained in vivo before occlusion of the anterior descending artery.* **(c)** *and* **(d):** *TE 30-msec images in the same planes showing apical dilitation, thinning, and intracavitary signal suggestive of static blood postocclusion. TE 30-msec images* **(e)** *and* **(f)** *show progressive signal enhancement in the infarct zone, 30 and 150 minutes after coronary occlusion.* **(g):** *TE 60-msec image at 1 hour.* **(h):** *The inversion recovery image 4 hours after occlusion.*

TABLE 1. T_1 and T_2 values (msec)

	Reperfusion (n = 7)				Nonreperfusion (n = 7)			
	T_1		T_2		T_1		T_2	
	Infarct	Control	Infarct	Control	Infarct	Control	Infarct	Control
Occlusion								
1–2 hours	*445 ± 32	350 ± 11	*52 ± 5	40 ± 2	*448 ± 51	351 ± 11	*51 ± 8	41 ± 2
2–3 hours	†555 ± 65‡	348 ± 12	†65 ± 8	39 ± 2	*460 ± 49	349 ± 12	*54 ± 10‡	40 ± 2
Day 5	*512 ± 55	349 ± 11	39 ± 8§	39 ± 2	†490 ± 64	350 ± 11	†63 ± 9§	39 ± 2
Day 21	*450 ± 47	351 ± 11	35 ± 7§	41 ± 2	*427 ± 43	349 ± 1	*55 ± 11§	40 ± 2

*$p < 0.05$, †$p < 0.01$ } versus control.
‡$p < 0.01$, §$p < 0.0025$ } reperfusion versus nonreperfusion.

TABLE 2. Extent of Signal Abnormality (% of Left Ventricle)

	Reperfusion ($n = 7$)	Nonreperfusion ($n = 7$)
Occlusion		
1–2 hours	*14 ± 8†	20 ± 11†
2–3 hours	‡22 ± 11	22 ± 11
Day 5	13 ± 6†	*25 ± 12†
Day 21	11 ± 5†	18 ± 11†
Pathology	10 ± 6†	18 ± 9†

†$p < 0.05$ reperfusion versus nonreperfusion.
‡$p < 0.01$, *$p < 0.05$ versus pathology.

values, measured on a 0.15-T system, increased progressively over the first few hours, peaked at 1 week following infarction, and returned toward normal values at 3 weeks when myocardial edema had largely resolved. With reperfusion, the breakdown in endothelial integrity that had already occurred by 2 hours led to an abrupt increase in tissue water and regional T_1 and T_2 changes, which peaked immediately after restoration of flow and gradually fell over the next 3 weeks. The extent of regional T_1 and T_2 abnormalities observed with MRI was compared with myocardial infarct size measured by pathology. Because early images (day of infarction and 1-week thereafter) overestimated the extent of infarction, it is presumed that increases in tissue water (edema) extend beyond the infarct zone initially and resolve by 3 weeks when a better approximation of infarct size was achieved (Table 2).

Clinically, several investigators have published studies attesting to the ability of MRI to detect recent myocardial infarction with regional increases in signal intensity and/or T_1 and T_2 in infarcts 2 to 30 days old.[7,8] However, chronic infarction more than 3 to 4 months old, in which tissue edema has completely resolved and is replaced by fibrous scar, produces a decrease in signal intensity and measured T_2 values.[9]

We have used MRI to assess the effect of thrombolytic therapy to reduce infarct size in a clinical study of 66 patients.[10] Using an increase in measured T_1 and/or T_2 values >2 SD above normal, we were able to demonstrate a significant reduction in infarct size to 3% of left ventricular mass in the streptokinase group versus 10% for the placebo group.

In the future, MRI may play an important role in monitoring the clinical effectiveness of interventions to reduce infarct size.

Transplant Rejection

Transplant rejection serves as a model of global changes that may occur in proton density and water content. Transplant rejection is essentially an inflammatory response to foreign tissue and is associated with considerable tissue edema, as well as lymphocytic infiltration and myocytolysis. We sequentially studied 25 patients who underwent cardiac transplant rejection up to 107 days after surgery (Figure 3).[11] In essentially all cases in which imaging was performed within 25 days of transplantation, T_1 and T_2 were markedly increased, even in the absence of rejection, because of edema secondary to the trauma of graft harvesting, transportation, and implantation. However, when rejection was not present, as assessed by endomyocardial biopsy, late MRI (>25 days after surgery) found that T_1 and T_2 values had normalized. In the presence of rejection, T_1 and T_2 abnormalities correctly predicted 14 of 15 abnormal biopsies. In the future, MRI may largely supplant the need for biopsies, which are prone to sampling errors because of the limited amount of tissue obtained. Furthermore, conditions such as myocarditis, also with widespread inflammation, may also be accurately identified by MRI.

Regional or Global Flow-Dependent Changes in Relaxivity Following Injection of Paramagnetic Tracers

Quantitation of coronary blood flow has long been a goal of those exploring the potential of a variety of noninvasive imaging modalities. Thus far, positron emission tomography may have come the closest to achieving this goal.

In regard to MRI, in the absence of infarction leading to changes in regional water content, changes in coronary blood flow alone produce no changes in myocardial tissue signal intensity or relaxivity. However, there may be changes in regional wall motion that develop in response to acute ischemia (decrease in wall thickening, enhanced signal from intracavitary blood due to relative stasis adjacent to hypokinetic/ akinetic myocardium). Fortunately, it may be possible to use tracers to allow flow quantitation through MRI. These tracers, paramagnetic agents that significantly reduce T_1 and T_2 and therefore enhance relaxivity in a tissue concentration–dependent manner, may be used to qualitatively and quantitatively assess coronary blood flow. McNamara et al.[12] and Runge et al.[13] have previously published the results of animal imaging experiments performed respectively in vitro and in vivo that demonstrated the ability to qualitatively assess acute myocardial ischemia within 60 minutes of coronary occlusion before tissue edema had developed, following the intravenous administration of gadolinium-DTPA, a paramagnetic agent. This agent is rapidly cleared from the intravascular space into tissue in a flow-dependent fashion. However, following first-pass clearance, particularly with a constant infusion, its tissue concentration is more a reflection of the extracellular volume. Thus, strategies to use gadolinium-DTPA as a quantitative flow tracer will require rapid measurement of tissue relaxivity (within 1 to 2 minutes) following its initial infusion.

As mentioned earlier, Larsson et al.[3] have recently published data on normal human volunteers using a "turbo FLASH" sequence, which literally takes only seconds to acquire, to measure regional blood flow. A modification of the Kety equation was used, which relates tissue concentrations of a given substance to 1) arterial concentrations of the substance; 2) its extraction fraction; 3) its tissue volume of distribution; and 4) flow. By assuming extraction efficiency to be 1) in these normal individuals (not necessarily a valid assumption nor necessarily one that applies under different tissue states, ie, acute ischemia, infarction, reperfusion), regional blood flows of 55 to 72 mL/min per 100 g tissue were obtained that would closely approximate the expected normal myocardial flows in humans.

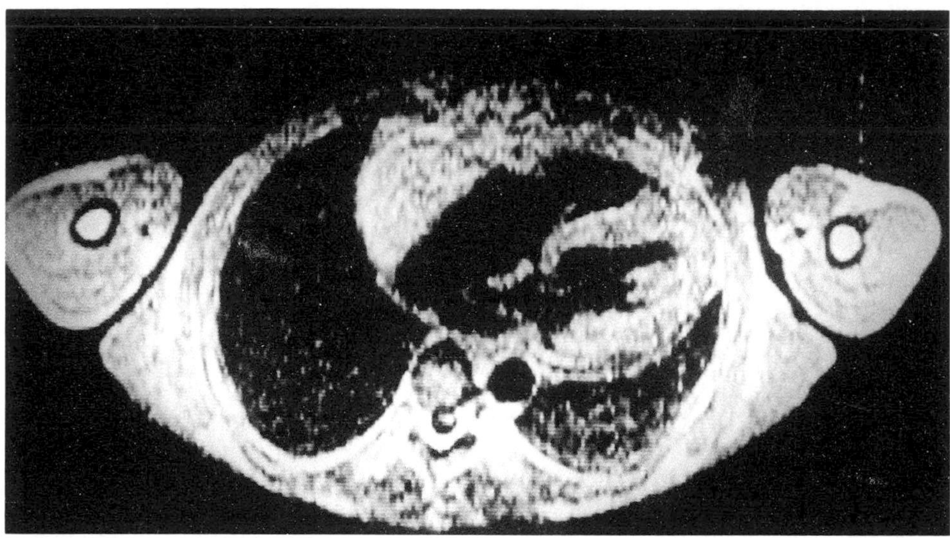

A

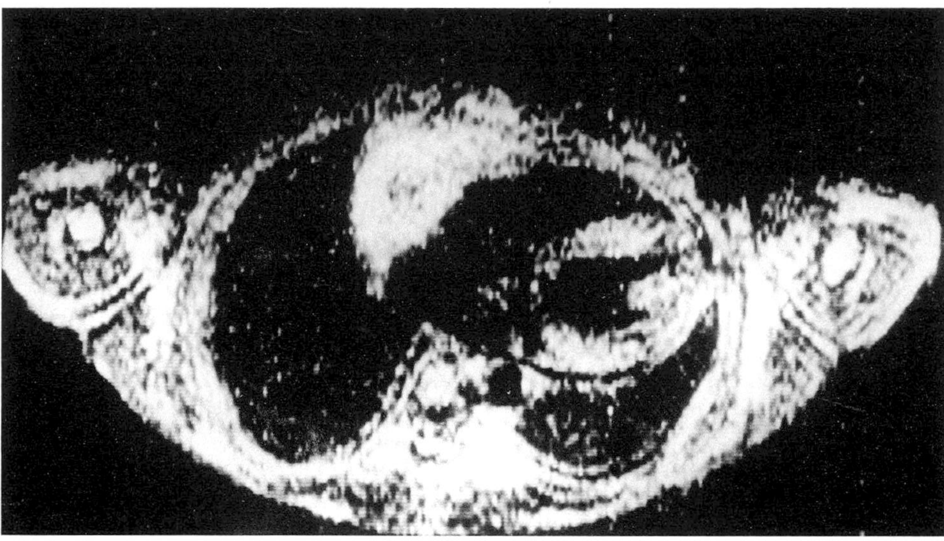

B

FIGURE 3. A: *30-msec; TR = 600-msec image.* **B:** *TE = 60-msec; TR = 600-msec image taken 57 days after cardiac transplantation. The increase in myocardial signal and wall thickness both suggest rejection, which was confirmed on biopsy. A pericardial effusion is also present. After adjustment of the immunosuppressive regimen in an attempt to treat rejection, a repeat set of images were obtained 107 days after transplantation.*

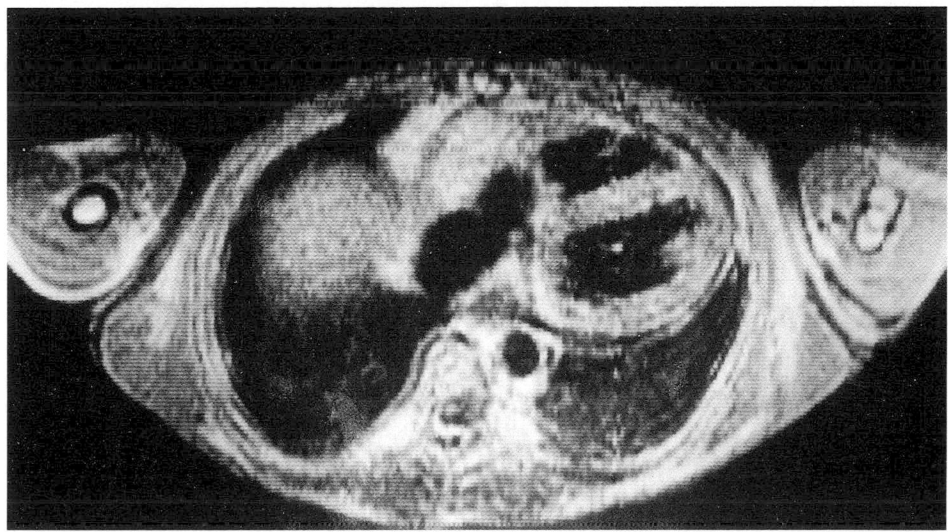

C

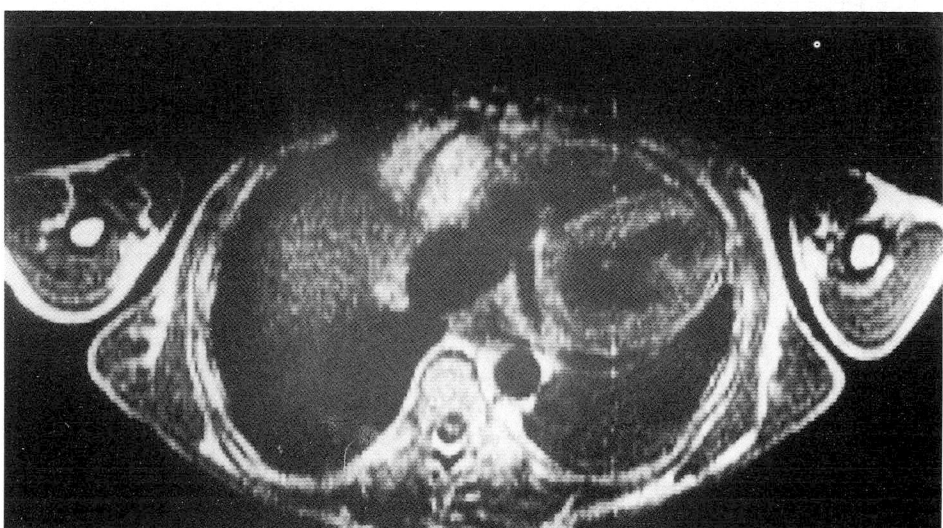

D

FIGURE 3. *Continued.* **C:** *TE = 30 msec; TR = 770 msec.* **D:** *TE = 60 msec; TR = 770 msec. There is a significant decrease in myocardial signal on the TE = 60-msec image, implying normalization of the T_2 value. Rejection was not identified on biopsy.*

In our laboratory, we have adopted a similar approach for measurement of blood flow using the following modified Kety equation:[14]

$$[Gd\text{-}DTPA]_i(t) = F_i \cdot E_i \int_0^t [Gd\text{-}DTPA]_a(y) \exp\left(-\frac{F_i \cdot E_i}{\lambda_i}(t-y)\right) dy$$

where $[Gd\text{-}DTPA]_i(t)$ is the concentration of *Gd-DTPA* at any time t in any region i of the myocardium, $[Gd\text{-}DTPA]_a$ is the arterial concentration of gadolinium-DTPA at any time y, E_i is the extraction efficiency in myocardial region i, λ_i is the partition coefficient or extracellular volume in milliliters per gram in myocardial region i, and F_i is the flow in milliliters per minute per gram in the myocardial region.

In a series of animal experiments, we have determined that:[15]

1. In normal myocardium, the F·E product was constant at about 0.5 to 0.6 for flows from 0.4 to 4.5 ml/min per gram. For determination of an absolute value of F_i, for flows above 0.4, an additional kinetic technique to noninvasively measure E will have to be developed, by deconvoluting the impulse retention function, and we are presently working on strategies to accomplish this.
2. In ischemic and infarcted myocardium, where $F_i < 0.4$ mL/min per 100 g, E is essentially 1. Therefore, solving the modified Kety equation does give F_i since $F_i \approx F_i \cdot E_i$.

Using a modified "turbo FLASH" sequence, it should be possible to measure both tissue and arterial blood relaxivity, dependent on gadolinium-DTPA concentration in the early minutes following infusion and thus, flow. At present, using a flash cine sequence, we are able to obtain images following a bolus of gadolinium-DTPA that allow differentiation between subendocardial and subepicardial regions, with markedly reduced flow in the former (Figure 4)[10] following occlusion with correspondingly reduced signal. Simultaneously, the flash cine images also provide data regarding regional function.

Regional or Global Changes in Vascular Permeability

Important in the evaluation of coronary disease, acute ischemia, and myocardial infarction, tissue characterization would be aided significantly by knowledge of the extracellular water content in addition to flow. As outlined in Table 3, four different tissue states may exist, and could be characterized by their flow and extracellular volume states. Normally perfused, noninfarcted myocardium would have both normal flow and normal volume. Acutely ischemic myocardium would have reduced flow but normal extracellular volume. Nonreperfused, recently infarcted tissue would have reduced flow and an increase in extracellular water content as well. Finally, reperfused myocardium would have normal flow and increased extracellular water. In the latter two cases, the increase in extracellular water content is due in large part to altered capillary permeability to a variety of solutes that carry with them extravascular water. Further, a breakdown of cellular integrity in infarcted tissue will also allow leaching of solutes and water out of cells.

Once cleared from the intravascular compartment, Gd-DTPA is largely

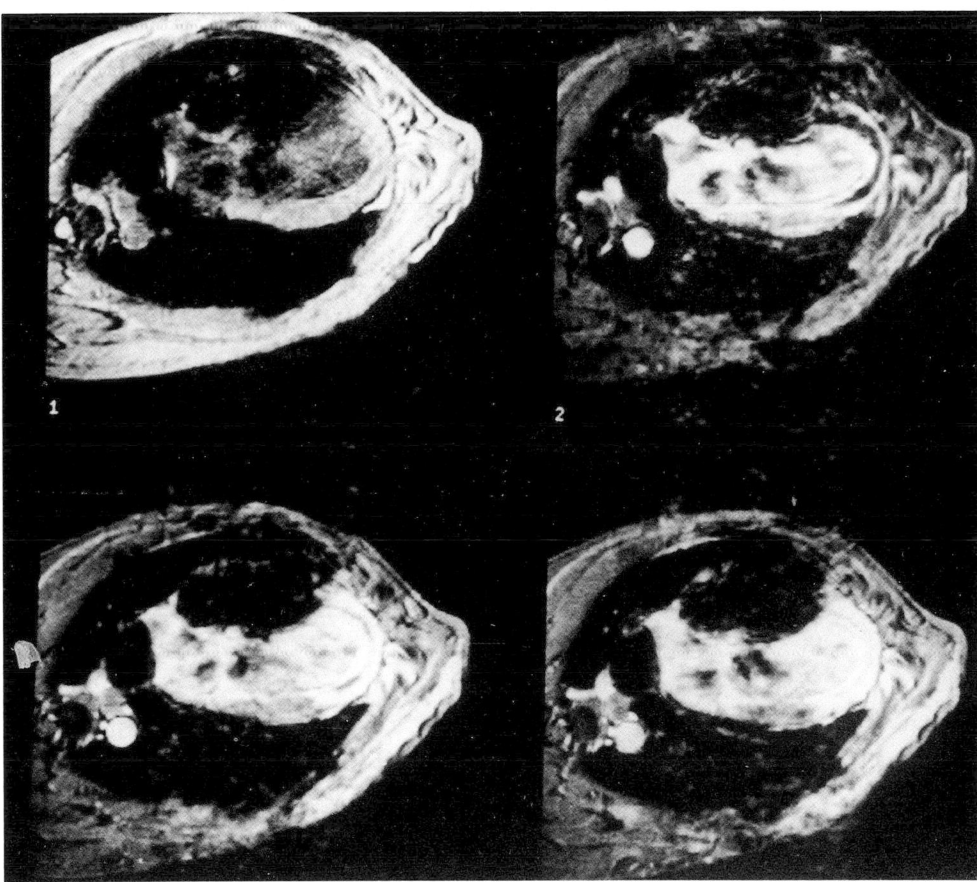

FIGURE 4. *Images of a canine heart 7 days after anterior descending coronary artery occlusion. All images represent the third frame of a 15-frame FLASH cine with TR = 37 msec; TE = 10 msec; tip angle = 40°; 256 × 256, two acquisitions per k-space line and 10-mm slice thickness. (Each image was taken 74 msec after the R wave). The artifact in the right side of the heart (to the top) corresponds to magnetic field distortion due to the presence of a temporary transvenous pacemaker.* Upper left: *Baseline image prior to gadolinium-DTPA injection.* Upper right: *2 minutes after start of constant infusion of gadolinium-DTPA (note the reduced signal in the subendocardial regions of the infarction zone).* Lower left: 37 minutes after start of constant infusion. Lower right: *80 minutes after start of infusion. By 80 minutes, the signal value in the subendocardial region had nearly reached that of the subepicardial zone.*

TABLE 3. Myocardial Tissue States

Tissue state	Flow	Extracellular water content
Normal	Normal	Normal
Acute ischemia	Reduced	Normal
Infarction	Reduced	Increased
Reperfused infarct	Normal	Increased

limited in its volume of distribution to the extracellular space. Wesbey et al.[17] demonstrated that at 90 seconds following a bolus of gadolinium-DTPA there was a marked reduction in T_1 and T_2 in normally perfused myocardium, whereas 24-hour-old infarcted myocardium changed minimally. However, at 5 minutes following bolus injection the pattern was reversed, with lower values in the infarct regions, presumably because of greater washout from normally perfused tissue, and progressive sequestration into infarcted tissue (Table 4) that in effect acts as a reservoir.

With a bolus followed by a constant infusion of gadolinium-DTPA, equilibrium can be achieved in terms of blood concentrations, as an infusion at a rate of 0.01 to 0.02

TABLE 4. Magnetic Resonance Contrast and Spectrometer Relaxation Times 90 Seconds After DTPA

	T_1 (msec)		T_2 (msec)		
Dog #	Normal myocardium	Infarct	Normal myocardium	Infarct	MR contrast (SE 500/56)
4	149.9	226.1	34.1	41.9	45%
5	139.0	330.0	33.5	53.3	36%
6	112.1	165.7	35.1	41.7	58%
Mean	133.6	241	34.2	45.6	46%
SD	19.4	83	0.8	6.6	11%

5 Minutes After Gd-DTPA

	T_1 (msec)		T_2 (msec)		
Dog #	Normal myocardium	Infarct	Normal myocardium	Infarct	MR contrast (SE 500/56)
7	212.7	135.5	39.6	38.7	23
8	222.3	139.4	38.1	41.2	33
9	181.6	153.6	37.1	40.2	23
10	220.2	139.4	38.4	40.8	40
11	216.4	167.4	40.5	42.5	31
Mean	210.6	147.1	38.7	40.7	30
SD	16.6	13.3	1.33	1.40	7.3

mM/kg approximates renal clearance of this agent in canines. With such an infusion, we have observed progressive changes in tissue signal in infarction. As shown in Figures 4 and 5, the initial image obtained minutes following gadolinium-DTPA infusion in essence reflects the flow-dependent tissue distribution of this compound. However, over the course of time during a continuous infusion, signal progressively increases in the subendocardial region as it eventually comes into equilibrium with the intravascular concentration.

We hope to use the modified Kety equation and knowledge of regional flow measured quantitatively following the first pass of gadolinium-DTPA to quantita-

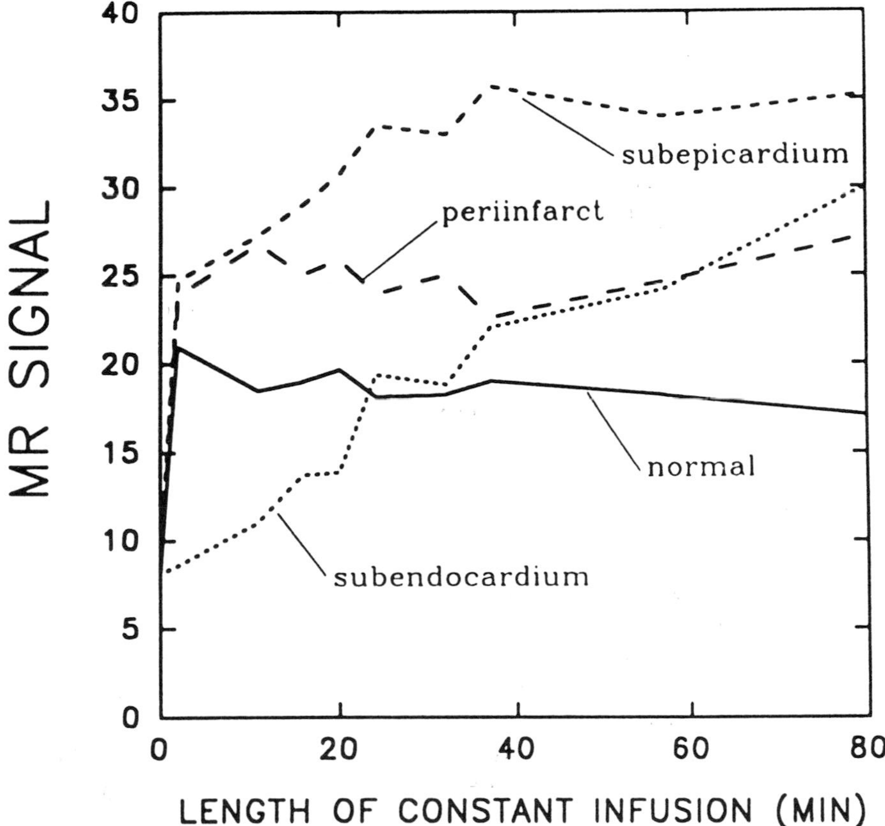

FIGURE 5. *Signal intensity changes over time obtained from images depicted in Figure 4. Normal myocardium maintains a stable signal value during the course of the infusion as does the peri-infarct region, but the latter at a slightly higher level. The subepicardial region slowly increases over the first 40 minutes and then stabilizes, implying equilibrium has been obtained between intravascular gadolinium-DTPA and that in the increased extracellular space in this infarcted region. In the subendocardial region, where flows were found to be markedly reduced, signal progressively increases over time, and appears not to have equilibrated by the completion of the 80-minute constant infusion.*

tively measure regional extracellular volume (partition coefficient) and thus differentiate the previously identified four tissue states.

In a clinical study, Eichstaedt et al.[18] demonstrated a differential response to a bolus of gadolinium-DTPA depending on the length of time following infarction. Whereas relative signal enhancement of infarcted tissue occurred on delayed imaging in patients within 7 days of the event, no significant enhancement occurred in patients with infarcts more than 3 weeks old in which edema had largely resolved, to be replaced by nonsequestering fibrous scar.

Altered Tissue Concentrations of Iron Increase Relaxivity

Iron deposition disorders such as those associated with hemochromatosis or repeated transfusions in patients with thalassemia will lead to increased myocardial tissue iron stores. Tissue relaxivity will increase proportional to tissue iron stores. These changes have recently been reported by Liu and associates.[19] In an iron overload murine model, a significant reduction in T_2 in hearts with excessive iron (19.4 ± 3.9 versus 54.2 ± 6.0 msec in control hearts) was demonstrated. Furthermore, $1/T_2$ correlated linearly with tissue iron stores as measured by flame atomic spectrometry. Liu et al.[20] have also used NMR to quantitate the degree of tissue iron in patients with renal failure and thalassemia and are currently using the technique to assess patients with hemochromatosis.

Further assessment of other infiltrative disorders, eg, amyloid, may allow NMR to more accurately identify the presence and severity of these disorders.

Summary

Since its inception, MRI has offered unique data regarding tissue composition. In the forthcoming years, we are likely to see greater clinical application of this technique for a variety of conditions, particularly myocardial infarction, in which differentiation between sustained coronary occlusion and reperfusion often remains difficult clinically. The monitoring of cardiac transplant rejection with MRI will likely be performed with greater frequency. Use of paramagnetic agents may allow the determination of both regional blood flow and tissue extracellular volume. Finally, infiltrative disorders such as hemochromatosis may be well characterized noninvasively by MRI.

References

1. Prato FS, Drost DJ, Keys T, et al: Optimization of signal-to-noise ratio in calculated T_2 images derived from two spin echo images. *Magn Reson Med* 1986;3:63–75.
2. Prato FS, Drost DJ, King M, et al: Cardiac MR spin-echo imaging employing a modified cardiac trigger to improve T_1 accuracy and precision. *Magn Reson Med* 1987;4:227–243.
3. Larsson HGW, Stubgaard M, Søndergaard L, et al: In vivo quantitation of myocardial perfusion using MRI and Gd-DTPA. *Proc Soc Magn Reson Med* 1991;10:1145.
4. Higgins CG, Herfkens R, Lipton MJ, et al: Nuclear magnetic resonance imaging of acute

myocardial infarction in dogs: alterations in magnetic relaxation times. *Am J Cardiol* 1983;52:184.

5. Pflugfelder PW, Wisenberg G, Prato FS, et al: Early detection of canine myocardial infarction by magnetic resonance in vivo. *Circulation* 1985;71:587
6. Wisenberg G, Prato FS, Carroll SE, et al: Serial nuclear magnetic resonance imaging of acute myocardial infarction with and without reperfusion. *Am Heart J* 1988;115:510.
7. McNamara MT, Higgins CB, Schechtmann N, et al: Detection and characterization of acute myocardial infarction in man with use of gated magnetic resonance. *Circulation* 1985;71:717.
8. Johnston DL, Thompson RC, Liu P, et al: Magnetic resonance imaging during acute myocardial infarction. *Am J Cardiol* 1986;57:1059.
9. McNamara MT, Higgins CB: Magnetic resonance imaging of chronic myocardial infarcts in man. *AJR* 1986;146:315.
10. Wisenberg G, Finnie KJ, Jablonsky G, et al: Nuclear magnetic resonance and radionuclide angiographic assessment of acute myocardial infarction in a randomized trial of intravenous streptokinase. *Am J Cardiol* 1988;62:1011.
11. Wisenberg G, Pflugfelder PW, Kostuk WJ, et al: Diagnostic applicability of magnetic resonance imaging in assessing human cardiac allograft rejection. *Am J Cardiol* 1987;60:130-136.
12. McNamara MT, Higgins CB, Ehman RL, et al: Acute myocardial ischemia magnetic resonance contrast enhancement with gadolinium-DTPA. *Radiology* 1984;153:157.
13. Runge VM, Clanton JA, Wehr CJ, et al: Gated magnetic resonance imaging of acute myocardial ischemia in dogs. Applications of multi-echo techniques and contrast enhancement with Gd-DTPA. *Magn Reson Imaging* 1985;3:255.
14. Diesbourg LD, Prato FS, Wisenberg G, et al: Quantitation of myocardial blood flow and extracellular volumes using a bolus injection of Gd-DTPA: kinetic modelling in canine ischemic disease. *Magn Reson Med* 1992;23:239–253.
15. Tong CY, Prato FS, Wisenberg G, et al: Towards the absolute measurement of myocardial perfusion and myocardial extracellular volumes using MRI and a bolus injection of Gd-DTPA: measurement of extraction efficiency for Gd-DTPA. *Proc Soc Magn Reson Med* 1991;10:245.
16. Robb RA, Hanson DP, Karwoski RA, et al: ANALYZE: a comprehensive, operator-interactive software package for multidimensional medical image display and analysis. *Comput Med Imaging Graphics* 1989;13(6):433–454.
17. Wesbey G, Higgins CB, McNamara MT, et al: Effect of Gadolinium-DTPA on the magnetic relaxation times of normal and infarcted myocardium. *Radiology* 1984;153:165.
18. Eichstaedt HW, Felix R, Dougherty FC, et al: Magnetic resonance imaging (MRI) in different stages of myocardial infarction using contrast agent gadolinium-DTPA. *Clin Cardiol* 1986;9:527.
19. Liu P, Hinkelman M, Joshe J, et al: Quantitation of tissue iron using NMR relaxation: validation in a thalassemia-iron overload murine model. *Proc Soc Magn Reson Med* 1991;10:692.
20. Liu P, Uldall P, Olivieri N, et al: Comparison of iron contents in patients with renal failure and thalassemia. *Proc Soc Magn Reson Med* 1990;5:93.

Chapter 12

Present Status of Contrast Agents to Assess Perfusion

Ronald M. Peshock, MD

Magnetic resonance imaging (MRI) is capable of providing extensive information regarding the cardiovascular system.[1] It can provide high-resolution images of cardiac structure and can be used to obtain precise measures of cardiac motion using techniques of myocardial tagging. Because MRI is sensitive to motion, it can be used to obtain quantitative information regarding blood flow and thus, a variety of potential MRI approaches are emerging for the evaluation of myocardial perfusion. Spectroscopic techniques can also be used to obtain important insights into aspects of cardiac metabolism.

Of all of these areas of interest, the assessment of myocardial perfusion by MRI may have the greatest impact on clinical practice. Magnetic resonance imaging has a number of potential advantages in the assessment of perfusion. First, it has high spatial resolution, typically on the order of 1–2 mm. This may allow the assessment of the transmural gradient of blood flow across the myocardial wall. Second, MRI is characterized by excellent soft tissue contrast with multiple contrast mechanisms. This provides multiple potential approaches to the assessment of myocardial perfusion. This potential was recognized early in the development of MRI, but its application was limited by the toxicity of contrast agents and the time required for imaging.[2,3] Recent developments in contrast agent design and high-speed imaging have made it possible to realize this potential.[4–6]

Thus, the purpose of this chapter is to briefly describe: 1) the general classes of MRI contrast agents; 2) the technical advances in MRI that have made the assessment of perfusion practical; and 3) to discuss some recent experimental and clinical developments in this area.

Background

It is important to realize that the use of contrast agents in MRI is fundamentally different than the use of contrast agents in any other standard imaging modality. This

Supported in part by Ischemic SCOR (HL-1776) and a grant from Toshiba America MRI, Inc.
From Pohost GM (ed.), *Cardiovascular Applications of Magnetic Resonance*. Mount Kisco, NY, Futura Publishing Co., Inc., © 1993.

is due to the fact that MRI contrast agents are not directly imaged. It is the interaction between the MRI contrast agent and the surrounding hydrogen nuclei that is observed. The contrast material is used to alter the relaxation times (T_1 and T_2) of the nearby hydrogen nuclei, yielding a change in image contrast that can be observed under appropriate conditions. To achieve this effect, relatively high concentrations of material (typically millimolar) are required. This is to be differentiated from radionuclide imaging, in which the concentration of the contrast material is much lower.

Given the fact that MRI contrast agents are detected indirectly necessitates careful design of the agent. One must choose a means of altering the local tissue relaxation times that minimizes the amount of material to be delivered and the potential toxicity of the agent while maintaining its efficacy. A means of targeting the agent to the tissue of interest must also be devised. Magnetic resonance contrast agents presently being used or in development fall into two general classes: 1) paramagnetic contrast agents and 2) magnetic susceptibility agents. Paramagnetic contrast agents take advantage of the magnetic properties of a metal ion that has an unpaired electron, such as copper, chromium, manganese, or gadolinium. This unpaired electron produces a large magnetic moment that provides an additional means of interaction with the magnetic moments of the hydrogen nuclei in water. This allows the nuclei to return to equilibrium more quickly. At low concentrations, this leads to an increase in signal intensity due to shortening of the T_1 relaxation time, while at higher doses it leads to a decrease in signal intensity due to a decrease in T_2.

Unfortunately, most paramagnetic metal ions are highly toxic and therefore must be chelated to prevent their interaction with proteins. The chelating agent (such as diethylene triamine pentaacetic acid or DTPA) binds the metal ion strongly to prevent it from binding with other proteins. However, it must also allow water hydrogen nuclei free access to the paramagnetic atom to achieve the desired change in relaxation times.

Susceptibility contrast agents take advantage of the magnetic behavior of larger groups of metal ions. Groups of metal ions (typically iron) introduce inhomogeneity in the local magnetic field on a macroscopic scale. This leads to a decrease in signal intensity due to a decrease in the observed T_2 of the hydrogen nuclei (T_2^* effect). If the groups of metal ions are large they will become permanently magnetized—this is thus termed a ferromagnetic contrast agent. If the groups of metal ions are smaller, they will not become permanently magnetized—termed a superparamagnetic contrast agent. Although these particles are not chelated, they are frequently associated with macromolecules such as albumin or dextran to reduce toxicity.

After choosing the general class of contrast agent as described above, one is then left with the problem of formulating the material to target it for a specific purpose. For the assessment of myocardial perfusion, there are a variety of potential approaches.[4] These include the use of extracellular agents, intravascular agents, and intracellular agents (Figure 1). A variety of agents falling into each of these classes are under investigation. Examples of extracellular agents include gadolinium-DTPA, gadolinium-DOTA, and gadolinium-DTPA-MBA. Intravascular or blood pool agents include gadolinium-DTPA, superparamagnetics, or ferromagnetic agents bound to albumin or polysaccharides.[7,8] Intracellular agents include manganese chloride, manganese-DPDT, and other agents. Each of these formulations could potentially be used for the assessment of perfusion. The use of a particular formulation will depend significantly on the general approach used for the assessment of perfusion.

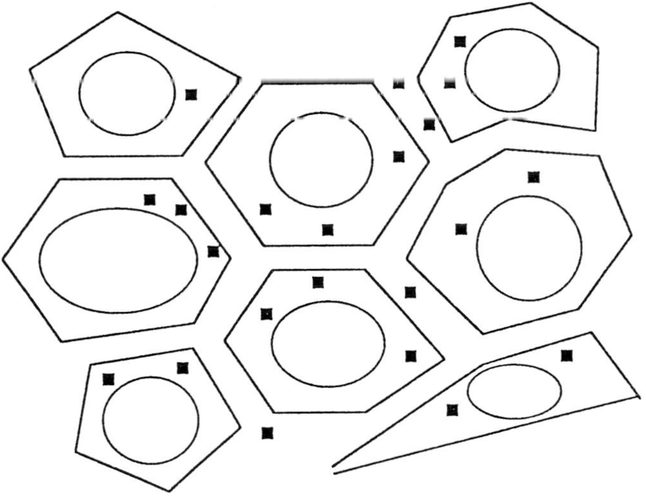

Extracellular

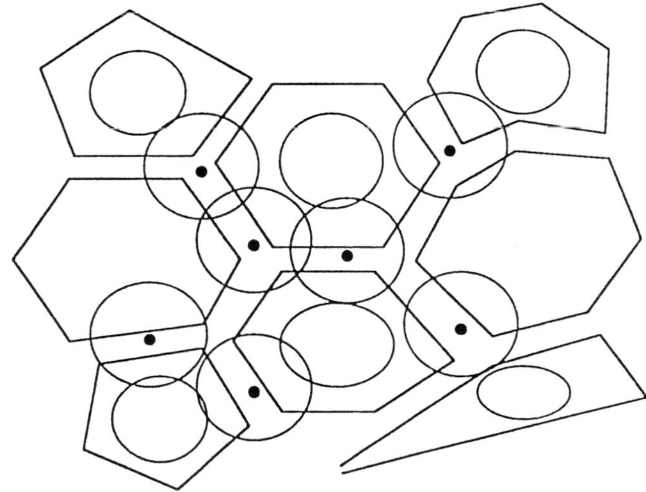

Intravascular Susceptibility Agent

FIGURE 1. *Schematic diagrams of the general approaches to the targeting of MRI contrast agents. Cells are indicated by ovals surrounded by the interstitium and capillary bed in each case.* **Top:** *An illustration of the distribution of a conventional extracellular agent (squares) such as gadolinium-DTPA with an agent in the capillaries and the interstitial space.* **Bottom:** *An illustration of the distribution of an intravascular susceptibility agent (circles) with the agent limited to the capillary space. Of note is the fact that the effect of the agent extends outside the capillary (indicated by the circles surrounding the individual particles). See text for details.*

The choice of a general approach is influenced by the time required to obtain a measure of the concentration of the agent. To examine the transit of a bolus of contrast material through the heart, one must be able to obtain measurements at least with every cardiac cycle, if not more frequently. There have been several recent developments that have significantly reduced the time required for imaging the heart using present MRI devices. These include the development of so-called "subsecond" scanning (also termed "turbo FLASH") and echo-planar imaging. A brief discussion of these techniques is relevant for an understanding of MRI assessment of perfusion.

To generate any magnetic resonance image, a certain amount of data must be acquired prior to Fourier transformation. In standard MRI, one single piece of this information is acquired with each repetition time or TR. This means that the total time for the image acquisition is the number of lines in the original data set times the TR. For example, if one wants an image with 256 lines of information at a TR of 1 second, then one must acquire 256 pieces of data so that total imaging time equals 256 seconds (total time $= 256 \times TR$). Given that a certain resolution is required, one cannot decrease the total number of data acquired to less than approximately 32 to 64 steps.

To reduce acquisition time further, one approach is to substantially reduce the TR. This is the approach taken in subsecond scanning, in which one reduces the TR to <10 msec, allowing one to acquire an entire 64-line image in 640 msec or less. The total imaging time is now comparable to the length of diastole in many patients, allowing one to obtain an entire image with each cardiac cycle. In this way, one can observe the dynamics of the passage of a bolus of contrast agent through the myocardium. An important feature of the "turbo FLASH" or subsecond scanning approach is that this imaging sequence can be performed using standard MRI devices and gradients.

This sequence can be made particularly sensitive to changes in T_1 by preceding the rapid pulses by a single inverting (180°) pulse (Figure 2). By adjusting the time between the inverting pulse and the imaging pulses one can zero or null the signal from blood. In this case, the signal from blood in the ventricular cavity is zero in each image. With the administration of a contrast that shortens T_1 (Figure 2, bottom), there is an increase in the blood signal intensity. As the blood containing the contrast agent is delivered to the left ventricle and myocardium it causes an increase in signal intensity that can be used to evaluate perfusion.

The second general approach involves the use of echo-planar imaging. In this imaging technique, all of the data required for the images are acquired with a single pulse. Acquisition times for echo-planar MRI vary from approximately 50 to 100 msec. One can adjust the imaging parameters so that one obtains either T_1- or

---

FIGURE 2. *Diagram illustrating the use of subsecond scanning or "turbo FLASH" for the assessment of myocardial perfusion.* **Top:** *Myocardial perfusion I. An inverting pulse is applied at the time of the QRS. After an appropriate delay to null the signal from blood, all of the pulses required for each image are acquired during diastole. This yields a complete image of the heart with each cardiac cycle in which the blood is dark.* **Bottom:** *Myocardial perfusion II. Using the same inverting and imaging pulses one obtains an image with dark blood with the first cardiac cycle. Administration of a contrast agent that decreases T_1 leads to an increase in signal intensity in the blood that can then be observed as the blood passes through the cardiac chambers and myocardium.*

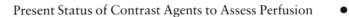

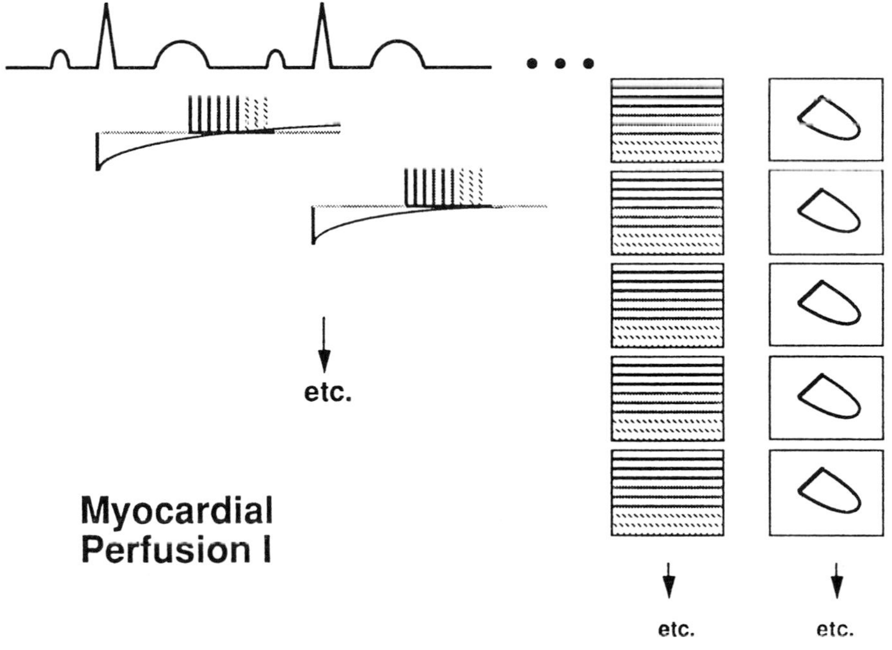
etc.
Myocardial
Perfusion I
etc.
etc.

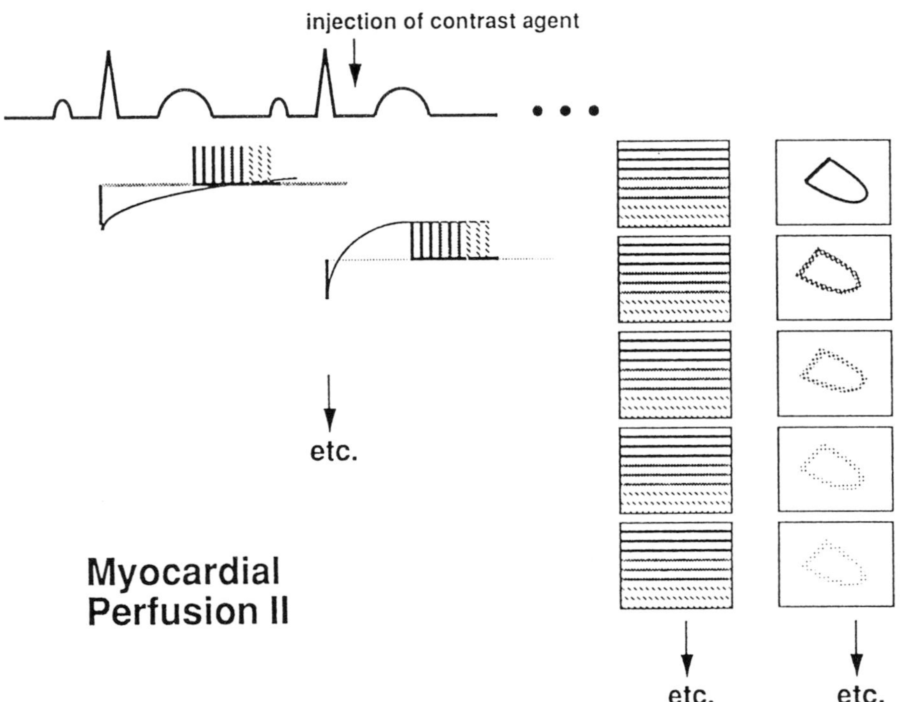
injection of contrast agent
etc.
Myocardial
Perfusion II
etc.
etc.

FIGURE 2.

T_2-weighted echo-planar sequences. In addition, these sequences are very sensitive to magnetic susceptibility differences. Thus they are particularly appropriate to studies using susceptibility agents. Unfortunately, echo-planar imaging requires specialized gradient systems that are not widely available. Thus, this limits the applicability of echo-planar imaging for the assessment of perfusion at the present time.

Assessments of Perfusion

There are two general approaches to the assessment of perfusion: 1) first-pass techniques that require the deposition of the contrast material in the tissue; and 2) washout techniques in which the rate of clearance of the agent from the tissue is measured after an equilibrium level is obtained.[9] The majority of interest now involves the evaluation of first-pass approaches. The ideal perfusion marker would 1) be distributed in the tissue only on the basis of blood flow; 2) be completely extracted on the first pass through the tissue; 3) remain in the tissue long enough for the measurement; and 4) be excreted rapidly to allow serial measurements. At present, the ideal agent does not exist. However, the combination of agents now in use or in development and fast MRI scanning have made first-pass studies feasible.

A number of groups have now demonstrated that subsecond scanning can be used to assess the transit of a bolus of gadolinium-DTPA through the heart.[10–12] A typical study performed in our laboratory is shown in Figures 3 and 4. In the precontrast agent image study, the imaging parameters (including an inverting pulse prior to the imaging sequence) were adjusted so that the signal from the intracavitary blood is nulled. With the administration of a contrast agent, the T_1 of the blood is decreased, yielding an increase in signal intensity. As the blood moves through the ventricular cavity and into the myocardium there is an increase in the signal intensity. Several groups have demonstrated that this technique can be used qualitatively to detect areas of complete occlusion in animals and in humans. Recent studies by Wilke et al.[13] in an animal model with partial coronary occlusion have illustrated that this technique can detect regions of partial coronary occlusion under conditions of dipyridamole stress. More importantly, they also found that by using an appropriate kinetics model these intensity data can be used to obtain a measure of quantitative myocardial perfusion.

An important feature of these studies is the fact that they use a contrast agent (gadolinium-DTPA) that has already been approved for other applications in humans. In addition, there are additional agents, gadolinium-HP-DO3A and gadolinium-DTPA-BMA, which are near approval for use in humans. Thus, if technical details of rapid imaging and the quantitation of blood flow can be resolved, potential contrast agents are already available.

However, these agents are also significantly limited in that their space of distribution is complex. In particular, it is well established that gadolinium-DTPA rapidly moves from the intravascular into the interstitial space. This complicates approaches to the quantification of blood flow. The kinetics of gadolinium-DTPA washin are a function of multiple factors, including the concentration of gadolinium-DTPA, coronary flow rate, diffusion into the interstitial space, relative tissue volume fraction, bolus duration, and recirculation.[14] One approach to this problem would be to design a contrast agent that remained in the intravascular space.

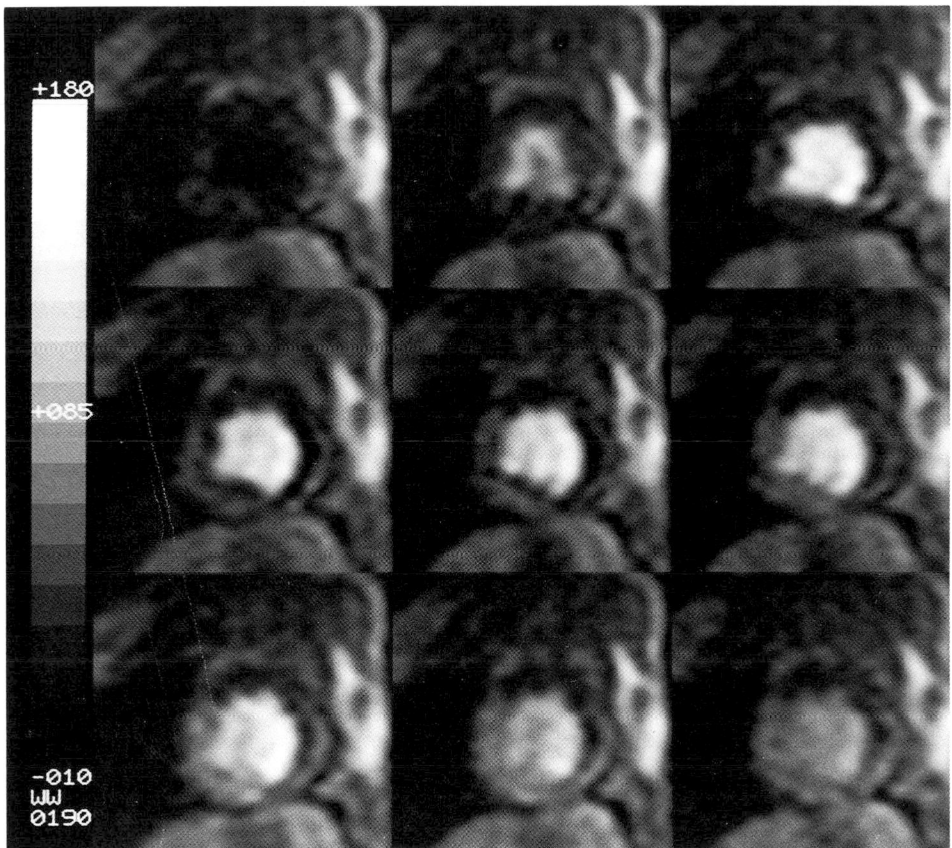

FIGURE 3. *Serial subsecond images illustrating the transit of a bolus of gadolinium-DTPA through the heart in a canine model of acute regional ischemia. Short-axis images acquired at 0.5 T (Toshiba America MRI, Inc.) every other heartbeat. The contrast material is seen arriving in the left ventricle in early frames followed by appearance of increased signal intensity in the myocardial wall. A region of hypoperfusion is noted in the anterior wall.*

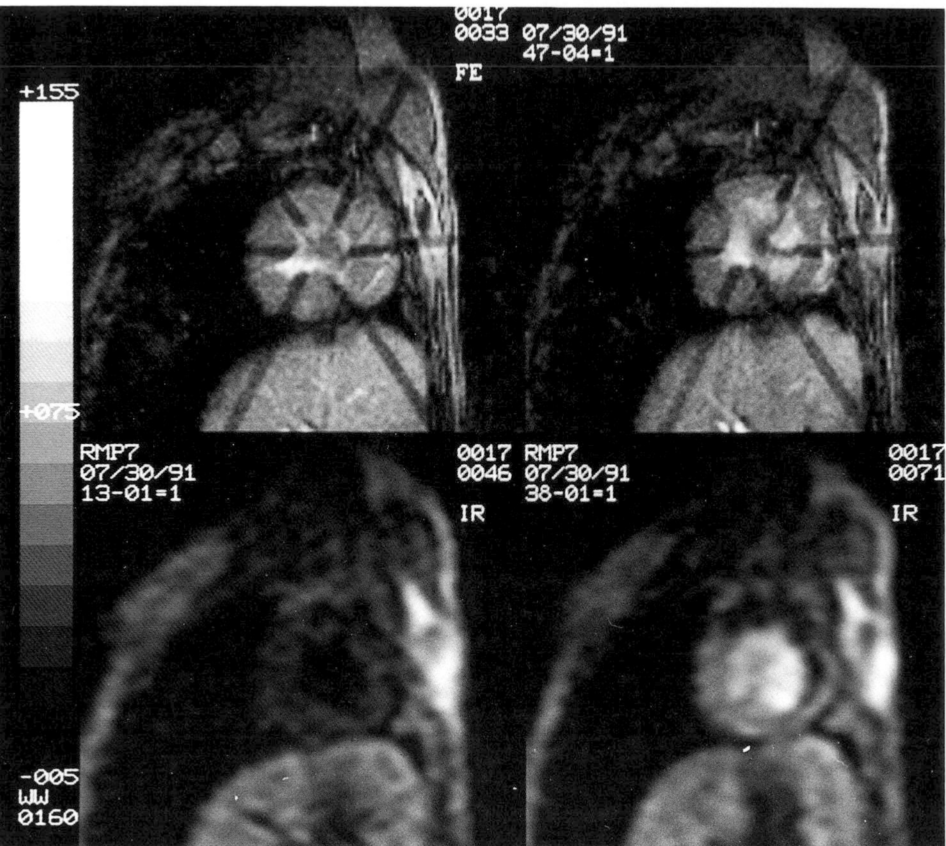

FIGURE 4. *Images obtained using myocardial tagging for the assessment of function and subsecond scan providing near simultaneous assessments of perfusion in a canine model of acute regional ischemia.* **Upper left:** *Systolic frame from a cine MRI sequence with radial tagging illustrating normal thickening.* **Upper right:** *Systolic frame from a cine MRI sequence with tagging after left anterior descending coronary artery occlusion illustrating loss of anterior thickening.* **Lower left:** *Subsecond scan prior to coronary occlusion without contrast agent for reference.* **Lower right:** *Subsecond scan after occlusion following administration of contrast agent demonstrating a perfusion defect. There is good correlation between the extent of perfusion abnormality and the region of abnormal thickening.*

Intravascular contrast agents have in general involved binding a standard extracellular agent to a larger macromolecule. As described above, a variety of macromolecules have been suggested, including albumin and polysaccharides. Initial studies in animals models using these agents are encouraging.[7,8] However, their potential efficacy and safety in humans have not been established. A variation on the intravascular agent approach is the intravascular susceptibility agents. These materials typically use a large macromolecule bound to a superparamagnetic or ferromagnetic particle. An advantage of this approach is that the superparamagnetic or ferromagnetic particle can have a wide-ranging affect on surrounding hydrogen nuclei in water. This can potentially allow the use of smaller doses of contrast material. Again, animal studies in this area have been encouraging. Intravascular susceptibility agents may have substantial application elsewhere in the body; thus their development for assessment of myocardial perfusion may be favored.

The final overall approach to the assessment of myocardial perfusion involves the use of intracellular agents. In fact, the first assessments of myocardial perfusion were performed in the 1970s using manganese chloride.[2] Manganese is taken up similar to thallium, thus allowing assessment of both perfusion and cell viability. Unfortunately, manganese is quite toxic. Efforts to produce agents that both enter the cell and are nontoxic have been reasonably difficult, although there are some encouraging potential agents.[15] An important advantage of the intracellular agent is that if the agent is completely extracted in the first pass and remains in or bound to the cell for a period of minutes to hours, then imaging does not need to proceed so rapidly.

Alternative Approaches

A variety of more unconventional approaches have also been suggested for the assessment of myocardial perfusion. These include the use of deuterium oxide (D_2O)[16] and oxygen-17–[17] and fluorine-19 containing compounds.[18] In addition, recent research suggests that it may be possible to detect changes in oxygen concentration in the brain on the basis of changes in the deoxyhemoglobin state in the brain.[19,20] If these approaches can be applied to the heart, it may be possible to obtain assessments of the adequacy of myocardial perfusion without the use of any contrast agent whatsoever.

Summary

At the present time, studies suggest that MRI with contrast agents can be used effectively in the assessment of myocardial perfusion. Through the use of subsecond scanning and other fast scanning techniques, it appears that currently approved MRI contrast agents are certainly capable of providing qualitative information and potentially providing quantitative information regarding myocardial perfusion. However, it is clear that the presently available contrast agents are not optimal for the assessment of perfusion. A variety of new contrast agents, both intravascular and intracellular, are presently undergoing early evaluation. However, the ideal agent has not yet been determined. Finally, advances in high-speed imaging may significantly impact the choice and development of MRI contrast agents for the assessment of myocardial perfusion.

Acknowledgments

The author would like to acknowledge the efforts of Cindy Miller, Maria Morgan, Jerri Payne, Christy Ward, and Bill Ennen in obtaining these studies and the efforts of H. Takai and Y. Ogikubo in the development of the pulse sequences for subsecond scanning. The author would also like to acknowledge the work of Cathy Starnes, Virginia Vaughn, Dorothy Gutekunst, and Alison Russell in the preparation of this manuscript.

References

1. *Cardiac Imaging—A Companion to Braunwald's Heart Disease*. Philadelphia, PA: WB Saunders Co., 1991.
2. Goldman MR, Brady TJ, Pykett IL, et al: Quantification of experimental myocardial infarction using nuclear magnetic resonance imaging and paramagnetic ion contrast enhancement in excised canine hearts. *Circulation* 1982;66(5):1012–1016.
3. Johnston DL, Liu P, Lauffer RB, et al: Use of gadolinium-DTPA as a myocardial perfusion agent: potential applications and limitations for magnetic resonance imaging. *J Nucl Med* 1987;28:871–877.
4. Wolf GL: Role of magnetic resonance contrast agents in cardiac imaging. *Am J Cardiol* 1990;66:59F–62F.
5. Brown JJ, Higgins CB: Myocardial paramagnetic contrast agents for MR imaging. *AJR* 1988;151:865–872.
6. Wolf GL, Rogowska J: Contrast agents for fast imaging? *Magn Reson Med* 1991;22:268–272.
7. Brasch RC: Rationale and applications for macromolecular Gd-based contrast agents. *Magn Reson Med* 1991;22(2):282–287.
8. Rozenman Y, Zou X, Kantor HL: Magnetic resonance imaging with superparamagnetic iron oxide particles for the detection of myocardial reperfusion. *Magn Reson Imaging* 1991;9:933–939.
9. Henkleman RM: Does IVIM measure classical perfusion. *Magn Reson Med* 1990;16:470–475.
10. Atkinson DJ, Burstein D, Edelman M: First-pass cardiac perfusion: evaluation with ultrafast MR imaging. *Radiology* 1990;174:757–762.
11. Larsson HBW, Stubgaard M, Sondergaard L, et al: In vivo quantitation of myocardial perfusion using MRI and Gd-DTPA (abstract). Proceedings of the Society of Magnetic Resonance in Medicine. 1991:1145.
12. van Rugge FP, Boreel JJ, van der Wall EE, et al: Cardiac first-pass and myocardial perfusion in normal subjects assessed by subsecond Gd-DTPA enhanced MR imaging. *J Comput Assist Tomogr* 1991;15(6):959–965.
13. Wilke N, Simm C, Engles G, et al: Contrast enhanced first pass myocardial perfusion imaging in man and dogs. *Radiology* 1991:181:56.
14. Burstein D, Taratuta E, Manning WJ: Factors in myocardial "perfusion" imaging with ultrafast MRI and Gd-DTPA administration. *Magn Reson Med* 1991;20:299–305.
15. Schaefer S, Lange RA, Kulkarni PV, et al: In vivo nuclear magnetic resonance imaging of myocardial perfusion using the paramagnetic contrast agent manganese gluconate. *J Am Coll Cardiol* 1989;14:472–480.
16. Mitchell MD, Osbakken M: Estimation of myocardial perfusion using deuterium nuclear magnetic resonance. *Magn Reson Imaging* 1991;9:545–552.
17. Kwong KK, Hopkins AL, Belliveau JW, et al: COMMUNICATIONS: proton NMR imaging of cerebral blood flow using H_2O. *Magn Reson Med* 1991;22:154–158.
18. Nunnally RL, Babcock EE, Horner SD, et al: Fluorine-19 spectroscopy and imaging investigation of myocardial perfusion and cardiac function. *Magn Reson Med* 1985;3:399–405.
19. Turner R, Le Bihan D, Moonen CTW, et al: Echo-planar time course MRI of cat brain oxygenation changes. *Magn Reson Med* 1991;22:159–166.
20. Wright GA, Hu BS, Macovski A: Estimating oxygen saturation of blood in vivo with MR imaging at 1.5T. *Magn Reson Imaging* 1991;1:275–283.

Chapter 13

Toward the Clinical Application of Magnetic Resonance Myocardial Perfusion Measurements

Graeme C. McKinnon, PhD,
André C. Eichenberger, MD,
C.A. von Weymarn, Walter A. Fuchs, MD,
and Gustav K. von Schulthess, MD, PhD

The diagnosis and evaluation of myocardial infarction and ischemia using magnetic resonance imaging (MRI) is a rapidly growing field, recently well reviewed by de Roos et al.[1] One area that has developed over the last 2 or 3 years,[2,3] largely through the increasing availability of rapid imaging sequences, involves the study of the perfusion dynamics after a bolus injection of gadolinium-DTPA.

The dynamics of myocardial gadolinium-DTPA perfusion require a time resolution of approximately two heart cycles, with measurements continuing over about 30 heart cycles. Further, to be really useful, approximately four to six short-axis slices should be acquired. To avoid motion blurring, the images should all be either obtained in approximately <50 msec or in end diastole, when the heart is reasonably stationary. These requirements place large demands on an MRI scanner. However, if "subsecond" MRI is to become competitive with isotope techniques, which currently represent the gold standard for the determination of myocardial perfusion, then this sort of performance should be the goal.

At present, a fast gradient-echo sequence is generally used, mainly because it is available as a standard sequence on most scanners, but also because it is very robust with respect to motion, flow, and (at short TE) susceptibility changes. Later in this chapter we describe how maximum gradient strengths and slew rates, a 64*40 fractional k-space acquisition, and imaging times of about 220 msec can be used to achieve a 20-cm field of view.

Echo-planar imaging[4] is another potential approach for myocardial perfusion assessment. However, with conventional gradients it is virtually impossible to image

From Pohost GM (ed.), *Cardiovascular Applications of Magnetic Resonance.* Mount Kisco, NY, Futura Publishing Co., Inc., © 1993.

the heart in a single shot, because the short transversal relaxation of the myocardial tissue and the long time required for the echo train.[5]

We are investigating an interleaved gradient echo-planar imaging sequence[6] whereby multiple acquisitions are performed. Approximately eight k-space lines are collected in each acquisition in an interleaved k-space manner. To obtain the same resolution as with the gradient-echo sequence, imaging times are approximately 90 msec.

Myocardial Perfusion Measurements

The perfusion dynamics of the myocardium can be followed using fast gradient-echo imaging.[2,3] The procedure involves intravenously injecting a bolus of gadolinium-DTPA and making images of the heart every one or two heart cycles. After approximately 16 heart cycles the gadolinium-DTPA causes signal enhancement in the myocardium. In infarcted or ischemic regions the signal enhancement is weaker or absent.

Figure 1 shows a series of short-axis equatorial plane images taken immediately following the application of gadolinium-DTPA. The images are measured every second heart cycle. The imaging time per image was just <500 msec. The field of view here is 20 cm and the resolution is 64*128.

The images presented in this section are from a patient with an infarcted region in the inferior myocardium at the equatorial level, with a region of ischemia in the apex. To date the images have not been analyzed quantitatively. In fact, they must be interpreted carefully, as the measurements were performed with a surface coil to prevent image "wrap around" and also to improve the signal-to-noise ratio. Thus, there is a natural decrease in image intensity from the superior to the inferior heart wall. We present them here merely to illustrate the measurement technique. In Figure 1 the temporal order is from left to right. The first image is shown at the top (left) and the last is shown at the bottom (right). On careful examination, it can be seen that the myocardial signal intensity has increased at about the eighth image, or after 16 heart cycles. It can also be seen that in the infarcted region the enhancement is almost absent. The importance of collecting images every 1 or 2 seconds is to enable the detection of regions with delayed perfusion.

Since an MRI treadmill exercise is not possible, ischemia must be detected under the influence of pharmacologically induced stress[7,8] with agents such as intravenous dipyridamole. This causes the healthy vessels to dilate. However, the presence of stenoses inhibits dilation. Thus, there is increased blood flow to the healthy myocardium, but generally reduced flow to the poorly perfused regions. By comparing two sets of measurements, one at rest and the other under stress, ischemia should be distinguishable from infarction, analogously to isotope studies. In the resting state an ischemic region will have enhanced signal intensity after the gadolinium-DTPA bolus; however, under stress there is very little increase in signal intensity in such a region. If successful, such measurements might replace myocardial perfusion studies that use thallium scintigraphy.

Figure 2 shows dynamic perfusion images from the apical plane before and after the administration of dipyridamole. The top two images show the heart in a resting

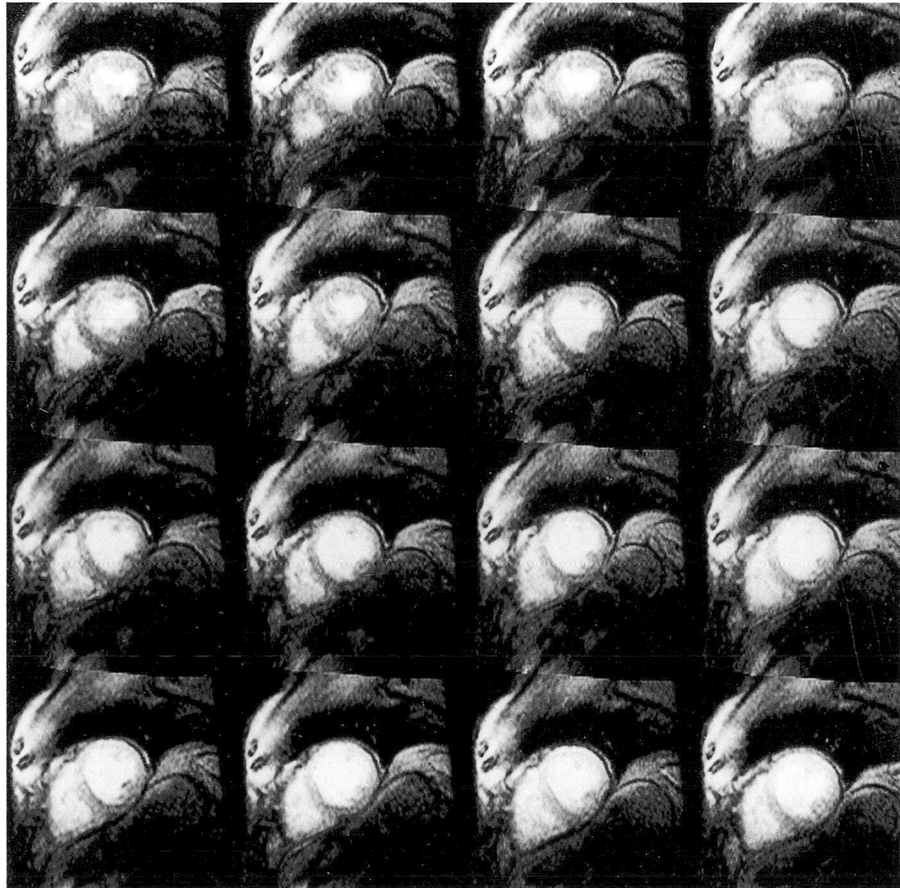

FIGURE 1. *Short-axis, equatorial plane images of the heart following the administration of a gadolinium-DTPA bolus. Two heart cycles between images.*

state, and the bottom two are measured with the heart in a stressed state. The left image is taken as the gadolinium-DTPA bolus is administered, and the right is that image 16 heart cycles later. The stressed series was measured 30 minutes after the resting series to allow the gadolinium-DTPA to wash out. In Figure 2 one can see that the signal enhancement in the inferior myocardial region is less in the stressed series compared with the resting series. This is indicative of an ischemic region.

Finally, to investigate the whole myocardium, multislice imaging is required. At present we measure three slices. Their temporal position with respect to the electrocardiogram is illustrated in Figure 3. Selective images from a multislice multiphase series are shown in Figure 4. The different slices represent, from left to right, the basal, equatorial, and apical planes, respectively. The time after the gadolinium-DTPA bolus increases from top to bottom. The images are eight heart phases apart. Even though three slices are a start, the ideal minimum number of slices to cover the heart from base to apex should be four to six.

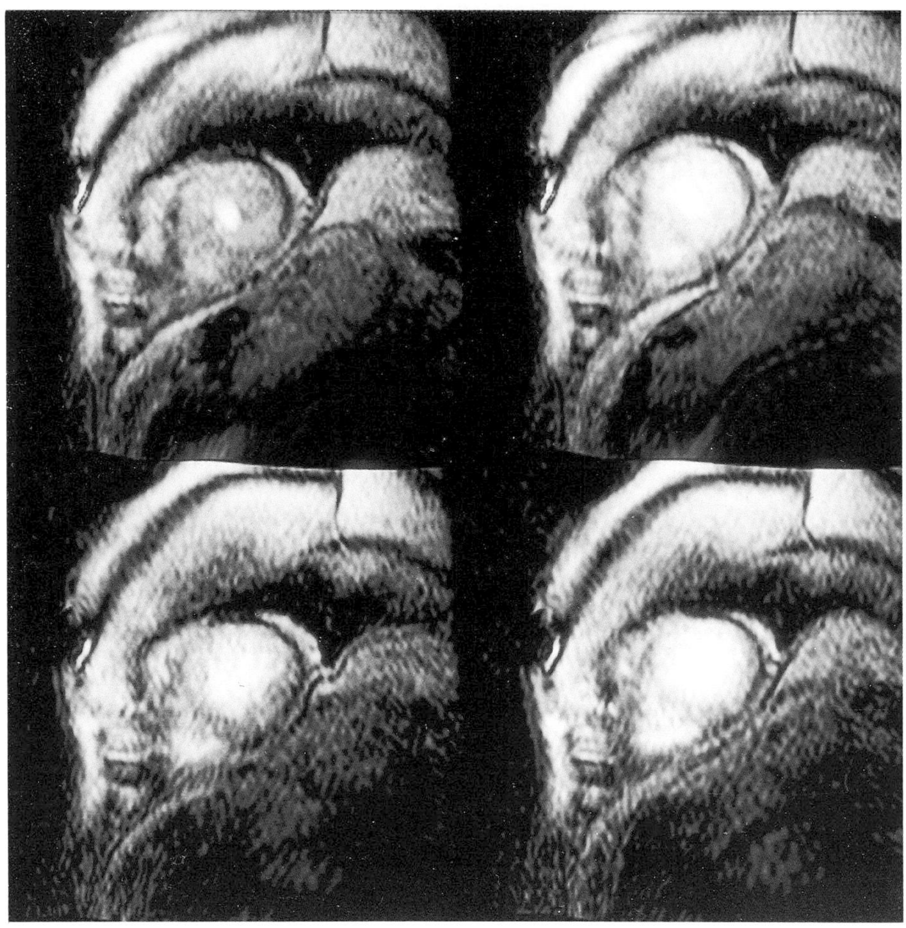

FIGURE 2. *Apical plane images before and 16 heart cycles after a gadolinium-DTPA bolus.* **Top:** *The heart in the resting state.* **Bottom:** *Heart stressed with dipyridomole.*

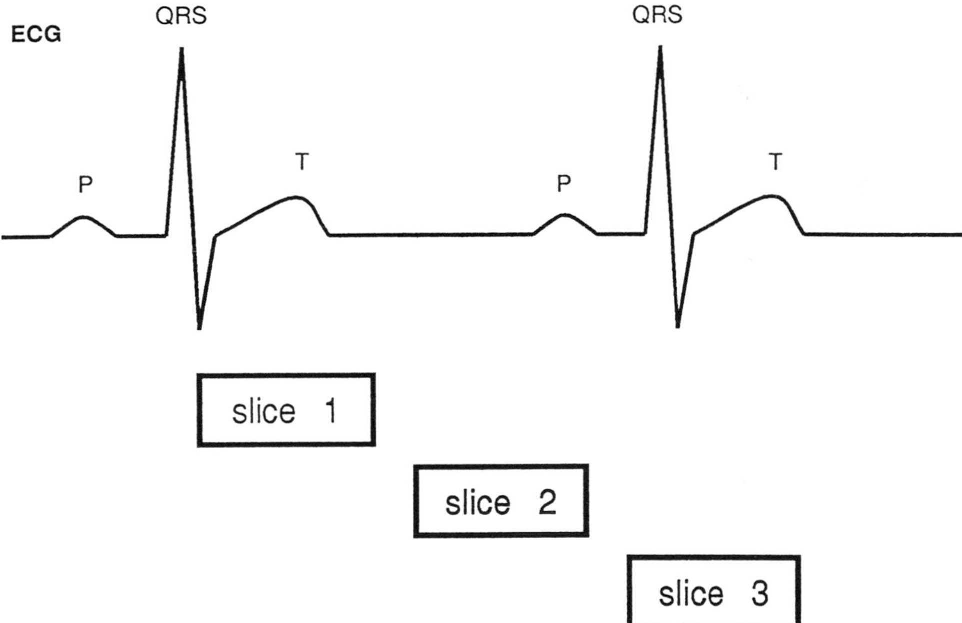

FIGURE 3. *Slice acquisition timing with respect to the electrocardiogram.*

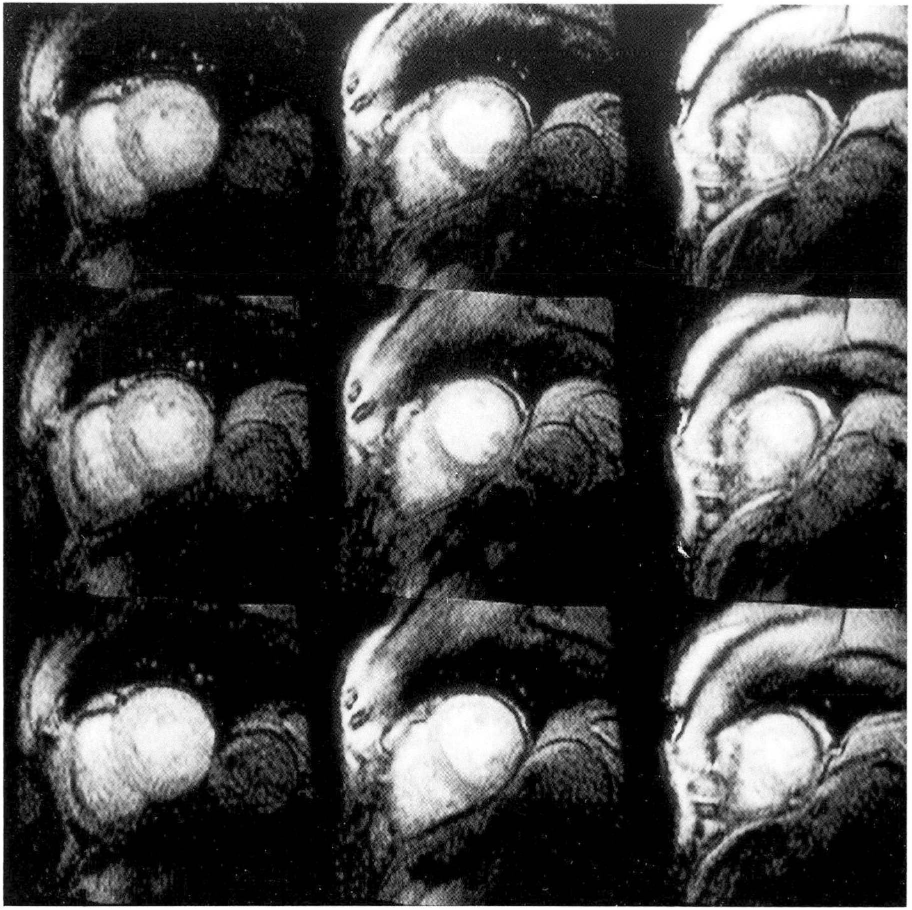

FIGURE 4. *Multislice, multiphase images following gadolinium-DTPA bolus. Left, basal plane; center, equatorial plane; right, apical plane.*

Fast Imaging Requirements

Figure 5 is a schematic diagram illustrating the heart volume changes in relation to the electrocardiogram. To obtain images not blurred by motion, measurements should be made during that interval in diastole when the ventricle is relatively stationary. This time period is dependent on the heart rate. For a patient with a heart rate of 80 beats per minute, the stationary period is about 400 msec. If one assumes that six slices are required to give good coverage of the whole myocardium, then with a time resolution of two heart cycles, the desired imaging time is around 140 msec.

Gradient-Echo Imaging

A schematic diagram of our fast gradient-echo sequence[9] is shown in Figure 6.[9] With a field of view of 20 cm and a scan resolution of 64*128, the TR was 7.5 msec.

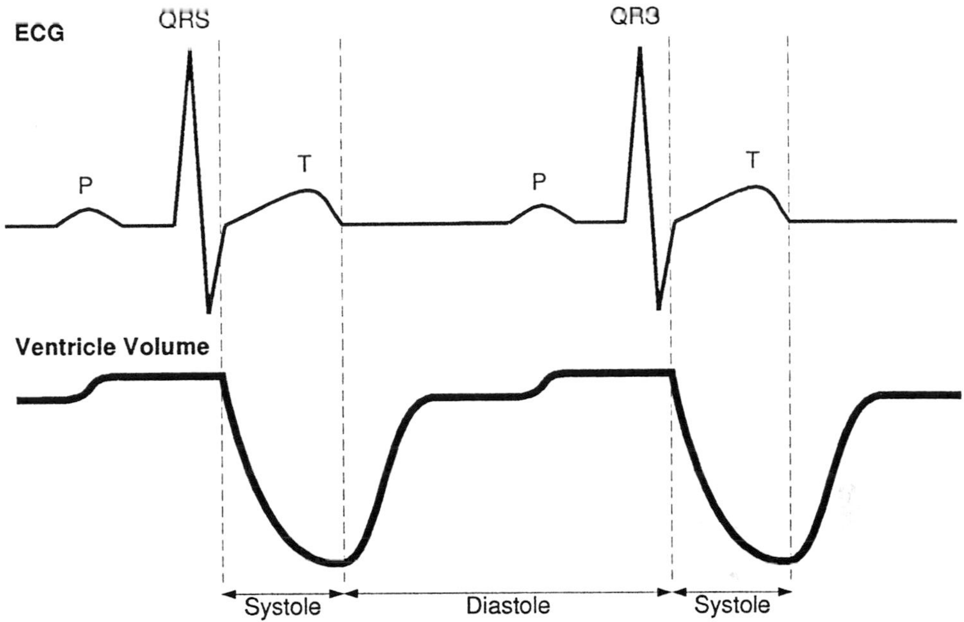

FIGURE 5. *Schematic diagram of ventricular volume changes in relationship to the electrocardiogram.*

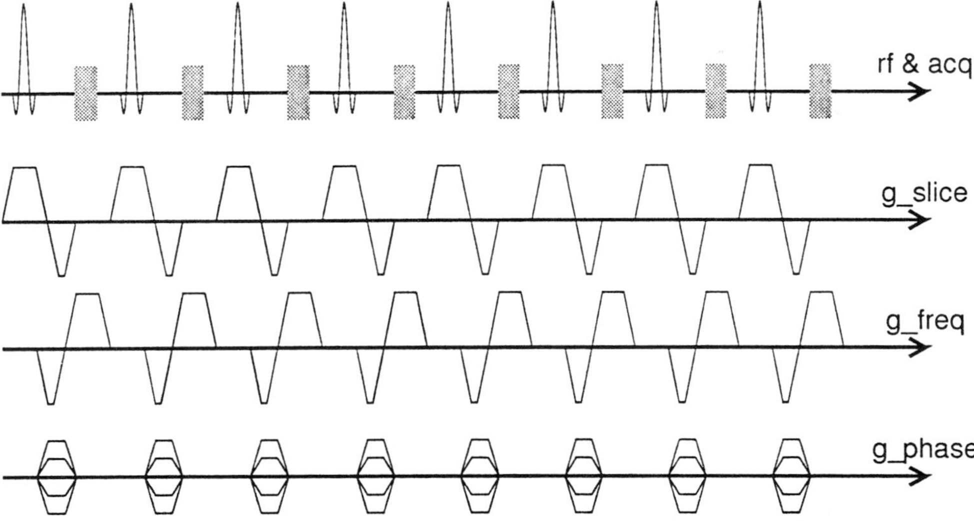

FIGURE 6. *Rapid gradient-echo imaging sequence.*

This gives an imaging time of 480 msec. Thus, with this sequence we are forced to image throughout the heart cycle, as illustrated in Figure 3. Furthermore, three slices is about the maximum obtainable in two heart cycles.

We have been able to improve the standard gradient-echo sequence somewhat by using maximum gradient strengths and slew rates, which are 10 mT/m and 20 mT/m per millisecond, respectively, for our scanner. For a field of view of 20 cm and a scan resolution of 64*64, the TR is 5.4 msec. This gives an imaging time of approximately 345 msec. A pair of such images is shown in Figure 7. The measurements for the image on the left were started on detection of the R wave of the electrocardiogram; those on the right, with a delay of 150 msec after the R wave. Notice that these images are measured doubly oblique. For images measured parallel to one of the principle gradient axes, the TR is 4.5 msec.

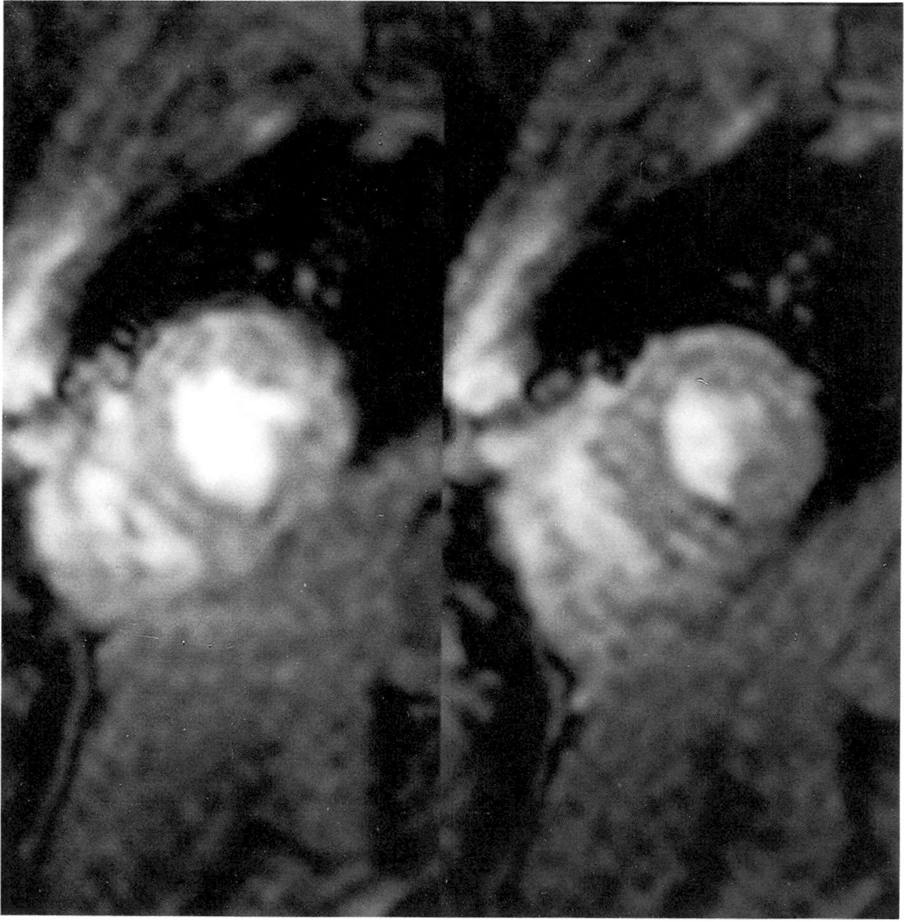

FIGURE 7. *Gradient-echo images: 220-msec acquisition time.*

Using fractional k-space acquisitions, for instance only 40 k-space lines, we are able to reduce the imaging time to 220 msec. Using the fractional k-space processing software provided by the scanner manufacturer, the image quality is only marginally reduced with respect to that obtained with the conventionally reconstructed 64*64 scan resolution images.

Thus, with these improvements we hope to be able to obtain four slices in two heart cycles measured during the stationary period of diastole.

Echo-Planar Imaging

An obvious candidate for very fast imaging of the heart is the echo-planar imaging method (Figure 8).[4] We have been evaluating echo-planar imaging on other scanners. However, without special gradients[10,11] the image quality is very poor, as discussed by others.[5]

Assuming a fractional k-space acquisition with eight k-space lines before the spin-echo point, then for the same resolution as discussed above the minimum TE is approximately 40 msec. Furthermore, for 40 k-space lines the echo train is approximately 80 msec long when standard gradients are used. For good imaging results the echo train length and TE should be short with respect to the tissue T_2^* and T_2, respectively. This is not the case with myocardium, which has relatively short transverse relaxation time constants.

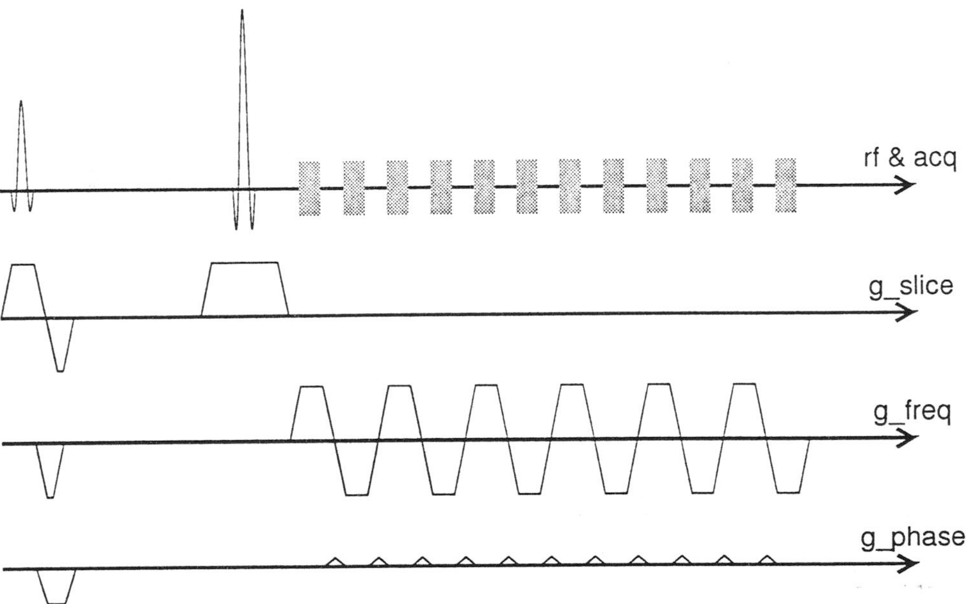

FIGURE 8. *Echo-planar imaging sequence.*

Hybrid Gradient Echo-Planar Imaging

If only a few k-space lines are collected, then the echo-planar TE and echo train length can be reduced sufficiently such that heart imaging becomes feasible on a conventional scanner. To obtain sufficient image resolution this shortened sequence must be repeated several times, each time collecting other k-space lines,[6] usually in an interleaved fashion. For rapid imaging the TR between sequences must be kept very short. Interleaved echo-planar imaging can be performed using gradient echoes or spin echoes. Neither seems to have been investigated in much depth.

We have developed an interleaved gradient echo-planar sequence (Figure 9). The sequence is a hybrid between a fast gradient-echo sequence and an echo-planar sequence. As implemented, eight k-space lines are collected each subsequence. For a field of view of 20 cm and a scan resolution of 64*64, the average TR per k-space line is 2.25 msec, which gives an imaging time of 144 msec. This imaging time is desirable for useful perfusion imaging. A pair of short-axis heart images obtained with this sequence is shown in Figure 10. The acquisition for the image on the left was started at the R wave, and that for the right image 150 msec later.

The image quality in Figure 10 is not as good as that in Figure 7. This illustrates some of the difficulties with the echo-planar–type sequences, which are more sensitive to field inhomogeneity than gradient-echo sequences. Also, with echo-planar–type sequences each k-space line must be individually phase corrected, which necessitates the measurement of reference data. At this stage data correction strategies are still being developed.

Despite the difficulties, we feel it is worth persevering with this sequence. Using a factional k-space acquisition, whereby 40 k-space lines are acquired, the imaging time is only 90 msec. This time is becoming comparable to that achieved by dedicated echo-planar scanners.

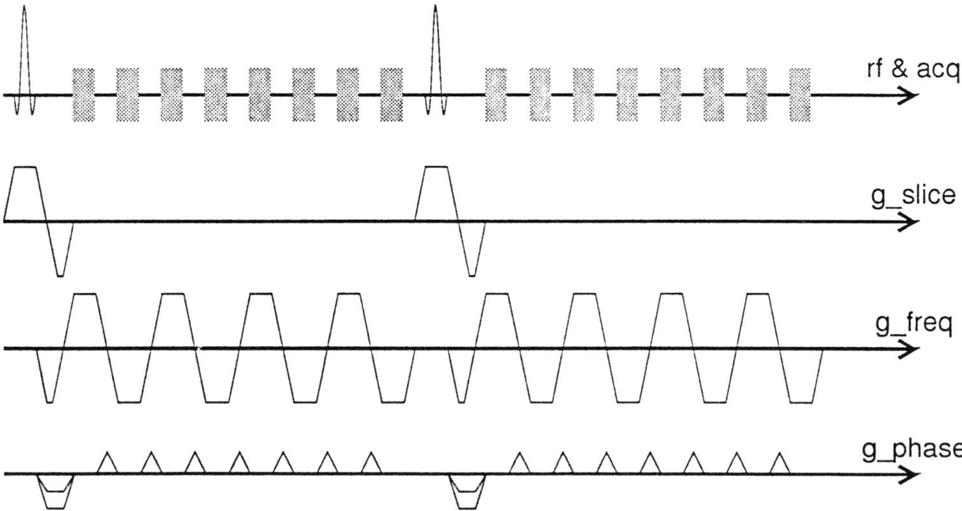

FIGURE 9. *Hybrid gradient echo-planar imaging sequence.*

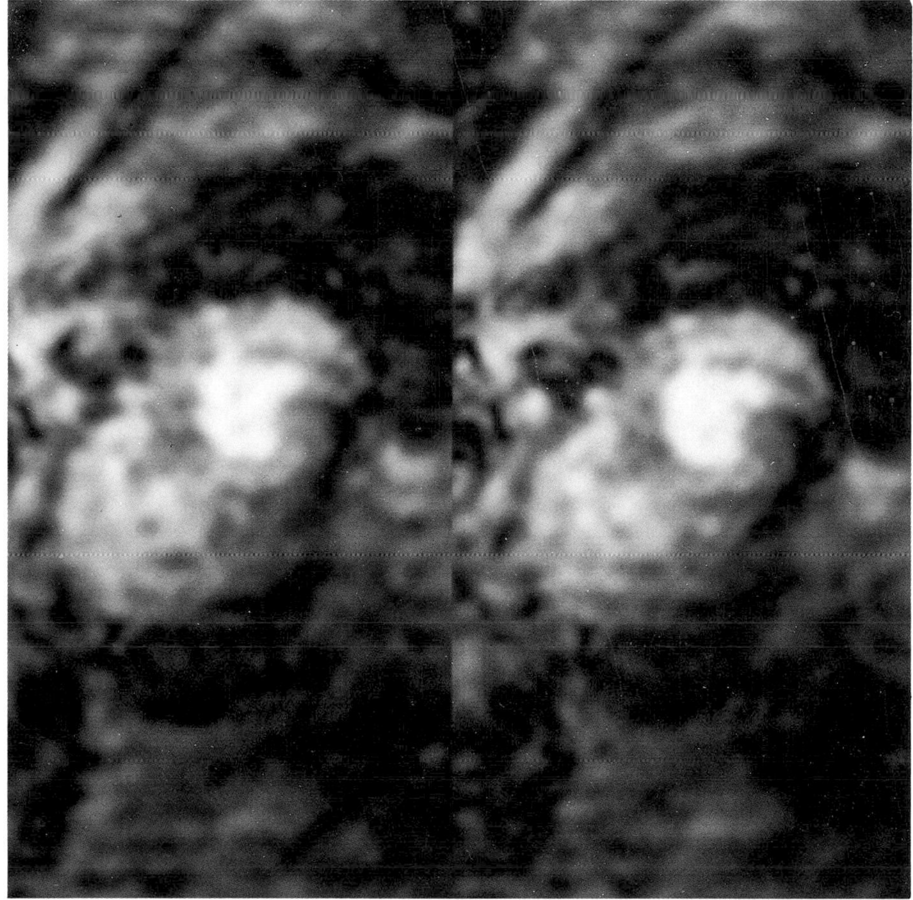

FIGURE 10. *Hybrid gradient echo-planar images: 144-msec acquisition time.*

The Future

Pulse sequences are tending to merge into hybrid arrangements of spin-echo, gradient-echo, and echo-planar–type sequences whereby the salient features of the canonical forms are combined in sequences optimized for particular requirements. This merging is made possible in part by the development of gradient systems that generate greatly reduced eddy current fields.

Now that optimization of image acquisition is fairly well understood, we have to reexamine the question of image signal to noise. When the imaging time is less than the longitudinal relaxation time, one should not use the "Ernst angle" for the excitation pulse. Instead variable (optimized) excitation angles should be applied.[12,13] These procedures can potentially increase the signal-to-noise ratio quite significantly. However, to date, they do not appear to have been applied clinically.

We have demonstrated that even with a standard scanner and the proper choice of sequence, one can achieve very short imaging times. It seems that the near future will see the proliferation of improved gradient systems with higher current capacity and reduced switching times.[11] Thus the trend appears to be away from dedicated fast imaging scanners toward high-performance multipurpose machines.

References

1. de Roos A, van der Wall EE, Bruschke AVG, van Voorthuisen AE: Magnetic resonance imaging in the diagnosis and evaluation of myocardial infarction. *Magn Reson Q* 1991;7:191–207.
2. Atkinson DJ, Burstein D, Edelman RR: First-pass cardiac perfusion: evaluation with ultrafast MR imaging. *Radiology* 1990;174:757–762.
3. van Rugge FP, Boreel JJ, van der Wall EE, et al: Cardiac first-pass and myocardial perfusion in normal subjects assessed by subsecond Gd-DTPA enhanced MR imaging. *J Comput Assist Tomogr* 1991;15:959–965.
4. Mansfield P: Multiplanar image formation using NMR spin echoes. *J Phys C: Solid State Phys* 1977;10:L55-L58.
5. Farzaneh F, Riederer SJ, Pelc NJ: Analysis of T_2 limitations and off-resonance effects on spatial resolution and artifacts in echo-planar imaging. *Magn Reson Med* 1990;14:123–139.
6. Farzaneh F, Riederer SJ, Maier JK, Vavrek R: View-interleaved EPI on a commercial scanner. (abstract) In: Proceedings of the Society of Magnetic Resonance in Medicine Annual Meeting. 1989;832.
7. Miller DD, Holmvang G, Gill JB, et al: MRI detection of myocardial perfusion changes by gadolinium-DTPA infusion during dipyridamole hyperemia. *Magn Reson Med* 1989;10:246–255.
8. Pennell DJ, Underwood R, Longmore DB: Detection of coronary artery disease using MR imaging with dipyridamole infusion. *J Comput Assist Tomogr* 1990;14:167–170.
9. Frahmn J, Merboldt KD, Bruhm H, et al: 0.3-second FLASH MRI of the human heart. *Magn Reson Med* 1990;13:150–157.
10. Pykett IL, Rzedzian RR: Instant images of the body by magnetic resonance. *Magn Reson Med* 1987;5:563–571.
11. Souza SP, Roemer PB, St. Peters RL, et al: Echo planar imaging with a non-resonant gradient power system. (abstract). In: Proceedings of the Society of Magnetic Resonance in Medicine Annual Meeting 1991; 217.
12. Frahmn J, Haase A, Matthaei D, et al: Rapid NMR imaging using stimulated echoes. *J Magn Reson* 1985;65:130–135.
13. Stehling MK: Optimised (incremented) rf-angle gradient-echo imaging: ORANGE. (abstract) In: Proceedings of the Society of Magnetic Resonance in Medicine Annual Meeting. 1990; 459.

Chapter 14

Magnetic Resonance Strategies to Assess Regional Myocardial Perfusion and Function

Leon Axel, PhD, MD

Magnetic resonance imaging (MRI) has the potential to assess both regional myocardial perfusion and regional function. When both kinds of regional assessment are obtained at one imaging session, the results can be overlaid in a common functional image display. This could provide new kinds of information, eg, possibly distinguishing infarcted from potentially reversibly damaged muscle with diminished function, but preserved or restored perfusion. This chapter briefly reviews the principal strategies currently available for MRI assessment of regional perfusion and function, with the emphasis on principles rather than specific implementation or results.

Strategies for Perfusion Studies

Most methods for assessing perfusion rely on following the passage of a tracer substance (indicator) through the tissue after it is administered via the blood. This methodology, known as indication-dilution, is well developed for use with other measurement techniques.[1] While there are some specific considerations to be kept in mind when applying indication-dilution methods to MRI as described below, the basic principles are the same and are briefly reviewed.

The essence of the indicator-dilution approach to the assessment of perfusion is to follow the time course of the concentration of the tracer in the blood draining the tissue or in the tissue itself after a known administration of the tracer (input function) (Figure 1). We can think of three idealized types of tracers, although real tracer substances will generally have characteristics intermediate between them: intravascular, freely diffusible, and extracted. A purely intravascular tracer will remain within the intravascular compartment as it passes through the tissue and will move through

Supported by NIH Grant # 1R01-Hl 43014-01A1.
From Pohost GM (ed.), *Cardiovascular Applications of Magnetic Resonance.* Mount Kisco, NY, Futura Publishing Co., Inc., © 1993.

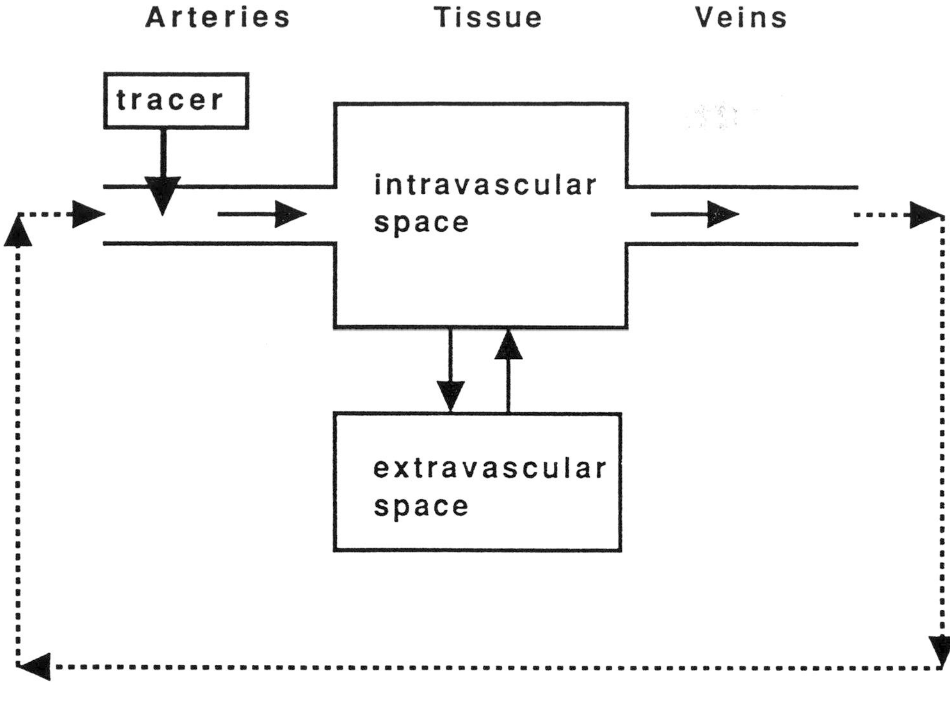

FIGURE 1. *Simple model of the transit of a tracer substance through tissue. After injection into the arteries (or further upstream), the tracer appears in the tissue capillaries. After possible exchange into the extravascular space it will be washed into the veins. After recirculation it may reappear in the arterial inflow to the tissue.*

the tissue rapidly. A freely diffusible tracer will freely move out of the vascular compartment as it passes through the tissue, mixing into the extravascular space, and will be washed out of the tissue more slowly than an intravascular tracer. Finally, an extracted tracer will leave the vessels and be "stuck" in the tissue and will have a relatively long residence in the tissue. The characteristic time for a tracer to transit through the tissue, the mean transit time (MTT), will depend on the ratio of the effective distribution volume of the tracer in the tissue to the blood flow through the tissue. If the MTT can be determined and the effective distribution volume in the tissue (V) is known or can also be determined, then the flow per unit volume of tissue (F) can be calculated as $F = V/MTT$. If the tracer is administered as an instantaneous bolus injection in the blood flowing into the tissue, the MTT can be found as the first moment (or centroid of the curve) of the function describing the concentration of tracer in the blood draining the tissue as a function of time after the injection. Rather than measuring the draining blood, in imaging studies it is often more convenient to measure the tracer remaining in the tissue, the "residue function." The MTT can be found as the area under the curve of the tissue concentration of tracer as a function of time after an instantaneous bolus injection, normalized to unity at the initial time.

In practice, the tracer cannot be administered as an ideal instantaneous bolus injection into the arterial inflow into the tissue. In addition to the finite duration of the injection itself, there will be further prolongation of the bolus and a delay between the administration in a site upstream and arrival at the tissue. This can be significant if the tissue relies on collateral blood supply. Injection of the tracer as an intravenous bolus will result in further prolongation of and delay in the arrival of the bolus at the tissue. Finally, recirculation of the tracer after a transit around the circulatory system will further distort the input function. The effect of a prolonged input of tracer into the tissue can be modeled by considering the input function as composed of a series of ideal bolus input functions of varying size. The tissue response (if the system is linear) is then found as a corresponding (superimposed) series of scaled ideal tissue response functions (Figure 2). Mathematically, this is described as the convolution of the actual input function with the ideal tissue impulse response. If both the actual input function and tissue response are known, then the ideal bolus tracer tissue transit can be calculated (at least, in principle) by the mathematical process of deconvolution.

(A)

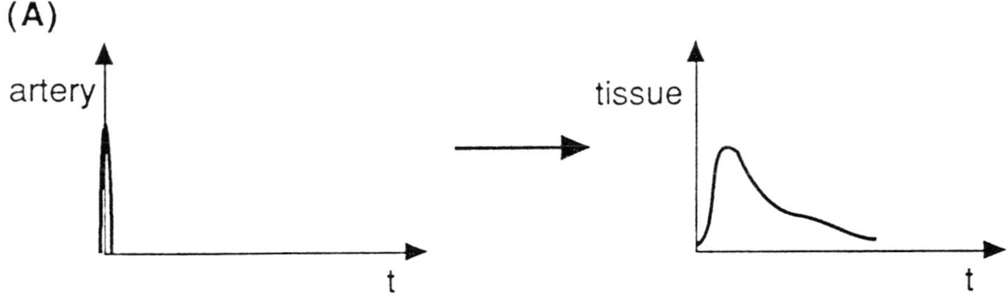

(B)

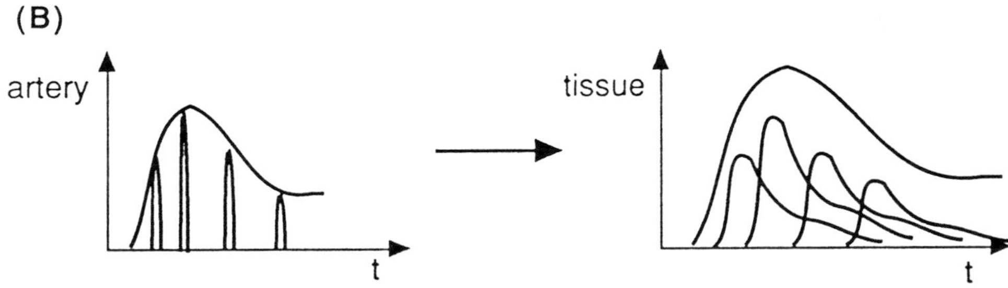

FIGURE 2. *Schematic model of the effect of a prolonged input of tracer on the observed transit through the tissue.* **A:** *With a bolus input to the tissue, the observed transit through the tissue (impulse response) is determined by the tissue blood volume, the flow rate, and any exchange with the extravascular space.* **B:** *With prolonged input to the tissue (eg, after intravenous administration), the observed transit will be correspondingly broadened. This can be modeled by considering the input as a series of boluses and the observed transit as a superimposition of their corresponding scaled and delayed impulse responses. This is equivalent to a mathematical convolution.*

In seeking to apply tracer methods for MRI measurements of perfusion, various additional difficulties can be encountered. The observed signal changes due to the passage of the tracer may not be simply related to the tracer concentration, but may depend on details of the imaging technique and the particular tracer used. The input function to the tissue, as derived from images of feeding blood vessels, may not be well defined, not only due to possible nonlinearity of the concentration–signal change relationship, but also due to possible volume averaging of the vessel with surrounding structures and possible delays and temporal blurring between the vessel measured and the tissue of interest. Imaging artifacts, eg, due to the changing signals caused by the tracer itself, may interfere with measurement of signal changes due to the tracer transit. In the analysis, the effective distribution volume of the tracer may not be well defined, eg, with partial extraction of tracer into the extravascular space during the transit through the tissue.

There are a variety of ways that tracers can induce signal changes in MRI and a variety of types of tracer agents that can be used. Many tracers, such as the contrast agents using gadolinium chelates, shorten both the T_1 and the T_2 relaxation times; the net effect on the observed signal will depend on the specific imaging techniques. Other agents, such as fine iron particles, produce very small-scale magnetic field gradients around themselves that can reduce the signal by shortening the effective T_2^*, particularly with gradient-echo imaging techniques. Such agents may also decrease the signal with conventional spin-echo imaging due to diffusion along these gradients. Note that paramagnetic agents, such as gadolinium chelates, may also create gradients around the vessels if they are confined largely to the intravascular space, with similar resulting effects on signal. Ferrite particles and large molecules will stay intravascular (although they may be rapidly cleared from the blood by the liver and reticuloendothelial system). Smaller molecules, such as gadolinium chelates, may initially be largely intravascular, but will generally rapidly mix into the extravascular, extracellular space. Water, either as ^2H_2O or $H_2{}^{17}O$ (which will shorten T_2), can serve as a freely diffusible tracer. Note that even though tracers may be restricted to the intravascular space, they may still affect the extravascular space, either through gradients around the vessels, as described above, or by exchange of water across the vessel walls.

In summary, there is much prior experience with the use of other kinds of tracer transit studies to measure perfusion that can be drawn on, but care must be taken in applying it to MRI.

Strategies for Function Studies

Conventional MRI, like other tomographic imaging techniques such as fast computed tomography, can provide three-dimensional analysis of global and regional wall motion. However, additional information on wall motion, such as nonradial components of wall motion or transmural differences in motion, can also be studied by exploiting the unique motion-sensitive aspects of MRI.

The tomographic nature of MRI, together with the good blood-tissue imaging contrast that MRI can provide, makes it possible to provide both global and some regional measurements of heart wall motion with conventional MRI.

The ability to trace the inner contour of the heart at multiple well-defined levels in space enables calculation of the volume of the heart. The change of the left ventricular volume during systole gives the stroke volume. The stroke volume multiplied by the heart rate gives cardiac output, and the ratio of the end-systolic and end-diastolic left ventricular volumes gives the ejection fraction, both useful measures of cardiac performance.

Measurement of regional motion is also possible, in principle, from the sucessive contours of the left ventricle. As with other cardiac imaging methods, however, there is the unresolved question of what to take as a reference point for the relative measurement of motion. In addition, there is uncertainty introduced by motion of the curved and roughly conical heart wall through the imaging plane, which can mimic motion within the plane.

The ability to define the inner and outer walls of the heart further permits measurement of wall thickening. This is a sensitive measure of function, as ischemia quickly leads to loss of contraction and thus of thickening. However, the "pull through" of the curved heart wall can again potentially cause problems with the measurement. In addition, subendocardial ischemia may result in a nontransmural loss of contraction that could be missed by a measurement of total wall thickness alone.

The additional MRI effects of heart wall motion that can be used to overcome some of the limitations of conventional MRI are the same as those used to study the flow of blood or cerebrospinal fluid: time-of-flight effects and phase shifts. In particular, the ability to create magnetic "tags" within the heart wall permits tracking the motion of individual regions of the heart wall by tracking the displacement of the corresponding visual tags.

Alternatively, the phase shifts produced by motion along magnetic field gradients permits following the velocity of different parts of the heart wall; the corresponding displacements can be found by integrating the velocities.

The production of magnetic tags within the heart wall can be done as a preliminary step triggered by the heartbeat, prior to conventional cardiac synchronized imaging, analogous to the inverting pulse used prior to image data acquisition in inversion recovery MRI. It is, in principle, straightforward to produce a tagging stripe by producing selective saturation of a slab of tissue oriented perpendicularly to the imaging plane.[2] However, it is inefficient to cover the heart in this way with a grid of tags. An alternative way to produce a grid of tags is with spatial modulation of magnetization (SPAMM), which uses nonselective radiofrequency pulses alternating with magnetic field gradient pulses.[3,4]

The measurement of heart wall velocity with phase shifts can be done just as for blood flow studies.[5] As in flow studies, a reference phase image must also be acquired in order to correct for phase shifts unrelated to motion. An alternative approach uses interference between a conventional spin echo and a stimulated echo with different motion sensitivity to combine the reference and motion-sensitized images.[6]

Having a map of displacements in the heart wall is useful by itself. However, analysis of the differential motion between adjacent regions, resulting in deformation or strain, is potentially even more useful.[7] By eliminating the need to choose a global reference frame, we can analyze the motion of each wall segment independently. The ability to study the transmural distribution of motion may enable the delineation of nontransmural dysfunction. The availability of new measures of heart wall motion may provide greater specificity of motion analysis. Preliminary results in normal subjects and patients with infarction or hypertrophy are encouraging.[8]

The large array of new measures of wall motion that MRI can provide leads to the need for efficiently created and easy to understand new displays. The recent development of new powerful and inexpensive computers makes this easier. The unique motion sensitive properties of MRI, together with its good blood-tissue contrast and spatial resolution and capability for three-dimensional imaging, make MRI a tool of great promise for the evaluation of cardiovascular function. In conjunction with measures of perfusion, MRI has the potential for an integrated examination of function and perfusion that could improve the ability to define areas of mismatch that may reflect potentially salvageable ischemic myocardium.

References

1. Lassen NA, Perl W: *Tracer Kinetic Methods in Medical Physiology*. New York, Raven Press, Publishers, 1979.
2. Zerhouni E, Parish WF, Yang A, et al: Human heart: tagging with MR imaging—a method for noninvasive assessment of myocardial motion. *Radiology* 1988;169:59–63.
3. Axel L, Dougherty L: MR imaging of motion with spatial modulation of magnetization. *Radiology* 1989;171:841–845.
4. Axel L, Dougherty L: Heart wall motion: improved method of spatial modulation of magnetization for MR imaging. *Radiology* 1989;172:349–350.
5. van Dijk P: Direct cardiac NMR imaging of heart wall and blood flow velocity. *J Comput Assist Tomogr* 1984;8:429–430.
6. Hennig J: Generalized MR interferography. *Magn Reson Med* 1990;16:390–402.
7. Axel L, Goņcalves R, Bloomgarden D: Two-dimensional analysis and functional imaging of regional heart wall motion with magnetic resonance imaging. *Radiology* 1992;183:745–750.
8. Clark NR, Reichek N, Bergey P, et al: Circumferential myocardial shortening in the normal human left ventricle: assessment by magnetic resonance imaging using spatial modulation of magnetization. *Circulation* 1991;84:67–74.

Chapter 15

New Approaches to the Assessment of Myocardial Function

Nathaniel Reichek, MD

Cardiac magnetic resonance imaging (MRI) is a promising investigative methodology for the assessment of myocardial function. While cardiac MRI does not currently play a major role in clinical research on myocardial function, over the next decade it is likely to do so. In part, this will reflect the well-documented ability of cardiac MRI to perform traditional volumetric analyses of ventricular function and planar analyses of endocardial motion and wall thickening in a reliable and noninvasive fashion.[1–6] However, even more important may be the recent development of a variety of methods for point tracking within the myocardium using MRI tissue tagging and several alternative methods.[7–11] Tissue-tagging methods have already played an important role in attracting recognition of the investigative value of cardiac MRI for local myocardial function. New and unique information on segmental myocardial performance in normal and diseased hearts has already emerged, both in experimental models and in humans. By comparison, conventional imaging methods for evaluation of segmental myocardial performance are far less informative, while other point tracking methods, such as sonomicrometry or roentgenographic tracking of implanted markers, are highly invasive.[12,13] This chapter surveys recent developments in the application of tissue tagging and related methods to the assessment of local myocardial function in normal and diseased hearts. Because the methods are new, much of the work has been published only in abstracts, which will necessarily be referenced herein.

The application of magnetic resonance tissue tagging using saturation planes orthogonal to the imaging plane was first described by Zerhourni and colleagues in 1988.[7] The original method used conventional preimaging saturation planes placed orthogonal to the imaging plane in a radial array centered on the center of the left

Supported in part by HL 42958; by a Focused Research Grant from the American Heart Association, Southeastern Pennsylvania Affiliate; and by a Commonwealth of Pennsylvania Health Services Contract for Cardiovascular Studies.
From Pohost GM (ed.), *Cardiovascular Applications of Magnetic Resonance*. Mount Kisco, NY, Futura Publishing Co., Inc., © 1993.

ventricular cavity (Figure 1). Electrocardiographic (ECG) gating of multiphase, multislice, compound oblique spin-echo images was required. Placement of the tags was relatively slow and asynchronous and provided only a relatively sparse set of tagged points, precluding a finely detailed analysis of intramyocardial motion. Axel and Dougherty[8] then applied spatial modulation of magnetization or SPAMM, a method they had previously evaluated for flow tracking, to the problem of myocardial point tracking in order to provide a denser, rectilinear matrix of tagged loci. Using ECG gating, SPAMM is produced over a 6-msec interval within a 13-msec interval between the electrographic QRS complex detection and acquisition of the first gated image in a spin-echo multiphase, multislice acquisition. Two sequences of nonselective radiofrequency pulses separated by magnetic field gradients are applied. In its most basic form, each sequence includes two radiofrequency pulses. The first turns some preexistent uniform longitudinal magnetization into transverse magnetization, initially all with the same phase. The gradient pulse "wraps" the transverse magnetization in the direction of the gradient, producing periodic spatial modulation of the phase. Modulated transverse magnetization is mixed with the longitudinal magnetization by the second radiofrequency pulse, resulting in modulated longitudinal magnetization. If the second radiofrequency pulse has the same flip angle as the first, then longitudinal magnetization returns to its initial value at the peaks of the modulation. The phase of the second radiofrequency pulse determines the relative phase of the spatial modulation pattern. The second sequence of radiofrequency pulses and gradients creates a similar effect orthogonal to the first sequence in three-dimensional space. The effect is to produce two orthogonal three-dimensional stacks of saturation planes perpendicular to the image plane. Within the image plane, this results in two orthogonal sets of in-plane saturation stripes of modulated magnetization (Figure 2).

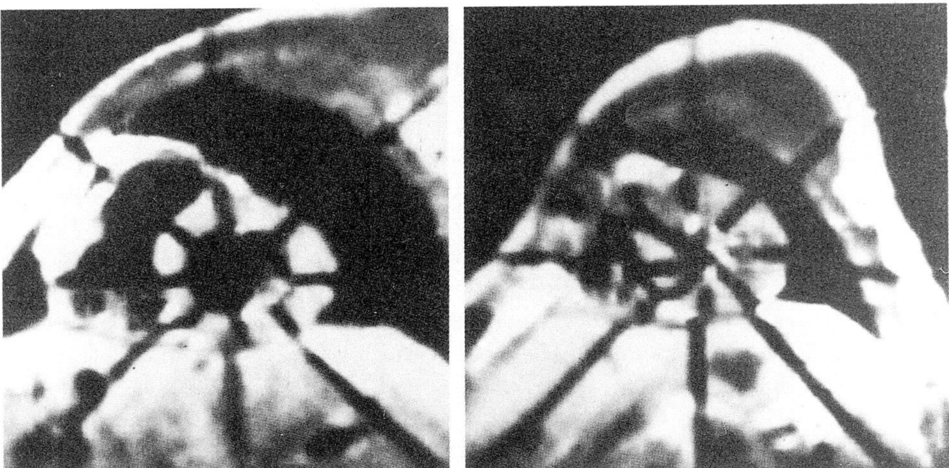

FIGURE 1. *Human end-systolic short-axis spin-echo images tagged with radial stripes. Basal* **(left)** *and apical* **(right)** *slices are shown. Myocardial stripes are not aligned with those outside the heart due to myocardial rotation and deformation. Rotation is counterclockwise on the apical slice relative to the basal slice. Reprinted from Reference 8 with permission.*

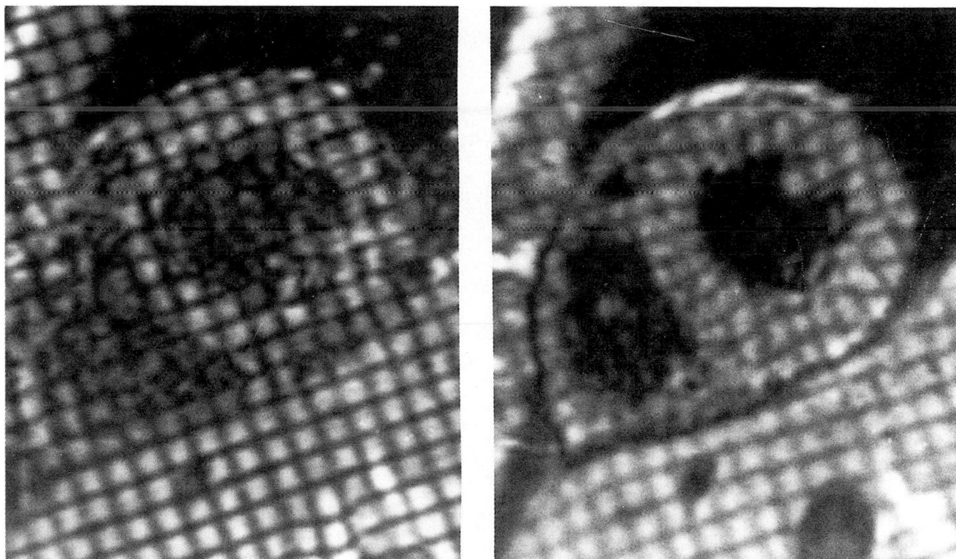

FIGURE 2. *Short-axis images using spatial modulation of magnetization (SPAMM) in normal human heart.* **Left:** *At end diastole, there is uniform stripe spacing at 7-mm intervals.* **Right:** *At end systole, chest wall stripes have not moved. However, stripes in myocardium have moved and are deformed. There is reduced separation of stripes perpendicular to the endocardium, as compared with end diastole, due to circumferential myocardial shortening. Such stripes converge at the endocardium, where circumferential shortening is maximal. Reprinted from Reference 19 with permission.*

The flip angle determines the extent of initial modulation of the magnetization, while the wrap gradient direction determines stripe orientation. The strength and duration of the wrap gradient is inversely proportional to stripe separation on the initial image.

Stripes move with myocardial motion during the cardiac cycle since they are caused by saturation of protons within the tissue. Imaging plane and the angular direction of stripes within the imaging plane can be varied as desired. Sharper-edged stripes are produced by using binomial pulse sequences.[9] The original pixel matrix used is $128(y)$ by $256(x)$, later interpolated to 256×256. Therefore, in order to obtain uniform resolution, orthogonal sets of black stripes are typically deposited along axes at 45° to the x and y image axes. The use of a pulse-sequence optimization approach can further enhance stripe sharpness.[14] Spacing of stripes can be specified at any value, independent of pixel matrix size and resultant resolution, but as a practical matter, the most useful spacing with 24-cm field of view is 7 mm or more center-to-center. Stripes fade over time due to T_1 relaxation, and respiratory motion also contributes to stripe degradation. If stripes do not persist to end systole, additional signal averaging may improve persistence. In addition, a second temporally overlapped acquisition on the same slices, with a delay in stripe deposition and imaging after electrographic QRS complex detection, may be used to reach end systole if needed. Stripes are further optimized if a 130° flip angle and flow compensation are used.

A typical ECG-gated multiphase, multislice spin-echo acquisition consists of five

5-mm-thick short-axis slices at five time points from beginning to end systole. This would take 16 minutes to acquire at a heart rate of 80 beats per minute, with one signal average. To time end systole, a single-slice cine MRI acquisition through the left ventricle and mitral valve plane is obtained before SPAMM imaging, with end systole defined as time of appearance of the smallest left ventricular cavity area. Spatial modulation of magnetization tissue tagging can also be applied with cine MRI, a retrospectively gated gradient-echo technique, and with echo-planar cardiac imaging.[15–17] Using cine MRI, only two or three slices can be simultaneously imaged, but enhanced stripe persistence and more time points over the entire cardiac cycle are gained. For three-dimensional point tracking, imaging can be performed in two orthogonal planes.

Tissue tagging permits tracking of fixed points within the myocardium over systole and early diastole, or with cine MRI or echo-planar MRI over the entire cardiac cycle. This allows analysis of myocardial motion at a given locus in one, two, or three dimensions. Thus, in-plane translational effects, transmural nonuniformity of myocardial function across the ventricular wall, and through-plane motion can be evaluated. Because tissue tagging is a unique capability of MRI, initial applications have stimulated much interest in the method. Until now, point tracking within the myocardium has been accomplished using surgical implantation of either sonomicrometry crystals or roentgenographic metallic markers within the myocardium.[12,13] Such methods are rarely suitable for application in humans, but quite useful in experimental animal models. Even in animal models, however, sonomicrometry and implanted markers cannot replicate the point-tracking density that can be achieved with MRI tissue tagging. Furthermore, the potential effects of local tissue trauma and tethering by sonomicrometry leads might alter the normal myocardial deformation pattern.

A variety of analytic approaches has been applied to tissue-tagging data. Data can be assessed using one-dimensional, two-dimensional, and three-dimensional approaches. Using SPAMM tagging, one-dimensional analysis can determine changes in stripe separation between adjacent pairs of parallel stripes or adjacent intersections of pairs of orthogonal stripes.[18] This approach is helpful for determination of circumferential segment shortening on images obtained in the short-axis plane. When applied to pairs of parallel stripes, it is best used where stripes are normal to the endocardium at end diastole. Using stripe analysis routines in the Volumetric Image Display and Analysis (VIDA™, University of Pennsylvania, Philadelphia, Pa) image analysis software package, the 0.9375×0.9375-mm SPAMM MRI image pixels are interpolated to 10^5 mm. The stripe separation measurement is readily made by displaying the image intensity profile along an operator-defined line perpendicular to the stripe pair interrogated (Figure 3). Because a trough in intensity exists at the center of dark stripes, the trough locations are readily identified in this fashion and stripe separation can be calculated. Stripe intersections forming a line parallel to the endocardium at end diastole can also be used to determine segment shortening using similar methods. These measurements can be made at the subendocardium, midwall, and subepicardium at a given location on the ventricular wall. Longitudinal shortening is determined in a similar fashion on long-axis images.

For two-dimensional analysis of myocardial motion and deformation from SPAMM data, several alternative approaches are feasible. First, small local elements

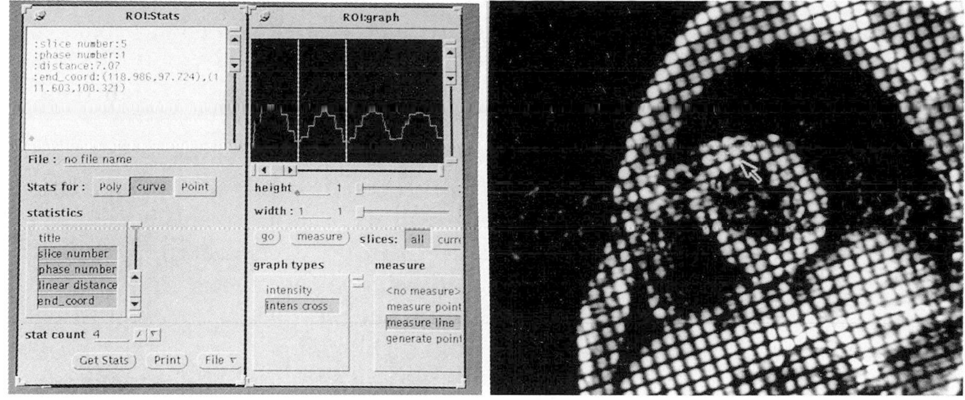

FIGURE 3. Left panel: *Digital display of signal brightness profile along a user-defined line normal to a row of stripes. At the nadirs of signal intensity on two adjacent dark stripes, cursors have been placed. Stripe separation is calculated in pixels.* **Right panel:** *Arrow denotes the myocardial region in which the line displayed in left panel was drawn. The line itself is located in the second set of stripes from endocardium to epicardium, parallel to the endocardium, and is itself perpendicular to stripes that are perpendicular to endocardium at end diastole. Changes in stripe separation from end diastole to end systole represent circumferential shortening. Reprinted from Reference 19 with permission.*

defined by stripe intersections or by all of the points along the bounding stripes can be evaluated. Thus, eg, triangular elements of myocardium can be defined by three adjacent stripe intersections at end diastole and sequentially identified over systole. From these data, in-plane principle strains and their direction and element rotation can be determined using the polar decomposition theorem.[19] In addition, in-plane translation of the centroid of each element can be determined. Alternatively, it may be more desirable to evaluate deformation in large elements for some applications. Because those strains determined in discrete small elements may have substantial statistical scatter, the determination of strain fields of large regions of the heart may have advantages.

The effect of through-plane motion on one- and two-dimensional analysis of SPAMM data must also be considered. In the short-axis plane, the myocardium evaluated at end systole was not in the image plane at end diastole, but is pulled into the image plane by systolic long-axis shortening. At first glance, this would imply that only three-dimensional analyses of deformation would have any validity. However, SPAMM stripes are laid down as symmetrical, uniformly spaced sets of saturation planes. They consist of two sets of such planes, orthogonal to each other and to the image plane. Because they are orthogonal to the image plane, stripe location and separation are constant throughout the myocardial volume at end diastole. Therefore, in a one-dimensional analysis, the initial stripe separation is uniform in all slices and the difference between that distance and the measured end-systolic stripe separation on a slice that is in-plane at end systole truly reflects myocardial shortening at that site. This is the case even if the end-systolic image depicts myocardium that was not in the image plane at end diastole. An analogous situation exists for in-plane strains and translation from two-dimensional analysis of small myocardial elements. To more directly eliminate the effect of through-plane motion, three-dimensional strains can be derived from multiplanar image sets.[19]

For the radial stripe approach, as developed by the Hopkins group, emphasis has been placed on myocardial "twist" and wall thickening. "Twist," or in-plane rotation of stripes, and differences in twist, or shear, between endocardium and epicardium and between basal and apical short-axis slices can readily be characterized with this approach.[20] The measurement incorporates both rotation and myocardial shortening, but increases with enhanced inotropic state. For wall thickening, a three-dimensional element approach has been developed to correct for obliquity of the image plane to the wall and for through-plane motion.[21] For full three-dimensional analysis, the short-axis radial stripes are used in combination with long-axis imaging with parallel stripes. Long-axis stripes are positioned to match radial stripe locations in the short axis, so that myocardial elements are defined by the intersections of radial and long-axis stripes.[22] Three-dimensional deformation can then be determined.

Applications of tagging methods are beginning to make important contributions to analysis of local myocardial function in the normal heart. In normal human left ventricle, we have used SPAMM tagging and one-dimensional analysis of circumferential and longitudinal segment shortening.[18,23] These studies have shown that short-axis circumferential shortening is maximal in the subendocardium, where shortening exceeds subepicardial shortening by a ratio of 2:1 (Figures 2 and 4).[18] There is also a long-axis gradient in circumferential shortening such that shortening normally is greater on more apical than more basal short-axis slices (Figure 5). The long-axis gradient is mainly present in the inferior wall and is not found in the anterior wall, lateral wall, or interventricular septum in humans. With respect to longitudinal shortening, a transmural gradient is found in the left ventricular free wall, but not the interventricular septum.[23] A long-axis gradient in longitudinal shortening also exists, with shortening maximal at the base. Thus, this gradient is opposite that found for circumferential shortening. It is noteworthy that gradients in shortening do not necessarily parallel fiber orientation. For example, in the circumferential plane the largest proportion of circumferential fibers is found in the midwall in canine heart,[24] while maximal circumferential shortening is found in the subendocardium in both canine and human hearts.[18,25] The physical basis for this apparent "cross-fiber shortening" remains to be elucidated.

In normal hearts, using radial stripes, left ventricular short-axis twist (viewed from the apex) is clockwise at the base and counterclockwise at the apex.[20] Similar observations have been made using SPAMM MRI, and it has also been shown that the left ventricular apex is essentially fixed in spatial location in systole, while both atrioventricular valve planes move toward the apex.[26] Because myocardial shortening is load dependent, it becomes important to evaluate effects of load alteration on normal segmental myocardial function. We have evaluated pharmacologic increases (phenylephrine) and decreases (nitroprusside) in afterload in normal canine left ventricle.[25,27] As expected, overall shortening fell with increased afterload and rose with decreased afterload. There was no change in the transmural gradient in shortening from endocardium to epicardium. However, regional heterogeneity of circumferential shortening did change in both long-axis and short-axis distribution. Thus, the long-

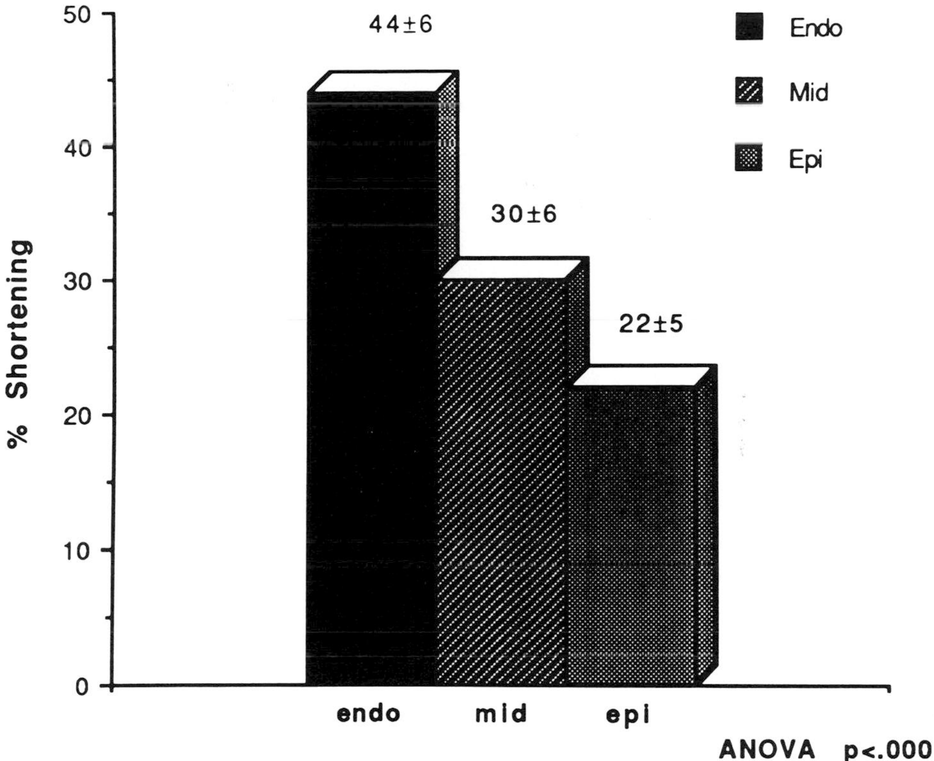

FIGURE 4. *Mean circumferential segment shortening in normal humans. Endocardial (endo), midwall (mid), and epicardial (epi) shortening are shown. A significant transmural gradient in shortening is found, with maximal shortening at the endocardium. Reprinted from Reference 19 with permission.*

axis gradient in circumferential shortening was abolished with increased or decreased afterload. Further, septal shortening increased markedly relative to other regions with afterload reduction. Moreover, under basal conditions the long-axis gradient in circumferential shortening parallels an inverse gradient in geometric determinants of ventricular wall stress. However, under increased or decreased load, this shortening gradient is abolished.[27]

Normal values for two-dimensional principle strains in normal human left ventricle have been developed by Axel et al.[19] They have also shown that the area of subendocardial myocardial elements is not constant over the cardiac cycle, as it would be if myocardial volume were constant. Rather, it falls significantly from end diastole to end systole. This probably reflects systolic reduction of subendocardial intramyocardial blood volume. One would hypothesize that such a change in blood volume might be abolished with ischemia.

In human hypertensive left ventricular hypertrophy with normal left ventricular ejection fraction, we have observed reduced circumferential and longitudinal shortening throughout the left ventricle.[23,28] Thus, intramural shortening appears to be more sensitive to altered myocardial function than is ejection fraction. The combination of

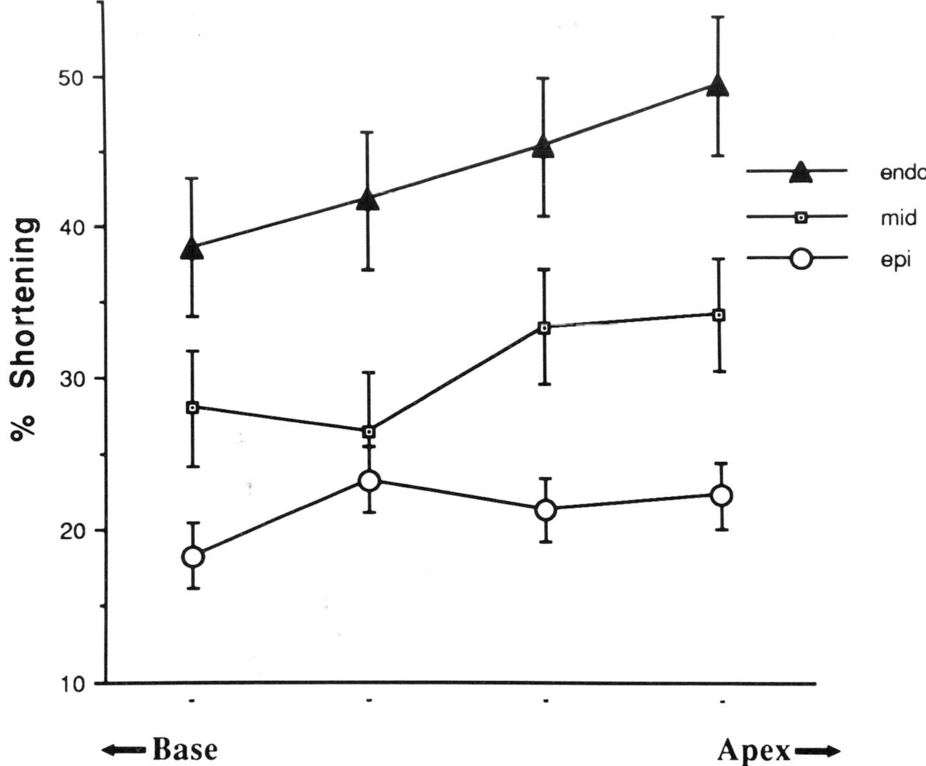

FIGURE 5. *Long-axis gradient in circumferential shortening from base to apex at endocardium, midwall, and epicardium. There is greater shortening at midwall ($p<0.05$) and at endocardium ($p<0.01$) on more apical slices. Reprinted from Reference 19 with permission.*

reduced intramural segment shortening with normal chamber pump function may at first seem counterintuitive. It may be possible only because absolute wall thickness is increased in such hearts. Thus, wall thickening, endocardial excursion, and resultant chamber emptying may remain normal despite less shortening per unit of myocardium. The basic mechanism of reduced segmental shortening in this setting remains undefined. Similar changes have been reported in abnormal myocardial regions in hypertrophic cardiomyopathy.[29]

Preliminary results of qualitative image analyses suggest that myocardial infarction, including nontransmural infarction, causes reduced segment shortening that is readily apparent using SPAMM MRI.[30] The potential ability to localize nontransmural infarction may prove particularly useful because existing clinical methods often show limited sensitivity in this setting. However, it is not practical to perform prolonged MRI studies in patients with acute infarction. Thus, full development of more rapid, real-time echo-planar imaging will likely be required to make magnetic resonance tissue tagging a useful tool for either large-scale clinical investigation or actual clinical use in that clinical setting.

Both infarction and myocardial stunning in animal models abolish circumferential shortening by myocardial tissue tagging.[31,32] In experimental acute infarction, similar reductions in function are found in portions of the ischemic zone showing actual diastolic thinning and in those that do not.[33] Such observations make it unlikely that, even with tissue-tagging methods, it will be possible to discriminate among infarction, stunning, and persistent ischemia using analyses of mechanical deformation alone. However, the combined use of contrast imaging and tissue tagging may distinguish infarcted or profoundly ischemic myocardium, characterized by loss of both contrast effect and mechanical deformation from stunned or less severely ischemic myocardium, characterized by loss of mechanical function with preserved contrast effect.[32,34] In chronic infarction, two-dimensional strain analysis of large apical infarction in an ovine model has been described.[35,36] Results indicate that at 1 week both magnitude and direction of principle strains are altered in the infarct region, consistent with passive circumferential stretching. Cyclical changes in the myocardial element area are diminished, which may reflect reduced local blood content due to diminished perfusion. Analogous changes are found in two-dimensional strain and one-dimensional segment shortening. Passive in-plane translation of myocardial elements was reduced as much as active deformation in the infarct region. Thus, it appears that tethering of the infarct to normally functioning myocardium does not produce appreciable passive motion in this model.

Validation of myocardial function analyses by MRI tissue tagging has been obtained in several studies by comparison with sonomicrometry. While sonomicrometry is a real-time method, conventional tagging sequences construct images from data acquired on hundreds of cardiac cycles. Lima et al.,[37] using the Zerhouni radial tag approach, demonstrated excellent correlation between sonomicrometry wall thickening and tagged MRI wall thickening by a three-dimensional analysis method in normal and ischemic myocardium. However, wall thickening was greater by MRI tagging than by sonomicrometry. In a comparison of SPAMM MRI tagging and sonomicrometry for circumferential segment shortening in normal and infarcted myocardium, excellent correlations were also found.[33,38] Again, however, shortening was greater by MRI than by sonomicrometry. Both studies indicated that tagged MRI distinguishes between normal and ischemic myocardium as effectively as sonomicrometry. Because myocardial tagging and sonomicrometry did not measure function on identical tissue in either study, it is unclear whether the systematic differences shown, which occur mainly in normal myocardium, are differences in method or in measurement location. One possibility is that local tissue injury and tethering occurs with sonomicrometry crystal implantation.

In addition to tissue tagging, several alternative MRI approaches to point tracking in myocardium have been proposed. The hope has been to overcome some of the limitations imposed by current pixel size and stripe fading due to T_1 relaxation and respiratory motion. Thus, magnetic resonance interferography has been used for tracking of velocity and acceleration within the myocardium.[10] With this method, contrast is not reduced by longitudinal relaxation as the cardiac cycle proceeds, but temporal resolution is worse than with tagging techniques. An innovative approach has been developed by Pelc[11] that uses gradient-echo phase contrast to determine myocardial velocity in two or three dimensions. Serial imaging over the cardiac cycle can then be used, by integrating myocardial velocity over time, to track the motion of fixed points in the myocardium. Again, T_1 relaxation effects are not limiting. The method is also free of the resolution-related limitations on tag spacing found with tissue tagging. However, a significant number of pixels must be averaged to obtain statistically reliable velocity data. Thus, effective spatial resolution may not exceed that of the SPAMM method. Moreover, through-plane motion may be a problem. Validation data for interferometry and velocity-tracking approaches have not yet been reported.

Thus, while most of the work discussed has not yet been published in full form, preliminary reports strongly indicate that MRI tissue tagging and similar methods have the potential to provide valuable new noninvasive approaches to the understanding of myocardial function in health and disease. With the wider availability of ultrafast and real-time MRI strategies, all of which are compatible with tissue tagging, the full impact of these methods should be realized.

References

1. Utz JA, Herfkens RJ, Heinsimer JA, et al: Cine MR determination of left ventricular ejection fraction. *AJR* 1987;149:839.
2. Markiewicz W, Sechtem U, Kirby R, et al: Measurement of ventricular volumes in the dog by nuclear magnetic resonance imaging. *J Am Coll Cardiol* 1987;10:170–177.
3. Buser PT, Auffermann W, Holt WW, et al: Noninvasive evaluation of global left ventricular function with use of cine nuclear magnetic resonance. *J Am Coll Cardiol* 1989;13:6.
4. Cranney GB, Lotan CS, Dean L, et al: Left ventricular volume estimation using intrinsic axis cine NMR: validation by calibrated ventricular angiography (abstract). *Circulation* 1988;78(suppl II):II431.
5. Blackwell GG, Dell'Italia LJ, Pearce DJ, et al: A new method for investigating the left ventricular pressure-volume relationship in an intact animal model using high-fidelity left ventricular pressure and cine NMR. (abstract) In: Proceedings of the Society of Magnetic Resonance in Medicine 9th Annual Scientific Meeting. 1990, 291.
6. Auffermann W, Wagner S, Holt WW, et al: Noninvasive determination of left ventricular output and wall stress in volume overload and in myocardial disease by cine magnetic resonance imaging. *Am Heart J* 1991;121:1750–1758.
7. Zerhourni EA, Parish DM, Rogers WJ, et al: Human heart tagging with MR imaging: a method for noninvasive assessment of myocardial motion. *Radiology* 1988;169:59–63.
8. Axel L, Dougherty L: MR imaging of motion with spatial modulation of magnetization. *Radiology* 1989;171:841–845.
9. Axel L, Dougherty L: Heart wall motion: improved method of spatial modulation of magnetization for MR imaging. *Radiology* 1989;172:349–350.
10. Hennig J, Krause T, Schopp D: The examination of heart wall motion in patients with transmural infarction by MR-interferography: a comparison of velocity measurement vs. acceleration measurements. (abstract) In: Proceedings of the Society of Magnetic Resonance in Medicine 10th Annual Scientific Meeting. 1991, 18.
11. Pelc NJ: Myocardial motion analysis with phase contrast MRI. (abstract) In: Proceedings of the Society of Magnetic Resonance in Medicine 10th Annual Scientific Meeting. 1991, 17.
12. Sasayama S, Franklin D, Ross J Jr, et al: Dynamic changes in left ventricular wall thickness and their use in analyzing cardiac function in the conscious dog. *Am J Cardiol* 1976;38:870.
13. Florenzano F, Glantz SA: Left ventricular mechanical adaptation to chronic aortic regurgitation in intact dogs. *Am J Physiol* 1987;252:H969.
14. Shinnar M, Bolinger L, Leigh J: The use of finite impulse response filters in pulse design. *Magn Reson Med* 1989;12:81–87.
15. Axel L, Dougherty L: Cine spatial modulation of magnetization imaging of heart wall motion. *Radiology* 1989;173:246-249.

16. Stehling MJ, Howseman AM, Ordidge RJ, et al: Whole body echo-planar MR imaging. *Radiology* 1989;170:257.
17. Blackband SJ, Chatham JC, Forder J, et al: Cardiac tagging and echo planar imaging. Application to the isolated perfused rabbit heart at 4.7 T. (abstract) In: Proceedings of the Society of Magnetic Resonance in Medicine 10th Annual Scientific Meeting. 1991:15.
18. Clark NR, Reichek N, Bergey P, et al: Circumferential myocardial shortening in the normal human left ventricle. Assessment by magnetic resonance imaging using spatial modulation of magnetization. *Circulation* 1991;84:67–74.
19. Axel L, Bloomgarden D, Chang CN, et al: MRI of normal regional heart wall motion. (abstract) In: Proceedings of the Society of Magnetic Resonance in Medicine 10th Annual Scientific Meeting. 1991:13.
20. Buchalter MB, Weiss JL, Rogers WJ, et al: Noninvasive quantification of left ventricular rotational deformation in normal humans using magnetic resonance imaging myocardial tagging. *Circulation* 1990;81:1236–1244.
21. Beyar R, Shapiro EP, Graves WL, et al: Quantification and validation of left ventricular wall thickening by a three-dimensional volume element magnetic resonance imaging approach. *Circulation* 1990;81:297–307.
22. Moore C, O'Dell W, McVeigh E, et al: Three dimensional myocardial strains in humans using bi-planar tagged MRI. (abstract) In: Proceedings of the Society of Magnetic Resonance in Medicine 10th Annual Scientific Meeting. 1991:14.
23. Palmon LC, Reichek N, Clark NR, et al: Long axis myocardial shortening in hypertensive left ventricular hypertrophy. (abstract) *Circulation* 1991;84(suppl II):II371.
24. Streeter DD Jr, Spotnitz HM, Patel DJ, et al: Fiber orientation in the canine left ventricle during diastole and systole. *Circ Res* 1969;24:339.
25. Palmon L, Reichek N, Tallant B, et al: Segmental circumferential myocardial function afterload alteration using magnetic resonance tissue tagging. (abstract) In: Proceedings of the Society of Magnetic Resonance in Medicine 10th Annual Scientific Meeting. 1991:19.
26. Hoffman EA, Rumberger J, Dougherty L, et al: A geometric view of cardiac "efficiency." *J Am Coll Cardiol* 1989;13(2):86A.
27. Palmon LC, Reichek N, Tallant B, et al: Heterogeneity of segment shortening in normal left ventricle: effects of load alteration. *Circulation* 1991;84(suppl II):II669.
28. Palmon LC, Reichek N, Yeon SB, et al: Abnormal segmental function in "compensated" concentric left ventricular hypertrophy. *Circulation* 1990;82(suppl IV):IV123.
29. Maier SE, Fischer SE, McKinnon G, et al: Evaluation of left ventricular segmental wall motion in normals and hypertrophic cardiomyopathies with MR tagging. (abstract) In: Proceedings of the Society of Magnetic Resonance in Medicine 10th Annual Scientific Meeting. 1991:167.
30. Clark NR, Reichek N, Bergey P, et al: Segment function in myocardial infarction. *Circulation* 1989;80(suppl II):II108.
31. Yeon SB, Reichek N, Palmon LC, et al: Myocardial segment shortening in canine myocardial infarction using spatial modulation of magnetization and sonomicrometry. (abstract) In: Proceedings of the Society of Magnetic Resonance in Medicine 9th Annual Scientific Meeting. 1990:270.
32. Clark NR, Tallant B, Palmon LC, et al: Segmental myocardial dysfunction in a canine model of "stunned myocardium" as depicted using spatial modulation of magnetization. (abstract) In: Proceedings of the Society of Magnetic Resonance in Medicine 10th Annual Scientific Meeting. 1991:862.
33. Yeon SB, Reichek N, Palmon LC, et al: Segmental shortening by magnetic resonance tagging in experimental myocardial infarction. *Circulation* 1990;82(suppl III):III763.
34. Yeon SB, Reichek N, Tallant B, et al: Imaging function and perfusion defects in myocardial infarction using magnetic resonance tagging and iron oxide contrast. (abstract) In: Proceedings of the Society of Magnetic Resonance in Medicine 10th Annual Scientific Meeting. 1991:371.
35. Lima J, Reichek N, Ferrari V, et al: Two-dimensional systolic deformation of infarcted myocardium by magnetic resonance with tissue tagging. *Circulation* 1991;84(suppl II):II670.

36. Lima J, Ferrari V, Palmon LC, et al: Myocardial rigid body translation with rotation by magnetic resonance tissue tagging before and after infarction. *Circulation* 1991;84(suppl II):II84.
37. Lima J, Jeremy R, Guier WH, et al: Accurate systolic thickening by 3-D MRI: correlation with sonomicrometers in normal and ischemic myocardium. *Circulation* 1990;82(suppl III):III762.
38. Yeon SB, Reichek N, Palmon LC, et al: Validation of circumferential segment shortening by magnetic resonance tagging. *Circulation* 1990;82(suppl III):III124.

Chapter 16

Magnetic Resonance Angiography and Quantitative Velocity Measurement

Charles L. Dumoulin, PhD

A rapidly growing specialty within the field of magnetic resonance imaging (MRI) is magnetic resonance angiography (MRA). This submodality exploits the properties of moving blood during magnetic resonance image acquisition. Magnetic resonance angiography is actually a collection of techniques, each having unique characteristics and each appropriate for addressing different clinical problems.

The earliest acceptance of MRA in the diagnosis and staging of vascular diseases occurred for applications in the brain and extracranial carotid arteries.[1–5] Neurovascular applications of MRA have grown during the past few years as the rapid pace of research has produced a variety of new techniques and instrumentation. Today, in many hospitals, MRA is used routinely as a screening test prior to x-ray angiography to assess carotid artery stenosis, as well as intercranial aneurysms, arteriovenous malformations, and vascular occlusions. In other clinical facilities, MRA has begun to replace x-ray angiography procedures for some applications. Magnetic resonance angiography of the intracranial arterial and venous circulation is the prototype for MRA of the peripheral arterial and venous circulation of the extremities, but differences in anatomy and blood flow physiology have necessitated the development of new methods specifically tailored to these new applications. To date, no MRA methods have been demonstrated to be viable for diagnostic coronary artery imaging, although work in this area is continuing.

Magnetic resonance angiography is not a single technique. Rather, it is a collection of methods, each having some unique features and limitations. Because of the relative strengths and weaknesses of each method and the complicated nature of blood flow in the body, different clinical applications are best served by different imaging protocols. In general, two broad classes of MRA are defined by the fundamental phenomena that give contrast in each case: 1) time-of-flight methods in which movement of longitudinal magnetization is detected; and 2) phase-sensitive

From Pohost GM (ed.), *Cardiovascular Applications of Magnetic Resonance.* Mount Kisco, NY, Futura Publishing Co., Inc., © 1993.

methods in which phase shifts induced by movement of transverse magnetization in the presence of a field gradient are detected. Many variations of both types of MRA have been described. Only a few of these, however, are widely used. These methods are described below.

Time-of-Flight Magnetic Resonance Angiography

In time-of-flight MRA, the contrast between blood and stationary tissue is determined by the inflow of unsaturated spins into the imaging volume and the saturation of stationary tissue in that same volume. Two methods are currently in use: three-dimensional time-of-flight (3D-TOF)[6,7] and two-dimensional time-of-flight (2D-TOF)[8] angiography. A new method, multislab three-dimensional time-of-flight angiography,[9] combines the best aspects of the two- and three-dimensional methods.

With 3D-TOF MRA, a three-dimensional image is acquired in a single scan as shown in Figure 1. A limited volume closely matched to the acquired field of view is excited by the radiofrequency pulses. This excitation volume is typically several centimeters thick. Blood from outside the excited volume enters the volume and initially gives a strong signal. Rapidly flowing unsaturated blood penetrates deeply into the volume and may traverse it entirely if the vessel is relatively straight. Slowly moving blood, however, is easily saturated and quickly becomes invisible in the angiogram. Blood flowing in tortuous vessels is forced to spend substantial time in the imaging volume and is also at risk of becoming saturated.

The choice of imaging parameters with 3D-TOF angiography is a compromise between the need to have strong blood signals in the volume of interest and the need to suppress the background as well as possible. The penetration problem in 3D-TOF procedures can be lessened by decreasing the acquisition volume. This is accomplished in the 2D-TOF procedure by acquiring data in thin planes perpendicular to the blood vessel as shown in Figure 2. Data from each plane is collected in a single scan. Additional planes are acquired on subsequent scans until a full three-dimensional matrix is obtained. Note that here the term "two-dimensional" refers to a single scan and not to the final data matrix.

Two-dimensional time-of-flight procedures are much more sensitive to slow flow than 3D-TOF procedures because of the decreased sensitivity to the penetration effect. An additional benefit is that the flip angle can be increased to more efficiently saturate the stationary tissue. Furthermore, increasing the field of view in the slice direction carries no penalty and long vessels are relatively straightforward to image. While 2D-TOF methods are much less sensitive to penetration effects than 3D-TOF methods, blood flow in vessels lying in the plane of data acquisition can be more difficult to image because of the more aggressive use of saturation.

Gradient and radiofrequency power limitations make the excitation of a slice that is thinner than 2.0 mm difficult. Consequently, 2D-TOF procedures typically have poorer resolution in the slice dimension than 3D-TOF procedures. Fortunately, this is rarely a problem for applications in the lower extremities, the neck, and the abdomen.

The primary shortcoming of 3D-TOF procedures is the penetration problem experienced by slowly moving blood. The primary shortcoming of 2D-TOF proce-

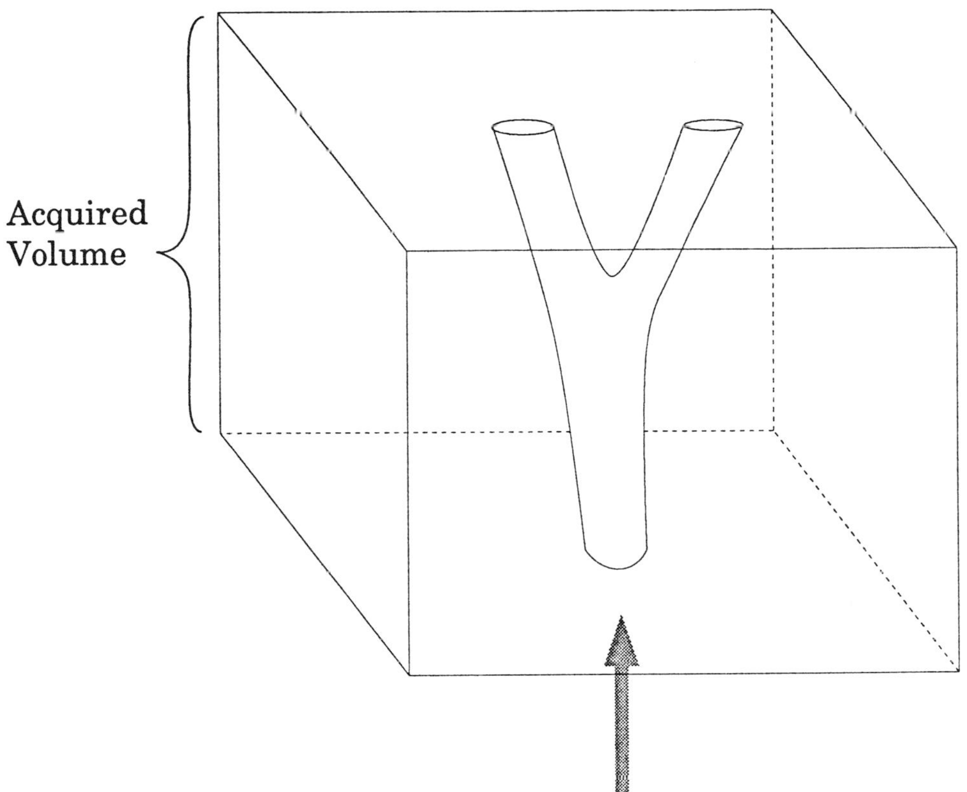

FIGURE 1. *Geometry of a typical three-dimensional time-of-flight procedure. In this procedure the entire volume of interest is subjected to the radiofrequency pulses and a full three-dimensional image is acquired. The frequent radiofrequency pulses cause the entire region to reach a state of partial saturation. Consequently, the saturated magnetization gives only a weak signal. Blood flowing into the region, on the other hand, has not experienced the radiofrequency pulses and is in a fully relaxed state. This causes the blood to give a relatively strong signal. Unfortunately, once the blood has experienced several radiofrequency pulses, it too becomes saturated and contrast between blood and the surrounding tissue is lost.*

dures (at least in neurovascular procedures) is the limited resolution in the third dimension. A hybrid technique (Figure 3) overcomes both problems by stacking adjacent volumes of 3D-TOF data. This technique is relatively new, but appears promising for neurovascular work. The potential for applications to the lower extremities is less certain, but worth investigating.

There are several important aspects of inflow-enhanced angiography. The first is that the blood is fully relaxed only before it reaches the region of interest. Once the blood is in the region of interest it is subjected to the same saturation effects that suppress the

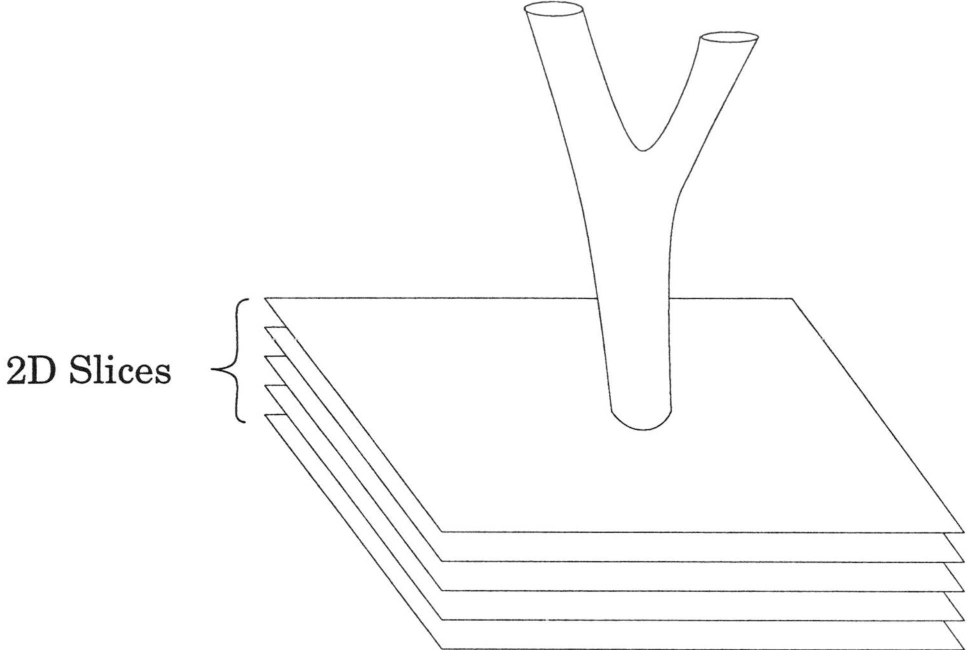

FIGURE 2. *Geometry of a typical two-dimensional time-of-flight procedure. In this procedure only the tissue in a thin slice is excited by the radiofrequency pulses. Consequently, the saturation region is limited to the slice. Blood entering the slice is not saturated and appears bright. A three-dimensional angiogram is generated by sequentially acquiring the slices until a full three-dimensional matrix is collected. Since the saturation region in this technique is much smaller than it is for a three-dimensional time-of-flight procedure, penetration of fully relaxed blood is more efficient and the contrast between blood and surrounding tissue is usually better. Image resolution in the third (ie, vertical) dimension, however, is usually less than with true three-dimensional methods due to instrument limitations.*

signals from the surrounding tissue. The blood loses its contrast after it experiences several radiofrequency pulses. Consequently, the penetration of detectable blood into the region of interest is limited by the velocity of the blood, the repetition rate of the radiofrequency pulses, the flip angle of the radiofrequency pulses, and the T_1 of blood.

The contrast mechanism of inflow-enhanced angiography is not flow. Rather, it is the different levels of saturation that can be obtained between flowing and nonflowing tissue. A compromise must be made to maximize the signal from blood and minimize the signal from the surrounding tissue. Consequently, surrounding tissue is difficult to fully suppress since the steps taken to suppress the tissue also act to limit the penetration of visible blood into the region of interest.

If all tissue in the body had the same T_1, the contrast generated by inflow effects would be unambiguous. Unfortunately, tissues having a short T_1 can appear artifactually bright in these images. For example, thrombus and mucus can appear isointense

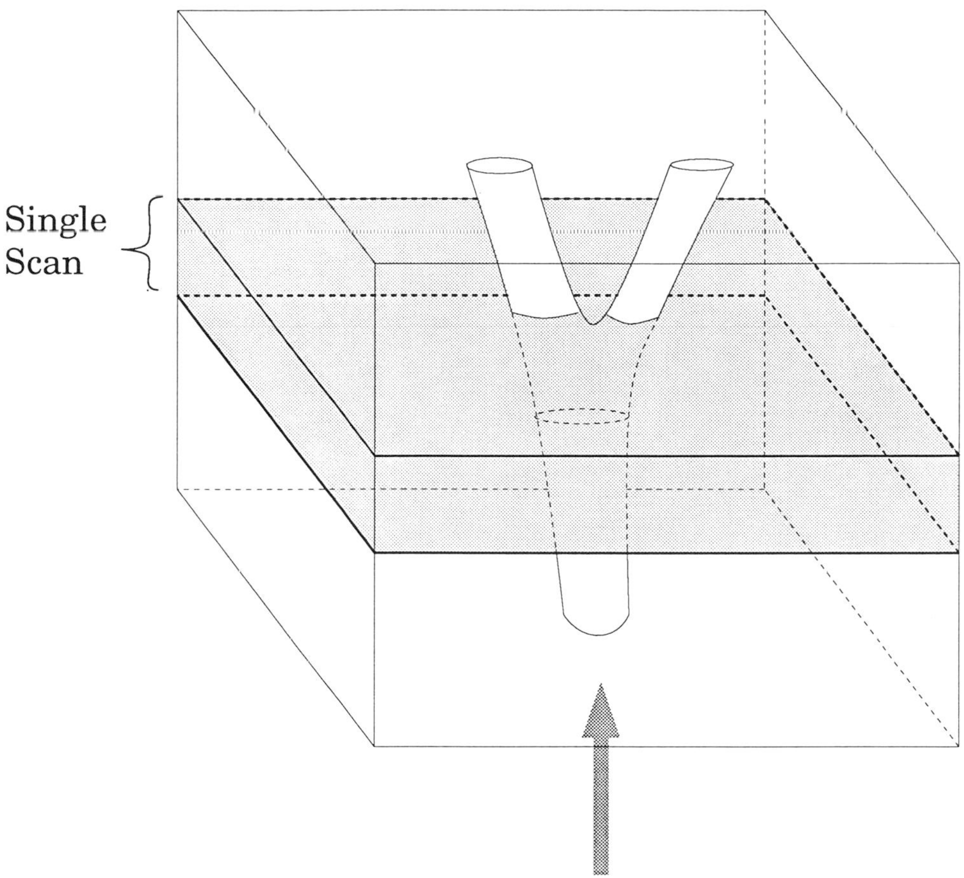

FIGURE 3. *Geometry of a typical multislab three-dimensional time-of-flight procedure. This method is a hybrid of three-dimensional and two-dimensional time-of-flight angiography. In this technique three-dimensional time-of-flight MRA images are collected at several locations over the region of interest. This minimizes the loss of contrast that occurs as the fully relaxed blood enters the region of the radiofrequency pulses and becomes saturated, without loss of resolution in the third dimension.*

with flowing blood in some imaging protocols. Care should be taken to avoid interpreting these tissues as patent vascular structures.

Phase Contrast Magnetic Resonance Angiography

The second magnetic resonance flow phenomenon that can be used to detect flow is the phase shift, which is induced in transverse spin magnetization moving along a magnetic field gradient. A fundamental aspect of magnetic resonance is that nuclei resonate at a frequency that is exactly proportional to the strength of the magnetic field. Consequently, when a magnetic field gradient is applied, the magnetic field is changed and transverse magnetization at different locations resonates at different frequencies. If the duration of the gradient is finite, a phase shift in the transverse magnetization that is directly proportional to position is induced. This phase shift is proportional to position, and thus encodes position.

The position-dependent phase shifts generated by a gradient pulse can be undone by applying a second gradient pulse of equal duration but opposite polarity. If the nuclei move during the interval between the first and second gradient pulses, however, the phase shifts induced by the first pulse will not be exactly canceled by those of the second pulse. The residual phase shift will be directly proportional to the distance that the nuclei traveled in the interval between the gradient pulses, and thus it will also be proportional to the flow velocity. This phase change, illustrated in Figure 4, is the key to phase-sensitive flow imaging procedures such as phase contrast MRA.

The phase shift induced by motion of transverse spin magnetization in the presence of a symmetric bipolar magnetic field gradient pulse pair, ϕ_{motion}, can be approximated by:

$$\phi_{motion} = \gamma VTA_g$$

where γ is the gyromagnetic ratio, V is the component of the spin's velocity parallel to the direction of the applied gradient, T is the time between the centers of the lobes of

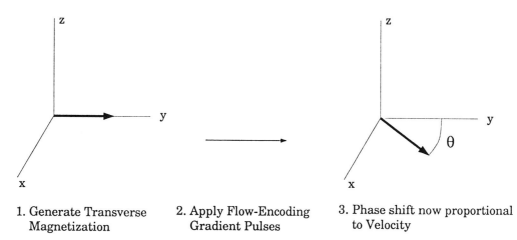

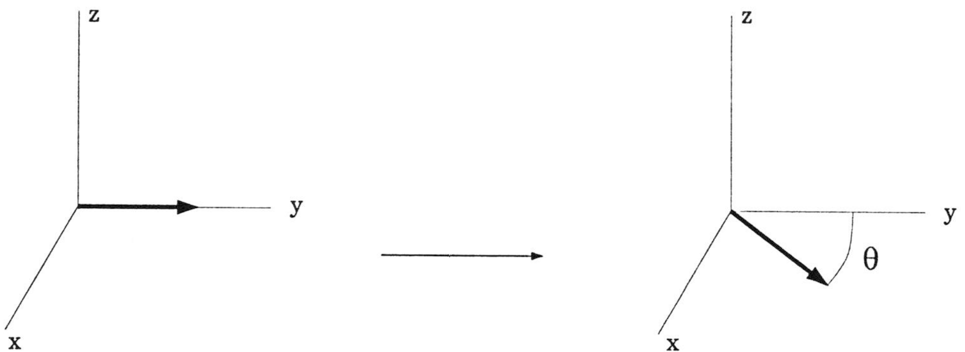

FIGURE 4. *Velocity-induced phase shifts in transverse spin magnetization. In the first step, transverse spin magnetization is created by generating longitudinal spin magnetization with a radiofrequency pulse. This transverse magnetization is represented as a vector in the XY plane. Then a flow-encoding gradient pulse is applied. This flow-encoding pulse induces a phase shift that is independent of the location of the spin within the magnet but is proportional to velocity. This phase shift, denoted as θ in step 3, is the angle of rotation that has been induced in the vector representing the transverse magnetization. Note that this effect is the fundamental phenomenon of phase-sensitive MRA methods.*

the gradient pulse, and A_g is the area (ie, the product of gradient strength and time) of one lobe of the bipolar pulse. Equation 1 ignores phase shifts that can arise from higher orders of motion such as acceleration and jerk. Motion-induced phase shifts can be made proportional to any combination of these orders by appropriately designed gradient waveforms. The most common flow-encoding gradient waveform is the simple bipolar gradient pulse described above and shown in Figure 5. This waveform induces a phase shift that is independent of position, but is proportional to velocity and all higher orders of motion.

In phase contrast procedures,[10–12] data are acquired first with flow-encoding gradients of one polarity and then with flow-encoding gradients of the opposite polarity. The complex difference of the acquired data is then taken. Signals from stationary tissue have no velocity-induced phase shift, and thus cancel upon subtraction. Signals from moving spins, however, combine additively and are preserved as illustrated in Figure 6. Suppression of background tissue in an ideal instrument is complete, and artifactually bright signals from short T_1 tissue does not occur. Furthermore, since the induced phase shift is directly proportional to velocity, quantitative flow information can be extracted.

The velocity sensitivity of a phase contrast angiogram is determined by the amplitude and duration of the flow-encoding gradient pulse. Since it is the phase shift that is proportional to velocity, the signal that is presented in a phase contrast angiogram

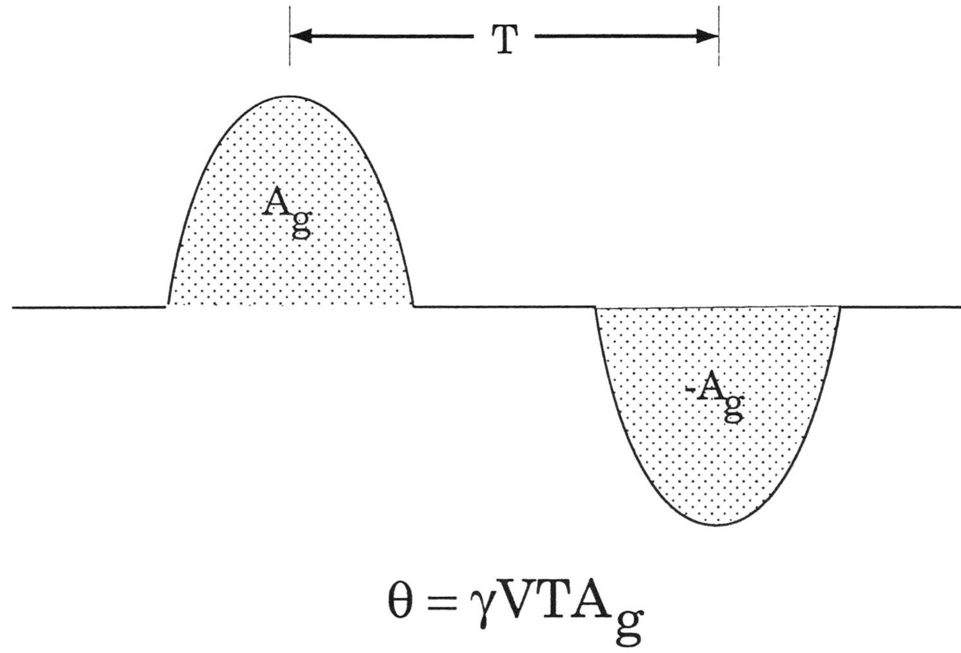

FIGURE 5. *The bipolar flow-encoding gradient pulse. The first lobe dephases transverse magnetization by an amount proportional to position. The second lobe rephases the magnetization. If the magnetization moves in the interval between the pulses, however, the cancellation of the induced phase shift is incomplete. The residual phase shift is proportional to velocity.*

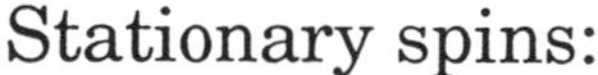

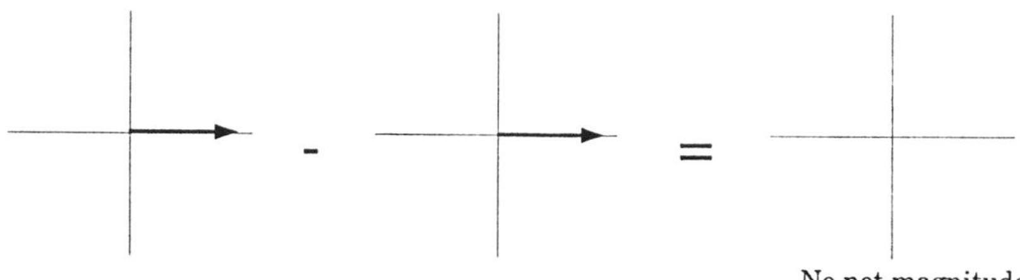

Moving spins:

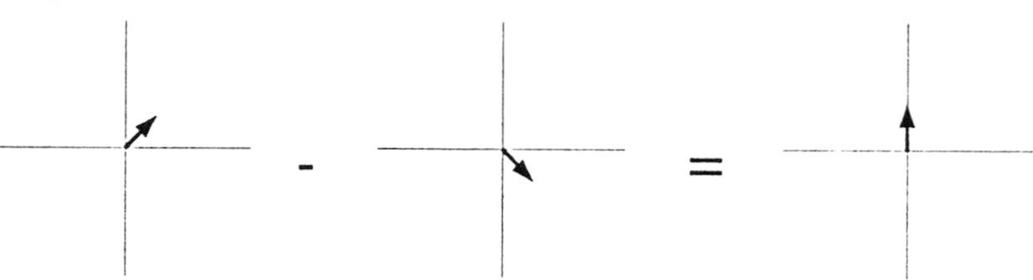

FIGURE 6. *Vector representation of the suppression of stationary tissue and the preservation of moving blood in phase contrast angiography. In a phase contrast procedure two sets of data are collected. The first data set is collected with a bipolar gradient pulse (eg, a positive lobe followed by a negative lobe) that induces a phase shift that is proportional to velocity (see Figure 5). The second data set is collected in an identical fashion except that the polarity of the bipolar gradient is reversed (eg, a negative lobe followed by a positive lobe). The difference of these two data sets is then calculated. Most of the transverse magnetization in the body is stationary and is not affected by the flow-encoding pulses since the flow-encoding pulses induce a phase shift that is proportional to velocity and the velocity of stationary tissue is 0. Consequently, the signals from stationary tissue are canceled upon subtraction of the detected signals, as illustrated in the top row of the figure. Signals from moving blood, on the other hand, undergo a phase shift that is proportional to the blood's velocity and that has a mathematical sign controlled by the gradient polarity. Consequently, when the difference is calculated, the signals from moving blood combine additively and appear in the angiogram.*

is approximately proportional to velocity only if the velocity induces a phase shift less than about 1 radian (ie, 57.29°). The velocity at which the pixel intensity is maximized, or in other words, the velocity giving a 90° phase shift, is frequently referred to as V_{enc}. The relationship between image pixel intensity and velocity is shown in Figure 7.

The ability to select the flow-encoding strength gives the operator a great deal of power. By the judicious choice of gradients the flow sensitivity can be set to detect very slow or very high flow velocities. Another advantage is that the detected phase shifts carry directional information that frequently proves to be diagnostically useful. Unlike time-of-flight methods, phase contrast methods are equally sensitive to flow in all directions and do not suffer from the penetration effect.

Phase contrast MRA procedures are created by incorporating flow-encoding

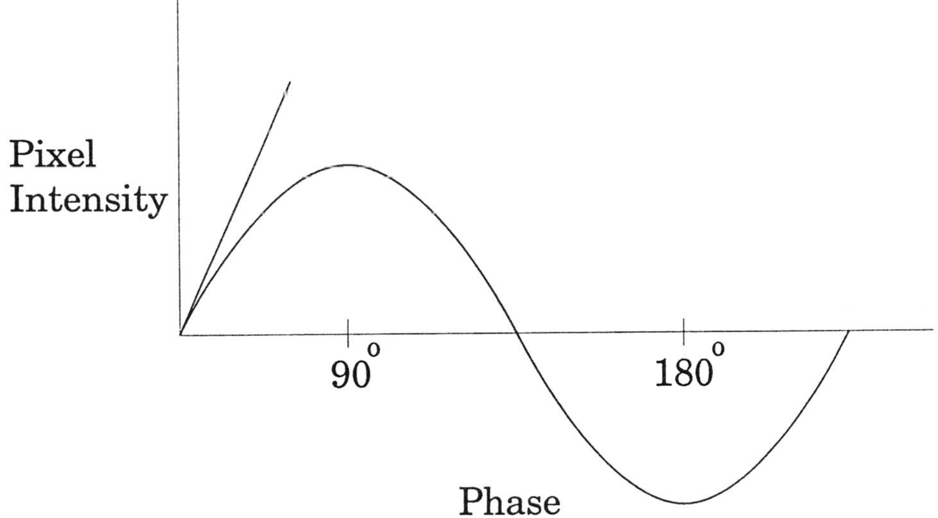

FIGURE 7. *The relationship between motion-induced phase shifts (and hence velocity) and image pixel intensity in phase contrast angiography. As the velocity of blood increases, the phase shift induced by a flow-encoding gradient increases. Unfortunately, if the phase shift increases too much it becomes indistinguishable from a smaller phase shift. For example, blood moving at a given velocity might induce a 45° phase shift. Blood moving three times faster would induce a $3 \times 45 = 135°$ phase shift. When the magnetic resonance image is formed, this 135° phase shift gives a signal intensity that is identical to the intensity generated by the 45° phase shift. To avoid this problem, the phase shift for the largest expected velocity should be limited to 90°. If the phase shift of the largest velocity is limited to about a radian (ie, 57°), the pixel intensity in the angiographic image is approximately proportional to velocity. If it were exactly proportional to velocity, the signal intensity would be given by the straight line.*

gradient pulses into conventional gradient recalled imaging procedures. Images containing only signals from flowing blood can be obtained using the same scan orientations and fields of view found in conventional MRI. Because the phase contrast mechanism efficiently suppresses signals from stationary tissue, however, angiographic images obtained from much larger volumes are possible. Thus, full projection angiograms can be obtained in the same scan time as a conventional image.

One problem with any projection technique is that the image voxel is highly anisotropic. The in-plane resolution of the image may be high, but each voxel has a depth that can be as large as the thickness of the anatomy being imaged. Overlapping vessels in a projection angiogram can share image voxels yet be physically in regions having different magnetic field strengths. If this happens, the signals from each vessel may have different absolute phases, and destructive interference of signals in the overlapping region is possible. Similarly, if overlapping vessels have very different flow or if a vessel is large enough to have a substantial variation of flow velocities in its projection, anomalous loss of signal is possible.

In normal blood flow to the extremities there is a triphasic pattern of flow that has a rapid forward flow component in systole, a slow reverse flow component at the beginning of diastole, and either stagnant flow or slow forward flow for the duration of diastole. Consequently, in nongated techniques, approximately two thirds of the data acquisition occurs when there is no significant flow. Cardiac gated, cine angiograms,[11] on the other hand, acquire images at multiple points during the cardiac cycle and some images are guaranteed to be acquired entirely during periods of flow. Because dynamic flow is found primarily in arteries rather than veins, it can be used to differentiate arteries from veins. This technique has proven particularly useful for applications in the pelvis and extremities where blood flow is highly dynamic.

An example of a time-resolved two-dimensional phase contrast angiogram is shown in Figure 8. This image combines 12 images obtained at different parts of the cardiac cycle. The total data acquisition time was approximately 6 minutes. Each image was obtained with a matrix size of 256 × 128 over a field of view of 24 cm. A 12-cm axial slab was excited and placed so that the myocardium was not excited. The projection direction was chosen to be 45° oblique to the subject's anterior/posterior axis so that the plane of the arch was coincident with the plane of the image. The image is a composite of all three orthogonal flow-sensitive flow directions.

Many of the problems of two-dimensional projection angiography can be overcome by obtaining the data directly in three dimensions.[12] Unlike a projection

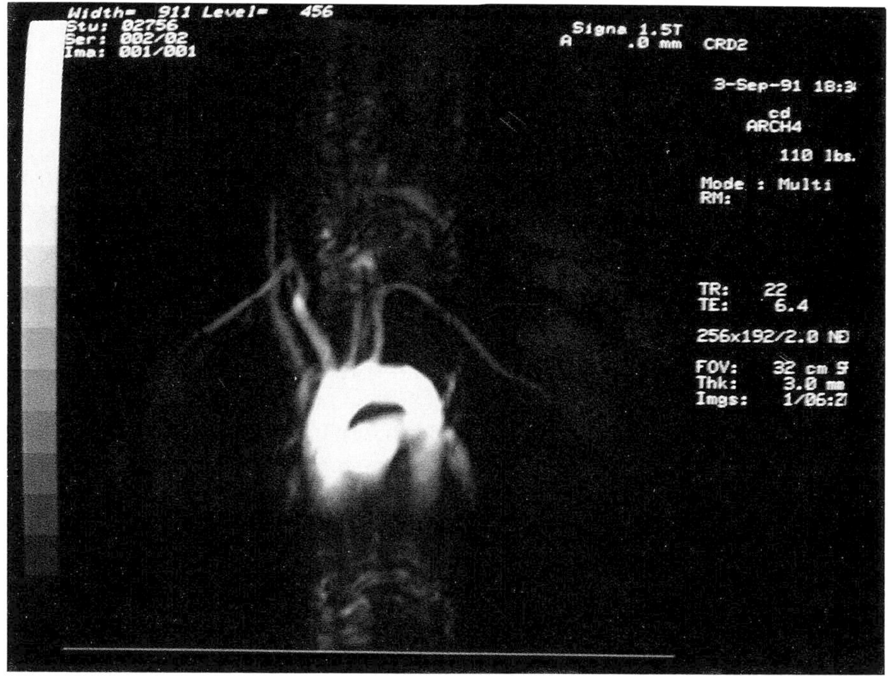

FIGURE 8. *Time-resolved two-dimensional phase contrast magnetic resonance angiogram of the aortic arch of a healthy subject. The image is a composite over the entire cardiac cycle and contains information from all three orthogonal flow directions.*

angiogram, a typical three-dimensional angiogram has approximately isotropic voxels. Phase variations across a voxel are minimized because the voxel dimensions are small. Perhaps the most significant advantage, however, is that the data can be analyzed retrospectively in a number of ways. For example, subvolumes of the acquired data set can be extracted to enhance the presentation of features of interest and cross sections of vessels can be generated.

Phase-sensitive MRA methods have a few limitations that should be recognized by the clinician. First, phase-sensitive methods demand high quality instruments, and phase stability is essential. Fortunately, most modern magnetic resonance scanners, when within their specifications, are adequate. A second limitation is that only a single flow dimension is obtained in each measurement. Consequently, a phase-sensitive acquisition can potentially be longer than an equivalent time-of-flight acquisition, but this is not always the case. An additional point that must be considered is the choice of the velocity sensitivity. Stronger flow-encoding gradient pulses induce larger phase shifts for lower velocities, but at the risk of aliasing phase shifts induced by higher velocities.

Quantitative Velocity Measurements

Flow-induced phase shifts can be used to obtain quantitative velocity information. The most straightforward method is to use the phase of each voxel to determine the average velocity within that voxel.[13–15] An alternative approach is the use of a Fourier transformation to obtain a velocity spectrum.

Fourier velocity encoding pulse sequences[16–20] are equivalent to conventional spin-warp imaging pulse sequences except that the spatially localizing phase encoding gradient pulses are replaced with bipolar flow-encoding gradient waveforms. Consequently, a Fourier velocity-encoded image has a phase-encoded dimension in which displacement of signal depends on spin velocity rather than on spin position. Additional spatial or velocity dimensions of data can be acquired by adding additional spatial or velocity phase-encoding gradient pulses, but this increases scan times.

Two Fourier velocity-encoding methods show particular promise for the study of in vivo and in vitro flow. The first method acquires a single spatial dimension, a single velocity dimension, and a temporal dimension that is gated to the cardiac cycle.[18] The second method also obtains data in a three-dimensional data matrix, but two of these dimensions are spatial and the third is velocity in a selected direction.[19] Higher dimensioned extensions of both of these methods can be easily envisioned, but are usually impractical with modern instrumentation due to scan time limits. In addition to the desire to obtain as much information as possible at a given position, it is frequently desirable to acquire data from a variety of positions within the subject, but this also increases scan times.

The velocity of an ensemble of spins can be quantitatively measured using Equation 1 if the motion-induced phase shift can be determined. Unfortunately, ensembles of spins frequently move with a distribution of velocities rather than a single velocity. This distribution can be broad enough to cause the phases of the component spin signals to cancel, resulting in a loss of signal.

The properties of the Fourier transform can be exploited to separate the constituent velocities and prevent signal loss. This can be done by sampling the moving spin magnetization with a progression of gradient lobe amplitudes or separations. Since the phase shift of moving spin magnetization is directly proportional to the lobe area, each velocity constituent will have a linear phase evolution as a function of the lobe area. Furthermore, the rate of phase change as a function of lobe strength will be directly proportional to velocity. Thus, spins moving with slow velocity will have a slow phase evolution (ie, they will be modulated at a low frequency), whereas spins moving at higher velocities will have faster phase evolutions (ie, higher modulation frequencies). Fourier transformation can then be used to separate the various velocity constituents by virtue of their modulation frequencies to give a data vector that presents signal intensity as a function of velocity.

Figure 9 shows two examples of Fourier velocity images. Velocity spectra were acquired from the descending aorta of two volunteers, the first having normal cardiac anatomy and the second having a bicuspid aortic valve. In both individuals the flow sensitivity was applied along the subject's inferior/superior axis. Data acquisition was synchronized to the subject's R wave. The data were reformatted to provide velocity versus position images. Note the differences in flow profiles over the cardiac cycle. In the normal individual the flow in the inferior vena cava is constant and has a broad distribution of velocities. In the individual with the bicuspid aortic valve, however, the flow in the inferior vena cava is pulsatile. Also note the pronounced retrograde flow during diastole in the individual with the bicuscpid valve.

The accuracy of velocity and flow measurements with Fourier velocity-encoding methods can be limited by instrument attributes. In particular, the performance characteristics of the gradient subsystem are important for accurate velocity measurements. Fortunately, modern instrumentation typically includes higher linear and precise gradient amplifiers that are essential to linear and well-characterized fields of view for conventional imaging. Since the mechanism of Fourier spatial encoding is essentially identical to the mechanism of Fourier velocity encoding, the precision and accuracy of velocity measurements are the same as that available for spatial measurement in conventional imaging. Consequently, flow quantitation is rarely limited by instrumental attributes.

Another potential limitation to the accuracy of flow measurement is the assumption that higher orders of motion such as acceleration and jerk are not present in the flow. Unless compensated for, these higher orders of motion will induce phase shifts that will be indistinguishable from phase shifts arising from velocity. Consequently, it is important to minimize the duration of flow-encoding gradient (ie, use strong gradient pulses).

Conclusions

Magnetic resonance angiography is still a relatively young field, and yet it has already found a place in diagnostic medicine. For some applications clinicians are beginning to routinely use MRA imaging in place of conventional x-ray angiography. Both time-of-flight techniques and phase contrast methods are finding use in a number of clinical applications for head, neck, abdominal, and peripheral vessels. Quantitative flow measurement using phase-sensitive magnetic resonance methods are also becoming useful. Direct phase measurements can be used with traditional MRI methods to

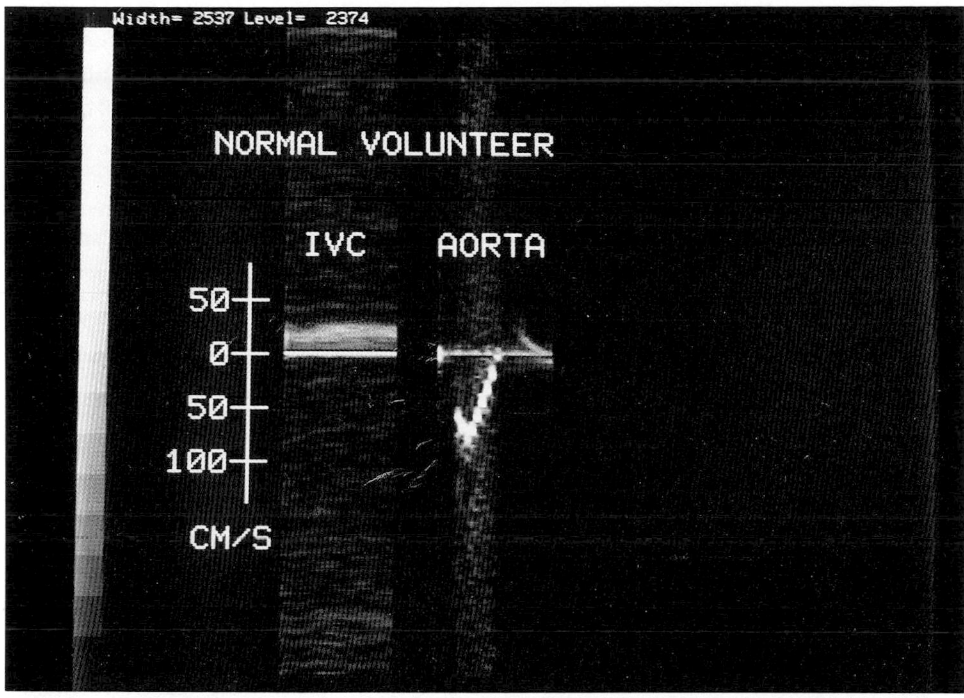

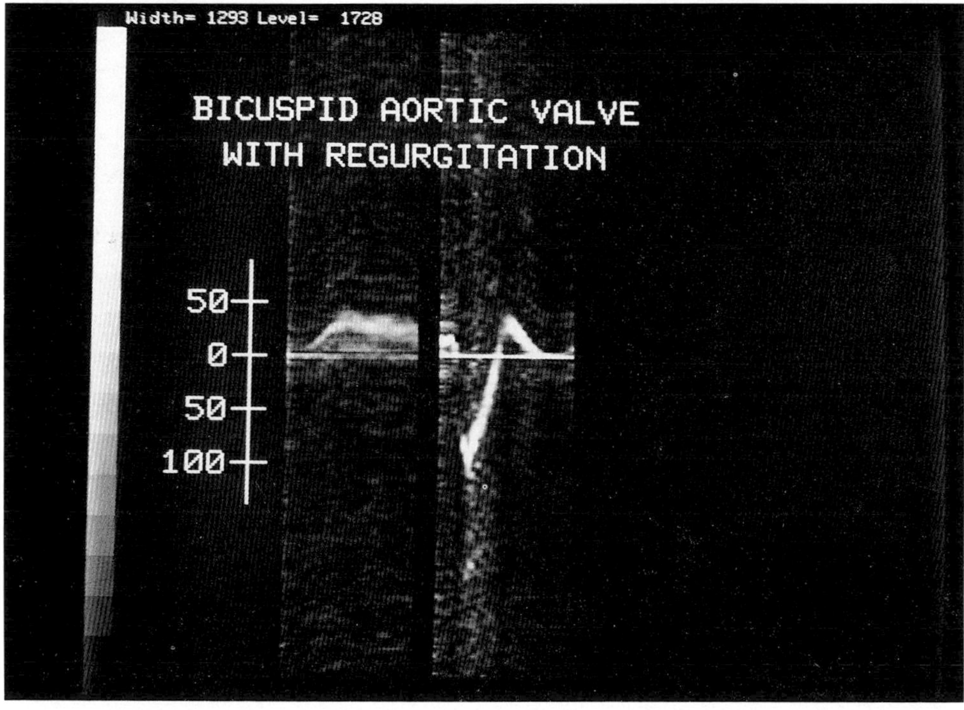

FIGURE 9. *Time-resolved quantitative velocity measurements of the descending aorta of two individuals.* **(Top):** *This volunteer has normal cardiac anatomy.* **(Bottom):** *This volunteer has a bicuspid aortic valve. Note the differences in velocity profiles between the two individuals and the broad distribution of velocities in the inferior vena cava.*

obtain average velocity within an image pixel. Alternatively, a velocity spectrum can be obtained using Fourier velocity-encoding methods. Quantitative methods can potentially address a number of clinical and physiologic problems. In the coming years advances in imaging technology are certain to expand the field of magnetic resonance flow imaging and flow measurement even further.

References

1. Masaryk TJ, Modic MT, Ruggieri PM, et al: Three-dimensional (volume) gradient-echo imaging of the carotid bifurcation: preliminary clinical experience. *Radiology* 1989;171:801–806.
2. Masaryk TJ, Modic MT, Ross JS, et al: Intracranial circulation: preliminary clinical results with three-dimensional (volume) MR angiography. *Radiology* 1989;171:793–799.
3. Pernicone JR, Siebert JE, Potchen EJ, et al: Three-dimensional phase-contrast MR angiography in the head and neck: preliminary report. *Am J Radiol* 1990;155:167–176.
4. Wagle WA, Dumoulin CL, Souza SP, et al: 3DFT MR angiography of carotid and basilar arteries. *Am J Neuroradiol* 1989;10:911-919.
5. Huston J, Rufenacht DA, Ehman RL, et al: Intracranial aneurysms and vascular malformations: comparison of time-of-flight and phase contrast MR angiography. *Radiology* 1991;181:721–730.
6. Ruggieri PM, Laub GA, Masaryk TJ, et al: Intracranial circulation: pulse-sequence considerations in three-dimensional (volume) MR angiography. *Radiology* 1989;171:785–791.
7. Dumoulin CL, Cline HE, Souza S, et al: Three-dimensional time-of-flight magnetic resonance angiography using spin saturation. *Magn Reson Med* 1989;11:35–46.
8. Gullberg GT, Wehrli FW, Shimakawa A, et al: MR vascular imaging with a fast gradient refocusing pulse sequence and reformatted images from transaxial sections. *Radiology* 1987;165:241–246.
9. Parker DL, Blatter DD, Robison R, et al: Proceedings of the 9th Annual Meeting of the Society of Magnetic Resonance in Medicine. 199:494.
10. Dumoulin CL, Hart HR: Magnetic resonance angiography. *Radiology* 1986;161:717.
11. Dumoulin CL, Souza SP, Walker MF, et al: Time-resolved magnetic resonance angiography. *Magn Reson Med* 1988;6:275-286.
12. Dumoulin CL, Souza SP, Walker MF, et al: Three-dimensional phase contrast angiography. *Magn Reson Med* 1989;9:139-149.
13. van Dijk P: Direct cardiac NMR imaging of heart wall and blood flow velocity. *J Comput Assist Tomog* 1984;8:429-436.
14. Bryant DJ, Payne JA, Firmin DN, et al: Measurement of flow with NMR imaging using gradient pulse and phase difference technique. *J Comput Assist Tomog* 1984;8:588–593.
15. Young IR, Bydder GM, Payne JA: Flow measurement by the development of phase differences during slice formation in MR imaging. *Magn Reson Med* 1986;3:175–179.
16. Redpath TW, Norris DG, Jones RA, et al: A new method of NMR flow imaging. *Phys Med Biol* 1984;29:891–895.
17. Feinberg DA, Crooks LE, Sheldon P, et al: Magnetic resonance imaging the velocity vector components of fluid flow. *Magn Reson Med* 1985;2:555.
18. Hennig J, Muri M, Brunner P, et al: Quantitative flow measurement with the fast Fourier flow technique. *Radiology* 1988;166:237.
19. Wendt RE, Nitz W, Murphy PH, et al: Characterization of fluid flow using low-spatial-resolution velocity spectra from NMR images. *Magn Reson Med* 1989;10:71–88.
20. Dumoulin CL, Souza SP, Hardy CJ, et al: Quantitative measurement of blood flow using cylindrically localized Fourier velocity encoding. *Magn Reson Med* 1991;21:242–250.

Chapter 17

Magnetic Resonance Imaging of the Coronary Arteries

Albert Macovski, PhD, Bob Hu, MD, Samuel J. Wang, MS, Craig Meyer, PhD, John Pauly, PhD, and Dwight G. Nishimura, PhD

The medical community has long sought methods for the noninvasive imaging of the coronary arteries. Coronary artery disease continues to represent the primary cause of death in all industrial societies. By virtue of its inherent nontoxic nature and lack of ionizing radiation, magnetic resonance is an ideal candidate for this task. This type of study can be repeated often to follow the progress of the disease or evaluate therapeutic procedures without any associated risk. However, efforts directed specifically at magnetic resonance coronary artery imaging must contend with a formidable set of challenges, including cardiac motion, respiratory motion, neighboring chamber blood, and small vessel size.

We have pursued two general methods for magnetic resonance coronary artery imaging: 1) a projective method with selective tagging of blood, and 2) a slice imaging method with fast spiral scanning. Both methods involve the use of breath-held fast scanning that mitigates problems associated with respiration. Before describing the specific coronary angiographic methods, we elaborate on our fast imaging work directed toward coronary imaging. We have developed and implemented two sequences suitable for breath-hold imaging: a fast version of two-dimensional Fourier transform imaging and an interleaved spiral scan sequence.

Fast Two-Dimensional Fourier Transform Imaging

This first method is a fast, cardiac gated version of the popular two-dimensional Fourier transform imaging sequence. During each cardiac cycle, we apply a rapid burst of N readout excitations to acquire N separate phase encodes (Figure 1). Because each excitation burst is separated by a pause until the next cardiac cycle, steady state is not achieved and thus care must be exercised to equalize the signal for all phase encodes.

From Pohost GM (ed.), *Cardiovascular Applications of Magnetic Resonance*. Mount Kisco, NY, Futura Publishing Co., Inc., © 1993.

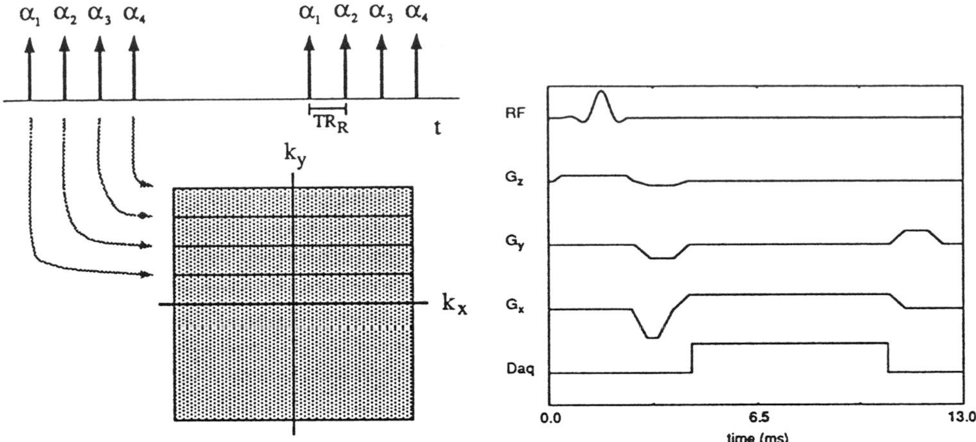

FIGURE 1.

As previously reported,[1,2] we progressively increase the tip angles over the readout excitation burst and reorder the phase encodes to avoid both ghosting artifacts and blurring in the phase encode direction. This multiple phase encode scheme is similar to the work of Tasciyan et al.,[3] including the so-called segmented k-space sequence.[4]

Each measurement in the two-dimensional Fourier transform imaging sequence is based on a gradient-echo acquisition with an offset echo readout and an offset radiofrequency excitation (Figure 1). These offsets reduce the gradient moments, thereby improving the coherence of the flow signal and shortening the echo time (TE) to <4 msec. Within each burst, the minimum repetition time (TR) between successive excitation pulses (TR_R) is constrained by the duration of each excitation/readout unit. Thus far, with 6-msec readouts, we have achieved a TR_R of about 13 msec. The overall imaging time for one image is $TR(N_{pe}/N)$, where N_{pe} is the total number of phase encodes. Typically, we use $N = 8$ and $N_{pe} = 96$, amounting to a scan of 12 heartbeats per image. Another important consideration for cardiac applications is the duration of an N-excitation burst. With $N = 8$ and $TR_R = 13$ msec, the duration is 104 msec, adequate for "freezing" the heart during the readout if synchronized to diastole.

Fast Spiral Scan Imaging

Instead of a conventional raster scan of k-space, another approach to fast scanning involves time varying gradients during signal readout. We have developed a sequence that uses a constant velocity (within gradient slew limits) spiral trajectory through k-space.[5,6] The spiral trajectory and the corresponding sequence timing diagram are depicted in Figure 2. We have implemented both a "square" and "round" spiral sequence, opting more recently for the round spiral because of its more efficient k-space coverage.

In principle, k-space can be traversed completely in a single readout. In practice, however, we collect an interleaved set of N spirals, each covering 1/N of k-space (Figure 2). Such interleaving reduces the gradient power requirements by a factor of $1/N^2$ and increases the signal-to-noise ratio (SNR) by $\sqrt{N}$ compared with a single readout scan, but still enables imaging within a reasonable breath-hold.

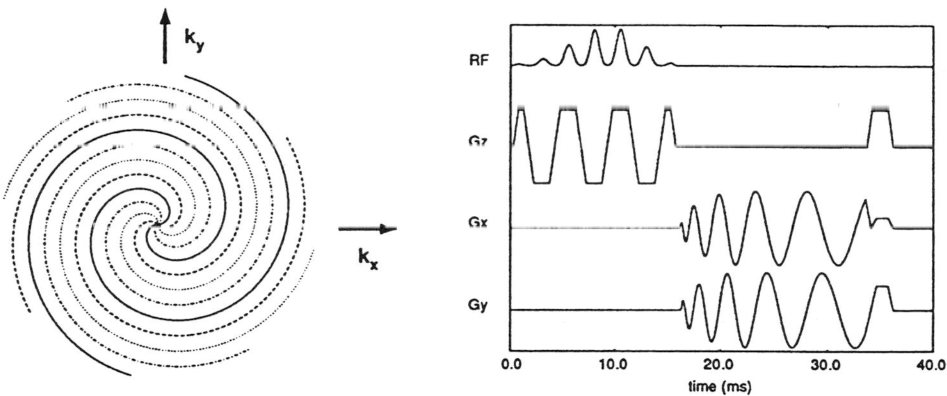

FIGURE 2.

Using a conventional gradient system with a maximum amplitude of 1 G/cm and slew rate of 2 G/cm per millisecond, the sequence evolved into a 20-interleave (hence a 20-heartbeat) spiral k-space scan for cardiac imaging, producing 20-cm field-of-view images with a 186 × 186 matrix. For cardiac imaging, the spiral scan sequence can be applied in various modes: single slice, multislice, or movie. When applied in movie mode, the spiral sequence provides temporal information in the same 20-heartbeat scan time.

Compared with echo-planar imaging, spiral scan imaging exhibits considerably better immunity to flow artifacts. The spiral sequence, with its k-space trajectory extending outward from the origin, possesses relatively small gradient moments near the k-space origin, resulting in insignificant loss of signal coherence due to flow.[6] Compared with the fast two-dimensional Fourier transform imaging method described above, which involves a burst of low tip angle excitations, spiral imaging allows the application of a 90° readout excitation for maximum signal. In addition, the duration of each spiral interleave is shorter than the overall duration per excitation burst of the fast two-dimensional Fourier transform imaging sequence. This shorter duration reduces artifacts due to heart motion during the signal acquisition.

The principal drawback of spiral scanning is its off-resonance behavior, which manifests as a blur rather than a shift as it does in two-dimensional Fourier transform imaging. However, we have addressed this concern in several ways. First, we use a novel spectral-spatial excitation pulse developed by our laboratory[7] that is simultaneously selective in space and temporal frequency. We use this pulse to excite only the water component in the slice of interest. This pulse, therefore, eliminates the fat component that would otherwise reconstruct blurred in the image. Second, we reduce the readout time per spiral interleave to 17.5 msec to minimize the amount of detrimental phase accrual. These two techniques significantly reduce the extent of off-resonance effects. In addition, we developed reconstruction algorithms that compensate for off-resonance effects when imaging with non-two-dimensional Fourier transform imaging k-space scanning sequences. One is a fast algorithm that relies on a separate field map scan to guide the reconstruction.[8] Another is an automatic deblurring algorithm[9] that does not require a separate field map scan; instead, it uses a focusing criterion based on minimizing the imaginary component over a local region after appropriate phase compensation.

Using these fast scan sequences, we have pursued two general methods for coronary angiography. These methods can be categorized as: 1) selective tagging, and 2) slice imaging with fast spiral scanning. While the first relies on time-of-flight effects, the second relies not on flow but on the nuclear magnetic resonance parameters of blood for improved contrast.

Selective Tagging

In this method, blood upstream to the region of interest gets tagged by a radiofrequency excitation. Two images, one with the tagging on and the other with the tagging off, are subtracted, leaving a difference signal from only the washed-in blood. Flow-related enhancement from fresh unexcited spins occurs for one of the two images; a second image set based on tagged blood allows subtraction of static material. The specific tagging method that we have pursued is called selective inversion recovery (SIR), which uses an inversion tagging excitation.[10,11]

When applied to vascular regions such as the carotid arteries, SIR produces high-resolution angiograms with good suppression of surrounding tissue and immunity to flow artifacts.[12] However, application of SIR to coronary arteries[13] involves a different set of considerations because of the more complex flow pathways, the presence of intervening heart chambers, and motion. Figure 3 illustrates the basic implementation. The inversion excitation tags the aortic root at end systole, since most coronary flow occurs during diastole, and then the readout excitations follow at end diastole.

To mitigate the problem caused by underlying chambers, we restricted the extent of projection to a slab and replaced the one-dimensional tagging excitation with a two-dimensional tagging pulse (Figure 3). This two-dimensional pulse, elegantly designed using the excitation Fourier space (k-space) interpretation developed by our laboratory,[14] tags a more limited region to minimize the amount of undesired blood leaking into the difference image.

To cope with respiratory motion, we modified SIR by using the fast two-dimensional Fourier transform imaging sequence with multiple readouts per cardiac cycle (Figure 3). Potential problems with subtraction were addressed by interleaving the acquisition of the two images; in addition, both the suspension of respiration and the brevity of the scan significantly improved the success of the subtraction.

The method is not tied to any specific imaging sequence. Although a two-dimensional Fourier transform imaging sequence is the standard choice, other sequences such as projection reconstruction, line scan, or a rapid k-space scan may be viable alternatives.

These changes led to dramatic improvements in image quality, as illustrated in Figure 4. These images were obtained on a standard 1.5-T imaging system (General Electric Signa System, Milwaukee, WI) with shielded gradients and conventional gradient amplifiers. They have a field of view of 20 cm and a spatial resolution of 0.78 mm $\times$ 2.1 mm (matrix size of 256 $\times$ 96). The inflow time (TI) ranged from 300 msec to 340 msec. A 14-cm diameter surface coil was placed on the chest of the supine subject. The scan times for the subtraction SIR angiograms were 24 heartbeats (12 heartbeats per image, 2 images for subtraction). We experimented with two cardiac gating systems: an electrocardiograph (ECG) and a photoplethysmograph. While a trigger from an ECG offers greater stability, the trigger point of a plethysmograph is closer to the point of tagging (Figure 3). The images presented here are plethysmograph gated, although we experienced success with both gating schemes.

Figure 4 (left) is a projection angiogram of an axial slab 3 cm thick showing the proximal portions of the left anterior descending coronary artery (LAD) and diagonal branch. For anatomical reference, Figure 4 (right) is an axial projection image of the same region. As can be inferred from Figure 4 (left), the two-dimensional cylindrical excitation is oriented in the superior inferior direction, perpendicular to the slab, and positioned to encompass the aortic root.

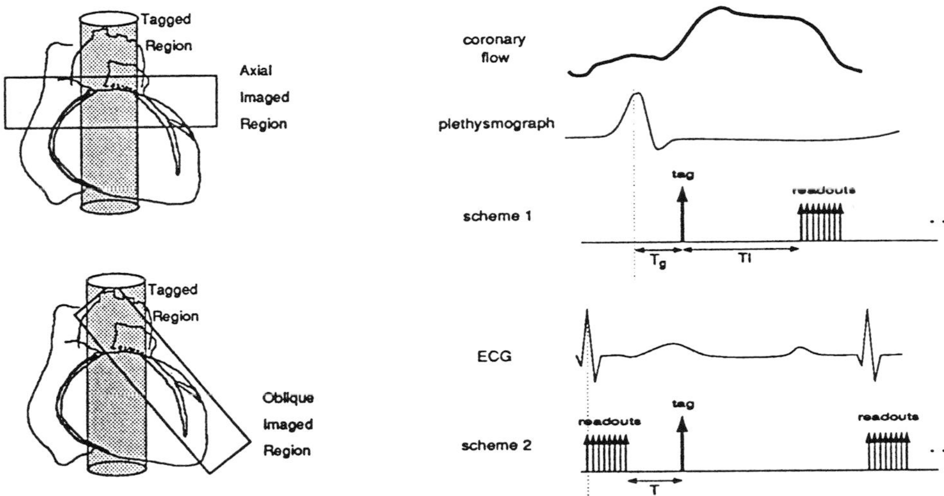

FIGURE 3.

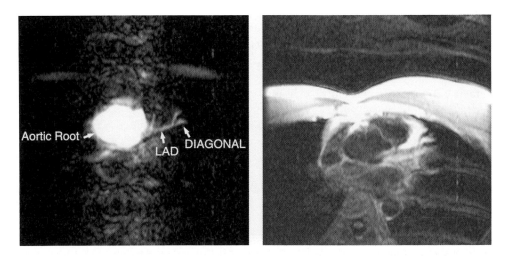

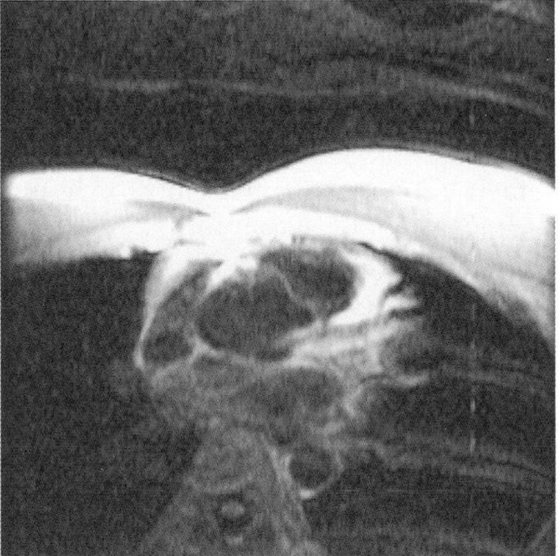

FIGURE 4.

Slice Imaging with Fast Spiral Scanning

This second general method, which uses the fast spiral scan sequence described earlier, can be subdivided into two areas: 1) sequential slice imaging with inflow enhancement and 2) flow-independent blood imaging.

Inflow-Based Signal Enhancement

This method relies on inflow enhancement and fast imaging of relatively thin slices. This method, similar to the two-dimensional time-of-flight method, involves collecting a set of contiguous thin slices, with subsequent postprocessing of this three-dimensional data set to extract and isolate the coronary artery component. For each slice, the cardiac gated acquisition is completed within a breath-hold to minimize respiratory artifacts and to avoid a prohibitively long scan time. The thin slice acquisition makes this method attractive for imaging more distal vessels with slower flow.

We implement this method using the interleaved spiral sequence. In one acquisition mode, we obtain a temporally resolved three-dimensional data set via a sequential two-dimensional slice scan in movie mode. Thus, for each slice, a train of partial tip angle excitations are applied throughout the cardiac cycle. The temporal information reveals the dynamics of the coronary vessels while the resulting three-dimensional acquisition alleviates problems with the surrounding heart chambers. For flow enhancement, thin-slice excitation using large tip angles renders inflowing blood bright in the coronary arteries compared with the relatively saturated tissue. Fat is suppressed by the spectral spatial excitation incorporated into the spiral sequence.

Flow-Independent Imaging

The basic idea of this method is to image the proximal portions of the coronary arteries with relatively few slices while minimizing the amount of competing signals from cardiac muscle, fat, and chamber blood. Because inflow is not a requirement, distal vessels with slow flow can be visualized and the slice thickness need not be as thin as the three-dimensional inflow method discussed above. Moreover, the preferred orientation of the slice is to provide a longitudinal view of the vessel to reduce the required number of slices. Proper orientation of the slice is greatly facilitated by the fast localization possible with the high-speed scanning. Although not dependent on flow effects, any inflow improves the blood contrast. We have studied several approaches of producing high-contrast coronary artery images using this flow-independent concept.

One approach uses the breath-held spiral imaging sequence with proper slice orientation. We have produced images showing substantial portions of the left main, LAD, right, posterior descending (PDA), and circumflex arteries. The spectral-spatial excitation pulse improves visualization considerably by suppressing surrounding epicardial fat.

Figures 5 through 7 are coronary images (3–10-mm slice thicknesses) obtained with the 20-interleave spiral scan sequence. All of these images were cardiac gated with a plethysmograph and have a spatial resolution of 1.1 mm. Figure 5 contains

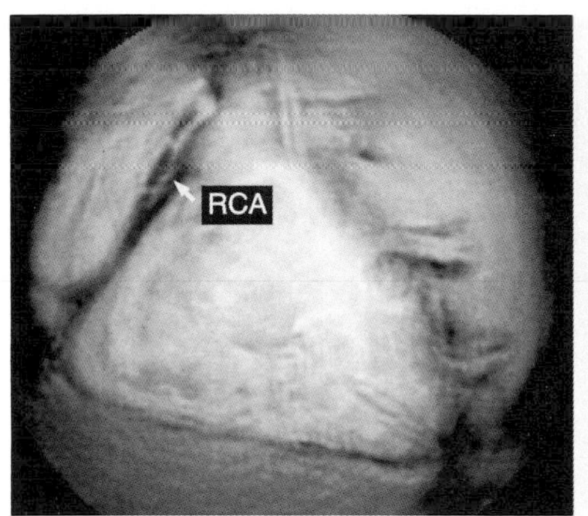

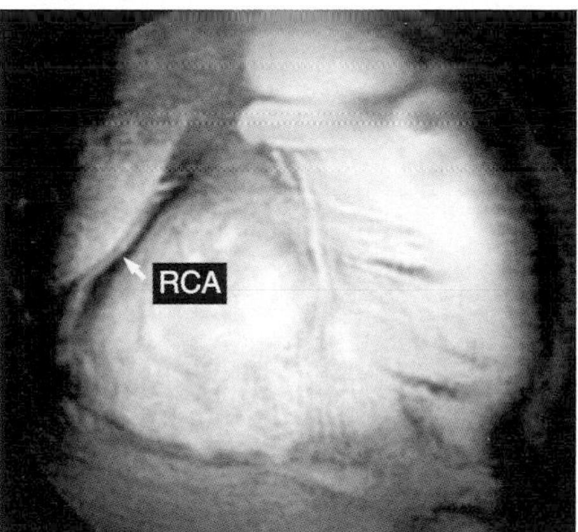

FIGURE 5.

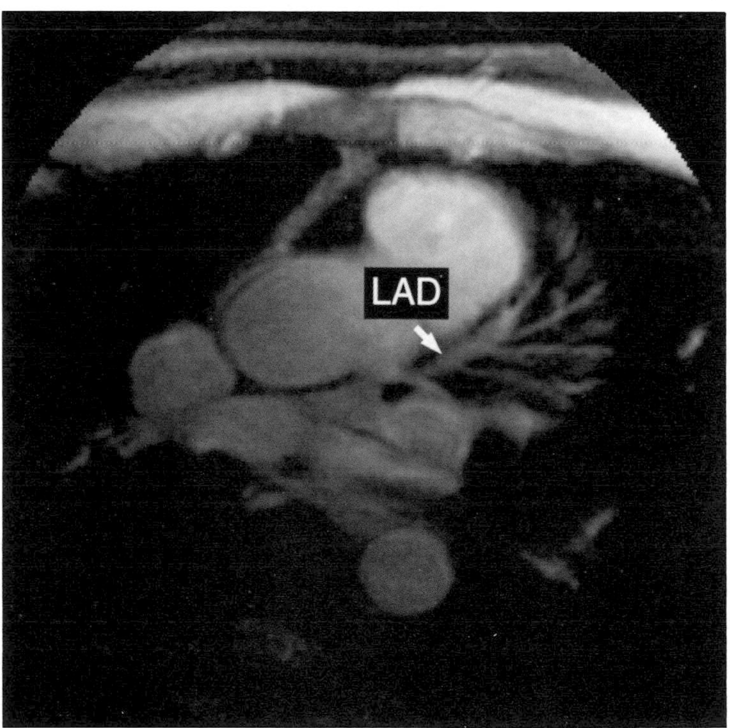

FIGURE 6.

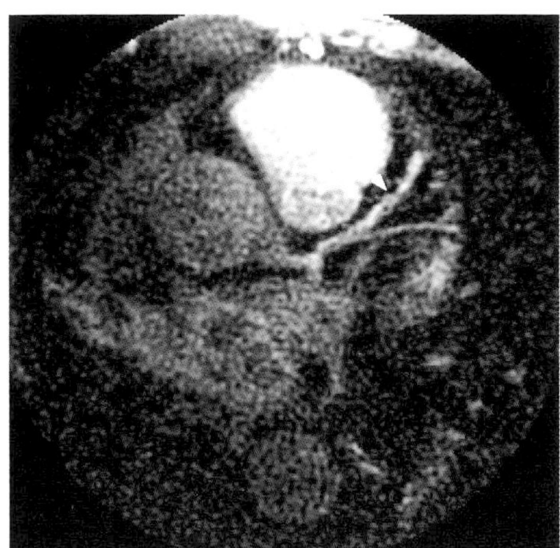

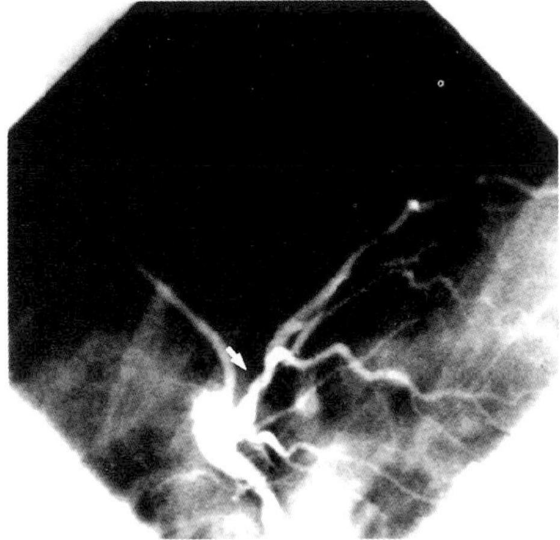

FIGURE 7.

right anterior oblique images of the right coronary artery (RCA). These images are two of five 7-mm slices obtained that reveal approximately 8 cm of the RCA. Figure 5 (left) shows the proximal segment while Figure 5 (right) shows the distal segment. In Figure 6, an oblique axial (Gruentzig) view, the LAD and diagonal are clearly visible. These spiral scan images illustrate the benefits of epicardial fat suppression by using the spectral-spatial pulse.

Figure 7 displays our initial clinical result with spiral coronary artery scanning. An axial spiral image (Figure 7, left) shows good correlation with the x-ray angiogram (Figure 7, right). A moderate stenosis in the LAD (see arrow) of this patient is apparent.

References

1. Wang SJ, Nishimura DG, Macovski A: Multiple readout selective inversion recovery angiography. *Magn Reson Med* 1991;17:244–251.
2. Wang SJ, Nishimura DG, Macovski A: Fast angiography using selective inversion recovery. *Magn Reson Med* 1992;23:109–121.
3. Tasciyan TA, Lee JN, Riederer SJ, et al: Fast limited flip angle MR subtraction angiography. *Magn Reson Med* 1988;8:261–274.
4. Chien D, Atkinson DJ, Edelman RR: 2D and 3D MR angiography using segmented k-space data acquisition (abstract). In: Proceedings of the 9th Annual Meeting of the Society of Magnetic Resonance in Medicine. 1990:62.
5. Meyer C, Macovski A, Nishimura DG: Square-spiral fast imaging (abstract). In: Proceedings of the 8th Annual Meeting of the Society of Magnetic Resonance in Medicine. 1989:362.
6. Meyer C, Macovski A, Nishimura DG: A comparison of fast spiral sequences for cardiac imaging and angiography (abstract). In: Proceedings of the 8th Annual Meeting of the Society of Magnetic Resonance in Medicine. 1989:403.
7. Meyer C, Pauly JM, Macovski A, et al: Simultaneous spatial and spectral selective excitation. *Magn Reson Med* 1990;15:287–304.
8. Noll DC, Meyer C, Pauly JM, et al: A homogeneity correction method for magnetic resonance imaging with time-varying gradients. *IEEE Trans Med Imaging* 1991; 10(4):629–637.

9. Noll DC, Pauly JM, Meyer C, et al: De-blurring for non-2D Fourier transform MR imaging. *Magn Reson Med* 1992;25:319–333.
10. Dixon WT, Du LN, Faul DD, et al: Projection angiograms of blood labeled by adiabatic fast passage. *Magn Reson Med* 1986;3:454–462.
11. Nishimura DG, Macovski A, Pauly JM, et al: MR angiography by selective inversion recovery. *Magn Reson Med* 1987;4:193-202.
12. Nishimura DG, Macovski A, Jackson JI, et al: Magnetic resonance angiography by selective inversion recovery using compact gradient echo sequence. *Magn Reson Med* 1988;8:96–103.
13. Wang SJ, Hu BS, Macovski A, Nishimura DG: Coronary angiography using fast selective inversion recovery. *Magn Reson Med* 1991;18:417–423.
14. Pauly JM, Nishimura DG, Macovski A: A k space analysis of small tip excitation. *J Magn Reson* 1989;81:43–56.

Chapter 18

Magnetic Resonance Angiography of Coronary Arteries

Robert R. Edelman, MD

Cardiovascular disease is the leading cause of mortality in the United States today, with more than 1.2 million myocardial infarctions and 600,000 deaths annually.[1] Approximately 500,000 diagnostic coronary artery catheterizations are performed each year for ischemic heart disease, with as many as 20% showing insignificant disease.[2] However, coronary catheterization has substantial drawbacks as a diagnostic tool.

Coronary catheterization is invasive, with substantial risks including local bleeding and pseudoaneurysm, coronary artery dissection, and contrast reaction.[3] Quantitation of the degree of stenosis is imprecise because the vessels cannot be imaged in cross section, nor is flow quantitation easy to obtain. Because of its invasive nature and cost (typically several thousands of dollars), coronary angiography is not suitable as a screening tool, nor is it ideal for early detection of restenosis after angioplasty. Unfortunately, no satisfactory alternative has been available.

Transesophageal echocardiography (TEE) can show the proximal coronary arteries and demonstrate left main disease.[4] However, isolated left main disease is uncommon, and TEE has not been widely applied for assessment of ischemic heart disease. Ultrafast computed tomography is promising, but currently suffers from drawbacks such as beam-hardening artifacts and contrast loads may be excessive. Moreover, ultrafast computed tomography scanners are not widely available.

The ideal coronary artery imaging technique would be entirely noninvasive, provide high-resolution images, allow measurement of blood flow, be widely available, and be inexpensive. Such a technique could be used for screening of high-risk patients, such as those with hypercholesterolemia, for assessing efficacy of medical therapy with cholesterol-binding agents, for follow-up after angioplasty, and for detection of coronary artery anomalies. Magnetic resonance angiography (MRA) has already proved useful for imaging blood vessels in other regions of the body.[5–14] Our group has developed methods for MRA of the coronary vessels that fulfill many of the above criteria.[15]

From Pohost GM (ed.), *Cardiovascular Applications of Magnetic Resonance*. Mount Kisco, NY, Futura Publishing Co., Inc., © 1993.

The potential value of magnetic resonance methods for the evaluation of cardiovascular disease has been recognized for several years. The introduction of electrocardiographic gating techniques[16] and cine gradient-echo pulse sequences[17] gave detailed views of cardiac anatomy and permitted dynamic assessment of cardiac function,[18] including measurements of blood flow,[19,20] chamber volumes,[21] ejection fraction,[22] demonstration of valvular stenosis and regurgitation,[23,24] and differentiation of the true and false lumens of an aortic dissection. Nonetheless, magnetic resonance has not come into widespread use for cardiac applications, in part because much of the same information can be provided more cheaply and readily by ultrasonography. The situation is different, however, for ischemic heart disease.

For the study of ischemic heart disease, one needs a method that can depict cardiac anatomy with high spatial resolution, demonstrate abnormal wall function, perfusion defects, myocardial metabolism, and coronary artery anatomy—this has been termed the "one-stop shop." Positron emission tomography is useful for evaluation of perfusion and metabolism, but not anatomy or function. Ultrasound can show anatomy and wall function, but not perfusion. Stress studies using thallium or the newer technetium agents accurately detect perfusion deficits, but spatial resolution is poor (>1 cm) and a radioactive substance must be administered.

An integrated study using magnetic resonance would be more cost effective and time efficient than using a combination of the above imaging methods. Cardiac anatomy and function are assessed by standard spin-echo and cine gradient-echo methods. First-pass studies obtained after bolus administration of a paramagnetic or superparamagnetic contrast agent show perfusion defects.[25,26] First-pass magnetic resonance studies require ultrafast imaging techniques such as "turboFLASH" or echo planar[27–29]; using these techniques, subsecond images can be acquired in which cardiac motion is mostly frozen. Thus, the remaining element of the one-stop shop is coronary MRA.

Several approaches for coronary MRA have been proposed. These include subtraction of thick-section images acquired with and without aortic presaturation,[30] spiral scan imaging, and gated three-dimensional imaging. These approaches have succeeded in showing portions of the proximal coronary arteries in healthy subjects. Our group has created the segmented k-space "turboFLASH" technique,[31,32] which allows us to portray not only the proximal coronary arteries but their distal portions and major branches in most subjects.

With standard cine techniques, one phase encoding step is acquired for each phase of the cardiac cycle during one R-R interval.[17] With the segmented acquisition method, a series of phase encoding steps (constituting one segment) are acquired. For eight lines per segment, scan time is reduced by a factor of 8. Using a short TR gradient-echo pulse sequence, the duration of a segment is kept short, typically 50–100 msec. For an acquisition with eight lines per segment, 16 segments (ie, 16 R-R intervals) would be required to create an image with 128 phase encoding steps. For an R-R interval of 800 msec, the total scan time per image is only 13 seconds, sufficiently short to allow breath-holding. We have found that breath-holding is essential to avoid excessive blurring from respiratory motion. Moreover, instead of one image, an entire cine study can be completed in the same scan time by concatenating a series of segments.

In order to improve signal-to-noise, the patient is placed in the prone position over a surface coil so that the heart falls forward and is superficially located. The excitation flip angle is incremented for each line in a segment; a typical flip angle series for eight lines per segment is 10°, 20°, 30°, 40°, 40°, 40°, 40°, and 40°. Flip angle incrementation avoids saturation of inflowing blood before the central phase encoding step is acquired; it is the central step that primarily determines image contrast. Finally, a chemical shift-selective radiofrequency pulse is applied shifted by 3.5 parts per million so as to suppress the signal intensity of fat. This maneuver greatly improves contrast between the coronary arteries and surrounding epicardial fat.

Initially, an axial plane of a section is used with a 2-mm section thickness and a 23 cm × 23 cm field of view. After localization of the proximal left and right coronary arteries, oblique views are acquired along the long axes of the right coronary, left main, left anterior descending, and left circumflex arteries. Only a few sections are required to encompass each artery, so that the total time for a coronary artery study is short, on the order of 15 minutes.

Flow velocity quantification is usually accomplished by acquiring two images in interleaved fashion.[19] One image is rephased, and the other is partially dephased so as to impart the appropriate degree of flow sensitivity. Alternatively, a velocity-dependent phase shift is imparted to each image, but of opposite polarity.[33,34] Complex image subtraction eliminates background phase shifts. Residual phase shifts are due to blood flow,[35] with the phase shift being proportional to velocity along the direction of gradient sensitization. By using the segmented k-space approach, scan times are reduced to a breath-hold; this is essential to reliable measurements of coronary artery flow velocities. Care must be taken to adjust the flow sensitivity correctly; an excessively low flow sensitivity gives poor vessel contrast; an excessively high flow sensitivity causes aliasing, which makes the measurement unreliable. Typical coronary artery flow velocities in our initial studies were on the order of 10–30 cm/s in healthy subjects.

In a series of healthy subjects and patients with coronary artery disease, 100% of the right coronary, left anterior descending, and left circumflex arteries, and 96% of the left main coronary arteries have been demonstrated, indicating the robustness of the imaging procedure (Manning WJ, Li W, Boyle N, and Edelman R, unpublished data). Although only a handful of patients with disease have been studied so far, all stenoses and occlusions have been shown. Further study is needed to determine the sensitivity and specificity of the procedure.

In conclusion, it is now feasible to image the coronary artery tree noninvasively using MRA with a segmented k-space acquisition method. Further improvements in image quality are expected with the introduction of better surface coils and faster and stronger magnetic field gradients. Although more development and testing are needed, clinical utility of coronary MRA appears near at hand.

References

1. American Heart Association: *Heart Facts*. Dallas, TX: American Heart Association; 1990:1.
2. Johnson L, Lozner E, Johnson D, et al: Coronary arteriography 1984–1987: a report of the registry of the Society for Cardiac Angiography and Interventions. I. Results and complications. *Cathet Cardiovasc Dis* 1989;17:5–10.

3. Davis K, Kennedy J, Kemp H, et al: Complications of coronary arteriography from the collaborative study of coronary artery surgery (CASS). *Circulation* 1979;59:1105.
4. Yoshida K, Yoshikawa J, Hozumi T, et al: Detection of left main coronary artery stenosis by transesophageal color Doppler and two-dimensional echocardiography. *Circulation* 1990;81:1271–1276.
5. Weeden V, Meuli R, Edelman RR, et al: Projective imaging of pulsatile flow with magnetic resonance. *Science* 1985;230:946–948.
6. Laub GA, Kaiser WA: MR angiography with gradient motion refocusing. *J Comput Assist Tomogr* 1988;12:377–382.
7. Laub G: Displays for MR angiography. *Magn Reson Med* 1990;14(2):222–229.
8. Edelman RR, Mattle MP, Atkinson DJ, Moogeoud HM: MR angiography. *AJR* 1990;154:937–946.
9. Finn JP, Edelman RR, Jenkins RL, et al: MR angiography: a prospective, blinded study with surgical validation in liver transplantation. *Radiology* 1991;179:265–269.
10. Keller PJ, Drayer BP, Fram EK, et al: MR angiography with two-dimensional acquisition and three-dimensional display. Work in progress. *Radiology* 1989;173:527–532.
11. Litt AW, Edelman EM, Pinto RS, et al: Diagnosis of carotid artery stenosis: comparison of 2DFT time-of-flight MR angiography with contrast angiography in 50 patients. *AJR* 1991;156:611-616.
12. Ruggieri PM, Masaryk TJ, Ross JS, Modie MT: Magnetic resonance angiography of the intracranial vasculature. *Top Magn Reson Imaging* 1991;3:23–33.
13. Masaryk TJ, Modic MT, Ross, JS, et al: Intracranial circulation: preliminary clinical results with three-dimensional (volume) MR angiography. *Radiology* 1989;171:793–799.
14. Masaryk AM, Ross JS, DiCello MC, et al: 3DFT MR angiography of the carotid bifurcation: potential and limitations as a screening examination. *Radiology* 1991;179: 797–804.
15. Edelman RR, Manning WJ, Burstein D, et al: Coronary arteries: breath-hold MR angiography. *Radiology* 1991;181:641–643.
16. Lanzer P, Botvinick EH, Schiller NB, et al: Cardiac imaging using gated magnetic resonance. *Radiology* 1984;150:121-127.
17. Glover G, Pelc N: A rapid gated cine MRI technique. In: Kresel HY (ed). *Magnetic Resonance Annual*. New York: Raven Press, Publishers; 1988:299–333.
18. Higgins CB: Functional evaluation of the heart with magnetic resonance imaging. *Magn Reson Med* 1988;6:121–139.
19. Underwood SR, Firmin DN, Klipstein RH, et al: MR velocity mapping: clinical applications of a new technique. *Br Heart J* 1987;57:404–412.
20. Klipstein RH, Underwood SR, Firmin DN, et al: Blood flow patterns in the human aorta studied by magnetic resonance. *Br Heart J* 1987;58:316–323.
21. Kondo C, Caputo GR, Semelka R, et al: Right and left ventricular stroke volume measurements with velocity-encoded cine MR imaging: in vitro and in vivo validation. *AJR* 1991;157:9–16.
22. Utz JA, Herfkens RJ, Heinsimer JA, et al: Cine MR determination of left ventricular ejection fraction. *AJR* 1987;148:839–843.
23. Mitchell L, Jenkins J, Watson Y, et al: Diagnosis and assessment of mitral and aortic valve disease by cine-flow magnetic resonance imaging. *Magn Reson Med* 1989;12:181-197.
24. Pflugfelder PW, Landzberg JS, Cassidy MM, et al: Comparison of cine magnetic resonance imgaing with Doppler-echocardiography for the evaluation of aortic regurgitation. *AJR* 1989;152:729–735.
25. Atkinson D, Burstein D, Edelman R: First-pass cardiac perfusion: evaluation with ultra fast MR imaging. *Radiology* 1990;174:757–762.
26. Manning WJ, Atkinson DJ, Grossman W, et al: First-pass nuclear magnetic resonance imaging studies using gadolinium-DTPA in patients with coronary artery disease. *J Am Coll Cardiol* 1991;18:959–965.
27. Mansfield P, Pykett IL: Biological and medical imaging by NMR. *J Magn Reson* 1978;29:355–373.

28. Pykett IL, Rzedzian RR: Instant images of the body by magnetic resonance. *Magn Reson Med* 1987;5:563-571.
29. Rzedzian RR, Pykett IL: Instant images of the human heart using a new, whole body MR imaging system. *AJR* 1987;149:245–250.
30. Wang SJ, Hu BS, Macovski A, Nishimura DG: Coronary angiography using fast selective inversion recovery. *Magn Reson Med* 1991;18:417–423.
31. Atkinson D, Edelman R: Cineangiography of the heart in a single breath hold with a segmented TurboFLASH sequence. *Radiology* 1991;178:357–360.
32. Chien D, Atkinson DJ, Edelman RR: Strategies to improve contrast in k-space coverage: reordered phase encoding and k-space segmentation. *J Magn Reson Imaging* 1991;1:63–70.
33. Dumoulin C, Souza S, Walker M, Wagle W: Three-dimensional phase contrast angiography. *Magn Reson Med* 1989;9:139–149.
34. Dumoulin CL, Yucel EK, Vock P, et al: Two- and three-dimensional phase contrast MR angiography of the abdomen. *J Comput Assist Tomogr* 1990;14:779–784.
35. Firmin DN, Naylor Gl, Kilner PJ, Longmore DB: The application of phase shifts in NMR for flow measurement. *Magn Reson Med* 1990;14:230–241.

Section 2

Magnetic Resonance and Myocardial Metabolism

Chapter 19

The Influence of Cardiac Work on the Electrical Potential Gradient Across the Mitochondrial Inner Membrane

Bang Wan, PhD, Chris Doumen, PhD, Jerzy Duszynski, PhD, Guy Salama, PhD, and Kathryn F. LaNoue, PhD

Cardiac oxygen consumption is tightly coupled to cardiac output, as demonstrated by the linear correlation between respiration and the product of heart rate and peak systolic pressure.[1,2] Thus, cardiac muscle depends on mitochondrially synthesized adenosine triphosphate (ATP) as a source of energy for muscle contraction, while mitochondria respond to an increased demand for ATP by increasing the synthesis of the high-energy phosphate. However, the signal transduction mechanism between the muscle fibers and the mitochondria has not been made clear.

Early studies of mitochondria from a variety of sources suggest a simple supply/demand solution to this problem. The addition of adenosine diphosphate (ADP) and phosphate to isolated mitochondria provided with sufficient substrates for the electron transport chain causes approximately a 10-fold increase in respiration.[3] Thus, a logical scheme for the coordination between muscle fiber ATP hydrolysis and mitochondrial respiration might be that ADP and phosphate generated at the muscle fiber diffuse to the mitochondria, where they stimulate respiration. In tissues such as the heart and brain, where rapid responses are required, the creatine kinase system might facilitate the transfer of ADP to the mitochondria.[4] This hypothesis can be tested in tissues that have high levels of cytosolic creatine kinase because free ADP (as calculated from the creatine kinase mass action ratio) should exhibit changes in concentration sufficient to account for changes in respiration. Moreover, these changes should be in the region of the Km of ADP for ATP synthesis by isolated mitochondria.

Supported by P01 HL18708.
From Pohost GM (ed.), *Cardiovascular Applications of Magnetic Resonance*. Mount Kisco, NY, Futura Publishing Co., Inc., © 1993.

Tests of the hypotheses using biochemical methods and the techniques of ^{31}P nuclear magnetic resonance to assess the components of the creatine kinase mass action ratio suggest that mitochondrial respiration is indeed controlled by the concentration of free ADP in tissues such as skeletal muscle[5–7] and neonatal cardiac tissue.[7,8]

However, similar experiments on adult mammalian hearts either in vivo[9] or in vitro[10,11] have not yielded positive results. Neither enzymatic nor nuclear magnetic resonance spectroscopic measurements have been able to detect an increase in ADP with increasing cardiac work. The apparent failure of the ADP hypothesis to explain the correlation between respiration and work has led to a search for an alternate messenger. An appealing candidate for this role is cytosolic free Ca^{2+}, as the concentration of this ion increases when work increases. Ca^{2+} is required to stimulate the interaction between myosin and actin that results in muscle fiber contraction and ATP hydrolysis. Moreover, studies carried out in the last 5 years show that three key mitochondrial dehydrogenases that generate NADH in mitochondria are regulated by Ca^{2+}.[12] Thus, rather than a serial control by free ADP, instead Ca^{2+} might regulate O_2 utilization and ATP hydrolysis in parallel, precluding a change in free ADP as ATP synthesis increased. In order to test this hypothesis and the more general one that substrate supply rather than ADP regulates respiration in adult hearts,[13] measurements were made of the mitochondrial electrical potential gradient, which would be expected to increase when the supply of electrons increases, but decrease when the supply of ADP increases.

Methods

Heart Perfusion

Isolated rat hearts were perfused for 1 hour in the retrograde mode without recirculation using Krebs-Henseleit solution as the perfusate. The perfusate solution contained either 11 mM glucose, 5 mM lactate, or 5 mM pyruvate. The lipophilic cation tritium-labeled tetraphenyl phosphonium ($[^3H]TPP^+$) (5 nM, 3.7 Ci/mM) was present during the first half hour of perfusion, but not during the second half hour. Hearts were perfused under conditions of either low, moderate, or high work. The low work condition was achieved by perfusing the heart at 60 mm Hg without an intraventricular balloon. The moderate-work condition was achieved by setting the perfusion pressure to 120 mm Hg and placing a balloon in the left ventricle. The volume of the balloon was adjusted so that left ventricular end-diastolic pressure (LVEDP) as measured by a pressure transducer was 15.5 ± 1.1 mm Hg. Under these conditions the left ventricular peak systolic pressure (LVPSP) was 137 ± 6 mm Hg. To achieve high work, hearts were perfused as described for moderate work load but isoproterenol (0.01 mM) was included in the perfusate. The LVEDP and LVPSP of the isoproterenol-treated hearts were -5.6 ± 4 and 225 ± 13 mm Hg, respectively, when glucose was the substrate and 6.1 ± 3.3 and 179 ± 7 mm Hg, respectively, when pyruvate was the substrate. Oxygen consumption was determined by measuring the O_2 tension in the influent and effluent perfusate and multiplying the difference by coronary flow.

Isolation of Ventricular Myocytes

Rat cardiac myocytes were isolated using the method described by Cheung et al.[14]

Assays

Oxygen tension was measured polarographically with a Clark electrode. The metabolites, NAD^+, ATP, ADP, adenosine monophosphate (AMP), and creatine phosphate were measured enzymatically using spectrophotometric techniques.[15] NADH was determined fluorometrically in neutralized potassium hydroxide extract.[16]

Determination of Mitochondrial Electrical Potential Gradients

The equilibrium distributions of the lipophilic cation $[^3H]TPP^+$ in and out of the hearts were determined kinetically and used to calculate the sum of the plasma and mitochondrial electrical potential gradients according to the Nernst equation:

$$\Delta\psi_m + \Delta\psi_c = 61.5 \times \log([TPP^+]_m / [TPP^+]_e)$$

where
$\Delta\psi_m$ = mitochondrial membrane electrical potential gradient
$\Delta\psi_c$ = sarcolemmal membrane electrical potential gradient
$[TPP^+]_m$ = concentration of free TPP^+ inside the mitochondria
$[TPP^+]_e$ = concentration of free TPP^+ in the perfusate at equilibrium

The details for obtaining $[TPP^+]_m$ from the equilibrium distribution of total cellular TPP^+ ($[TPP^+]_t$) and extracellular TPP^+ concentration ($[TPP^+]_e$) have been described previously.[17] Early experiments showed that a part of the TPP^+ accumulation in cells was due to passive binding in the cytoplasm and mitochondria, which occurred even in the absence of membrane potential. At the concentrations studied, these "binding sites" did not saturate and the binding affinity of cytosolic components, outer mitochondrial surface, and inner mitochondrial surface were different. The strategy used to obtain $[TPP^+]_m$ was to first calculate the content of TPP^+ inside the mitochondria from the total myocardial TPP^+ content by subtracting: 1) extracellular TPP^+ content, which is the product of the extracellular volume and $[TPP^+]_e$; 2) cytosolic free TPP^+ content, which is the product of cytosolic volume and free TPP^+ concentration ($[TPP^+]_c$) determined by the Nernst equation from the measured $[TPP^+]_e$ and time-averaged plasma membrane potential; and 3) cytosolic bound TPP^+, which is calculated as the sum of the products of $[TPP^+]_c$ and binding constants for cytosol and outer mitochondrial surface. The $[TPP^+]_m$ was then calculated from the relationship that the product of $[TPP^+]_m$ and the sum of matrix volume and binding constant for inner mitochondrial surface equals the intramitochondrial TPP^+ content. The relationship between $[TPP^+]_m$ and the measured $[TPP^+]_t$, $[TPP^+]_e$, and $\Delta\psi_c$ is defined by the following equation adapted from Rottenberg[18] and LaNoue et al.[17] and was used in the present experiment:

$$[TPP^+]_m = \frac{[TPP^+]_t - (10^{\Delta\psi_c/61.5} - [TPP^+]_e) \times (V_c + K_o + K_c) - [TPP^+]_e \times V_e}{V_m + K_i}$$

where
$\Delta\psi_c$ = time-averaged plasma membrane potential (mV)
$[TPP^+]_t$ = total TPP^+/g dry wt in the heart at equilibrium (cpm/g dry wt)
K_i = binding constant for mitochondrial inner surface (ml/g dry wt)
K_o = binding constant for mitochondrial outer surface (ml/g dry wt)
K_c = binding constant for plasma membrane and cytosolic components. (ml/g dry wt)
V_m = mitochondrial matrix volume (ml/g dry wt)
V_c = cytosolic volume (ml/g dry wt)
V_e = interstitial fluid volume (ml/g dry wt)

Values of K_i, K_o, and V_m are from LaNoue et al.[19] Values of V_c and V_e used are from Idell-Wenger et al.[20] Both $\Delta\psi_c$ and $(K_i+K_o+K_c)$ were determined in the present study.

The equilibrium distribution was not attained in these hearts, but rather was calculated by determining of the first-order rate constant of efflux (k_{out}) divided by the first-order rate constant of uptake (k_{in}). Since at equilibrium influx is equal to efflux:

$$k_{in}\,[TPP^+]_e = k_{out}\,[TPP^+]_t$$

$$K_{eq} = \frac{k_{out}}{k_{in}} = \frac{[TPP^+]_e}{[TPP^+]_t}$$

The equilibrium concentration of $[TPP^+]_e$ at the measured $[TPP^+]_t$ was calculated as the product of $[TPP^+]_t$ and K_{eq}. The rate of uptake of $[^3H]TPP^+$ was determined in the first half hour of perfusion from the product of the difference between radioactivity in the influent and effluent and the coronary flow. The approach to equilibrium was so slow that this value was constant when measured for as long as 2 hours. The k_{in} was calculated as:

$$\frac{(\text{cpm in coronary influent} - \text{cpm in coronary effluent}) \times \text{coronary flow}}{\text{cpm in coronary influent}}$$

In the second half hour, the perfusion was carried out with a TPP^+ free solution. The radioactivity in the coronary influent and effluent and in the potassium hydroxide extract of the subsequently freeze-clamped hearts were determined and used to calculate k_{out}:

$$\frac{(\text{cpm in coronary effluent} - \text{cpm in coronary influent}) \times \text{coronary flow}}{\text{cpm in the heart}}$$

The rate of efflux was again constant during the second half hour of the perfusion. The measured value of $[TPP^+]_t$ and the calculated value of $[TPP^+]_e$ at equilibrium were then inserted into Equation 2 to obtain free $[TPP^+]_m$. This value, $[TPP^+]_m$, was then used in Equation 1 to obtain $\Delta\psi_m + \Delta\psi_c$.

Measurement of Sarcolemmal Electrical Potential Gradient ($\Delta\psi_c$)

The sarcolemmal potential was measured in rat hearts perfused under conditions similar to those used for measurement of [^{3}H]TPP$^+$ accumulation in the tissues. Changes of $\Delta\psi_c$ with time were monitored fluorometrically using the potential-sensitive dye di-4-ANNEPS. The hearts were stained with the dye by perfusing the heart with Krebs-Henseleit medium containing 11 mM glucose and 10 mM di-4-ANNEPS for 10–15 minutes. The dye binds to the sarcolemmal membrane under these conditions without entering the cell. The optics and imaging system used have been described previously.[21] Previous studies have shown that the intensity of the fluorescent light from the membrane-bound di-4-ANNEPS excited at 520–590 nM and emitted at 665 nM is a linear function of $\Delta\psi_c$. Light from five small areas near the center of the left ventricle were simultaneously monitored for approximately 5 minutes at low-work, 5 minutes at moderate-work, and 5 minutes at high-work conditions, to obtain sarcolemmal potentials with excellent time resolution. The potentials were averaged over time to obtain the average $\Delta\psi_c$, which was used in Equation 1 to determine $\Delta\psi_m$.

Results

Determination of Binding Constants for [^{3}H]TPP$^+$

Total passive binding of TPP$^+$ to cardiac cells was determined in freshly isolated rat cardiac myocytes incubated in high K$^+$ medium containing a K$^+$ ionophore (valinomycin) to eliminate the sarcolemmal potential and a H$^+$ ionophore (1799) to eliminate the mitochondrial potential. Various concentrations of [^{3}H] TPP$^+$ were included and samples were taken at different time points to determine the equilibrium concentration of [^{3}H]TPP$^+$ in the media and the amount of [^{3}H]TPP$^+$ associated with cells. A plot of the cell-associated [^{3}H]TPP$^+$ against the media [^{3}H]TPP$^+$ concentrations is shown in Figure 1. The binding constant ($K_i + K_o + K_c$) in rat cardiac myocytes from linear least-square-fitting of the data was 54.6 ml/g protein.

When rat hearts were perfused with a similar solution containing (in millimoles) 123.9 KCl, 1.2 $MgSO_4$, 1.2 KH_2PO_4, 25 $NaHCO_3$, 15 glucose, 25 mU insulin, 0.05–0.1 μM valinomycin, 7 μM oligomycin, and 0.12–0.36 DNP with and without 20 2,3-butanedione monoxime, coronary flow decreased from 12–15 to 2 ml/min and the kinetically determined 1/keq by the protocol described in *Methods* was 51.6 ± 7.7 ml/g ($n = 3$). The value of the sum of $\Delta\psi_m + \Delta\psi_c$ calculated from Equations 1 and 2 using the binding constant obtained from isolated cardiac myocytes was 9.3 ± 5.6 mV ($n = 3$). The inference drawn from the remarkable agreement of the total binding constants measured kinetically from the perfused hearts and thermodynamically from the cardiac myocytes was that coronary flow and the capillary barrier did not significantly alter the kinetically determined equilibrium distribution of TPP$^+$ in and out of the myocardium, at least in the de-energized hearts.

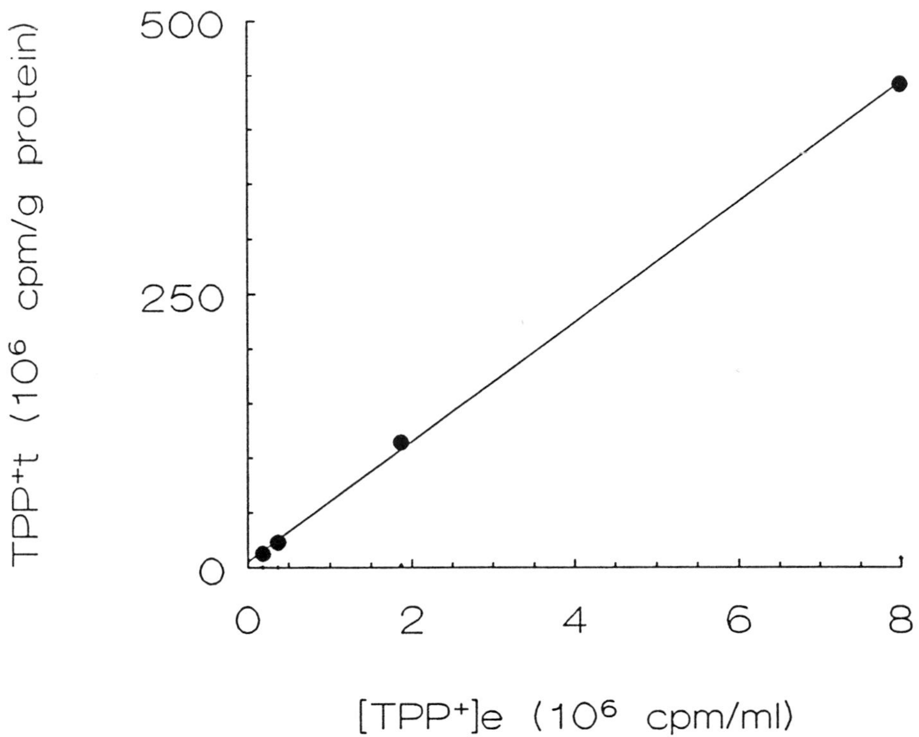

FIGURE 1. *Total TPP^+ binding to KCl and valinomycin depolarized rat cardiac myocytes. Freshly isolated rat cardiac myocytes (1.5 mg/ml) were incubated in solution containing (in millimoles) 125 KCl, 20 HEPES, 1.2 $MgSO_4$, 1.2 KH_2PO_4, 0.05 EGTA, 20 2,3-butanedione monoxime, and 15 glucose (pH 7.4) at 37°C for 10 minutes. Valinomycin and 1799 were then added to a final concentration of 0.1 μM and 75 μM, respectively. Also added were $[^3H]TPP^+$ to give final concentrations of 5 nM (45 Ci/mM), 10 nM (45 Ci/mM), 50 nM (9 Ci/mM), and 200 nM (2.25 Ci/mM). Samples were taken from the incubation at 5, 10, 20, 40, 60, 90, and 120 minutes. Cells were separated from the incubation media by rapid centrifugation through silicone oil. A solution of 50% formic acid below the oil quenched the cells. Pellet and supernatant fractions were counted to obtain the data shown. Total TPP^+ binding ($K_I + K_O + K_C$) of 54.6 ml/g was obtained from the slope of the plot. Each point represents mean ± SEM of seven determinations.*

The Effect of Substrates on $\Delta\psi_m$

Hearts were perfused with 5 nM [^{3}H]TPP$^+$ under low-work conditions with either glucose, lactate, or pyruvate in order to measure $\Delta\psi_m$ and $\Delta\psi_c$. At the end of the 1-hour perfusion, during which k_{in} and k_{out} were measured, the hearts were freeze-clamped with Wollenberger tongs and a part of each heart extracted with perchloric acid. The ATP, ADP, AMP NAD$^+$, and creatine phosphate were measured in the neutralized extracts. Another portion of each frozen heart was extracted with alcoholic potassium hydroxide and used to measure NADH and [^{3}H]TPP$^+$ per gram of dry weight. Separate studies using the potential-sensitive dye di-4ANEPPS indicated that the time-averaged plasma membrane potential was 72 mV.

This value was used in Equation 1 to determine $\Delta\psi_m$. The carbon substrates provided did not change the rate of oxygen consumption, but pyruvate-perfused hearts had higher creatine phosphate and NADH levels and greater $\Delta\psi_m$ than the glucose- or lactate-perfused hearts. This confirms reports by other workers that pyruvate is a better substrate for the heart than glucose.[22,23] The values for the ratio of total heart NADH/NAD$^+$, the nucleotide levels, and the $\Delta\psi_m$ are shown in Tables 1 and 2. The concentration of free ADP was calculated assuming creatine kinase was in equilib-

TABLE 1. The Effects of Substrate on Metabolites in Perfused Rat Hearts.

Substrate	ATP	CrP	ADP	Free ADP (μM)	NADH/NAD$^+$
	μmol/g dry				
Glucose	21.2 ± 1.3	23.1 ± 2.5	6.1 ± 0.5	89 ± 10	0.0141 ± 0.0064
Lactate	23.9 ± 0.4	30.1 ± 1.6	5.7 ± 0.4	65 ± 6	0.0633 ± 0.0032
Pyruvate	22.0 ± 1.1	41.6 ± 2.4	3.6 ± 0.1	30 ± 3	0.0375 ± 0.0017

Rat hearts were perfused at low work with 11 mM glucose, 5 mM lactate, or 5 mM pyruvate and freeze-clamped for 1 hour. Myocardial high-energy phosphates, NAD$^+$, and NADH were assayed enzymatically in PCA or KOH extracts as described in *Methods*. Free cytosolic ADP concentration was calculated from the creatine kinase equilibrium constant ([ATP][Cr]/[ADP][H+][CrP] = 1.66×10^{-9} M^{-1},[24] using a cytosolic pH value of 7.05,[22] a myocardial creatine (Cr) plus creatine phosphate (CrP) content of 68.5 ± 6.6 μmoles/g dry wt [25] and a cytosolic volume of 3.234 ml/g dry.[20] Data represent mean ± SEM of four experiments.

TABLE 2. The Effect of Substrate on the Free Energy of Cytosolic Phosphorylation Potential ΔGp and Mitochondrial Membrane Potential.

Substrate	ΔGp (Kcal)	ΔGp/nF	$\Delta\psi_m$	$\Delta\psi_m$ + (RT/nF)ΔpH	ΔpH
		(mV)			
Glucose (11 mM)	12.96	141	118	158–178	0.67–1.00
Pyruvate (5 mM)	14.98	162	145	185–205	0.67–1.00

Cytosolic phosphorylation potentials in hearts perfused with glucose or pyruvate at low work were calculated from the ATP and free ADP values listed in Table 1 using a $\Delta G_0'$p value of 7.0 Kcal/mol,[26] and P_i concentrations of 9.9 and 1 μmol/g dry weight for glucose- and pyruvate-perfused hearts, respectively.[22] For comparison with $\Delta\psi_m$, the mV equivalent of ΔGp (ΔGp/nF) was calculated using the caloric Faraday constant and an ATP/H$^+$ ratio (n) of 4.[27,28] Also listed are the measured $\Delta\psi_m$ and the proton motive force calculated as $\Delta\psi_m$ + (RT/nF)ΔpH and assuming a ΔpH ranging from 0.67 to 1.0.

rium. In Table 2, the value of ΔGp, the free energy available from the phosphorylation potential exhibited by adenine nucleotides, is compared with $\Delta\psi_m$, which together with ΔpH is the force available for formation of ATP and maintenance of ΔGp. Estimates of the values of ΔpH in the heart range from 0.67 to 1.0 (40 to 60 mV). Inspection of the table reveals that ΔGp/nF is significantly lower than $\Delta\mu H^+ = \Delta\psi_m + (RT/nF)\Delta pH$, as one would expect if $\Delta\mu H^+$ is the driving force for ΔGp and if they are far from equilibrium with each other. However, the higher value of $\Delta\psi_m$ obtained with pyruvate compared with glucose-perfused hearts is similar to the higher value of ΔGp comparing pyruvate with glucose, again as one would anticipate from the direction of energy flow. The data lend credence to the measurements of $\Delta\psi_m$. Additional evidence for the validity of the measurements comes from a comparison of the $\Delta\psi_m$ values obtained from the intact heart with those obtained from isolated rat heart mitochondria using [^{3}H]TPP$^+$.[19,29] The value of $\Delta\psi_m$ obtained in pyruvate-perfused hearts (145 mV) are similar to those obtained with isolated heart mitochondria metabolizing pyruvate in the absence of added ADP (139 mV). Addition of excess ADP to isolated mitochondria in the presence of pyruvate increases respiration 10-fold and lowers $\Delta\psi_m$ to 121 mV.[29]

The Effect of Cardiac Work on $\Delta\psi_m$

In order to determine the directional change of $\Delta\psi_m$ with increasing work, hearts were perfused at three levels of work as described in *Methods*. The oxygen consumption of hearts working at the highest work load was twice that of hearts undergoing moderate work and four times higher than hearts operating at the low work load. The rates of oxygen consumption of the low-work Langendorff hearts were similar to values previously reported (50 nanoatoms per minute per gram of dry weight) for these hearts. When converted to oxygen consumption per milligram of mitochondrial protein (from a knowledge of milligram mitochondrial protein per gram of dry weight), the low-work rates are about twice those observed with isolated cardiac mitochondria metabolizing pyruvate in the absence of added ADP (state 4).

As reported by others,[2,22] respiration was not influenced by the carbon substrate provided in the perfusate, nor were we able to make a positive correlation between free ADP and respiration, as illustrated in Figure 2. In general, NADH/NAD$^+$ increased when comparing low with moderate work. However, this ratio either remained the same (pyruvate) or decreased (glucose) when comparing moderate with high work. It was difficult to interpret these ratios confidently in terms of their influence on mitochondrial respiration because the measured NADH and NAD$^+$ included both mitochondrial and cytosolic pools and because directional changes of perfusate lactate/pyruvate ratios (a measure of cytosolic NADH) were similar to those of the total NADH/NAD$^+$ (Figure 3).

The changes in $\Delta\psi_m$ with work are illustrated in Figure 4. Although the value of $\Delta\psi_m$ is clearly influenced by the nature of the perfusate substrate, high cardiac work decreased $\Delta\psi_m$ independent of the nature of the substrate used.

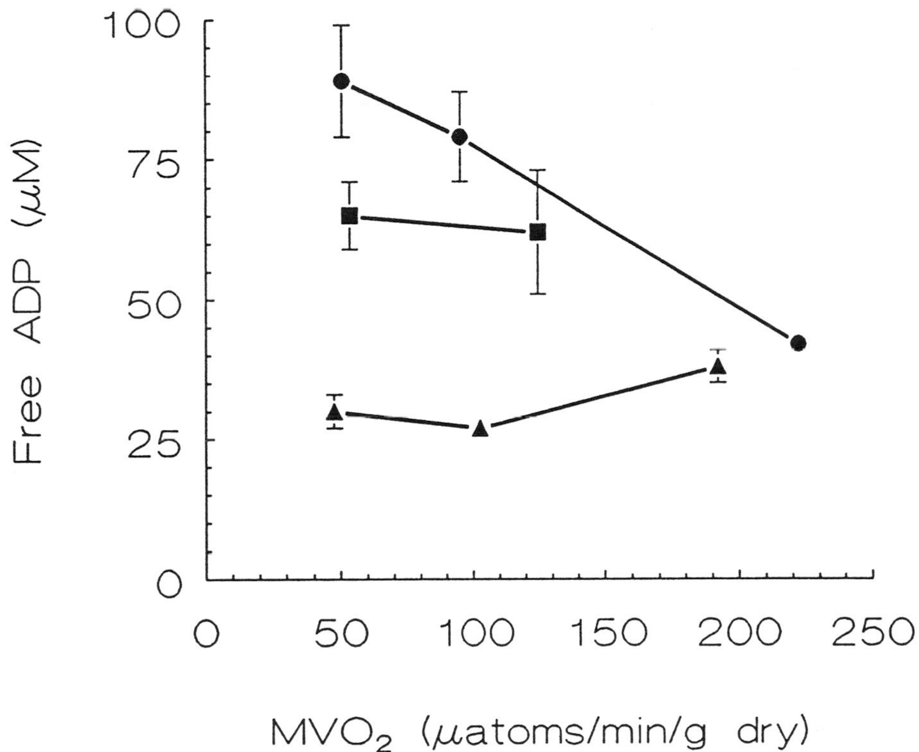

FIGURE 2. *The effect of cardiac work on free cytosolic adenosine diphosphate (ADP). Rat hearts were perfused with 11 mM glucose (solid circle), 5 mM lactate (solid square), or 5 mM pyruvate (solid triangle). The MVO_2 was varied by changing the work load as described in* **Methods**. *Creatine phosphate and adenosine triphosphate (ATP) were determined in perchloric acid extracts of hearts freeze-clamped for 1 hour and used to calculate the free cytosolic ADP concentration from the creatine kinase equilibrium constant as described in the legend for Table 1. Each point represents mean ±SEM of three to eight experiments.*

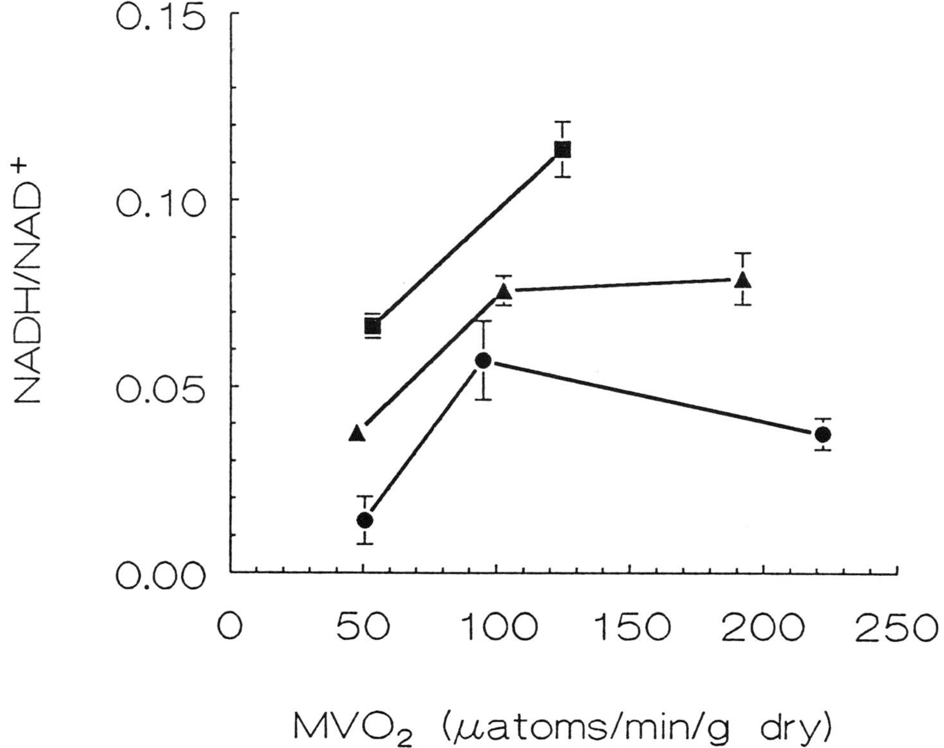

FIGURE 3. *The effect of cardiac work on total tissue NADH/NAD$^+$. Rat hearts were perfused with 11 mM glucose (solid circle), 5 mM lactate (solid square), or 5 mM pyruvate (solid triangle) as described in the legend for Figure 2. Total tissue NADH and NAD$^+$ were determined in potassium hydroxide and perchloric acid extracts, respectively, as described in* **Methods**. *Each point represents mean ± SEM of three to eight experiments.*

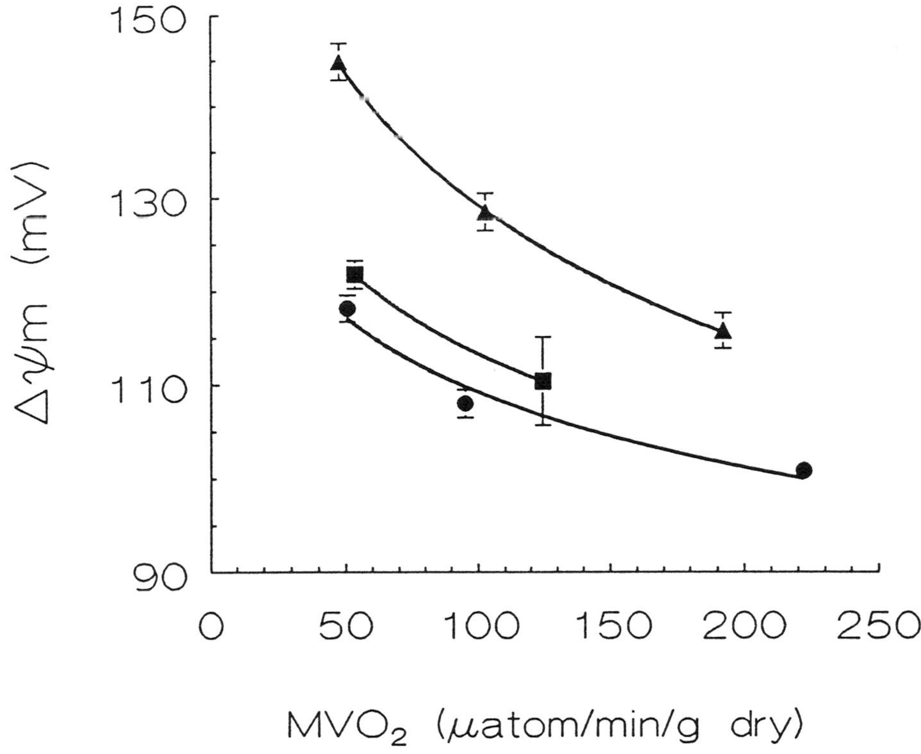

FIGURE 4. *The effect of work on the electrical potential gradient across the mitochondrial membrane. Rat hearts were perfused with 11 mM glucose (solid circle), 5 mM lactate (solid square), or 5 mM pyruvate (solid triangle) as described in the legend for Figure 2.* $\Delta\psi_m$ *was determined kinetically from the equilibrium distribution of* $[^3H]TPP^+$ *in and out of the myocardium as described in* **Methods**. *Each point represents mean ± SEM of three to eight experiments.*

Discussion

A scheme illustrating the control of energy metabolism in the working heart is shown in Figure 5. Variable conductances of energy flow from the energy available from the citric acid cycle intermediates, through the production of NADH to $\Delta\psi_m$ to ATP and on to muscle contraction, are shown as pistons changing the diameter of the pipe that acts as the conduit of energy flow. One can measure pressure at various points in the conduit as wells of NADH, $\Delta\psi_m$, or ATP. The level of fluid in the wells indicates pressure. A decrease in pressure is illustrated as one moves in the direction of flow along the conduits. Clearly, oxygen influences the flow of electrons from NADH and effects the buildup of NADH and its conversion to $\Delta\psi_m$. Likewise, ADP and P_i influence conduction between $\Delta\psi_m$ and ATP affecting the build-up of $\Delta\psi_m$ and its utilization for ATP synthesis. The Ca^{2+} is shown as potentially acting simultaneously at two sites, one at actomyosin adenosine triphosphatase (ATPase) affecting the flow

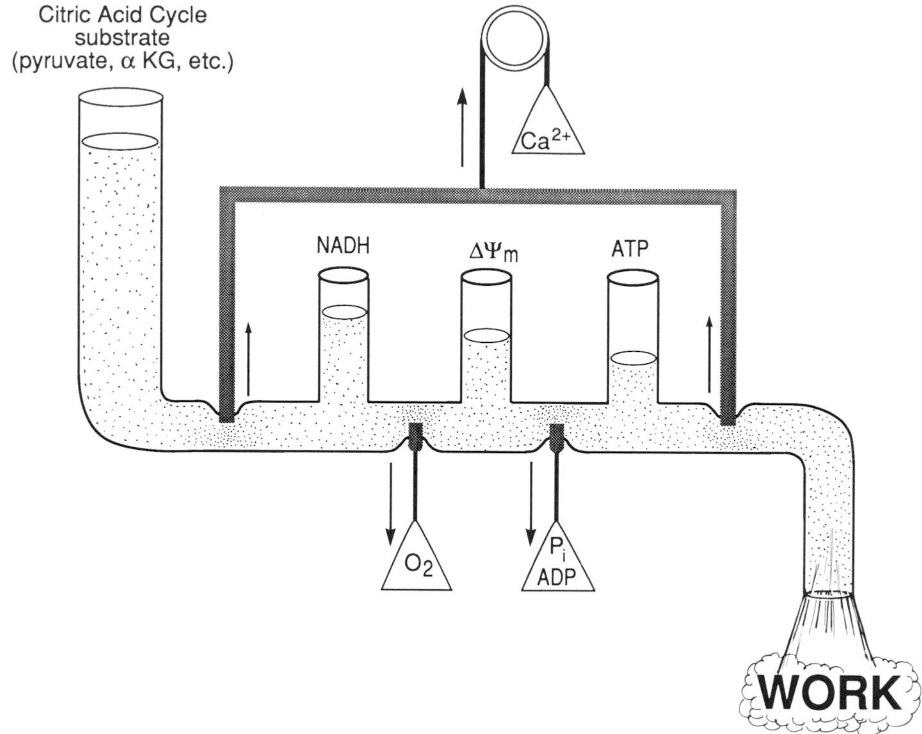

FIGURE 5. *Schematic diagram illustrating the current knowledge of the control of energy flow from citric acid cycle substrate to muscle contraction. Details of the figure are described in the text.*

of energy between ATP and muscle contraction and another conductance site (of unknown strength) acting between the citric acid cycle intermediates and NADH generation. The rationale of the present study was that measurement of the sites of potential energy buildup along the conduit might allow one to say which conductors (Ca^{2+}, oxygen, or ADP and P_i) were important in the control of flow.

The results of the study are clearly puzzling in light of this diagram. As work increases $\Delta\psi_m$ decreases, whereas the data suggest that NADH remains constant or increases. The putative pressure buildup might be the result of oxygen limitation as flow increases. The known regulation of conductance between $\Delta\psi_m$ and ΔGp in the conduit are ADP and P_i, but measurements made in the present study and by others[13] suggest that measured changes in ADP and P_i are too small to account for the increase in flow. It seems, therefore, that there may be a regulator that has not yet been identified, or our ability to estimate free ADP in the vicinity of the mitochondria is poor. This putative cryptic ADP must be free, unavailable to the bulk of the creatine kinase, and presumably generated by myosin ATPase.

We have difficulty in visualizing the nature of such a pool. However, several laboratories have reported data that suggest that the mitochondrial ATP synthase may be controlled by Ca^{2+}.[30,31] Although we have not been able to demonstrate such a control with isolated mitochondria, the possibility clearly exists that such a control requires components present in the intact cell, but not in isolated mitochondria, and is responsible for the observed changes in $\Delta\psi_m$ as net ATP synthesis increases.

Acknowledgments

The dye di-4-ANNEPS was generously provided by Dr. Leslie Loew of the University of Connecticut. The uncoupling agent 1799 was provided by Peter Heytler of the E.I. du Pont-de Nemours Co., Wilmington, Delaware.

References

1. Reimer KA, Jennings RB: Myocardial ischemia, hypoxia, and infarction. In: Fozzard HA, Haber E, Jennings RB, et al. (eds). *The Heart and Cardiovascular System*. New York: Raven Press Publishers; 1986;1133–1201.
2. Kobayashi K, Neely JR: Control of maximal glycolysis in rat cardiac muscle. *Circ Res* 1979;44:166–175.
3. Chance B, Williams GR: The respiratory chain and oxidative phosphorylation. *Adv Enzymol* 1956;47:65–134.
4. Meyer FA, Sweeney HL, Kushmerrick MJ: A simple analysis of the "phosphocreatine shuttle." *Am J Physiol* 1984;246:C365–C377.
5. Crow MT, Kushmerrick MJ: Chemical energetics of slow- and fast-twitch muscles of the mouse. *J Gen Physiol* 1982;79:147–166.
6. Kushmerick MJ, Meyer RA: Chemical changes in rat leg muscle by phosphorus nuclear magnetic resonance. *Am J Physiol* 1985;248:C542–C549.
7. Chance B, Leigh JS Jr, Kent J, et al: Multiple controls of oxidative metabolism in living tissues as studied by phosphorus magnetic resonance. *Proc Natl Acad Sci U S A* 1986;83:9458–9462.
8. Portman MA, Heineman FW, Balaban RS: Developmental changes in the relation between phosphate metabolites and oxygen consumption in the sheep heart in vivo. *J Clin Invest* 1989;83:456–464.
9. Katz LA, Swain JA, Portman MA, et al: Relation between phosphate metabolites and oxygen consumption of heart in vivo. *Am J Physiol* 1989;256:H265–H274.
10. Neely JR, Denton RM, England PJ, et al: The effect of increased heart work on the tricarboxylate cycle and its interactions with glycolysis in the perfused rat heart. *Biochem J* 1972;128:147–159.
11. From AHL, Petein MA, Michurski SP, et al: ^{31}-P-NMR studies of respiratory regulations on the intact myocardium. *FEBS Lett* 1986;206:257–261.
12. McCormack JG, Halestrap AP, Denton RM: Role of calcium ions in regulation of mammalian intramitochondrial metabolism. *Physiol Rev* 1990;70:391–425.
13. Heineman FW, Balaban RS: Control of mitochondrial respiration in the heart in vivo. *Annu Rev Physiol* 1990;52:523–542.
14. Cheung JY, Thompson IG, Bonventre JV: Effects of extracellular calcium removal and anoxia on isolated rat myocytes. *Am J Physiol* 1982;243:C184–C190.
15. Bergmeyer HV: *Methods of Enzymatic Analysis*. Second English edition. New York; Academic Press, Inc., 1974.
16. Williamson JR, Corkey BE: Assays of intermediates of the citric acid cycle and related compounds by fluorometric enzyme methods. *Methods Enzymol* 1969;13:434–513.
17. LaNoue KF, Strzelecki T, Strzelecka D, et al: Regulation of the uncoupling protein in brown adipose tissue. *J Biol Chem* 1986;261:298–305.
18. Rottenberg H: Membrane potential and surface potential in mitochondria: uptake and binding of lipophilic cations. *J Membr Biol* 1984;81:127–138.

19. LaNoue KF, Jeffries FMH, Radda GK: Kinetic control of mitochondrial ATP synthesis. *Biochemistry* 1986;25:7667–7675.
20. Idell-Wenger JA, Grotyohann LW, Neely JR: Coenzyme A and carnitine distribution in normal and ischemic hearts. *J Biol Chem* 1978;253:4310–4318.
21. Salama G, Lombardi R, Elson J: Maps of optical action potentials and NADH fluorescence in intact working hearts. *Am J Physiol* 1987;252:H384–H394.
22. From AHL, Zimmer SD, Michurski SP, et al: Regulation of oxidative phosphorylation rate in the intact cell. *Biochemistry* 1990;29:3731–3743.
23. Katz LA, Korestsky AP, Balaban RS: Activation of dehydrogenase activity and cardiac respiration: a ^{31}P-NMR study. *Am J Physiol* 1988;255:H185–H188.
24. Lawson JWR, Veech RL: Effects of pH and free Mg^{2+} on the kEq of the creatine kinase reaction and other phosphate hydrolyses and phosphate transfer reactions. *J Biol Chem* 1979;254:6528–6537.
25. Williamson JR: Glycolytic control mechanisms II. Kinetics of intermediate changes during the aerobic-anoxic transition in perfused rat heart. *J Biol Chem* 1966;241:5026–5036.
26. Slater EC, Rosing J, Mol A: The phosphorylation potential generated by respiring mitochondria. *Biochim Biophys Acta* 1973;292:534–553.
27. Lemasters JJ: The ATP-to-oxygen stoichiometries of oxidative phosphorylation by rat liver mitochondria. An analysis of ADP-induced oxygen jumps by linear nonequilibrium thermodynamics. *J Biol Chem* 1984;259:13123–13129.
28. Freedman JA, Lemaster JJ: Thermodynamics of reverse electron transfer across site 1: ATP/2e$^-$ is greater than one. *Biochem Biophys Res Commun* 1984;125:8–13.
29. Berkich DA, Williams GD, Masiakos PT, et al: Rates of various reactions catalyzed by ATP synthase as related to the mechanism of ATP synthesis. *J Biol Chem* 1991;266:123–129.
30. Yamada EW, Huzel NJ: The calcium-binding ATPase inhibitor protein from bovine heart mitochondria. Purification and properties. *J Biol Chem* 1988;263:11498–11503.
31. Das AM, Harris DA: Regulation of the mitochondrial ATP synthase in intact rat cardiomyocytes. *Biochem J* 1990;266:355–361.

Chapter 20

^{13}C Nuclear Magnetic Resonance Methods for the Analysis of Citric Acid Cycle Metabolism in the Heart

Craig R. Malloy, MD, A. Dean Sherry, PhD, and F. Mark H. Jeffery, PhD

The obvious long-term goal of developing ^{13}C nuclear magnetic resonance (NMR) is for diagnostic studies in humans. Studies in simpler preparations, however, are also important because they address current questions in cardiac metabolism. Although methods for detecting ^{14}C- or ^{11}C-enriched tracers are quite sensitive, timely metabolic questions are difficult to investigate with these techniques because of the limited amount of data provided. If a substrate is metabolized through a linear pathway (as is the case for glucose uptake or glycolysis), then data analysis is relatively straightforward. Conversely, once the tracer enters the citric acid cycle, interpretation becomes rather intricate because it is a cyclic pathway (Figure 1). Information about fluxes into the cycle must be derived from a limited number of experimental measurements such as total ^{11}C content in the heart or $^{14}CO_2$ release. ^{13}C NMR generally provides more information about the fate of a tracer and is now used in several laboratories for analysis of the citric acid cycle.[1–5]

The central objective in many tracer studies of the heart is the estimation of the respiratory fuel. The heart normally uses a mixture of fatty acids, lactate, and ketones, but the contribution of each to acetyl-CoA depends on the prevailing conditions. The sources of acetyl-CoA in the heart during ischemia or reperfusion may be important in the identification of myocardial ischemia by positron tomography.[6] It has been suggested that kinetics of fatty acid or acetate metabolism during or after ischemia may identify viable myocardium,[7] yet studies with radioisotope methods find both increased[8] and decreased[9] oxidation of fatty acids during or after ischemia. Studies with

Supported in part by a Research Associate Award and Merit Review from the Department of Veterans Affairs, NIH HL34557, SCOR HL17669, and a Biomedical Research Initiative from the Meadows Foundation.
From Pohost GM (ed.), *Cardiovascular Applications of Magnetic Resonance*. Mount Kisco, NY, Futura Publishing Co., Inc., © 1993.

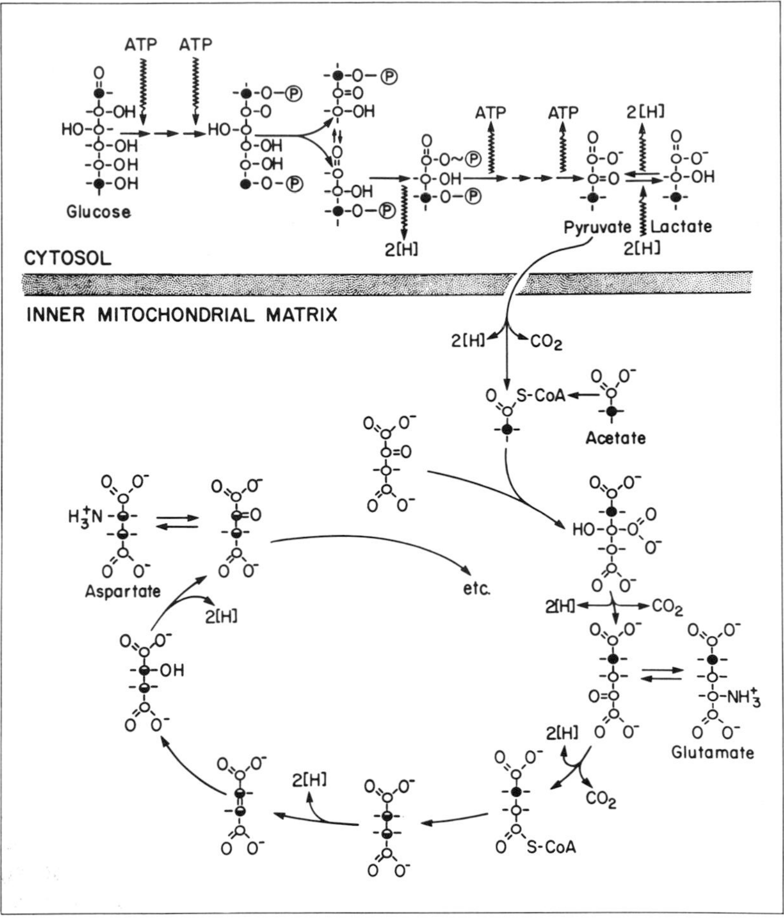

FIGURE 1. *Carbon flow in the citric acid cycle. The distribution of ^{13}C during one turn of the cycle is shown. In this example, ^{13}C may originate in [1,6-^{13}C]glucose, [3-^{13}C]lactate, or [2-^{13}C]acetate. Reprinted from Reference 30 with permission.*

traditional radiotracers are unlikely to resolve these important issues. Quantitation of fatty acid oxidation by ^{14}C methods is unreliable because of uncertainty about the intracellular fate of long-chain fatty acids and the extent to which a fatty acid undergoes complete β-oxidation.[10,11] The choice of [1-^{11}C]palmitate is also poor because one round of β-oxidation removes the entire label, and hence, shorter chain fatty acids could accumulate without being detected.

Sources of carbon for acetyl-CoA may also influence tolerance to ischemia. In animal models, suppression of fatty acid utilization improves mechanical function during reperfusion after ischemia.[12,13] Long-chain fatty acids are known to reduce myocardial efficiency, ie, oxygen consumption is somewhat increased for a given level of work,[14–16] and suppressing fatty acid utilization could have beneficial effects. Simple quantitative methods to measure fatty acid oxidation during ischemia and early after reperfusion could prove quite useful in a better understanding of ischemia and its therapy.

^{13}C is nearly ideal for NMR studies of intermediary metabolism. Because it is a stable isotope, complex enrichment patterns in physiologically relevant substrates may be produced. For example, uniformly enriched fatty acids are available, in contrast to the limitation of ^{11}C to carbonyl carbons. Thus, the fate of the "interior" carbons of fatty acids may be analyzed. ^{13}C also has the great advantage of low natural abundance, approximately 1.1%. Because ^{12}C cannot be detected by NMR, a metabolic pathway may be investigated using ^{13}C in a manner analogous to ^{11}C or ^{14}C by providing a substrate enriched in the appropriate site. The chemical shift range of ^{13}C (200 ppm) is a further advantage because structurally similar compounds are generally resolved and assignments are simple. The sensitivity of ^{13}C is approximately 1.6% compared with ^{1}H for an equal number of nuclei. Most protonated carbons in small molecules gain a factor of 2 to 3 in signal when protons are irradiated (nuclear Overhauser enhancement effect). This effect gives ^{13}C a sensitivity for detection of about 4–5% of ^{1}H in intact tissues that nearly equals the sensitivity of ^{31}P.

The most widely studied pathways so far have been related to glycogen storage and mobilization.[17–21] We have chosen to use ^{13}C NMR to examine a variety of biochemical reactions involving the Krebs citric acid cycle. The objective of this brief review is to present and compare various approaches to the analysis of citric acid cycle metabolism by ^{13}C NMR.

Analysis Based on Fractional Enrichment

Relative enrichment in various sites in a molecule can be measured easily by ^{13}C NMR. Several groups have taken advantage of this feature and used enrichment in various carbons of product molecules, analogous to ^{14}C tracer studies.[22–24] In these studies glutamate was selected as a convenient indicator of labeling patterns in the citric acid cycle (Figure 1) because it is in exchange with α-ketoglutarate and it is easily detected in most tissue. An important study reported by Chance et al.[22] in 1983 used ^{13}C NMR and traditional analytical methods to measure the fractional enrichment in carbons of glutamate as a function of time after providing a ^{13}C labeled substrate to the heart. Citric acid cycle flux could be calculated from these kinetic observations because the sizes of the major exchanging pools were included in the analysis. If pool sizes are not known, ^{13}C NMR estimates of citric acid cycle kinetics must be interpreted cautiously because the rate at which ^{13}C enters the C2 or C3 pools versus the C4 pool of glutamate will depend on the sizes of all other citric acid cycle intermediate pools.

A conceptually different approach was introduced in the early 1980s and has come to be known as isotopomer analysis.[25,26] Entry of ^{13}C into the citric acid cycle inevitably produces intermediates enriched with ^{13}C nuclei in more than a single site within the same molecule (^{13}C isotopomers). This complicates the ^{13}C NMR spectrum as a result of spin-spin coupling between adjacent ^{13}C nuclei, but it also provides valuable biochemical information. Patterns of ^{13}C enrichment in product molecules can be determined by observing multiplets in the ^{13}C NMR spectrum that are due to ^{13}C-^{13}C coupling.[27,28] Our analysis of the citric acid cycle exploits the additional information in a ^{13}C NMR spectrum to conveniently measure relative activities of numerous pathways intersecting in the cycle.[29–33]

Direct C4 Analysis

The glutamate C4 resonance from a tissue sample that has oxidized a combination of [1,2-^{13}C]acetate (or a uniformly enriched fatty acid mixture) and [3-^{13}C]lactate typically appears as a nine-line resonance consisting of four multiplet components (Figure 2) including a singlet (C4S), two doublets with differing one-bond coupling constants (C4D34 and C4D45), and a quartet (C4Q). The fraction of the acetyl-CoA pool that is doubly labeled (F_{c3}, [1,2-^{13}C]acetyl-CoA) versus the fraction that is singly labeled (F_{c2}, [2-^{13}C]acetyl-CoA) is simple to determine from the C4 resonance. The sum of the C4S + C4D34 resonance areas versus the C4D45 + C4Q resonance areas directly reports the relative utilization of [3-^{13}C]lactate versus [1,2-^{13}C]acetate, ie, F_{c2}/F_{c3}.

This analysis is direct and unambiguous. The data are obtained from a single ^{13}C resonance and hence are applicable to a variety of experimental conditions in which comparisons between different resonance areas may be problematic; eg, some in vivo

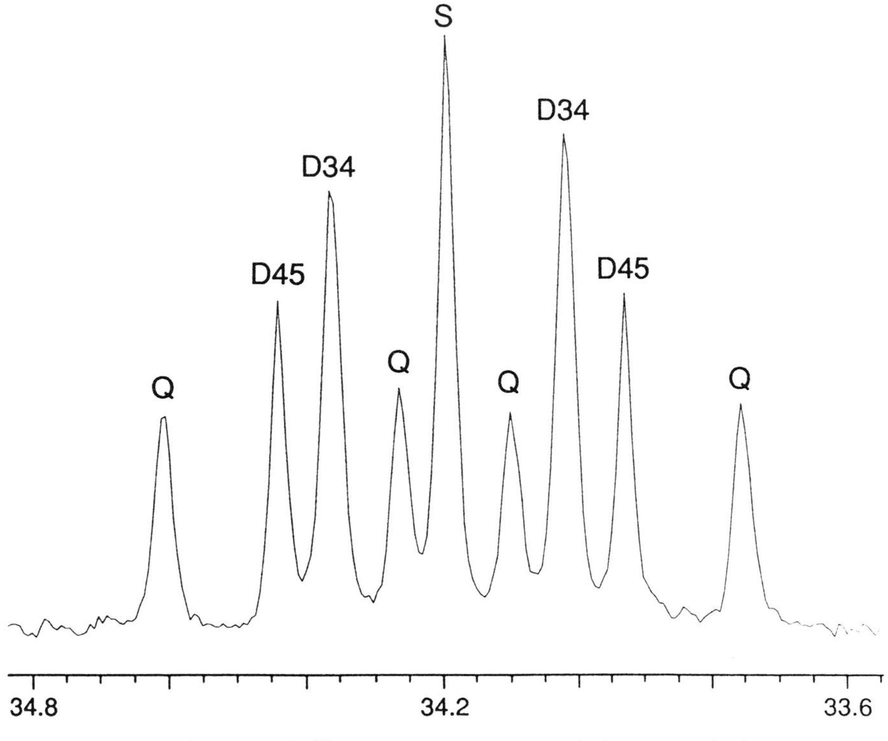

FIGURE 2. *Proton-decoupled ^{13}C NMR spectrum of the C4 of glutamate (tissue extract). The areas of the four multiplets (S, D34, D45, and Q), that make up the C4 resonance are proportional to the pools of glutamate isotopomers. (S, singlet in the C4 spectrum; D34, doublet due to J_{34}; D45, doublet due to J_{45}; Q, quartet or doublet of doublets.)*

spectra may have fatty acid resonances that overlap the glutamate C3 resonance or have differences in T_1 or nuclear Overhauser enhancement values that may unknowingly compromise a quantitative comparison of resonance areas. Relative substrate utilization may be obtained from either C4S/C4D45 (these components only arise when C3 is not enriched) or from C4D34/C4Q (these components only arise when C3 is enriched). This direct analysis does not require isotopic steady-state conditions, nor is it affected by entry of either labeled or unlabeled substrate into the citric acid cycle pools via an anaplerotic reaction or changing pool sizes. Since the measurement reflects entry of the various acetyl-CoA isotopomers into the glutamate C4 position averaged over the period of time required to collect an NMR spectrum in an intact heart, it would not be sensitive to alterations in flux between acetyl-CoA and glutamate (the first span of the citric acid cycle) that might occur during collection of the NMR data. One can reasonably assume that a given mixture of acetyl-CoA isotopomers (derived from various labeled substrates made available to the heart) arrive in the glutamate pool in exactly the same proportion as those that entered the cycle via the citrate synthase reaction.

This technique is quite valuable for detecting changes in relative substrate utilization between two differently labeled materials, but it does not measure either anaplerosis or the contribution of unlabeled exogeneous or endogeneous substrates to acetyl-CoA.

Nonsteady-State Analysis

Under many conditions we want to know the contribution of unlabeled substrates to acetyl-CoA, eg, after an ischemic or hypoxic interval, during changes in workload, or after administration of a drug. Recently, a ^{13}C NMR method for determining relative substrate utilization was reported that could be applied to in vivo situations in which the magnetic field homogeneity may not be sufficient to resolve ^{13}C-^{13}C coupling.[33] It was shown that $(C4D34)(C4/C3) = F_{c2}$ and $(C4Q)(C4/C3) = F_{c3}$, where C4/C3 is the ratio of total signal in the C4 and C3 carbons. This analysis is quite reliable in most cases, but suffers when the C4/C3 ratio is large (ie, C3 enrichment is low). Typically, this occurs during the first few minutes after introducing an enriched substrate as the citric acid cycle turns over. This method may also be of limited use in vivo, where there may be other resonances that overlap the C3 resonance. The direct C4 method presented above obviates that problem, but does not allow measurement of absolute F_{c2} and F_{c3} values.

Nonsteady-State Analysis With Homonuclear ^{13}C Decoupling

Recently, we investigated homonuclear ^{13}C decoupling for simplification of the ^{13}C spectrum. The ^{13}C-^{13}C coupling constants J_{23} and J_{34} are nearly equal in glutamate. Consequently, [2,3-^{13}C]glutamate cannot be distinguished from [3,4-^{13}C]glutamate in the C3 resonance. Information about the relative concentration of these isotopomers can be recovered by single-frequency homonuclear ^{13}C decoupling of the C2 or C4 resonance. If the C2 is irradiated, the (normally) five-line C3 collapses into a triplet. This triplet has a very simple relation to acetyl-CoA labeling patterns: $C3D\{C2\} = F_{c2} + F_{c3}$, and $C3S\{C2\} = F_{c0} + F_{c1}$ ({C2} indicates single-frequency irradiation of the C2 resonance of glutamate).

This method is useful because the nonsteady-state analysis allows measurement of F_{c0} only if the ratio C4/C3 in glutamate can be determined. Early after exposure to enriched substrates, however, enrichment in C3 is low relative to C4, and this ratio is difficult to determine accurately. Multiplet analysis of the C3 during C2 irradiation removes this limitation, and has the advantage of improving peak height/ noise. This method could prove valuable in vivo when other resonances may overlap the C4.

Steady-State Analysis

The metabolic pathways that feed carbon skeletons into the cycle have been called anaplerotic sequences by Krebs and Kornberg.[34] The activity of these pathways relative to citrate synthase have for historical reasons been given the variable y. Continuous synthesis of citric acid cycle intermediates occur largely via pyruvate carboxylation and propionate carboxylation.[35] There are many instances when one would like to completely evaluate substrate utilization including partitioning of pyruvate into carboxylation versus decarboxylation reactions. Like other isotope tracer methods, the most complete analysis of the glutamate spectrum requires steady-state metabolic and isotopic conditions, normally achieved in normoxic Langendorff or working hearts in about 20–25 minutes. A typical extract spectrum is shown in Figure 3. Under these conditions the relative concentrations of glutamate isotopomers are unchanging, and the fuel of oxidation, the relative activity of anaplerotic versus oxidative pathways, and the ^{13}C enrichment of molecules entering these pathways may all be determined by an isotopomer analysis. The assumptions for this steady-state model are typical of prior metabolic models. Recently, we have found some evidence that the assumption of full scrambling of label in the succinate and fumarate pools may not be valid in yeast,[36] but this phenomenon does not appear to influence analysis of the ^{13}C NMR spectrum of the heart.

The steady-state isotopomer analysis is based on the relation between each isotopomer of α-ketoglutarate and relative fluxes. The probability that any isotopomer will be replaced by the same or another isotopomer can be written as the product of the probabilities of a pathway at a metabolic branch point, and solution of the matrix will yield the relative concentration of each isotopomer in terms of the physiologic variables (F_{c1}, y, etc.). The mathematical relation between each isotopomer and the variables is quite complex, but this is not a real limitation because the concentration of an individual isotopomer is not provided by ^{13}C NMR. However, the spectrum does measure the relative concentrations of groups of isotopomers, and it is quite fortunate that these groups of isotopomers (the multiplets in the ^{13}C spectrum) have a relatively simple relation to physiologic variables. For example, if the heart is provided with [2-^{13}C]acetate and other unlabeled substrates, then we can assume that $F_{c2} = F_{c3} = 0$,

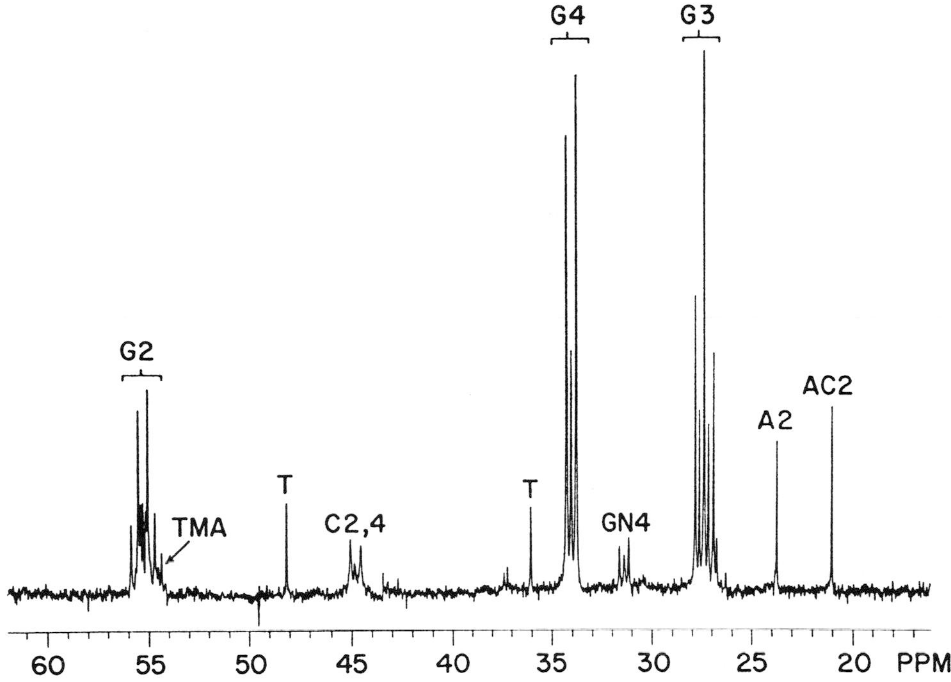

FIGURE 3. *Proton-decoupled ^{13}C NMR spectrum of the protonated carbons of glutamate (tissue extract). A2, carbon 2 of acetate; AC2, carbon 2 of acetylcarnitine; C2,4, carbons 2 and 4 of citrate; G2–C4, carbons 2–4 of glutamate; GN4, carbon 4 of glutamine; T, taurine; TMA, trimethyl amino group of acyl carnitine.*

$y > O$, and $F_{a0} = 1$. Under these boundary conditions the relations between multiplets and variables is quite simple. For example,

$$C3S = F_{c0}(F_{c0} + y)/(y + 1)$$
$$C3T = F_{c2}{}^2/(y + 1)$$
$$C4D34 = F_{c2}/(2y + 1)$$

Complete equations for other conditions are published elsewhere.[28] These equations may be used to predict the steady-state glutamate spectrum under assumed metabolic conditions or to analyze the glutamate spectrum in terms of metabolic fluxes.

The steady-state analysis is limited in vivo because steady-state conditions may be difficult to achieve due to the expense of administering high concentrations of highly enriched substrates for a prolonged period. Under these conditions, the nonsteady-state methods described above are appropriate.

Currently, isotopomer analysis does not provide a critical measurement of myocyte function:absolute citric acid cycle flux. However, it does yield relative fluxes into the cycle in a simple and convenient analysis, and some measurements, such as anaplerotic flux, are difficult by conventional radiotracer techniques. Nuclear magnetic resonance spectroscopic methods are complementary and may be used to analyze all major aspects of myocyte metabolism (Figure 4).

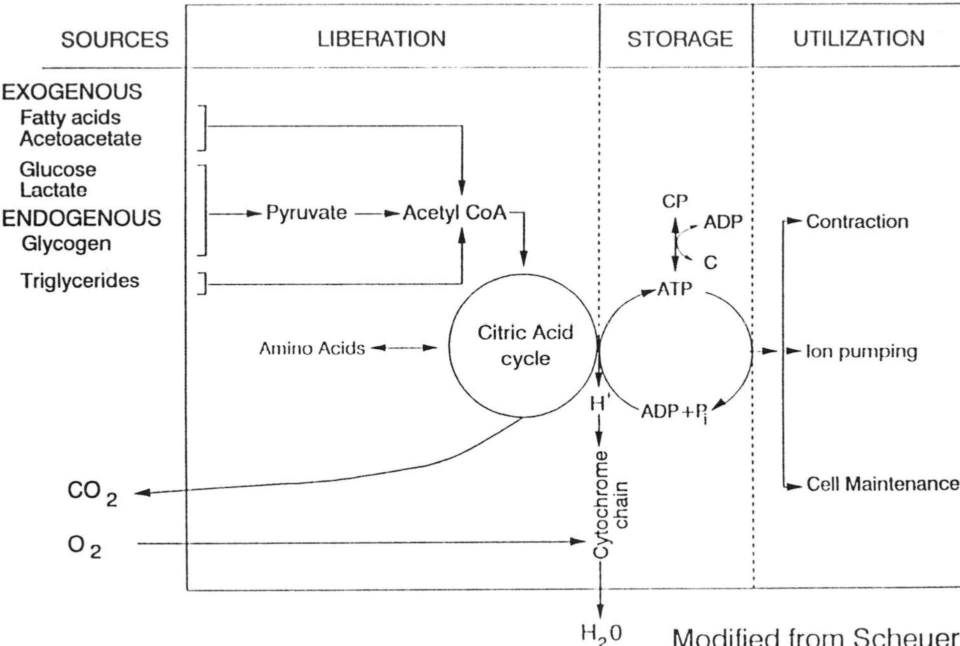

FIGURE 4. *Overview of cardiac cell metabolism. Modified from Reference 37 with permission.*

References

1. Damico LA, Closter J, Jan L, Clark BJ: The ontogeny of substrate choice in the neonatal piglet heart (abstract). In: Proceedings of the 9th Annual Meeting of the Society of Magnetic Resonance in Medicine 1990:179.
2. Buchthal SD, Ugurbil K, Zimmner SD, From AHL: Observation of changes in the anaplerotic flux of the post ischemic myocardium (abstract). In: Proceedings of the 9th Annual Meeting of the Society of Magnetic Resonance in Medicine 1990:906.
3. Lewandowski D, Johnston DL: Reduced substrate oxidation in postischemic myocardium: ^{13}C and ^{31}P NMR analyses. *Am J Physiol* 1990;258:H1357-H1365.
4. Lewandowski D, Johnston DL: The use of ^{13}C as a tracer in studies of intermediary metabolism (abstract). In: Proceedings of the 9th Annual Meeting of the Society of Magnetic Resonance in Medicine. 1990;905.
5. Nunnally RL, Redding EH, Germann MJ, et al: Metabolic regulation in mammalian heart *in vivo*: a ^{13}C NMR study (abstract). Proceedings of the 9th Annual Meeting of the Society of Magnetic Resonance in Medicine 1990;907.
6. Lerch RA, Ambos HD, Bergmann SR, et al: Localization of viable ischemic myocardium by positron emission tomography with ^{11}C palmitate. *Circulation* 1981;64:680–699.
7. Armbrecht JJ, Buxton DB, Schelbert HR: Validation of [1-^{11}C]acetate as a tracer for noninvasive assessment of oxidative metabolism with positron emission tomography in normal, ischemic, postischemic, and hyperemic canine myocardium. *Circulation* 1990;81:1594–1605.
8. Liedtke AJ, DeMaison L, Eggleston A, et al: Changes in substrate metabolism and effects of excess fatty acids in reperfused myocardium. *Circ Res* 1988;62:535–542.
9. Myears DW, Sobel BE, Bergmann SR: Substrate use in ischemic and reperfused canine myocardium: quantitative considerations. *Am J Physiol* 1987;253:H107-H114.

10. Veerkamp JH, van Moerkerk HTB, Glatz JFC, et al: $^{14}CO_2$ production is no adequate measure of [^{14}C] fatty acid oxidation. *Biochem Med Metab Biol* 1986;35:248–259.
11. Chatzidakis C, Otto DA: Labeled oxidation products from [1-^{14}C], [U-^{14}C], and [16-^{14}C] palmitate in hepatocytes and mitochondria. *Lipids* 1987;22:620–626.
12. Kjekshus JK, Mjos OD: Effect of inhibition of lipolysis on infarct size after experimental coronary artery occlusion. *J Clin Invest* 1973;52:1770–1778.
13. Mjos OD: Effect of free fatty acids on myocardial function and oxygen consumption in intact dogs. *J Clin Invest* 1971;50:1386–1390.
14. Challoner DR, Steinberg D: Oxidative metabolism of myocardium as influenced by fatty acids and epinephrine. *Am J Physiol* 1966;210:280–286.
15. Severeid L, Conner WE, Long JP: The depressant effect of fatty acids on the isolated rabbit heart. *Proc Soc Exp Biol Med* 1969;131:1239–1243.
16. Drake-Holland AJ, Elzinga G, Noble MIM, et al: The effect of palmitate and lactate on mechanical performance and metabolism of cat and rat myocardium. *J Physiol* 1983;339:1–15.
17. Brainard JR, Hutson JY, Hoekenga DE, Lenhoff R: Ordered synthesis and mobilization of glycogen in the perfused heart. *Biochemistry* 1989;28:9766–9772.
18. Jue T, Rothman DL, Tavitian BA, Shulman RG: Natural-abundance ^{13}C NMR study of glycogen repletion in human liver and muscle. *Proc Natl Acad Sci U S A* 1989;86:1439–1442.
19. Jue T, Rothman DL, Tavitian BA, Shulman RG: Direct observation of glycogen synthesis in human muscle with ^{13}C NMR. *Proc Natl Acad Sci U S A* 1989;86:4489–4491.
20. Shulman GI, Rothman DL, Chung Y, et al: ^{13} NMR studies of glycogen turnover in the perfused rat liver. *J Biol Chem* 1988;263:5027–5029.
21. Shulman GI, Rothman DL, Jue T, et al: Quantitation of muscle glycogen synthesis in normal subjects and subjects with non-insulin-dependent diabetes by ^{13}C nuclear magnetic resonance spectroscopy. *N Engl J Med* 1990;322:223–228.
22. Chance EM, Seeholzer S, Kobayashi K, Williamson JR: Mathematical analysis of isotope labeling in the citric acid cycle with applications to ^{13}C NMR in perfused rat hearts. *J Biol Chem* 1983;258:13785–13794.
23. Lewandowski ED, Johnston DL: Reduced substrate oxidation in postischemic myocardium: ^{13}C and ^{31}P NMR analyses. *Am J Physiol* 1990;258:H1357-H1365.
24. Weiss RG, Chacko VP, Glickson JD, Gerstenblith G: Comparative ^{13}C and ^{31}P NMR assessment of altered metabolism during graded reductions in coronary flow in intact rat hearts. *Proc Natl Acad Sci U S A* 1989;86:6426–6430.
25. Walker TE, Han CH, Kollman VH, et al: ^{13}C nuclear magnetic resonance studies of the biosynthesis by *Microbacterium ammoniaphilum* of L-glutamate selectively enriched with carbon-13. *J Biol Chem* 1982;257:1189–1195.
26. Cohen SM: Simultaneous ^{13}C and ^{31}P NMR studies of perfused rat liver. *J Biol Chem* 1983;258:14294–14308.
27. Sherry AD, Nunnally RL, Reshock RM: Metabolic studies of pyruvate and lactate perfused guinea pig hearts by ^{13}C NMR. *J Biol Chem* 1985;260:9272–9279.
28. Malloy CR, Sherry AD, Jeffrey FMH: Evaluation of carbon flux and substrate selection through alternate pathways involving the citric acid cycle of the heart by ^{13}C NMR spectroscopy. *J Biol Chem* 1988;263:6964–6971.
29. Malloy CR, Sherry AD, Jeffrey FMH: Analysis of the tricarboxylic acid cycle of the heart using ^{13}C isotope isomers. *Am J Physiol* 1990;28:H987-H995.
30. Jeffrey FMH, Rajagopal A, Malloy CR, Sherry AD: ^{13}C NMR: a simple yet comprehensive method for analysis of intermediary metabolism. *Trends Biochem Sci* 1991;16:5–10.
31. Malloy CR, Sherry AD, Jeffrey FMH: Substrate metabolism in the citric acid cycle of the heart by NMR. In: Schaefer S, Balaban RS (eds) *Cardiovascular NMR*. Kluwer Inc.; 1992:153-168.
32. Malloy CR: Analysis of substrate utilization by ^{13}C NMR spectroscopy. In: Srere PA (ed) *Structural and Organizational Aspects of Metabolic Regulation*. New York: Alan R. Liss, Inc.; 1990;363–374.
33. Malloy CR, Thompson JR, Jeffrey FMH, Sherry AD: Contribution of exogenous sub-

strates to acetyl CoA: measurement by ^{13}C NMR under nonsteady-state conditions. *Biochemistry* 1990;29:6756–6761.

34. Krebs HA, Kornberg HL: Energy transformations. In: *Living Matter*. Berlin: Springer-Verlag; 1957.
35. Sherry AD, Malloy CR, Roby RE, et al: Propionate metabolism in the rat heart by ^{13}C NMR spectroscopy. *Biochem J* 1988;254:593–598.
36. Sumegi B, Sherry AD, Malloy CR: Channeling of TCA cycle intermediates in cultured *Saccharomyces cerevisiae*. *Biochemistry* 1990;29:9106–9110.
37. Scheuer J, Penpargkul S: Myocardial metabolism. In: Willerson JT, Sanders CA (eds) *Clinical Cardiology*. New York: Grune & Stratton; 1977:47–63.

Chapter 21

Nuclear Magnetic Resonance Studies of Anoxia in Animal Hearts

Robert G. Shulman, PhD

Cardiac muscle stores glycogen in the cytosol at concentrations of ~50 mM, similar to the levels in skeletal muscle. In the latter, glycogen serves as a fuel during sustained work under both anaerobic and aerobic conditions in a generally understood fashion. During intense anaerobic exercise, skeletal muscle glycogen is reduced to negligible levels within several minutes. The possibility that glycogen might serve as a reserve fuel in the heart has developed very slowly since the suggestion by Evans in 1934 that "... glycogen is reserved for hypoxic emergencies ...".[1] Rapid utilization of cardiac glycogen during anoxia has been reported,[2–4] and the role of glycogen in myocardial survival has been demonstrated.[5–7] However, the absence of quantitative studies linking glycogen consumption to survival has inhibited widespread acceptance of this mechanism. In this chapter, the results from a series of in vivo nuclear magnetic resonance (NMR) studies that elucidate the role of glycogen during anoxia in rat and guinea pig hearts are reviewed.[8–13]

Our ^{31}P NMR studies of anoxia in vivo[9] followed numerous ^{31}P NMR studies of the effects of ischemia and hypoxia in the perfused heart.[14–20] In Figure 1, our results show a rapid decrease in phosphocreatine (PCr) with $t_{1/2} = 54.5 \pm 2.5$ s and an even faster recovery upon reoxygenation of $t_{1/2} = 38.2 \pm 3.3$ s. In these experiments adenosine triphosphate (ATP) was observed to stay constant for at least 7 minutes of spectral accumulation during terminal anoxia, whereas the hearts stopped beating after 12 to 14 minutes. In the perfused rat heart several experiments have shown that ATP declines much sooner after the start of anoxia. From the findings in this chapter, the shorter survival of the perfused heart could be caused by lower initial glycogen levels, possibly caused by excising the heart.

Supported by NIH grants DK27121 and DK43146.

From Pohost GM (ed.), *Cardiovascular Applications of Magnetic Resonance*. Mount Kisco, NY, Futura Publishing Co., Inc., © 1993.

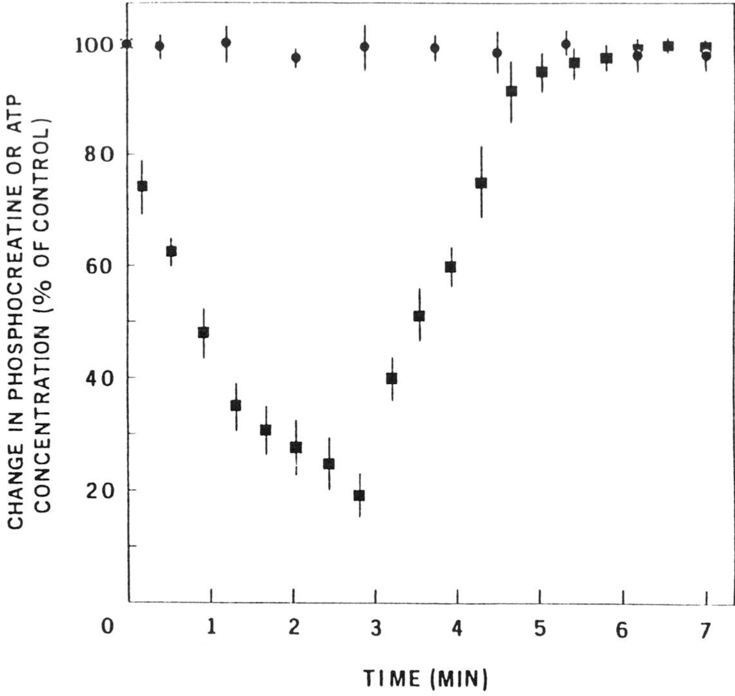

FIGURE 1. *(●), Time dependence of the intensity of the phosphocreatine resonance during 3 minutes of anoxia and subsequent reventilation. Data points are midpoints of 20.5-second accumulations and represent the average of five animals (±SEM). (■), Time dependence of the β-ATP signal during terminal anoxia. Data points are midpoints of 48-second accumulations (±SEM, N=4). There is a 2-second delay between consecutive spectra due to filing of individual spectra on floppy disk in an automated sequence. Reproduced from Reference 10 with permission.*

Results

Rates are calculated from published data with the limitation of not being able to make any additional measurements. It is shown how the published results support a hypothesis about the role of glycogen in the heart during anoxia. The hypothesis is that after PCr is consumed (in approximately 1 minute) cardiac pumping is sustained by glycogen consumption and that the heart stops beating when the glycogen is exhausted. The author believes that enough support for this hypothesis is indicated to encourage the planning of more quantitative experiments. In this approximate analysis, rat and guinea pig data are combined. Starting concentrations are assumed to be [PCr] = 8 mM, [ATP] = 7 mM, as discussed in conversation with K. Ugurbil (1990), and [glycogen] ≃40 mM, which are generally accepted values. During the initial period of anoxia, PCr decreased, whereas ATP remained constant. From the results shown in Figure 1

$$\frac{d[PCr]}{dt} = \frac{[PCr]}{54.5s} = 9\mu mol/gwwmin$$

Since each PCr generates one ATP, the consumption of ATP is also 9 μmol/gww minutes since the ATP stays constant. During anaerobic glycolysis, ATP is generated solely by substrate-level phosphorylation from glycogen. In this case, since each glucose moiety of glycogen makes three ATP molecules, the rate of glycogen consumption needed to supply ATP at 9 μmol/gww minutes is 3 μmol/gww minutes. At this rate, where constant ATP needs are met, ~40 mM glycogen will sustain the ATP consumption for approximately 13 minutes, which agrees with the time that the heart continues to beat.

In the guinea pig, the effects of anoxia upon the concentration of ^{13}C-labeled glycogen were measured by direct ^{13}C NMR.[11] As shown in Figure 2, from the direct ^{13}C spectra after a delay of approximately 1 minute, the rate of decrease of the labeled glycogen becomes constant. Estimates of the net GPase rate need to be corrected for the percentage enrichment, but the data are not complete enough to calculate that rate exactly. Only an estimate can be made. These ^{13}C measurements were made after the heart glycogen had been loaded with ^{13}C-enriched glucose during 50 minutes of infusion, during which time in the rat 12 μmol/gwwmin of total glycogen had been synthesized. From Figure 2 we see that in the guinea pig, after the same infusion protocol, all of the labeled glycogen has vanished at 6 minutes. If we assume that the last glycogen in is the first out, this will give the lowest rate of glycogen degradation during this period. This lower limit is 12 μmol/gww per 6 minutes, or 2 μmol/gwwmin. This is a lower limit because it assumes that the label is being degraded at the same fractional enrichment at which it was synthesized. Any departure from a strict last-in-first-out model will give a larger rate of glycogen degradation.

In one experiment, the activity of GSase (I form) was measured in rats as 0.23 ± 0.10 μmol/gwwmin under in vivo conditions of glycogen synthesis. The activity of GPase, measured under the same conditions of glycogen synthesis, was anomalously high at 3.8 ± 2.4 μmol/gwwmin. This high value of GPase would have prevented net glycogen synthesis, which in fact we observed. Similar anomalously high values of GPase activity had been noted previously. A possible functional use of this excess GPase activity is shown by the present results, which show that during anoxia, the GPase rate is approximately 30 μmol/gwwmin, while the direct ^{13}C NMR shows a rate >2 μmol/gwwmin. These values are at least an order of magnitude greater than the value during synthesis, which must be less than the GSase rate of 0.23 μmol/gwwmin from the agreement between in vitro and in vivo GSase rates. These results suggest that the reserve capacity of GPase is activated during anoxia, which is a time of great need. The present estimates show values that are close to the in vitro value of 3.8 μmol/gwwmin. Figure 2 shows that the GPase activity increases, to approach its in vitro value, by more than one order of magnitude in a period of ~ 1 minute. The mechanism for this activation could be studied further during this delay period by interventions intended to change the delay.

The rapid response of GPase to anoxia suggests that some activation mechanism exists. Its time course is similar to the $t_{1/2} = 54$ s of PCr decay and suggests there is a linkage between GPase activations and the energetic state. While P_i is a possible candidate, since it is expected to increase as PCr decreases, it should be operating as an

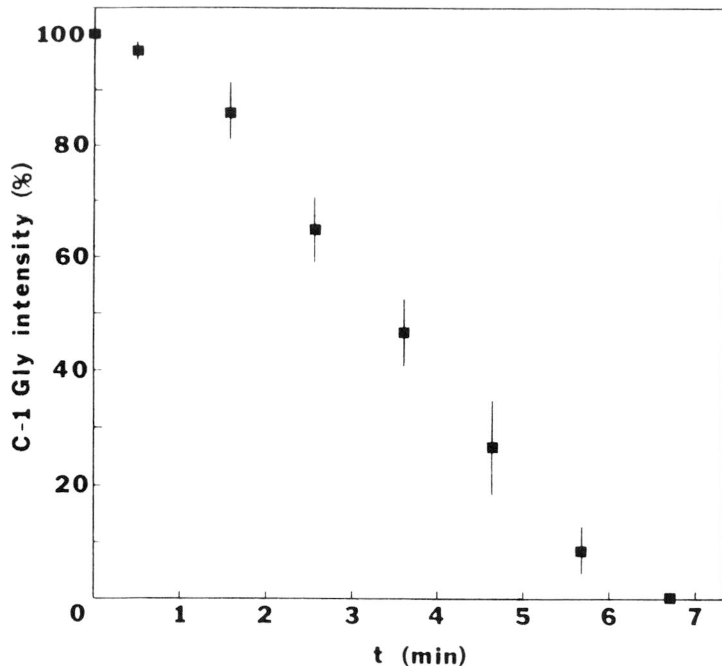

FIGURE 2. *Time course of the degradation of the 1-^{13}C-labeled myocardial glycogen during anoxia in guinea pig heart in vivo. Data points represent averages of seven experiments (±SEM). In each experiment, the respirator was turned off at time 0 and the peak height of the C1 glycogen resonance was measured from serially acquired 1-minute proton-decoupled ^{31}C NMR spectra. Reproduced from Reference 11 with permission.*

activator, not as a substrate, because GPase is well known from the original studies by the Coris not to be at equilibrium. The author does not believe that P_i has been shown to be an allosteric effector of GPase.

To make the present information more quantitative, it would be desirable to devise an experimental method for eliminating the uncertainties presently attendant upon the fractional enrichment. Certainly ^{1}H NMR of glycogen promises to help in this kind of assessment.[21] Another way this could be done would be to deplete glycogen anaerobically, then, while the animal was still alive, to refill the glycogen pool by infusing ^{13}C labeled glucose of known fractional enrichment, along with oxygen, so as to revive the animal and to replenish the glycogen to a known and uniform fractional enrichment. A subsequent period of anoxia would give ^{13}C NMR spectra whose intensities could be converted to net glycogen levels and rates.

Summary

The experiments reviewed seem consistent with two hypotheses:

1. During anoxia, the heart maintains its ATP levels and continues to beat by anaerobic glycolysis as long as the glycogen supply lasts.

2. During anoxia there is rapid stimulation of GPase activity by one order of magnitude so that it approaches the in vitro rate. This supplies a function for the excess GPase activity previously observed in vitro, but the mechanism of activation remains undetermined.

References

1. Evans G: The glycogen content of the rat heart. *J Physiol* 1934;82:468–480.
2. Opie LH: Relative rates of aerobic and anaerobic energy production during myocardial infarction and comparison with effects of anoxia. *Circ Res* 1976;(suppl I):I52–I68.
3. Capasso JM, Lemma TM, Zimmerman JA: Post-anoxic recovery of myocardial performance in senescent mice. *Exp Gerontol* 1981;16:261–269.
4. Liedtke AJ: Alterations of carbohydrate and lipid metabolism in the acute ischemic heart. *Prog Cardiovasc Dis* 1981;23:321–336.
5. Scheuer J, Stezoski SW: Protective role of increased myocardial glycogen stores in cardiac anoxia in the rat. *Circ Res* 1970;27:835–849.
6. Hearse DJ, Chain EB: The role of glucose in the survival and recovery of the anoxic isolated perfused rat heart. *Biochem J* 1972;128:1125–1133.
7. Rovetto MJ, Whitmer JT, Neely JR: Comparison of the effects of anoxia and whole heart ischemia on carbohydrate utilization in isolated working rat hearts. *Circ Res* 1973;32:699–711.
8. Neurohr KJ, Barrett EJ, Shulman RG: In vivo ^{31}P NMR reveals lowered ATP during heat shock of *Tetrahymena*. *Science* 1983;219:1223–1225.
9. Neurohr KJ, Gollin G, Barrett EJ, et al: In vivo ^{31}P NMR studies of myocardial high energy phosphate metabolism during anoxia and recovery. *FEBS Lett* 1983;159:207–210.
10. Neurohr KJ, Shulman RG: ^{13}C and ^{31}P NMR studies of myocardial metabolism in live guinea pigs. In: Dahalla HS, Hearse DJ (eds). *Advances in Myocardiology*. 1985:185–193.
11. Neurohr KJ, Gollin G, Neurohr JM, et al: ^{13}C NMR studies of myocardial glycogen metabolism in live guinea pigs. *Biochemistry* 1984;23:5029–5035.
12. Laughlin MB, Petit WA, Dizon JM, et al: In vivo NMR measurement of myocardial glycogen metabolism. *J Biol Chem* 1988;263:2285–2291.
13. Laughlin MR, Petit WA, Shulman RG, et al: Measurement of myocardial glycogen synthesis in diabetic and fasted rats. *Am J Physiol* 1990;258:E184-E190.
14. Gadian DG, Hoult DI, Radda GK, et al: Phosphorus nuclear magnetic resonance studies on normoxic and ischemic cardiac tissue. *Proc Natl Acad Sci U S A* 1976;73:446–448.
15. Hollis DP, Nunnally RL, Taylor GJ, et al: Phosphorus nuclear magnetic resonance studies of heart physiology. *J Magn Reson* 1978;29:319–330.
16. Garlick PB, Radda GK, Seeley PJ: Studies of acidosis in the ischemic heart by phosphorus nuclear magnetic resonance. *Biochem J* 1979;184:547–554.
17. Nunnally RL, Bottomley PA: Assessment of pharmacological treatment of myocardial infarction by phosphorus-31 NMR with surface coils. *Science* 1981;211:177–180.
18. Matthews PM, Radda GK, Taylor DJ: A ^{31}P NMR study of metabolism in the hypoxic perfused rat heart. *Biochem Soc Trans* 1981;9:236–237.
19. Bailey IA, Radda GK, Seymour AML, et al: The effects of insulin on myocardial metabolism and acidosis in normoxia and ischemia: a ^{31}P NMR study. *Biochim Biophys Acta* 1982;720:17–27.
20. Flaherty JT, Weisfeldt ML, Bulkley BH, et al: Mechanisms of ischemic myocardial cell damage assessed by phosphorus-31 nuclear magnetic resonance. *Circulation* 1982;65:561–570.
21. Zang LH, Howseman AM, Shulman RG: Assignment of the ^{1}H chemical shifts of glycogen. *Carbohydr Res* 1991;220:1-9.

Chapter 22

Lipid Metabolism: Basic Concepts and Nuclear Magnetic Resonance Studies

Jeanie B. McMillin, PhD

Oxidation of long-chain fatty acids is a primary source of metabolic energy in the working heart. Availability of fatty acids is considered to be critical for support of high levels of cardiac work.[1] Enzymological and metabolic analyses of the various steps involved in the pathways of long-and short-chain fatty acid metabolism suggest potential rate limitation of the oxidative pathway both by cytosolic and mitochondrial factors. Based on biochemical studies of isolated steps in the β-oxidation pathway, consideration of conditions under which rate control may be exerted will be discussed (Figure 1). Nuclear magnetic resonance (NMR) spectroscopy of the intact heart provides the opportunity to establish the physiologic conditions under which these controls may be expressed.

Control of Long Chain Acylcarnitine Production by Cardiac Malonyl-CoA

In order for long-chain fatty acids to gain access to the enzymes of β-oxidation, transfer of the activated fatty acids from the cytosolic to the intramitochondrial compartment must occur. This transfer is accomplished by conversion of long-chain acyl-CoA (LCA-CoA) to acylcarnitine by mitochondrial carnitine palmitoyltransferase I (CPT-I) and re-esterification to matrix CoA by the sequential action of a second enzyme located on the inner half of the inner membrane, CPT-II. Formation of LCA-CoA that is catalyzed by CPT-II enters into the β-oxidation pathway. The co-identity of CPT-I and CPT-II is controversial. (For a review, see McGarry et al.[2]) Therefore, recent work has focused on molecular biological approaches to resolve the biochemical data. Because CPT-II has been isolated as a pure protein, its molecular weight and amino acid composition are known. Based on partial amino acid sequences

Supported in part by a grant from the National Institutes of Health, RO1-HL 38863.
From Pohost GM (ed.), *Cardiovascular Applications of Magnetic Resonance.* Mount Kisco, NY, Futura Publishing Co., Inc., © 1993.

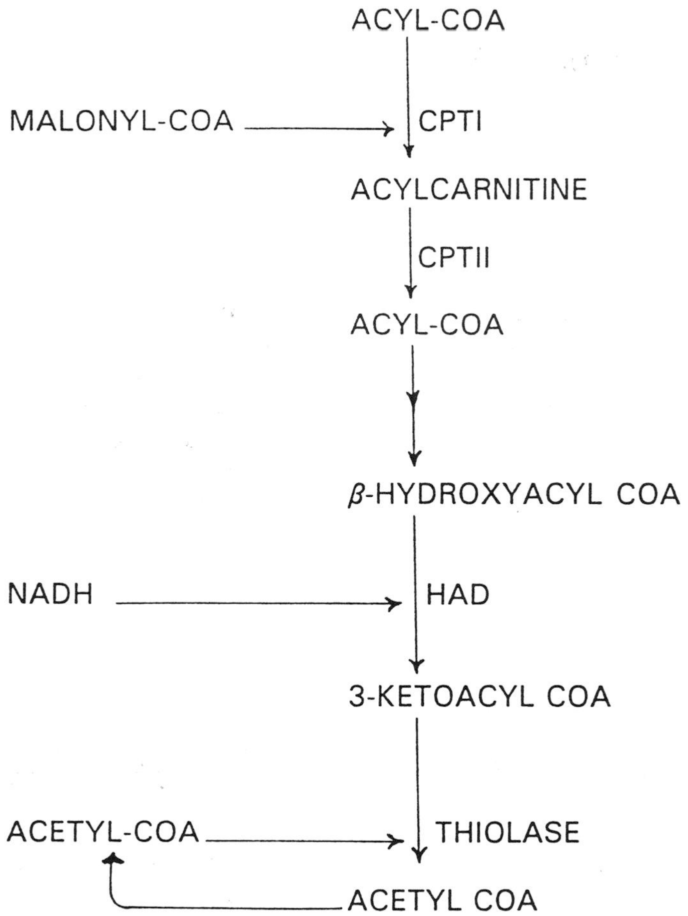

FIGURE 1. *Sites of proposed rate limitation in long-chain fatty acid oxidation in the heart. Rate control has been suggested for each of the following steps in β-oxidation: CPT-I; CPT-II; HAD; and thiolase. CPT, carnitine palmitoyltransferase; HAD, β-hydroxyacyl CoA dehydrogenase.*

of isolated CPT-II peptides, a rat liver cDNA library was screened using P^{32}-5′ end-labeled oligonucleotides. Clones of liver CPT-II have been isolated and the cDNA derived from these clones has been sequenced.[3] We have demonstrated that this cDNA hybridizes to a 2.4-kB fraction of RNA isolated from cultures of neonatal cardiac myocytes, suggesting that the primary structure of this protein is probably conserved between different organs. In contrast to expectations for the overtly expressed protein CPT-I, the nucleotide sequence of CPT-II contains a 5′ region coding for amino acids that have properties requisite to mitochondrial leader sequences.[3] Because of the proposed regulatory properties of CPT-I and observed differences in affinity of CPT-I for its effector, malonyl-CoA, it is tempting to speculate that this protein might be expected to be synthesized as isoenzymes dependent on the species and tissue of origin.

The activity of the overt CPT-I, which is in communication with the cytosol, is decreased by the lipogenic substrate malonyl-CoA.[2] Modulation of LCAcarnitine synthesis in the liver coordinates lipogenesis with fatty acid oxidation. In peripheral organs such as the heart, CPT-I is very sensitive to inhibition by malonyl-CoA. Malonyl-CoA is present in the heart, its levels responding to feeding and fasting.[2] Recently, discovery of a cardiac isoenzyme of acetyl-CoA carboxylase[4,5] provided additional support for the idea that CPT-I may participate in the regulation of acylcarnitine production and, subsequently, β-oxidation (Figure 1). To date, there are no physiologic studies that specifically address the relationship between variations in tissue levels of malonyl-CoA and flux of long-chain fatty acids through β-oxidation. However, there are some preliminary suggestions[6] that rate control at CPT-I may be expressed in the heart. When hearts are perfused with lactic acid, long-chain fatty acid uptake and metabolism by the heart is inhibited.[6] The site of this inhibition appears to be at CPT-I based on analyses of cardiac levels of LCA-CoA, triacylglycerides (increase), and LCAcarnitine (decrease).[7] An apparent action of lactic acid to activate acetyl-CoA carboxylase and to thereby increase malonyl-CoA production has been reported for the liver enzyme.[8] Although similar information is not available for the heart, activation of the cardiac isoform of acetyl-CoA carboxylase by increased tissue production of lactic acid should elevate malonyl-CoA in the heart with resultant inhibition of CPT-I.

Rate Limitation at CPT-II

At present, there is no biochemical evidence that LCA-CoA production from LCAcarnitine is limited by CPT-II (Figure 1), and this enzyme is apparently insensitive to inhibition by malonyl-CoA.[1] However, in the isolated, perfused working heart there is a suggestion that flux through β-oxidation is limited at a step subsequent to CPT-I but prior to transesterification of LCAcarnitine to LCA-CoA.[9] In hearts producing increased levels of contractile activity (120 mm Hg), LCA-CoA levels decreased and long-chain fatty acid carnitine increased, and these changes were associated with higher rates of fatty acid extraction and oxidation.[9] Increased oxidative metabolism of long-chain fatty acids was also demonstrated by drastically reduced levels of acetyl-CoA, the end product of β-oxidation. Using ^{31}P NMR to investigate the regulatory role of cytosolic adenosine diphosphate (ADP) in the regulation of the rate of oxidative phosphorylation in the Langendorff perfused rat heart, From et al.[10]

suggested that palmitate could not generate the high levels of NADH and acetyl-CoA achieved with octanoate perfusion, the latter substrate being metabolized independently of the carnitine pathway. These results support the observation that rate limitation of long-chain fatty acid utilization exists at either CPT or at the carnitine-acylcarnitine exchange. The carnitine exchange is, however, believed to be present in the mitochondrial inner membrane in excess concentrations, so that rate limitation of the transport of acylcarnitine across the inner membrane should not occur in most physiologic settings.

Physiologic Consequences of Short- Versus Long-Chain Fatty Acid Oxidation

The importance of fatty acid chain length on levels of contractile performance has also revealed important differences between hearts that were perfused with long-chain fatty acids versus medium-chain substrates. Where the carnitine-dependent metabolism of long-chain fatty acids results in various degrees of accumulation of the esters of the LCFA, oxidation of short- to medium-chain fatty acids bypasses the sequential reactions at CPT-I and CPT-II. Although β-oxidation of long-chain fatty acids can generate high levels of NADH and acetyl-CoA, these end products of metabolism do not appear to reach pathway saturation.[9] On the other hand, medium-chain fatty acids achieve and maintain high levels of acetyl-CoA, even at high degrees of cardiac work.[11] The observed limitation in flux of long-chain fatty acids through β-oxidation during increased contractility is compensated by increased flux of the acetyl-CoA produced through the citric acid cycle, with consequent increases in the rates of oxidative phosphorylation. Thus, under aerobic conditions no decrease in either adenosine triphosphate (ATP) production or contractile performance is observed in the presence of long-chain fatty acids.[11]

In contrast to the aerobic heart, contractile depression is observed when hearts are perfused with long-chain fatty acids following a 20–25-minute period of transient ischemia.[12,13] Under the same conditions, reperfusion of rat heart with 11 mM glucose results in complete mechanical recovery. Although glucose oxidation is suppressed when palmitate is added to the reperfusion medium, the biochemical explanation for decreased contractility is not obvious since ATP production is not compromised in these hearts. The apparent preference of cardiac mitochondria for fatty acid over glucose as substrate is well known in aerobic hearts[11] and has been further verified by C-13 NMR spectroscopy.[13] The contribution of long-chain fatty acids to ATP production in the reperfused, ischemic heart (90%) is not significantly different from control (93.8%) so that fatty acids also appear to be the preferred substrate during reperfusion.[12,13] Furthermore, the preferred oxidation of long-chain fatty acids by ischemic porcine heart during reperfusion has also been reported.[14] In the hearts reperfused with long-chain fatty acids, there is an increased accumulation of tissue LCAcarnitine,[12] again suggesting the appearance of rate limitation at CPT-II (see above). Myocardial utilization of glucose can be increased by perfusing drugs that inhibit CPT-I (thereby decreasing long-chain fatty acid utilization). Under these conditions, functional recovery of the postischemic heart may be improved.[12] Whereas the deleterious effect of long-chain fatty acids on contractile function has been attributed to the membrane-active properties of long-chain fatty acid esters,[15] a decrease in mechanical coupling of oxygen consumption to cardiac work may also reflect the lower ATP:O ratios achieved with fatty acids as substrate both in vitro[16] and in vivo.[10]

Using P^{31} and C^{13} NMR spectroscopy to examine the ability of reducing equivalents generated by β-oxidation to support contractile recovery in postischemia, Lewandowski et al.[17] perfused rabbit hearts with the short-chain fatty acid C^{13} butyrate. In bypassing the carnitine pathway, physiologic complications due to generation of amphipathic esters of long-chain fatty acids could be avoided. When butyrate was compared to acetate, which enters the tricarboxylic acid cycle (TCA) directly, either substrate supported contractile function of aerobically perfused hearts. However, in postischemic hearts, β-oxidation of butyrate improved contractile recovery when compared with acetate.[17] No differences in the high-energy phosphate spectrum between postischemic hearts perfused with acetate or butyrate were observed. These investigators concluded that by providing fatty acids directly to β-oxidation and by minimizing synthesis of long-chain fatty acyl-CoA and long-chain fatty acyl carnitine, functional recovery of postischemic myocardium may be improved.

Control of Fatty Acid Flux Through β-Oxidation

The enzymatic steps of the β-oxidation spiral have been well delineated. The specific steps involved in the regulation of fatty acid oxidation have been proposed based on both biochemical studies with isolated mitochondria and purified enzymes of β-oxidation, as well as a physiologic model, the isolated, perfused working heart. Unlike the liver, which stores lipid as triglyceride and fatty acids in the fed state, the primary fate of lipid in the heart is β-oxidation that changes in response to the level of cardiac work. Changes in cardiac triglyceride synthesis and accumulation occur with anoxia and ischemia, and these changes are mentioned below. Three possible sites of rate control of β-oxidation have been examined. The first step in β-oxidation, the FAD^+-linked dehydrogenation of acylCoA, might be anticipated to exert rate control depending on the rate of oxidation of $FADH_2$. However, in early work, Bremer and Wojtczak[18] concluded that the flavoprotein-linked oxidation of palmitoyl-CoA was not easily suppressed. In contrast, the NAD^+-dependent oxidation of β-hydroxyacylCoA responded to physiologically meaningful alterations in the mitochondrial $NADH/NAD^+$ (Figure 1). The TCA cycle metabolite succinate promoted accumulation of β-hydroxypalmitoylcarnitine by elevating the mitochondrial $NADH/NAD^+$ ratio at low-energy states (resting respiration).[18] Studies with the purified β-hydroxyacyl-CoA dehydrogenase also demonstrated strong inhibition of activity by NADH.[19] In the absence of other substrates, eg, succinate, addition of acetoacetate to oxidize NADH during resting respiration has no effect on the rates of palmitoylcarnitine oxidation.[19] These data suggest that NAD^+ in the mitochondrial matrix is present in sufficient concentrations to support β-hydroxyacyl-CoA dehydrogenase activity, even at low-energy states. It was concluded that the $NADH/NAD^+$ ratio may become important to flux of fatty acids through β-oxidation only when other substrates (eg, succinate) support the reduction of matrix NAD^+ at low-energy states. Thus, in the normoxic heart, tissue concentrations of β-hydroxy fatty acids are low.

However, under ischemic conditions when mitochondrial NADH is very high, palmitate-perfused hearts rapidly accumulate β-hydroxy fatty acids.[20] Thus, β-oxidation appears to be slowed at the β-hydroxyacyl-CoA dehydrogenase when NADH is pathologically elevated.

The importance of the energy demand to rates of β-oxidation of long-chain fatty acids has been demonstrated by studies in the isolated, perfused heart in which Neely and co-workers[9] concluded that β-oxidation at low-work levels is limited by acetyl-CoA disposal through the TCA cycle. When cardiac work is increased with long chain fatty acids as substrate, acetyl-CoA concentrations drop, concomitant with high rates of oxygen consumption.

In heart mitochondria oxidizing long-chain fatty acids, high rates of oxygen uptake coupled to ATP synthesis are associated with lower ratios of both NADH/NAD^+ (see discussion above) and acetyl-CoA/CoA.[21] In this situation, the rate of β-oxidation cannot keep pace with the rate of acetyl-CoA oxidation. In contrast, production of acetyl-CoA from octanoate (independent of controls exerted by the CPT pathway) leads to saturation of the TCA cycle even during high cardiac work when rates of oxygen uptake and ATP production are high.[11] Under these conditions, TCA cycle intermediates are also high,[22] suggesting that electron transport coupled to ATP synthesis limits flux through β-oxidation and TCA cycle.

Since increases in the matrix acetyl-CoA/CoA ratio are associated with decreased rates of β-oxidation, one group has[19,23] sought to correlate the changes in acetyl-CoA–dependent rates of β-oxidation with the activity of a specific enzyme in the terminal step of β-oxidation, β-ketoacyl-CoA thiolase (Figure 1). This enzyme was found to be strongly inhibited by acetyl-CoA, especially at low concentrations of CoA. Carnitine stimulates β-oxidation in intact mitochondria at both low- (state 4) and high- (state 3) energy states by producing a dramatic decrease in the acetyl-CoA/CoA ratio.[19] These investigators conclude that the rates of β-oxidation are geared to the rates of oxidative phosphorylation via control of thiolase activity by acetyl-CoA/CoA. Thus, when the TCA cycle slows, disposal of acetyl-CoA decreases. The increased matrix concentration of acetyl-CoA, at the expense of free CoA, then inhibits thiolase and slows β-oxidation.

Triacylglycerol Synthesis

The liver regulates the distribution of long-chain fatty acids between β-oxidation and lipogenesis by control mechanisms dependent on the hormonal and nutritional status of the animal. Less is known concerning the degree to which similar controls operate in the heart. However, it is known that the myocardium possesses an active pathway for triglyceride synthesis so that activated fatty acids derived from either exogenous or endogenous sources are esterified to glycerol-3-phosphate. In the heart, the rate of triglyceride synthesis appears to be regulated primarily by availability of acyl-CoA and glycerol-3-phosphate (for a review on these aspects of triacylglycerol metabolism, see Stam et al.[24]). In the normal heart, there is a close coupling between the rate of triglyceride breakdown and the rates of glycogenolysis producing triose phosphates to support triglyceride synthesis.[24] Triglyceride homeostasis is significantly altered in myocardial ischemia, in which turnover and/or content may be increased. In early ischemia (up to 90 minutes of no-flow ischemia in the rat heart), there are no measurable changes in the content of triacylglycerol, even though tissue concentrations of glycerol increase.[25] Production of glycerol is a direct measure of triglyceride breakdown since the heart does not contain glycerokinase activity. The lack of a significant decrease in tissue triglyceride suggests that synthesis of triglyceride de novo must increase to keep pace with degradation. In early studies with anoxic cardiac subcellular fractions, we observed enhanced radiolabeled fatty acid incorporation into myocardial triglyceride that was dependent on the availability of glycerol-3-phosphate.[26] These results are compatible with the suggestion that increased glycerol-3-phosphate production in the ischemic heart enhances triacylglycerol long-chain fatty acid cycling by mass action.[25] In prolonged ischemia (4 hours or longer), the endogenous content of triacylglyceride increases,[27] a probable consequence of increased release of endogenous long-chain fatty acids.[25]

The glycerol that accumulates during the brief ischemic interval is released at the onset of reperfusion. Thereafter, glycerol release returns to the levels observed at preischemic steady state.[25] In [C^{14}]palmitate-perfused hearts, radiolabel incorporated into triglycerides doubled when compared with the preischemic control. This enhanced activity occurred in the absence of any change in tissue triglyceride content.[12] These data are consistent with the observed delay in clearance of the positron label C^{11} palmitic acid in reperfused canine heart following a 3-hour occlusion of the left anterior descending coronary artery.[28] Using H^1 NMR chemical shift imaging of the ischemic, stunned heart, methylene resonances initially increase and then decrease following 4 hours of myocardial reperfusion (Balshai, Hetherington, and Pohost, personal communication). In contrast, reperfusion of transiently ischemic hearts in the presence of norepinephrine increases the resonance intensities of the myocardial methylene residues. This increase may be a consequence of increases in plasma long-chain fatty acids due to stimulation of tissue lipolysis.

Conclusions

In summary, it is anticipated that multinuclear NMR spectroscopy can begin to provide answers to the question of rate control of lipid metabolism in the intact beating heart. The presence of four potential regulatory sites suggests that the quantitative importance of each may be variable and depend on the physiologic state of the heart.

Acknowledgment

The cDNA derived from clones of rat liver CPT-II was kindly provided to us by Dr. Denis McGarry from the University of Texas Southwestern Medical School, Dallas, Texas.

References

1. Crass MF III, McCaskill ES, Shipp JC: Effect of pressure development on glucose and palmitate metabolism in perfused heart. *Am J Physiol* 1969;216:1569–1576.

2. McGarry JD, Woeltje KF, Kuwajima M, Foster DW: Regulation of ketogenesis and the renaissance of carnitine palmitoyltransferase. *Diabetes Metab Rev* 1989;5:271–284.
3. Woeltje KF, Esser V, Weis BC, et al: Cloning, sequencing and expression of a cDNA encoding rat liver mitochondrial carnitine palmitoyltransferase II. *J Biol Chem* 1990;265:10720–10725.
4. Thampy KG: Formation of malonyl-CoA in the heart. *J Biol Chem* 1989;264:17631–17634.
5. Bianchi A, Evans JL, Iverson AJ, et al: Identification of an isozymic form of acetyl-CoA carboxylase. *J Biol Chem* 1990;256:1502–1509.
6. Rose CP, Goretsky CA: Constraints on the uptake of labelled palmitate by the heart. *Circ Res* 1977;41:534–540.
7. Bielefeld DR, Vartz TC, Neely JR: Inhibition of carnitine palmitoyltransferase activity and fatty acid oxidation by lactate and oxfenicine in cardiac muscle. *J Mol Cell Cardiol* 1985;17:619–625.
8. Beynen AC, Buechler KF, Van der Molen AJ, et al: The effects of lactate and acetate on fatty acid and cholesterol biosynthesis by isolated rat hepatocytes. *Int J Biochem* 1982;14:165–169.
9. Oram JF, Bennetch SL, Neely JR: Regulation of fatty acid utilization in isolated perfused rat hearts. *J Biol Chem* 1973;248:5299–5309.
10. From AHL, Zimmer SD, Michurski SP, et al: Regulation of the oxidative phosphorylation rate in the intact cell. *Biochemistry* 1990;29:3731–3743.
11. Neely JR, Rovetto MJ, Oram JF: Myocardial utilization of carbohydrates and lipids. *Prog Cardiovasc Dis* 1972–1973;15:289–329.
12. Lopaschuk GD, Spafford MA, Davies NJ, et al: Glucose and palmitate oxidation in isolated working rat hearts reperfused after a period of transient global ischemia. *Circ Res* 1990;66:546–553.
13. Johnston DL, Lewandowski ED: Fatty acid metabolism and contractile function in the reperfused myocardium. Multinuclear NMR studies of isolated rat hearts. *Circ Res* 1991;68:714–725.
14. Renstrom B, Nellis SH, Liedtke AJ: Metabolic oxidation of glucose during early myocardial reperfusion. *Circ Res* 1989;65:1094–1101.
15. Liedtke AJ, Nellis SH, Neely JR: Effects of excess free fatty acids on mechanical and metabolic function in normal and ischemic myocardium in swine. *Circ Res* 1978;43:652–661.
16. Bremer J, Davis EJ: Phosphorylation coupled to acyl-coenzyme A dehydrogenase-linked oxidation of fatty acids by liver and heart mitochondria. *Biochim Biophys Acta* 1972;275:298–301.
17. Lewandowski ED, Chari MV, Roberts R, et al: NMR studies of β-oxidation and short-chain fatty acid metabolism during recovery of reperfused hearts. *Am J Physiol* 1991;261:H354–H363.
18. Bremer J, Wojtczak AB: Factors controlling the rate of fatty acid β-oxidation in rat liver mitochondria. *Biochim Biophys Acta* 1972;280:515–530.
19. Wang HY, Baxter CF, Schulz H: Regulation of fatty acid β-oxidation in rat heart mitochondria. *Arch Biochem Biophys* 1991;289:274–280.
20. Van der Vusse GJ, Prinzen FW, Van Bilsen M, et al: Accumulation of lipids and lipid-intermediates in the heart during ischaemia. *Basic Res Cardiol* 1987;82(suppl 1):157–168.
21. Hansford RG, Johnson RN: The steady state concentrations of coenzyme A-SH and coenzyme A thioester, citrate and isocitrate during tricarboxylic acid cycle oxidation in rabbit heart mitochondria. *J Biol Chem* 1975;250:8361–8375.
22. Sundquist KE, Peuhkurinen KJ, Hiltunen JK, et al: Effect of acetate and octanoate on tricarboxylic acid cycle metabolite disposal during propionate oxidation in the perfused rat heart. *Biochim Biophys Acta* 1984;801:429–436.
23. Olowe Y, Schulz H: Regulation of thiolases from pig heart. Control of fatty acid oxidation in heart. *Eur J Biochem* 1980;109:425–429.

24. Stam H, Schoonderwoerd K, Hulsmann WC: Synthesis, storage and degradation of myocardial triglycerides. *Basic Res Cardiol* 1987;82(suppl 1):19–28.
25. Van Bilsen M, Van der Vusse GJ, Willemsen PHM, et al: Lipid alterations in isolated, working rat hearts during ischemia and reperfusion: its relation to myocardial damage. *Circ Res* 1989;64:304–314.
26. Wood JM, Hutchings AE, Brachfeld N: Lipid metabolism in myocardial cell-free homogenates. *J Mol Cell Cardiol* 1972;4:97–111.
27. Bruce TA, Meyers JT: Myocardial lipid metabolism in ischemia and infarction. *Recent Adv Stud Cardiac Struct Metab* 1973;3:773–780.
28. Schwaiger M, Schelbert HR, Ellison D, et al: Sustained regional abnormalities in cardiac metabolism after transient ischemia in the chronic dog model. *J Am Coll Cardiol* 1985;6:336–347.

Chapter 23

Pathophysiology of Ischemic Heart Disease

Sanford P. Bishop, DVM, PhD

Sudden occlusion of a major coronary artery due to thrombosis of a vascular lesion that may have been developing for many years remains the major cause of ischemic heart disease today. When the lesion has developed slowly over many months or years, there is often significant collateral development, which may reduce or delay the extent of cell necrosis following major vessel occlusion. With the advent of early reperfusion techniques, including coronary artery bypass and angioplasty methods, it is often possible to salvage at least portions of the myocardium if irreversible injury has not already occurred. Identification of such reversibly damaged, and thus salvageable, myocardium would greatly enhance the prognostic capability of the interventional cardiologist. The purpose of this chapter will be to describe the morphologic changes that occur during stages of reversible and irreversible injury associated with ischemic heart disease.

Reversible and Irreversible Injury

The simplest definition of reversible and irreversible injury is the distinction between tissue that will or will not recover a normal functional state when returned to a viable environment. In the case of ischemic injury, this includes such elements as the duration of ischemia, the metabolic rate, which is of the tissue influenced by such factors as temperature, heart rate, and thyroid status, and the extent of blood flow and oxygen reduction. The latter is determined by the degree of occlusion of the blood vessel and the extent of collateral development.

The issue of whether injury may occur as a result of the return to a normal environment, or reperfusion injury, has received much discussion in recent years.[1–4] It is certain that if tissue subjected to conditions below that needed for continuing survival does not receive sufficient oxygen to survive before death of the cell has

Supported in part by Research Grants HL-36892, HL-38070, and HL-17667 from the National Heart, Lung, and Blood Institute, National Institues of Health, Bethesda, Maryland.
From Pohost GM (ed.), *Cardiovascular Applications of Magnetic Resonance.* Mount Kisco, NY, Futura Publishing Co., Inc., © 1993.

occurred, there is no chance for recovery of the tissue. However, the manner in which normal blood flow is returned to the tissue may influence the ability of the tissue to survive, much as a diver who has been at great depths must ascend slowly to normal atmosphere to avoid debilitating injury. Although the existence of reperfusion injury is accepted by many as a certainty, the issue remains a difficult one to test, since there are few available methods with which to identify reversibly damaged tissue in the patient or individual animal during life and prior to the initiation of reperfusion. The issue of whether reperfusion actually damages tissue previously only reversibly injured could be tested if a reliable procedure were available to label all reversibly injured tissue prior to the initiation of the reperfusion procedure. For patient studies, such a procedure would require that the labeled tissue be able to be sufficiently resolved in the intact patient.

Collateral Circulation

The coronary vascular system in the human heart is able to transform from a system that in young individuals consists mainly of end arteries with virtually no collateral circulation to one in which extensive epicardial and endocardial communications have developed between the major vascular beds. The pioneering studies of Schaper[5] demonstrated that slowly developing occlusions, such as experimentally produced with ameroid constrictors, are able to provide sufficient collateral circulation within 2 weeks to completely prevent the development of tissue necrosis when the vessel finally becomes completely occluded. Sudden occlusive thrombosis of a coronary vessel in which there has been little previous vascular narrowing results in rapidly developing transmural ischemic necrosis extending from the endocardium toward the epicardium with increasing time.[6] The lateral borders of the infarct are very sharply defined as there is no intermixing of blood between adjacent vascular beds.[7,8] However, it is commonly observed at autopsy that patients with a history of slowly progressive vascular disease may have complete occlusion of one or more major coronary arteries with no evidence of ischemic necrosis. Collateral circulation develops in the human heart in response to slowly progressive narrowing and is able to completely protect a vascular bed from the loss of the major source of blood supply.

The choice of an experimental animal model to use to study human myocardial ischemia is influenced by the extent of collateral circulation present in the animal model and the stage of coronary disease in humans to be mimicked. The canine model has been widely used for studies of ischemic myocardial disease but has been criticized because of the variability of epicardial coronary collateral vessels, which ranged from very extensive in some animals to nearly none in others. This results in a wide variation in infarct size in canine studies, with area of necrosis due to occlusion of the same anatomical location in different animals ranging from none to small subendocardial lesions to transmural necrosis involving more than 40% of the left ventricular mass. It could be as easily argued that those dogs with poorly developed collaterals are typical of young patients with no preexisting coronary disease, and thus no collaterals, while the majority of dogs with moderate to extensive collaterals are more typical of patients with preexisting disease, progressive narrowing, and more extensive collateral development.

Other animal models that have been used to study myocardial ischemia include the pig, which has virtually no collateral circulation and thus develops large transmural infarcts following vascular occlusion, similar to that of young patients with no preexisting disease.[9] The rat also has virtually no collateral circulation, and thus nearly always develops transmural infarcts with sharp lateral borders when a major coronary vessel is occluded. On the other hand, the guinea pig has a very well-developed coronary collateral circulation that completely protects against ischemic necrosis when a major coronary vessel is occluded, similar to older patients with extensive preexisting, gradually occlusive vascular disease.[10]

Transmural Distribution of Blood Flow in Normal and Ischemic Myocardium

The regional transmural distribution of myocardial blood flow has been studied with a number of techniques in both normal and ischemic myocardium. The radioactive tracer microsphere method has become widely accepted as a reproducible method that allows the study of regional myocardial blood flow in experimental animals.[11] The technique allows precision to within a few millimeters or 2–300 mg of tissue, but is destructive to the animal. Nondestructive clinical techniques including thallium-201 gamma imaging, microbubble echocardiography, positron emission tomography (PET) scan procedures, and emerging magnetic resonance methods hold much promise, but currently lack the precision of the microsphere technique.

Distribution of blood flow within the myocardium measured with virtually all methods has demonstrated an increased blood flow in the inner half of the myocardium relative to the outer, or epicardial half, in normal animals and humans. Most studies with microspheres in closed-chest animals report a 10–25% increase in blood flow to the subendocardial third of the wall relative to the subepicardial third. Anesthesia, open chest, and a number of pharmacologic interventions may alter this relationship. Blood flow in the right ventricular myocardium is consistently slightly less than that in the left ventricle.

Occlusion of a major epicardial coronary artery in an animal or patient with no existing collateral circulation results in a transmural cessation of blood flow in the ischemic bed. However, most dogs, as well as many humans, have some collateral flow due to preexisting epicardial connections between vascular beds, and therefore maintain variable degrees of residual flow. However, flow is most severely reduced in the subendocardial regions and is progressively greater toward the epicardial regions.[12–14] Survival of tissue with permanent vascular occlusion is dependent on the extent of collateral flow as well as a number of other factors mentioned above. In normal animals, the percentage of normal preischemic area flow that must be maintained to prevent eventual development of irreversible damage is variably measured between 20% and 50% in different studies.

Nontotal Coronary Vascular Obstruction

Patients with severe narrowing of two or more major coronary arteries, but without acute thrombotic occlusion of a major vessel, often present with unstable angina, electrocardiographic (ECG) evidence of myocardial ischemia, cardiac hypertrophy, and congestive heart failure, but no enzymatic evidence of acute myocardial injury. At autopsy there is cardiac hypertrophy and subendocardial replacement fibrosis, but no major loss of myocardial mass.[15] Histologically, small focal areas of coagulation necrosis with only mild inflammatory exudate may be present and vacuolar degeneration of myocytes characterized by loss of contractile proteins, but intact nuclei, are present. The pathogenesis of such lesions appears to be a gradual degeneration and slow loss of muscle fiber with fibrous replacement occurring over time, probably the result of repeated short periods of sharply reduced blood flow that is not sustained long enough to cause large areas of myocardial necrosis. While partial or complete occlusion of a major coronary artery due to atherosclerotic coronary artery disease is the most common cause of myocardial ischemia, relative reduction of blood flow to portions of the myocardium may also occur with alterations to the intramyocardial resistance vessels, such as occurs with severe cardiac hypertrophy due to hypertension. Reduced coronary reserve, especially in the subendocardial regions, has been demonstrated in experimental canine studies with renal mechanisms of hypertension,[16] banding of the proximal aorta soon after weaning and study 1 year later,[17,18] and in patients with hypertension-induced cardiac hypertrophy.[19] In these studies, myocardial stress, such as that induced by exercise or by pharmacologic vasodilation, resulted in a decreased ability to increase blood flow from the basal resting level. Although not actually demonstrated, this loss of coronary reserve would theoretically produce multiple short transient periods of relative ischemia to the subendocardial regions when these hearts are subjected to daily activities. Such intermittent ischemic periods would be expected to result in variable amounts of reversible and irreversible damage to the affected myocardial tissue.

Morphologic Changes of Reversible and Irreversible Injury

With reduction of blood flow below the critical level necessary to maintain normal function and concomitant with the cessation of contractile function, biochemical and morphologic changes disrupt the normal architecture of the myocyte (Figure 1). Several functional, biochemical, and structural features characteristic of reversible and irreversible injury are listed in Table 1. With the loss of oxygen supply, mitochondria immediately lose their ability to produce adenosine triphosphate (ATP) by oxidative phosphorylation, and within several beats, creatine phosphate (CrP) starts to drop, soon followed by ATP. Contraction ceases, but CrP and ATP continue to drop due to the demands of maintaining basal metabolism in the cell.[20–23] Glycogen is used by the anaerobic metabolic pathways since glucose in no longer available. One of the earliest microscopic changes of ischemia is the loss of glycogen, which may be recognized by special stains such as periodic acid Schiff's test at the light microscopic level, or by loss of glycogen granules by electron microscopy (Figure 2). Lactate, NADH, hydrogen ions, and other products of glycolytic intermediary metabolism as well as inorganic phosphate, adenosine monophosphate (AMP), adenosine, inosine, and other adenine nucleosides accumulate because these normal metabolic products are not able to be used in the absence of oxygen or to be carried away from the cell.[24] The decrease in

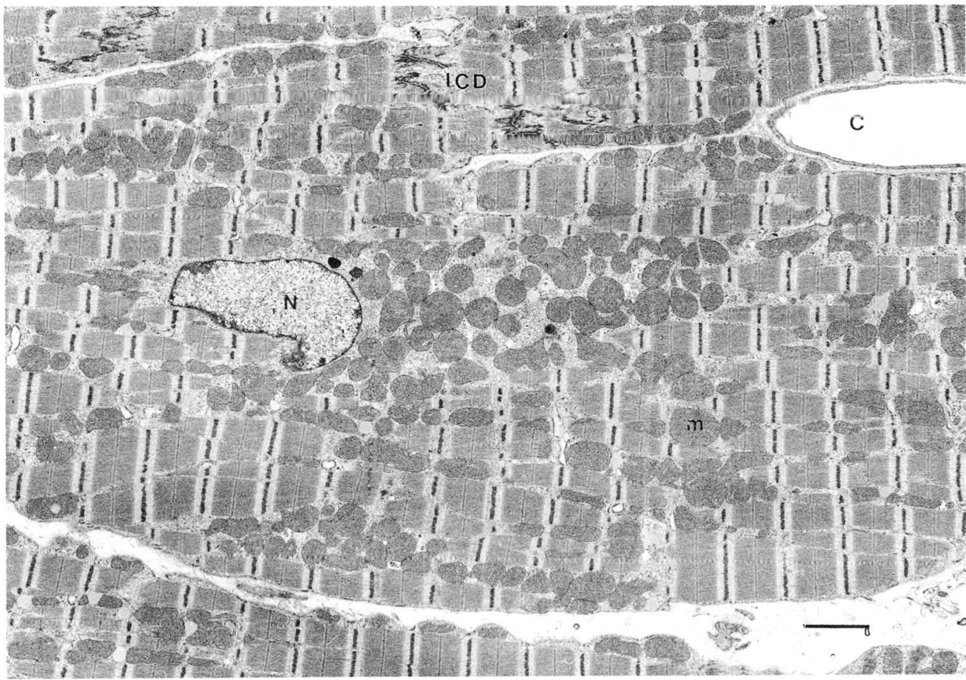

FIGURE 1. *Electron micrograph of normal canine myocardium perfusion fixed with 2% glutaraldehyde. Note the relaxed but not overstretched state of the sarcomeres and the normal appearance of mitochondria. Glycogen granules are barely visible at this magnification between mitochondria. Nuclear chromatin is evenly dispersed. m, mitochondria; N, nucleus; C, capillary; ICD, intercalated disc. Bar = 2.0 μm.*

TABLE 1. Development of Functional, Metabolic, and Structural Changes in Ischemic Myocardial Injury

Functional change	Metabolic change	Structural change
Reversible Injury		
↓ contraction	↓ ox. phosphorylation	glycogen loss
↓ dias. function	↑ lactate	marginated chromatin
↑ LA pressure	↑ $[H^+]$, Na^+	edema
↑ ST seg ECG	↑ Pi	mitochondrial swelling
	↓ ATP, CrP	lipid accumulation
Irreversible Injury		
↑ serum enzymes	enzyme leakage	membrane blebs
↑ antimyosin uptake	protein uptake	sarcolemmal breaks
↑ $Tc\text{-}^{99m}$ PYP	depleted ATP, CrP	cytoskeletal damage
	Ca^{2+} uptake	mito dense granules
	DNA loss	nuclear disruption
	collagen	contraction bands
		scar

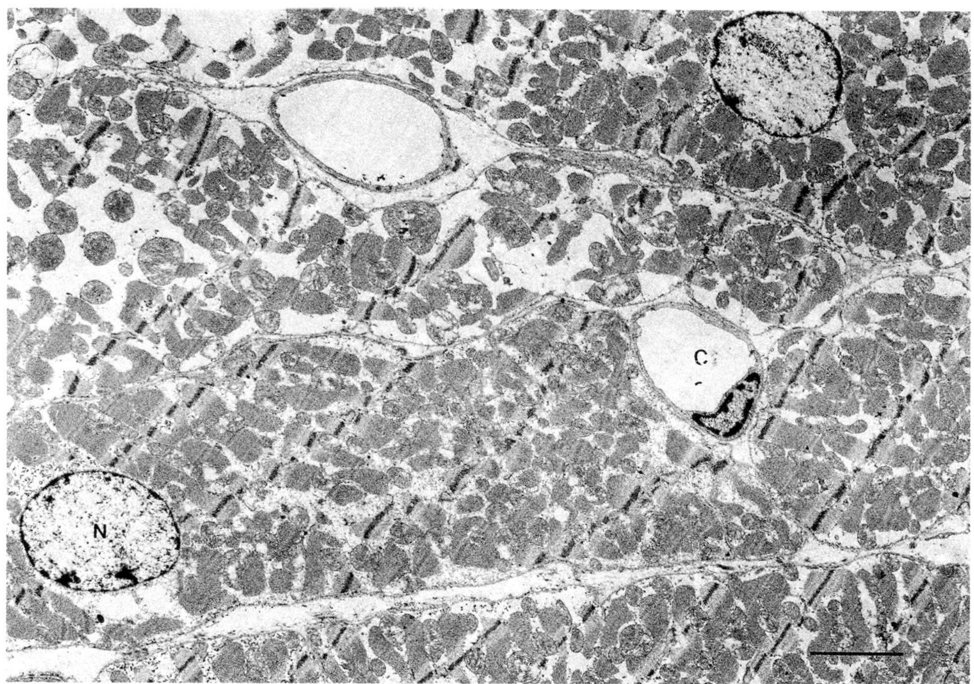

FIGURE 2. *Electron micrograph of canine myocardium with 15 minutes of ischemia, illustrating reversible changes of partial glycogen loss and early edema separating the myofibrils and causing mild mitochondrial swelling. There is mild clumping of nuclear chromatin. N, nucleus; C, capillary. Bar = 2.0 μm.*

high-energy phosphates results in the failure of ion pump mechanisms in the cell membrane, resulting in accumulation of intracellular sodium ion and water, producing cellular edema. Mitochondria lose their normal matrix granules, become swollen with edema, and may actually rupture the outer membranes. There is marginal clumping of nuclear chromatin. The sarcomeres become elongated with wide I-bands because they are no longer able to contract and are passively stretched by hemodynamic forces. These changes all occur within the first 10–30 minutes, depending on residual flow and other metabolic factors, and are fully reversible with return of normal blood flow.

With the continuation of tissue ischemia, high-energy phosphates drop to very low levels, and additional changes occur that result in irreversible damage to the cell and cell necrosis.[23] Additional fluid accumulation occurs with further separation of cellular elements, perhaps resulting in physical disruption of cytoskeletal elements and membranes. Intracellular proteases likely contribute to cellular destruction as well. Membrane blebs appear on the sarcolemma, lifting the glycocalyx from the membrane and producing actual physical defects in the membrane (Figure 3). The increased leakiness of the cell allows massive influx of sodium as well as calcium ions, and the mitochondria rapidly accumulate the calcium. The first densities to appear by electron microscopy in the mitochondria are flocculent, moderately translucent, and appear to consist of protein material. Soon, however, dense mitochondrial densities appear that contain calcium ions; these are considered to be the hallmark of irreversible injury to

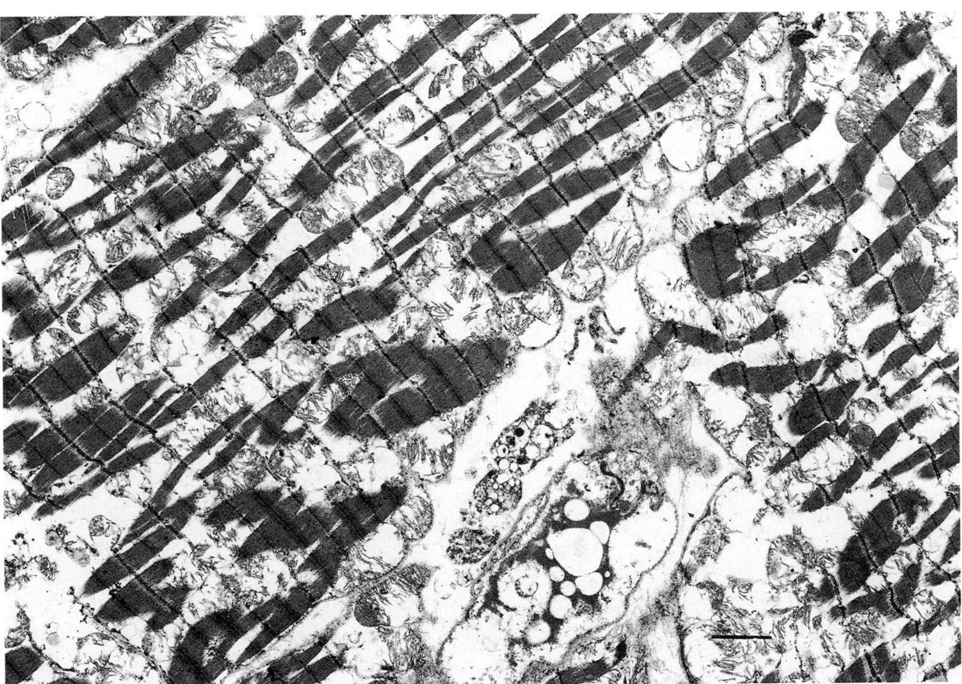

FIGURE 3. *Myocytes from canine myocardium with 30 minutes of ischemia. Intracellular edema is prominent, separating myofibrils, mitochondria are swollen and disrupted, and there are numerous membrane blebs present. Bar = 2.0 μm.*

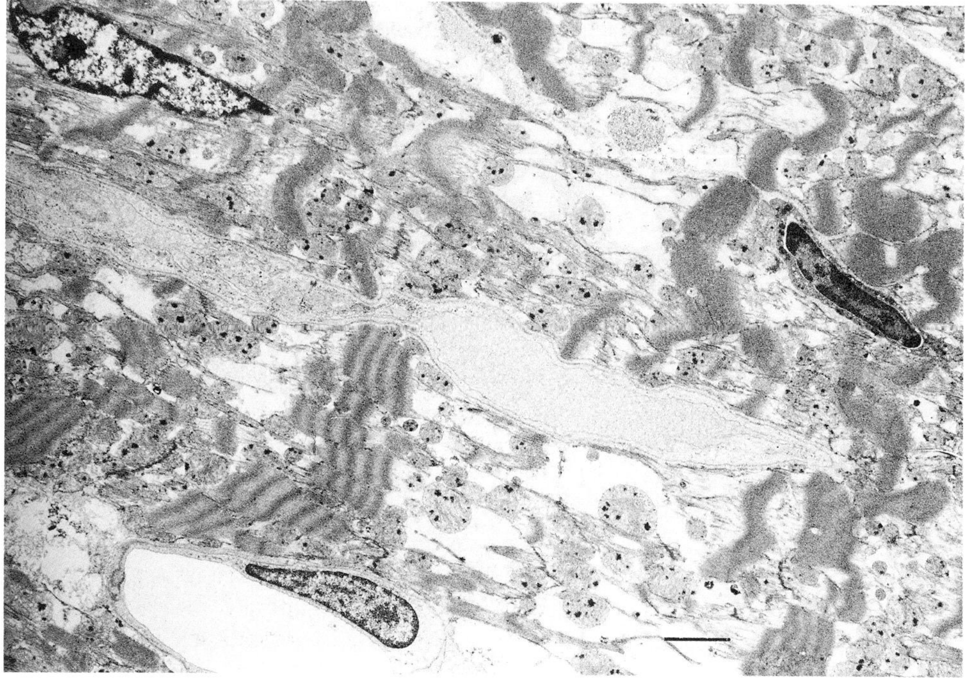

FIGURE 4. *Canine myocardium after 90 minutes of ischemia and 24 hours of reflow, illustrating numerous dense granules in the mitochondria due to rapid uptake of calcium ions. The dark vertical bands in the myocytes are multiple severely contracted sarcomeres characteristic of contraction band necrosis. Bar = 2.0 μm.*

the cell (Figure 4). Severe mitochondrial swelling and rupture, nuclear membrane rupture, loss of cytoskeletal components, and plasmalemmal rupture are all features of the irreversibly injured cell.[25–27] Reflow to this tissue will not result in recovery, but may hasten the healing process with formation of fibrous scar tissue.

The increased leakiness of irreversibly damaged cells also allows the escape of intracellular substances, such as the enzymes lactate dehydrogenase, creatine kinase, and many others, as well as myoglobin and other intracellular proteins. In addition, the permeable membrane will allow entry of serum substances, such as serum proteins. This makes the addition of specific markers to the blood possible, such as antibodies to myoglobin, which may be tagged to aid in identification of necrotic tissue.[28]

The sarcomeres undergo a series of changes during cellular ischemic injury, starting with elongation due to loss of ATP, and perhaps physical stretching of the cell as described above (Figure 3). Patients with sudden death due to ischemic damage often have wavy fibers in histologic sections of acutely ischemic myocardium. The wavy fibers are the result of this sarcomere elongation and the inability of the fibers to contract normally. When these fibers are compressed by the surrounding tissue during systole or rigor mortis, they are forced into wavy folds (Figure 5). With increasing time of ischemia, contracture of myocardial tissue occurs[20,29] with a shortening of

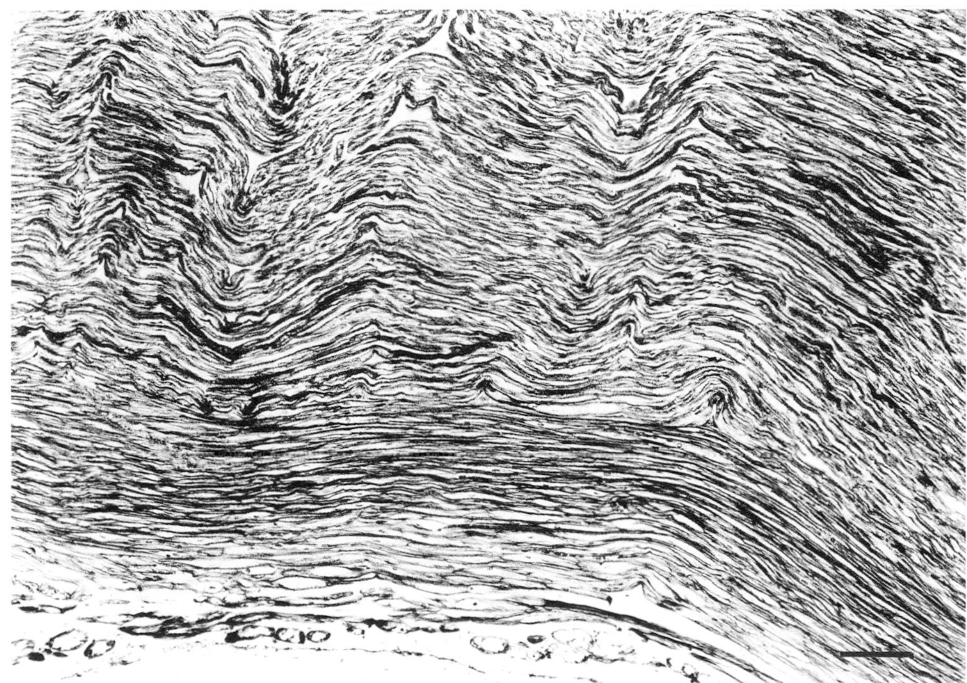

FIGURE 5. *Wavy fibers present in canine myocardium following 90 minutes of complete coronary artery occlusion. Normal fibers are present in the lower portion of the photograph adjacent to the endocardium. Gomori aldehyde fuchsin trichrome stain. Bar = 100 μm.*

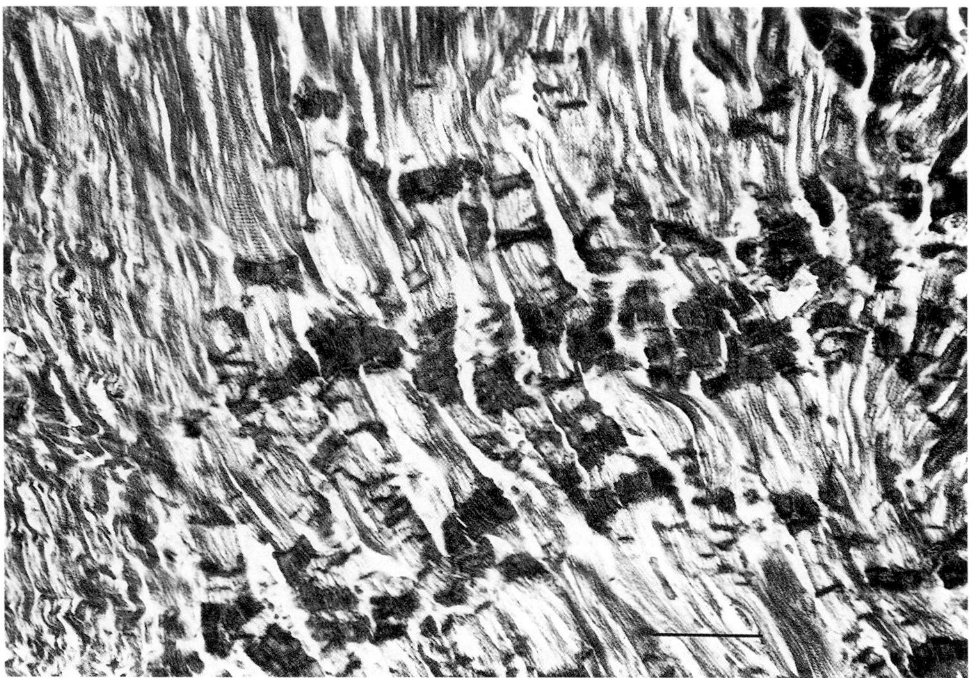

FIGURE 6. *Light micrograph of contraction band necrosis at the edge of an infarct in canine myocardium after 90 minutes of ischemia. Gomori aldehyde fuchsin trichrome stain. Bar = 50 μm.*

sarcomere lengths to their physiologically shortest length, approximately 1.5 μm. In globally ischemic (nonbeating) hearts, this contracture results in an increase in intraventricular pressure. Around the periphery of infarcted tissue where there is some diffusion of calcium and other ions from viable tissue, or if reflow occurs to necrotic tissue, a rapid influx of calcium occurs and there is super contraction of sarcomeres, resulting in severe shortening such that six to 10 sarcomeres are compressed to 2–3 μm, and large regions of cytoplasm remain with no contractile elements (Figures 4 and 6). These changes are referred to as contraction band necrosis, a definite lesion of irreversible injury.[30]

Lipid Accumulation in Ischemic Tissue

The accumulation of lipid in moderately ischemic tissue surrounding an area of infarction was previously recognized in pathologic studies.[31–35] The recent demonstration of myocardial lipid accumulation around the periphery of infarcts in experimental animals using NMR methods[36,37] suggests the possibility that this lesion may be useful in identifying margins of ischemic tissue in intact animals or patients. Lipid may accumulate in ischemic tissue by the following processes: 1) accelerated accumulation from elevated serum free fatty acids usually present following myocardial infarction, related to action of elevated catecholamines; 2) action of phospholipases on cell membranes; and 3) decreased utilization of fatty acids due to shutdown of oxidative phosphorylation, resulting in accumulation of triglycerides in the cytoplasm.[38] Lipid accumulation in totally ischemic tissue is limited to movement of lipids from the membrane pool to the cytoplasmic pool because no source of external lipids is available. In tissue with severe reduction in blood flow, but still sufficient to prevent cell necrosis, a partial shutdown of oxidative metabolism is the most plausible explanation for the triglyceride droplets that accumulate in the zone of viable tissue surrounding the outer periphery of the infarct zone (Figure 7). Lipid accumulation in this peripheral tissue has been shown to occur within 1 hour of coronary artery occlusion.[39] Studies in our laboratory have demonstrated a good correlation of NMR spectroscopically detectable lipid in myocardial samples from the infarct periphery with moderately reduced blood flow measured with radioactive tracer microspheres in canine experimental myocardial infarction (unpublished data). This peri-infarct lipid correlates well with high-signal regions identified in experimental animal infarcts by NMR imaging techniques, suggesting a method for identifying peripheral margins of necrotic myocardium in the intact animal.[36,37]

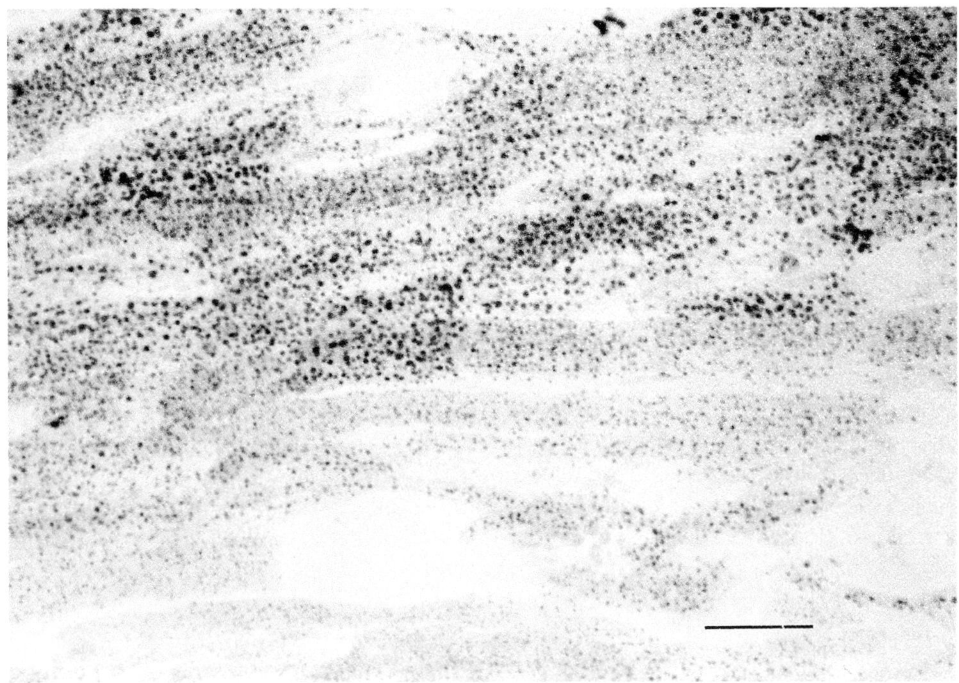

FIGURE 7. *Lipid droplet accumulation in viable tissue peripheral to the zone of cell necrosis in canine myocardium 24 hours after permanent coronary artery occlusion. Cells with fewer droplets at bottom of micrograph are toward normally perfused tissue. Frozen section; Oil Red O. Bar = 25 μm.*

Reflow to Reversibly Injured Tissue

Jennings, Reimer, and co-investigators[6,40,41] demonstrated that if reflow is established to ischemic myocardium in a pentobarbital-anesthetized, open-chest canine within 15–20 minutes after occlusion of a coronary artery, complete structural recovery of the tissue occurred within 15 minutes to 1 hour. This period of time to maintain fully reversible changes may be extended if anesthetic regimens with slower heart rates are used, collateral flow is greater, or other means to reduce metabolic activity, such as hypothermia, are used. Recovery of the adenine nucleotide pool and complete functional recovery, however, takes considerably longer, up to 1–2 days.[1,22] This stunned myocardium eventually returns to completely normal function and structure, indicating that there are no persistent residual effects of reversibly injured tissue.

Healing of Irreversibly Injured Tissue

If no reflow is established to the ischemic myocardium, a zone of inflammatory cells accumulates around the border of the necrotic and viable myocardium within 12–18 hours, and the peripheral necrotic tissue is characterized by extensive contraction band formation. Within the center of the necrotic tissue, the sarcomeres remain elongated, and in the absence of blood flow to the tissue the contractile proteins are slow to be removed, resulting in a preserved appearance to the tissue by light microscopy that has been termed "mummification."[42] Cross striations remain evident for days to weeks or longer, though nuclei are not present and there are severe ultrastructural alterations of the tissue. Vascular invasion from viable tissue at the periphery of the infarct, macrophage activity to remove tissue debris, and fibroblastic activity to replace the dead tissue with a viable scar eventually result in healing by scar formation.

In summary, reversible changes in myocardial structure occur within minutes after occlusion of a coronary artery, which are converted to irreversible changes if blood flow is not restored. Changes start at the subendocardial region of the ischemic area and spread with time toward the epicardium. The time required for irreversible changes to occur depends on a variety of factors, including collateral blood flow and metabolic activity. Specific features that may allow identification of endangered or necrotic tissue by clinical tools such as NMR include fluid accumulation, intracellular increase in ions such as sodium and calcium, changes in intracellular high-energy phosphates, increased lactic acid or inorganic phosphates, and increased triglycerides in viable myocytes adjacent to the necrotic tissue. The refinement of these tools will also provide the opportunity to more closely examine the sequence of metabolic and pathologic changes that occur during development of ischemic injury, and the effects of specific interventions such as early blood reperfusion.

References

1. Jennings RB, Schaper J, Hill ML, et al: Effect of reperfusion late in the phase of reversible ischemic injury: changes in cell volume, electrolytes, metabolites, and ultrastructure. *Circ Res* 1985;56(2):262–278.

2. Chapell SP, Lewis MJ, Henderson AH: Myocardial reoxygenation damage: can it be circumvented. *Cardiovasc Res* 1985;19:299–303.
3. Jennings RB, Reimer KA, Steenbergen C: Myocardial ischemia revisited. The osmolar load, membrane damage, and reperfusion. *J Mol Cell Cardiol* 1986;18:769–780
4. Opie LH: Reperfusion injury and its pharmacologic modification. *Circulation* 1989;80(4):1049–1062.
5. Schaper W: *The Collateral Circulation of the Heart.* New York: Elsevier Science Publishing Co., Inc., 1971.
6. Reimer KA, Lowe JE, Rasmussen MM, Jennings RB: The wavefront phenomenon of ischemic cell death. I. Myocardial infarct size vs. duration of coronary occlusion in dogs. *Circulation* 1977;56:786–794.
7. Okun EM, Factor SM, Kirk ES: End-capillary loops in the heart: an explanation for discrete myocardial infarctions without border zones. *Science* 1979;206:565–572.
8. Murdock RH Jr, Harlan DM, Morris JJ III, et al: Transitional blood flow zones between ischemic and nonischemic myocardium in the awake dog. *Circ Res* 1983;52:451–459.
9. Fugiwara H, Ashraf M, Sato S, Millard RW: Transmural cellular damage and blood flow distribution in early ischemia in pig hearts. *Circ Res* 1982;51:683–693.
10. Schaper W: Experimental infarcts and the microcirculation. In: Hearse DJ, Yellon DM, eds. *Therapeutic Approaches to Myocardial Infarct Size Limitation.* New York: Raven Press Publishers; 1984:79–89.
11. Bishop SP: How well can we measure coronary flow, risk zones and infarct size? In: Hearse DJ, Yellon DM, eds. *Therapeutic Approaches to Myocardial Infarct Size Limitation.* New York: Raven Press Publishers; 1984:139–162.
12. Bishop SP, White FC, Bloor CM: Regional myocardial blood flow during myocardial infarction in the conscious dog. *Circ Res* 1976;38:429–439.
13. White FC, Sanders M, Bloor CM: Regional redistribution of myocardial blood flow after coronary occlusion and reperfusion in the conscious dog. *Am J Cardiol* 1978;42:234–243.
14. Jugdutt BI, Hutchins GM, Bulkley BH, Becker LC: Myocardial infarction in the conscious dog: three-dimensional mapping of infarct, collateral flow and region at risk. *Circulation* 1979;60:1141–1150.
15. Geer JC, Crago CA, Little WC, et al: Subendocardial ischemic myocardial lesions associated with severe coronary atherosclerosis. *Am J Pathol* 1980;98:663–680.
16. Marcus ML, Harrison DG, Chilian WM, et al: Alterations in the coronary circulation in hypertrophied ventricles. *Circulation* 1987;75(2):PI19–PI25
17. Alyono D, Anderson RW, Parrish DG, et al: Alterations of myocardial blood flow associated with experimental canine left ventricular hypertrophy secondary to valvular aortic stenosis. *Circ Res* 1986;58:47–57.
18. Hittinger L, Shannon RP, Bishop SP, et al: Subendomyocardial exhaustion of blood flow reserve and increased fibrosis in conscious dogs with heart failure. *Circ Res* 1989;65(4):971–980.
19. Marcus ML, Doty DB, Hiratzka LF, et al: Decreased coronary reserve: a mechanism for angina pectoris in patients with aortic stenosis and normal coronary arteries. *N Engl J Med* 1982;307:1362–1366.
20. Anderson PG, Bishop SP, Digerness S: Transmural progression of morphologic changes during ischemia and reperfusion in the normal and hypertrophied rat heart. *Am J Pathol* 1987;129:142–167.
21. Jennings RB, Ganote CE: Structural changes in myocardium during acute ischemia. *Circ Res* 1974;34(suppl III):156–172.
22. Reimer KA, Hill ML, Jennings RB: Prolonged depletion of ATP and of the adenine nucleotide pool due to delayed resynthesis of adenine nucleotides following reversible myocardial ischemic injury in dogs. *J Mol Cell Cardiol* 1981;13:220–239.
23. Jennings RB, Hawkins HK, Lowe JE, et al: Relation between high energy phosphate and lethal injury in myocardial ischemia in the dog. *Am J Pathol* 1978;92:187–214.
24. Neely JR, Grotyohann LW: Role of glycolytic products in damage to ischemic myocardium: dissociation of ATP levels and recovery of function of reperfused ischemic hearts. *Circ Res* 1984;55:816–824.

25. Steenbergen C, Hill ML, Jennings RB: Cytoskeletal damage during myocardial ischemia: changes in vinculin immunofluorescence staining during total in vitro ischemia in canine heart. *Circ Res* 1987;60(4):478–486.
26. Schaper J, Mulch J, Winkler B, Schaper W: Ultrastructural, functional, and biochemical criteria for estimation of reversibility of ischemic injury: a study on the effects of global ischemia on the isolated dog heart. *J Mol Cell Cardiol* 1979;11:521–541.
27. Schaper J: Ultrastructural changes of the myocardium in regional ischaemia and infarction. *Eur Heart J* 1986;7(suppl B):3–9.
28. Khaw BA, Strauss HW, Moore R, et al: Myocardial damage delineated by indium-111 antimyosin Fab and technetium-99m pyrophosphate. *J Nucl Med* 1987;28(1):76–82.
29. Humphrey SM, Vanderwee MA: Factors affecting the development of contraction band necrosis during reperfusion of the isolated isovolumic rat heart. *J Mol Cell Cardiol* 1986;18:319–329.
30. Ganote CE: Contraction band necrosis and irreversible myocardial injury. *J Mol Cell Cardiol* 1983;15:67–74.
31. Mallory CK, White PD, Salcedo-Salgar J: The speed of healing of myocardial infarction. A study of the pathologic anatomy in seventy-two cases. *Am Heart J* 1939;18:647–671.
32. Sommers HM, Jennings RB: Experimental acute myocardial infarction. Histologic and histochemical studies of early myocardial infarcts induced by temporary or permanent occlusion of a coronary artery. *Lab Invest* 1964;13:1491–1503.
33. Wartman WB, Jennings RB, Yokoyama HO, Clabaugh GF: Fatty change of the myocardium in early experimental infarction. *Arch Pathol* 1956;62:318–323.
34. Buja LM, Tofe AJ, Kulkarni PV, et al: Sites and mechanisms of localization of technetium-99m phosphorus radiopharmaceuticals in acute myocardial infarcts and other tissues. *J Clin Invest* 1977;60:724–740.
35. Bilheimer DW, Buja LM, Parkey RW, et al: Fatty acid accumulation and abnormal lipid deposition in peripheral and border zones of experimental myocardial infarcts. *J Nucl Med* 1978;19:276–283.
36. Bouchard A, Doyle M, Wolkowicz PE, et al: Visualization of altered myocardial lipids by 1H NMR chemical-shift imaging following ischemic insult. *Magn Reson Med* 1991;17(2):379–389.
37. Reeves RC, Evanochko WT, Canby RC, et al: Demonstration of increased myocardial lipid with postischemic dysfunction ("myocardial stunning") by proton nuclear magnetic resonance spectroscopy. *J Am Coll Cardiol* 1989;13(3):739–744.
38. Katz AM, Messineo FC: Lipid-membrane interactions and the pathogenesis of ischemic damage in the myocardium. *Circ Res* 1981;48:1–16.
39. Burton KP, Templeton GH, Hagler HK, et al: Effect of glucose availability on functional membrane integrity, ultrastructure and contractile performance following hypoxia and reoxygenation in isolated feline cardiac muscle. *J Mol Cell Cardiol* 1980;12:109–133.
40. Herdson PB, Sommers HM, Jennings RB: Comparative study of the fine structure of normal and ischemic dog myocardium with special reference to early changes following temporary occlusion of a coronary artery. *Am J Pathol* 1965;46:367–386.
41. Jennings RB, Sommers HM, Smyth GA, et al: Myocardial necrosis induced by temporary occlusion of a coronary artery in the dog. *Arch Pathol Lab Med* 1970;70:68.
42. Kloner RA, Fishbein MC, Lew H, et al: Mummification of the infarcted myocardium by high dose corticosteroids. *Circulation* 1978;57:56–63.

Chapter 24

Emission Tomography of the Heart

Thomas F. Budinger, MD, PhD
and Gerald M. Pohost, MD

Nuclear medicine techniques involving imaging the heart after an injection of radioactive isotopes for evaluation of heart muscle perfusion and cardiac ejection fraction have been the traditional diagnostic techniques for ischemic heart disease. Over the past 10 years tomographic methods with radioisotopes have become commonplace, with reported specificity and sensitivity for diagnosis of ischemic heart disease somewhat better than that of conventional projection techniques. The two major approaches to emission (radionuclide) tomography are single-photon emission tomography (SPECT) and positron emission tomography (PET). Both techniques give images that reflect the spatial distribution of flow or metabolism in the myocardium as illustrated in Figure 1. The status of these techniques will be discussed after reviewing the basic physiologic concepts.

Basic Physical and Physiologic Concepts

Emission tomography involves detection of the concentration of specific radionuclides that accumulate in tissue in proportion to flow or metabolism or receptor concentration. These tracers, which are transported into tissue and pool in the cells in proportion to the amount delivered but do not readily wash out of the tissue are sometimes known as "molecular microspheres." A typical flow tracer in SPECT is ^{201}Tl, which is believed to behave like potassium in that it enters into cells and other pools with a large potassium concentration. The washout of thallium is low; thus, after injection of this tracer the amount of thallium in different portions of the myocardium gives a measure of relative flow. Other chemical ligands labeled with ^{99m}Tc have been developed. These agents provide improved radionuclide imaging potential over ^{201}Tl. The flow tracers for PET include ^{13}N-labeled ammonia, ^{82}Rb, and ^{15}O-labeled water. Ammonia generally follows flow, but its accumulation can be governed by the

From Pohost GM (ed.), *Cardiovascular Applications of Magnetic Resonance*. Mount Kisco, NY, Futura Publishing Co., Inc., © 1993.

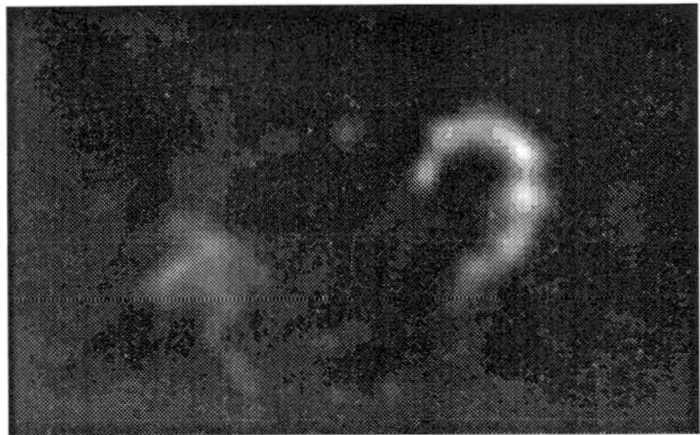

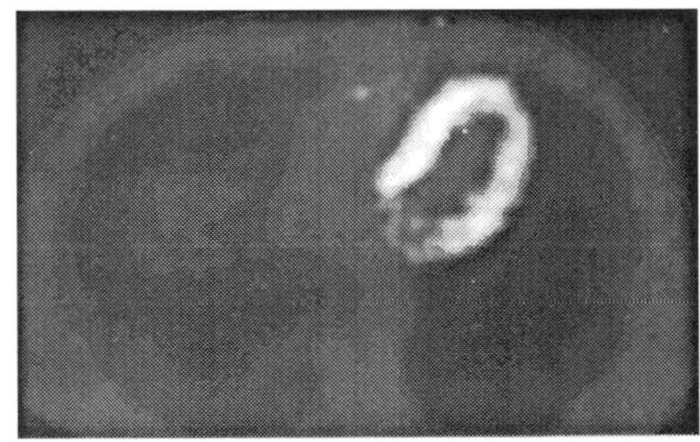

SPECT
NO Attenuation Correction

PET
Attenuation Correction

FIGURE 1. *Comparison of SPECT (^{99M}Tc-MIBI) and PET (^{82}Rb-C1) in transverse section of the same heart. The absence of septal activity is the result of not applying attenuation compensation. Liver activity is seen for ^{99M}Tc-MIBI. Transmission data (blue, right panel) used in PET for attenuation correction shows the heart, blood pools, lungs, and dome of the liver on the right side of the patient.*

metabolic status of enzymes. Rubidium-82 is an analogue of potassium and behaves somewhat similarly to ^{201}Tl, but its extraction decreases more dramatically as flow increases.[1] Ammonia is obtained from a cyclotron; ^{82}Rb is conveniently obtained from a portable generator. These tracers (^{201}Tl, ^{99m}Tc, ^{13}N-labeled ammonia, and ^{82}Rb) act like microspheres to a first approximation and can be modeled as in Figure 2A.

The simplest and most widely used model for tracer kinetics is a single compartment model in which flow (F) and extraction (E) are inferred from the accumulation divided by the integral of the input function:

$$FE = \frac{Q(\tau)}{\int^{\tau} A(t)dt} \tag{1}$$

The numerator represents the quantity Q(τ) and is the measured activity in the myocardium and the denominator is the area under the arterial concentration A(t) curve from the time of injection to time τ. The simplifying assumption is that there is no appreciable washout during the time of observation. The washout rate for ^{201}Tl is about 30 times the washin, whereas for other myocardial perfusion tracers the difference is close to 10.

For situations wherein washout is appreciable, such as with diffusible tracers (eg, ^{15}O-labeled water) the flow information is derived from a mathematical fit to a washin/washout kinetic model as shown in Figure 2B.[1,2] Here, k_1 and k_2 give tissue perfusion with the difference between k_1 and k_2 being the difference in distribution volumes between tissue and blood—the partition coefficient. Oxygen-15 water studies are performed either by injection of $H_2{}^{15}O$ or by inhalation of $C^{15}O_2$ that is efficiently converted to $H_2{}^{15}O$ by carbonic anhydrase in the lungs.[3] Interestingly, C-11 acetate studies also use this model but in this case k_1 is the delivery parameter that is dependent on flow and extraction and k_2 represents the loss of C-11 in the form of

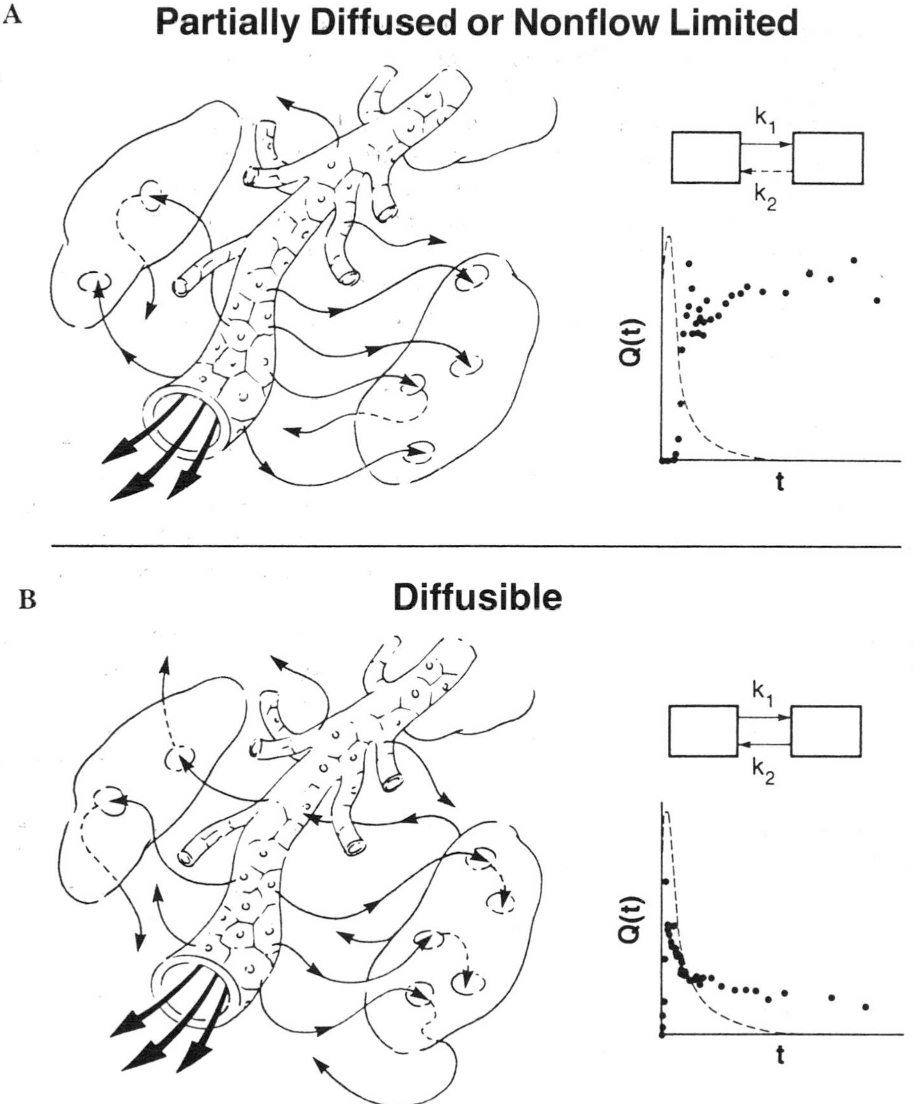

FIGURE 2. *Diffusible and partially diffusible flow tracers.* **A**: *Two-compartment model wherein the washout k_2 is negligible between compartments.* **B**: *Two-compartment model with a tracer freely diffusing.*

CO_2. The rate of loss is related to the rate of β-oxidation.[4,5] A fit to the mathematical model for these tracers involves collecting tomographic data for the arterial input, A(t), and for the myocardium accumulation (washin and washout), Q(τ):

$$Q(\tau) = k_1 \int^{\tau} A(t)e^{-k_2(\tau - t)}\,dt \tag{2}$$

Positron emission tomography of the heart allows simultaneous measurement of the myocardial activity and the blood pool activity as both regions of interest are available in the same tomographic slices. Thus, both A(t) and Q(γ) are measured using dynamic PET. These considerations extend to fast scan magnetic resonance imaging (MRI) of the heart wherein a paramagnetic contrast agent (eg, gadolinium-DTPA) is injected and the observed MRI signal is tailored to reflect changes in regional relaxation rates. However, in the case of MRI, the volume of distribution is not the myocyte but the vascular and interstitial fluid spaces of the myocardium. Thus, in MRI some estimate of extracellular volume and a knowledge of the variation of extraction with flow is necessary. Since extraction (E) is usually related to the permeability surface product (PS) as:

$$E = (1 - e^{-PS/F}) \tag{3}$$

and $k_1 = FE$, the model of Equation 2 will not give a measure of flow directly. An exception is studies with labeled water, wherein extraction is 1.0, and k_2 is approximately the same as k_1 because the distribution volume for water is about the same in tissue and blood. The major limitation for PET, SPECT, and MRI are the available statistics.

The physiologic principles behind measurement of cardiac metabolism (eg, fatty acid, glucose metabolism) or adrenergic receptor concentrations using radionuclide tracer techniques frequently involve somewhat more complex models than those of Figure 2. However, to date, all of the clinical science applications of these techniques have relied on visual comparisons of the relative changes from one portion of the myocardium to another in making clinical decisions. For example, the most commonly used metabolic tracer for the heart is ^{18}F-deoxyglucose (FDG), and the diagnosis of viable versus nonviable tissue is made by a visual inspection of the images that reflect the accumulation of FDG (Figure 3). Anaerobic metabolism is thought to be the mechanism for accumulation of glucose in myocardial tissue with reduced perfusion.[6] Below we discuss the relationships between the FDG PET studies and the potentials of SPECT and PET perfusion for determination of myocardial viability.

Single-Photon Emission Computed Tomography of Cardiac Perfusion

Since the mid-1970s, the mainstay of cardiac perfusion studies has been ^{201}Tl injected during exercise or pharmacologic (dipyridamole- or adenosine-induced) coronary dilation. It was discovered in the late 1970s that a defect seen during cardiac stress would fill in in a large percentage of patients.[7] This defect fill in phenomenon usually is partial or complete 2 to 4 hours after initial thallium injection. The phenomenon was termed "redistribution" or the "reversible defect." Those patients without fill in were diagnosed as having a fixed defect corresponding to recent or previous myocardial infarction. Over the past 15 years this phenomenon has been

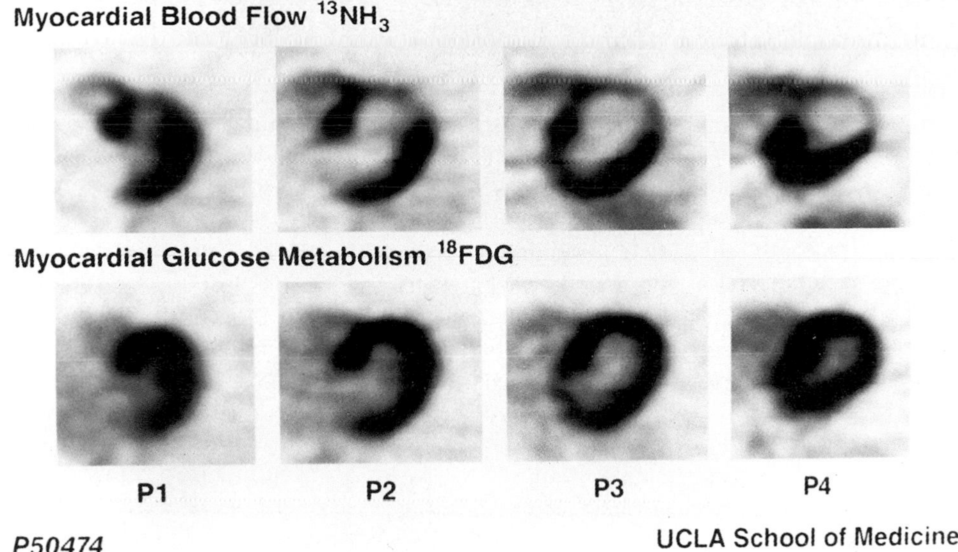

FIGURE 3. *Comparison of myocardial blood flow ($^{13}NH_3$) and glucose metabolism (^{18}FDG). Note the increased accumulation of FDG relative to flow in the anterior myocardium. Reprinted from H.R. Schelbert, UCLA with permission.*

useful for diagnosis and risk stratification in patients with suspected ischemic heart disease versus myocardial infarction and is the major diagnostic technique in most clinical nuclear medicine departments throughout the world. But the mechanism of redistribution is still not known and is the subject of intense theoretical and experimental investigations wherein kinetic models and even local tissue diffusion have been called on to provide an explanation. An important motivation for the intense interest in seeking the mechanism for redistribution is the fact that as many as 50% false-negative diagnoses for viability were found in some clinical studies.

Positron emission tomography studies using FDG compared with $^{13}NH_3$ perfusion images (Figure 3) demonstrated a positive accumulation of this glucose analogue in the segment thought to be infarcted by ^{201}Tl because there was little or no redistribution.[8] It was this discovery that led to worldwide interest in clinical cardiac PET and provided an argument for incorporation of PET FDG studies in patients with ischemic heart disease. As explained below, the particular ^{201}Tl protocol and inferior SPECT reconstruction might explain the majority of the false-positive diagnoses of fixed defects.

A Model That Explains Redistribution and False-Positives

In 1986 we evaluated the work on redistribution mechanisms and sought to explain the false-positive diagnosis of fixed defects.[9] This evaluation led to an explanation of the redistribution phenomenon that has a strong impact on the relative roles of cardiac SPECT and cardiac PET as well as the potential future role of nuclear magnetic resonance (NMR) perfusion studies using contrast agents.

We found that a lack of sustained blood pool activity can explain false-positive diagnoses for many of the fixed defects.[9,10] This was confirmed by investigations involving reinjection of ^{201}Tl.[11,12] Reinjection of ^{201}Tl enhances the blood pool concentration and this has been shown to improve detection of reversible defects that would otherwise have been diagnosed as fixed defects due to the fact that in some cases there is a low blood pool concentration of thallium after the initial injection.

More recently, through application of our two-compartment model to the particular experimental conditions of animal and human studies we found that the majority, if not all, of the results can be explained in a consistent manner.[13] In particular, we find the model helps us to understand the phenomenon of redistribution. The work on late redistribution was able to significantly reduce the false-positive rate by imaging subjects as long as 48 hours after injection.[14] Interest in redistribution from injection at rest stems from the fact that in some patients who could not be exercised and in experimental laboratory animal studies[15] there was an accumulation of activity in ischemic tissues, whereas normal tissues had a progressive washout of activity.

Key to our understanding of thallium kinetics is the discovery that the release of thallium from ischemic tissue is low, unlike the washout of potassium. For thallium, the ratio of washin to washout can be nearly equal for normal and ischemic conditions, based on our analysis of animal and clinical studies. The ratio of k_1 to k_2 of about 30 explains both human and canine sequential biopsy data and in vivo imaging data. The two-compartment model, similar to Figure 2B, shows that the equilibrium or steady-state value of the ratio of tissue to blood pool concentration is the ratio of washin to washout rates. If the ratios for tissue concentration in ischemic and normal tissues to the common blood concentration are similar at rest and postexercise, the time to reach equal concentrations in the tissues will be given as $3/k_2$. For k_2 of 0.03 minute^{-1} to 0.01 minutes^{-1}, the corresponding times to reach equilibrium range from 1.6 hours to 5 hours, and this explains the apparent delay in accumulation in an ischemic region or the redistribution phenomenon either from an injection at rest or an injection with exercise. A slight difference between the ratios in normal and ischemic tissue explains late redistribution that will occur as long as there is sustained activity in the blood pool (Figure 4).

Single-Photon Emission Computed Tomography: Diagnostic Accuracy

Single-photon emission computed tomography has been used in an attempt to improve the detection sensitivity of ^{201}Tl for many years, and although the specificity and sensitivity have sometimes been shown to be better than conventional projection imaging, the methodology that is currently used can lead to serious artifacts and false-positive diagnoses because attenuation compensation is rarely applied properly. The recent development of ^{99m}Tc-labeled ligands promises to overcome the statistical limitations of ^{201}Tl studies (five times more dose can be injected) and these radiopharmaceuticals have led to renewed interest in cardiac perfusion imaging using SPECT.

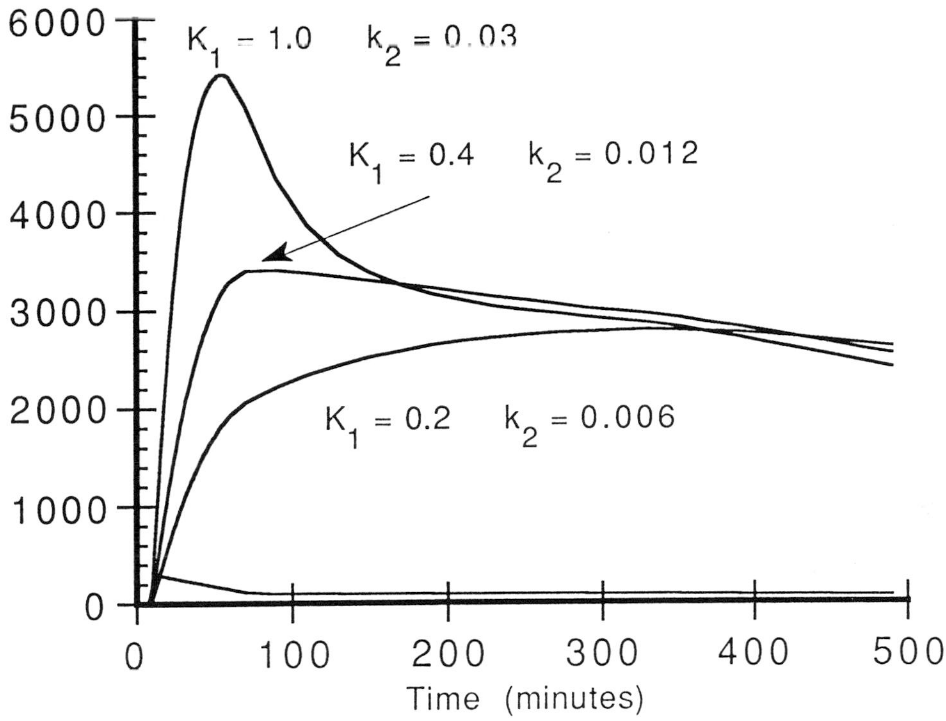

FIGURE 4. *Simulation of expected myocardial activity for different conditions of washin (k_1) and washout (k_2). The ratio k_1:k_2 is 33. Curves show that the time required for a similar tissue concentration to be reached for the low- and high-flow conditions is 4 to 8 hours. Ordinate axis is in arbitrary units.*

But the blood pool concentration of these ligands falls to low levels at a rapid rate in contrast to ^{201}Tl. Thus, the evaluation of myocardial viability using exercise or pharmacologic methods to induce coronary vasodilation requires two separate injections, but thallium has sufficient residual blood pool concentration to provide a "self-reinjection" during the interval between the initial and later injections of ^{201}Tl.

Thus, even with modification of protocols, new ligands, and new SPECT instruments, the potentials of SPECT imaging for accurate differentiation between viable and nonviable myocardium has not been realized.

Dynamic Single-Photon Emission Computed Tomography

As is the case with PET, it is possible to acquire cardiac SPECT blood pool data with 360° of angular sampling at 5-second intervals using a three-headed gamma camera instrument.[16] Whereas this approach was thought to be excluded by difficulties with available statistics, use of ^{99m}Tc ligands and new instrumentation make such measurements feasible.

After collection of preliminary data from laboratory animal studies and mathematical simulations, data were collected after 20 mCi Tc-MIBI was injected intravenously over a 40-second interval in two patients with 90° angles of data collection at 4° increments. The data acquisition protocol consisted of 5-second intervals for 200 seconds followed by 180-second intervals. Regions of interest over the heart chambers and myocardium are readily placed for the input function and residue function in order to calculate flow times extraction (Equation 1) or k_1 and k_2 for a two-compartment model shown in Equation 2 (Figure 1, right panel).

The first results give a flow × extraction of 0.3 ml/min per milliliter, which relates well to a normal flow of 0.9 ml/min per milliliter based on expected values of the extraction coefficient of 0.3 determined from laboratory animal studies. Results of kinetic analysis for patients with coronary artery disease showed a twofold decrease. One can expect similar results from fast-scan MRI with the cautions expressed previously.

The results can be obtained without additional patient time. The procedure is applicable to cardiac perfusion agents with higher washout rates than Tc-MIBI. Thus, in situations in which a second injection rather than redistribution would suffice, the most reliable study requires correction for attenuation made by separate transmission study. Reliable attenuation correction is still a major obstacle in cardiac SPECT (Figure 5).

At the present time, the new technetium-based ligands in SPECT, perfusion agents with PET, and contrast agents with MRI require two injections: one at exercise and one at rest.

Positron Emission Tomography

The attributes of PET for cardiac studies are better sensitivity and the availability of tracers of metabolic activity (eg, fatty acids, sugars, amino acids).

The sensitivity of PET relative to SPECT assuming the SPECT detectors surround the body is:

$$\frac{\text{PET}}{\text{SPECT}} = \frac{150\,\text{mm}}{d(\text{mm})} \tag{4}$$

where d is the resolution at which the two instruments are being compared.[17] Thus, at the practical resolution of 7.5 mm for both modalities, PET is 20 times more sensitive than SPECT for the same concentration of radionuclide activity. The radiopharmaceuticals available for PET include flow tracers such as $^{13}NH_4$,[18–20] $H_2{}^{15}O$,[2,3] and ^{82}Rb[21–23]; and metabolic ligands such as ^{18}F-deoxyglucose,[6] ^{11}C acetate,[4,5] ^{11}C-labeled palmitic acid, and neuroreceptor ligands specific for the adrenergic and cholinergic cardiac receptors.[24,25]

The practical problems of PET mainly revolve around cost and to some extent the need for a cyclotron. Improvements in cyclotrons and automation of radiophar-

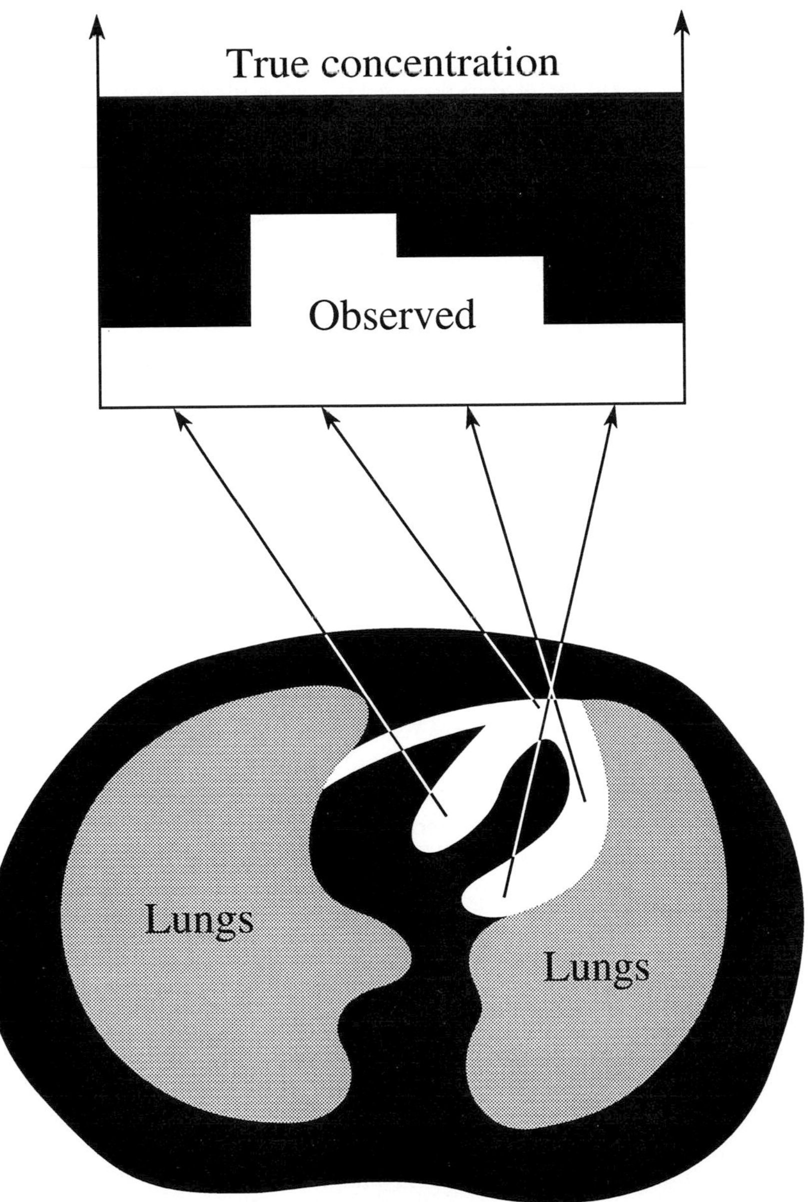

FIGURE 5. *The effect of attenuation of photons will be largest from the posterior septal region (right arrowhead) in single-photon tomography. Whereas accurate compensation methods are known, practical implementation is not yet readily available.*

maceutical synthesis have to a great extent overcome the burdens of operating PET systems. However, the start-up costs remain high. Yet PET can be performed using ^{18}F-radiopharmaceuticals ($\tau^{1/2}$ = 1.98 hours) delivered from cyclotrons as far away as 100 miles and generator-produced positron emitters such as rubidium ($\tau^{1/2}$ = 76 seconds) produced from a small "table top" device by merely eluting the parent Sr-82 ($\tau^{1/2}$ = 25 days) using a physiologically acceptable sodium chloride solution.

^{18}F-Deoxyglucose has become an important tracer of ischemic but viable tissue. Yet the clinical future of FDG in staging ischemic heart disease is still not clear. One of the problems is the question of the mechanism for glucose transport into the ischemic myocardium. An important variable is the dependence of accumulation of FDG on the nutritional status of the subject (Figure 5). Without insulin and glucose, very little FDG enters the myocardium. The differential uptake of FDG between ischemic and normal myocardium depends on both specific and nonspecific transport as well as accumulation in metabolically active granulocytes. The relative importance of all these factors is not yet understood for each patient condition. Nevertheless, an FDG PET study is useful in the patient in whom serial images demonstrate no thallium redistribution, but in whom there is reason to believe viable myocardium exists in the defect area.

Advances in Positron Emission Tomography Flow Studies

Automated procedures for quantitative evaluation of the change in washin of PET and SPECT perfusion tracers between the resting and stressed, or vasodilated, conditions are now available. In the past, we used visual qualitative comparisons of the activity differences for different regions of the myocardium before and after stress. The capability of emission tomography to provide quantitative data through Equation 1 or 2 has led to the clinical research question: will quantitative evaluation of the washin parameter improve our ability to detect ischemia over visual observations? An example of the application of the method is shown in Figure 6.

Studies of myocardial adrenergic receptors after myocardial infarction are presently underway and have promise for evaluation of patients at risk for sudden death.[25] A strength of PET, and to some extent SPECT, is the capability to assess the nanomolar concentrations of neuroreceptor tracers. Herein lies a distinct advantage of emission studies over magnetic resonance studies. However, the detection of the local concentration of radionuclides does not allow one to deduce chemical composition—a unique strength of NMR.

The high-resolution capabilities of PET have the potential to study relationships that might be found between the central nervous system and cardiovascular pathologies based on the conjecture that the balance of α_2-adrenergic receptor systems of the *locus ceruleus*, *nucleus tractus solatarius*, and forebrain cortex will be related to ischemia and possibly hypertension. Positron emission tomography has the potential to image at 2-mm resolution tracers sensitive to alterations in brain neurochemistry related to the circulatory system, and it is in this area where the unique capabilities of PET are best exemplified.[26]

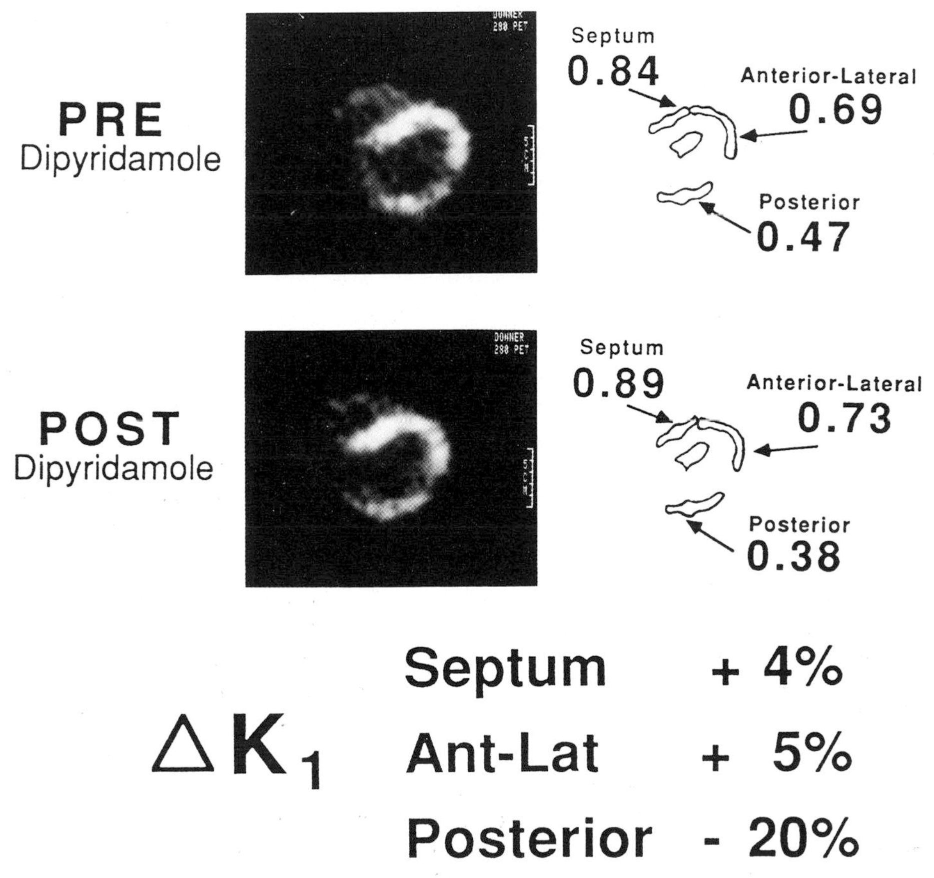

FIGURE 6. *Rb-82 PET, transverse section of the myocardium have been analyzed for flow using a two-compartment model. The values for washin at rest (PREdipyridamole) and after pharmacologic stress (POSTdipyridamole) give a quantitative assessment of pharmacologically induced flow changes.*

Synopsis and Perspective on Positron Emission Tomography Versus Single-Photon Emission Computed Tomography Versus Magnetic Resonance Imaging

For approximately 20 years, the clinical evaluation of ischemic heart disease has included radionuclide studies with a principle focus on imaging myocardial perfusion. From the mid-1970s to the present, the major radionuclide has been ^{201}Tl and the protocol involved studying the patient by perfusion imaging at rest and during exercise or pharmacologic stress. Positron emission tomography instrumentation improved in the late 1980s, and FDG PET was found to distinguish patients with viable myocardium in populations missed by the ^{201}Tl study. But in 1990, through modification of the SPECT protocols including reinjection of ^{201}Tl, many misleading persistent defects were properly diagnosed. By 1991, there were at least 13 radiopharmaceuticals under evaluation for assessment of perfusion and for the effects of detection of coronary artery disease (Table 1). Of these agents, markers of metabolism (eg, FDG)[6] and hypoxic tissues (eg, misonidazole)[27] have promise for direct labeling of injured myocardial tissue. Though no large-scale comparative studies have been made with misonidazole, studies comparing FDG to ^{201}Tl with reinjection[12] have resulted in some skepticism regarding the singular importance of PET FDG for detection and have led us to question whether perfusion studies alone will provide sufficient information to sensitively distinguish between viable and nonviable myocardium. Indeed, using cyclotron-produced ^{13}N-labeled ammonia or generator-produced ^{82}Rb as myocardial perfusion imaging agents, the sensitivity is 90% and specificities range from 78% to 100% for detection of coronary artery disease. One study directly compared PET to ^{201}Tl SPECT and demonstrated similar specificities, but improved sensitivities, from 76% for ^{201}Tl to 93% for ^{82}Rb PET.[23] This and one other study[28] did not use state-of-the-art PET versus state-of-the-art SPECT instruments. Thus, it is premature to conclude superiority of one methodology over another in myocardial perfusion assessments. One would expect that the ease of correction for photon attenuation, the somewhat superior resolution, and the speed of modern PET instruments would give PET the advantage. Clearly, if attenuation correction is not used in SPECT, false-positive diagnoses of septal and other defects will be high as shown in Figure 6. Attenuation compensation methods for SPECT that are computationally practical are not yet available for clinical studies.

It may be that properly performed single-photon imaging studies at rest and exercise are as accurate as the more involved FDG or hypoxic tissue marker PET or SPECT studies for assessment of viability. Despite the good results of radionuclide studies to assess perfusion and viability, magnetic resonance strategies should be developed and investigated. Since magnetic resonance can generate high-resolution imaging of the heart to assess morphology and function and has the potential to image coronary artery flow, the addition of perfusion and metabolic assessment would provide the patient with a "one-stop shop" for heart disease assessment.

Such a scenario would involve the bolus injection of a paramagnetic contrast agent such as gadolinium-DTPA and serial high-speed MRI. The injection would

TABLE 1. Agents for Ischemic Heart Disease Using Emission Tomography

$^{13}NH_3$	perfusion
$H_2{}^{15}O$	perfusion
^{60}Cu PTSM	perfusion
^{62}Cu PTSM	perfusion
^{81}Rb	perfusion
^{82}Rb	perfusion
^{68}Ga-BAT-TECH	perfusion
^{122}I-ligands	perfusion
^{99m}Tc sesta MIBI (SP)	perfusion
^{99m}Tc teboroxime (SP)	perfusion
^{201}Tl (SP)	perfusion
[^{11}C-]acetate	hypoxic tissue
[^{11}C-]palmitic acid	hypoxic tissue
[^{18}F-]fluorodeoxyglucose	metabolism
[^{123}I]-(----) nitazole (SP)	
[^{18}F-]fluoromisonidazole	metabolism

(SP) = single-photon method

be made during the infusion of dipyridamole or adenosine. Phosphorus-31 myocardial NMR spectroscopy might allow assessment of viability by comparing the relative content of PCr and ATP between the segment(s) in question and the functioning (control) segment(s).

Beyond clinical characterization of patients with possible ischemic heart disease, we look to PET might allow assessment of myocardial metabolism in cardiomyopathies and other applications such as characterization of atheroma using probes such as radiolabeled lipoproteins and radiolabeled peptides thought to be useful for assessment of smooth muscle or endothelial processes involved in the development of active atherosclerosis.

References

1. Budinger TF, Huesman RH: Ten precepts for quantitative data acquisition and analysis. *Circulation* 1985;72(suppl IV):53–62.
2. Bergmann SR, Herrero P, Markham J, et al: Noninvasive quantitation of myocardial blood flow in human subjects with oxygen-15-labeled water and positron emission tomography. *J Am Coll Cardiol* 1989;14:639–652.
3. Araujo L, Lammerstam A, Rhodes C, et al: Noninvasive quantification of regional myocardial blood flow in coronary artery disease with oxygen-15-labeled carbon dioxide inhalation and positron emission tomography. *Circulation* 1991;83:875–885.
4. Henes CG, Bergmann SR, Walsh MN, et al: Assessment of myocardial oxidative metabolic reserve with positron emission tomography and carbon-11 acetate. *J Nucl Med* 1989;30(9):1489–1499.
5. Armvrecht JJ, Buxton DB, Schelbert HR: Validation of [1–11C] acetate as a tracer for noninvasive assessment of oxidative metabolism with positron emission tomography in normal, ischemic, post-ischemic and hyperemic canine myocardium. *Circulation* 1991;81(5):1594–1605.
6. Schelbert HR, Buxton DB: Insights into coronary artery disease gained from metabolic imaging. *Circulation* 1988;78:496–515.

7. Pohost GM, Zir LM, Morre RH, et al: Differentiation of transiently ischemic from infarcted myocardium by serial imaging after a single dose of thallium-201. *Circulation* 1977;55:294–302.
8. Bruken RC, Kottou S, Nienaber CA, et al: PET detection of viable tissue in myocardial segments with persistent defects at Tl-201 SPECT. *Radiology* 1989;172:645–673.
9. Budinger TF, Pohost GM: Thallium "redistribution"—an explanation (abstract). *J Nucl Med* 1986;27(6):996.
10. Budinger TF, Knittel BL: Cardiac thallium redistribution and model (abstract). *J Nucl Med* 1987;28:588.
11. Dilsizian V, Rocco T, Freedman N, et al: Enhanced detection of ischemic but viable myocardium by the reinjection of thallium after stress-redistribution imaging. *N Engl J Med* 1990;323:141–146.
12. Bonow R, Dilsizian V, Cuocolo A, Bacharach S: Identification of viable myocardium in patients with chronic coronary artery disease and left ventricular dysfunction: comparison of thallium scintigraphy with reinjection and PET imaging with F-18-fluorodeoxyglucose. *Circulation* 1991;83(1):26–27.
13. Budinger TF, Pohost GM: General thallium redistribution model explains false negatives, late redistribution, redistribution at rest, early and late redistribution after reinjection *J Nucl Med* 1992;33:915.
14. Kiat H, Berman DS, Maddahi J, et al: Late reversibility of tomographic myocardial thallium-201 defects: an accurate marker of myocardial viability. *J Am Coll Cardiol* 1991;12:1456–1463.
15. Beller GA, Watson DD, Ackell P, Pohost GM: Time course of thallium-201 redistribution after transient ischemia. *Circulation* 1980;61:791–797.
16. Budinger T, Araujo L, Ranger N, et al: Dynamic SPECT feasibility studies (abstract). *J Nucl Med* 1992;32:955.
17. Budinger TF: Advances in emission tomography instrumentalion: quo vadis? *J Nucl Med* 1990;31:628–631.
18. Schelbert HR, Wisenberg G, Phelps ME, et al: Noninvasive assessment of coronary stenoses by myocardial imaging during pharmacologic coronary vasodilation. VI. Detection of coronary artery disease in man with intravenous N-13 ammonia and positron computed tomography. *Am J Cardiol* 1982;49:1197–1207.
19. Hutchins G, Schwaiger M, Rosenspire K, et al: Noninvasive quantification of regional blood flow in the human heart using N-13 ammonia and dynamic positron emission tomographic imaging. *J Am Coll Cardiol* 1990;15(5):1032–1042.
20. Bellina C, Parodi O, Camici P, et al: Simultaneous in vitro and in vivo validation of nitrogen 13-ammonia for the assessment of regional myocardial blood flow. *J Nucl Med* 1990;31:1335–1343.
21. Goldstein RA, Mullani NA, Wong W-H, et al: Positron imaging of myocardial infarction with rubidium-82. *J Nucl Med* 1986;27:1824–1829.
22. Demer LL, Gould KL, Goldstein RA, et al: Assessment of coronary artery disease severity by positron emission tomography. Comparison with quantitative arteriography in 193 patients. *Circulation* 1989;79:825–835.
23. Go R, Marwick T, MacIntyre W, et al: A prospective comparison of rubidium-82 PET and thallium-201 SPECT myocardial perfusion imaging utilizing a single dipyridamole stress in the diagnosis of coronary artery disease. *J Nucl Med* 1990;21:1899–1905.
24. Schwaiger M, Kalff V, Rosenspire K, et al: Noninvasive evaluation of sympathetic nervous system in human heart by positron emission tomography. *Circulation* 1990;82(2):457–464.
25. Delforge J, Janier M, Syrota A, et al: Noninvasive quantification of muscarinic receptors in vivo with positron emission tomography in the dog heart. *Circulation* 1990;82(4):1494–1504.
26. Budinger TF, Derenzo SE, Huesman RH, et al: High resolution positron emission tomography for medical science studies. *Acta Radiol Suppl* 1991;376:15–23.

27. Shelton M, Dence C, Hwang D, et al: In vivo delineation of myocardial hypoxia during coronary occlusion using fluorine-18 fluoromisonidazole and positron emission tomography: a potential approach for identification of jeopardized myocardium. *J Am Coll Cardiol* 1990;16(2):477–485.
28. Tamaki N, Yonekura Y, Senda M, et al: Value and limitation of stress thallium-201 single photon emission computed tomography: comparison with nitrogen-13 ammonia positron tomography. *J Nucl Med* 1988;29:1181–1188.

Chapter 25

^{31}P Nuclear Magnetic Resonance Studies of Experimental Myocardial Ischemia

Robert J. Bache, MD, Arthur H.L. From, MD, Jianyi Zhang, MD, PhD, and Kamil Uğurbil, PhD

During normal conditions, left ventricular systolic wall stress and, therefore, myocardial oxygen demands and blood flow, are greatest in the subendocardium.[1] In contrast, when arterial inflow is insufficient to meet myocardial needs, the limited blood flow is delivered preferentially to the outer myocardial layers, which results in hypoperfusion that is most severe in the subendocardium.[2,3] These inhomogeneities of myocardial perfusion and contractile function might be expected to result in parallel inhomogeneities of metabolic activity. Consequently, there has been great interest in the development of methodologies for assessment of the metabolic state of the heart that are capable of providing spatially localized information across the wall of the left ventricle. ^{31}P nuclear magnetic resonance (NMR) spectroscopy provides a nondestructive method for repetitive determination of phosphorus-containing compounds in biologic tissue.[4] Localization of the phosphorus signal to discrete transmural layers of the myocardium is possible using the FLAX-ISIS technique.[5,6] Application of this technique to the heart has the potential for allowing assessment of transmural inhomogeneities of myocardial energy metabolism in the intact beating heart both during normal conditions and in the presence of ischemia.

Supported by U.S. Public Health Service Grants HL21872 and HL34701 from the National Heart, Lung, and Blood Institute and by a Research Fellowship from the Minnesota Affiliate of the American Heart Association.
From Pohost GM (ed.), *Cardiovascular Applications of Magnetic Resonance*. Mount Kisco, NY, Futura Publishing Co., Inc., © 1993.

Relationships Between Perfusion, Contractile Function, and High-Energy Phosphate Content During Experimental Myocardial Ischemia

The transmural responses of myocardial perfusion, function, and high-energy phosphate compound content produced by progressively more severe flow-limiting coronary artery stenoses have been the subject of several studies.[7,8] Adult mongrel canines were anesthetized with sodium pentobarbital (30–35 mg/kg IV), intubated, and ventilated with a respirator.[7,8] Catheters were placed in the left ventricle and ascending aorta for pressure measurement and blood sampling, while a catheter in the left atrium allowed administration of radioactive microspheres for measurement of regional myocardial blood flow. To allow production of variable degrees of coronary stenosis, the proximal left anterior descending coronary artery was instrumented sequentially with a hydraulic occluder and an indwelling microcatheter for measurement of distal coronary pressure. To allow measurement of myocardial contractile performance, in some of the animals a pair of 5-MHz piezoelectric microcrystals were implanted in the inner third of the left ventricular wall in the region that became cyanotic during transient occlusion of the anterior descending coronary artery. The ultrasonic crystal pairs were separated by a distance of 10 to 15 mm and were oriented circumferentially in a plane parallel with the subendocardial myocardial fibers to allow measurement of myocardial segment shortening.

^{31}P Nuclear Magnetic Resonance Techniques

A 28-mm NMR surface coil encased in silicone rubber that included a reference standard consisting of 15 μl of 3 M phosphonoacetic acid was sutured to the area of the anterior left ventricular wall, adjacent to the piezoelectric crystals and in the region perfused by the anterior descending coronary artery. The surface coil leads were connected to a balanced tuned circuit external and perpendicular to the thoracotomy incision, and the animals were placed in a 40-cm bore 4.7-T magnet interfaced with a CSI-II console. ^{31}P and ^{1}H resonant frequencies were 81 and 200.1 MHz, respectively. Spectra were recorded in late diastole using respiratory and cardiac gating with a pulse repetition time of 6–7 seconds.[9] This repetition time yields full relaxation for adenosine triphosphate and P_i with approximately 95% relaxation of the phosphocreatine (PCr) resonance. Phosphocreatine resonances were corrected for this minor saturation. The H_2O signal detected at 200.1 MHz was used to homogenize the magnetic field and to adjust the position of the animal so that the coil was at or near the magnet and gradient isocenters. Chemical shifts were measured relative to PCr, which was assigned a chemical shift of -2.55 ppm relative to phosphoric acid.

Spatial localization across the left ventricular wall was accomplished with the FLAX-ISIS technique.[5,6] Signal origin was restricted to a 17×17 mm-column coaxial to the surface coil (perpendicular to the epicardial surface). Within the column, the signal was localized to five voxels centered approximately 45°, 60°, 90°, 120°, and 135° spin-rotation increments, respectively. Fourier coefficients and the multiplication factors used to construct the voxels were those reported by Robitaille et al.[6] The position of the voxels relative to the coil was set using the B_1 strength at the coil center, which was determined by measuring the 90° pulse length for the reference located at the coil center. The voxels were positioned along the column so that the capillary at the coil center experienced a 158° rotation for the incremented square pulse when $n = 1$.

The 17 × 17-mm column was defined using sech/tahn-modulated, 1.5- to 2-msec long, adiabatic inversion pulses and 2.5–3.0 G/cm B_0 gradients. The adiabatic excitation pulse that follows the adiabatic inversion pulses in FLAX-ISIS was based on optimized NOM (sin/cos; v:0.2–20) functions and was typically 1 msec in duration. Complete localized transmural spectra were acquired in two 13-minute data sets that were subsequently added to enhance the signal-to-noise ratio. A total of 116 scans were accumulated in each 13-minute block. The number of scans for each term in the 12-term FLAX-ISIS series is reported by Robitaille et al.[6]

Spectra were integrated using GEMSCI software, and integrals were normalized to those obtained during control conditions. Adenosine triphosphate content was taken as the average of the ATPγ and ATPβ resonances. The ATPα resonance was corrected for a small contribution from NAD/NADH. Because of off-resonance problems, ATPβ is not suitable for assessing transmural ATP content. Although ADPα and ADPβ overlap with the respective ATP resonances, adenosine diphosphate content is approximately three orders of magnitude less than ATP. Nucleoside monophosphates such as adenosine monophosphate (AMP) and inosine monophosphate (IMP) that can accumulate during ischemia resonate in the phosphomonoester region, downfield from the P_i peak and are consequently distinct from the resonances of interest.

Experimental Measurements

Aortic, left ventricular, and mean left anterior descending coronary pressures, systolic segment shortening, and ^{31}P NMR spectra were first obtained during basal conditions. Spectra were acquired in two consecutive 13-minute data sets. Because of electrical interference between the piezoelectric crystals and the radiofrequency transmitter/detector, segment shortening was measured at discrete intervals before, midway through, and at the end of spectra acquisition. Microspheres were administered for measurement of myocardial blood flow between the two spectra acquisition periods. After completion of the control measurements, the coronary occluder was partially inflated to decrease distal coronary pressure to 60 mm Hg. After a 2- to 4-minute stabilization period, segment shortening was measured followed by acquisition of spectra; microspheres were administered and segment shortening was measured as previously described. After completion of the measurements, the stenosis was released and the heart allowed to recover for at least 10 minutes. The coronary occluder was then inflated to reduce distal coronary pressure to 50 mm Hg and all measurements repeated. After another recovery period, coronary pressure was reduced to 40 mm Hg and all measurements repeated.

As shown in Figure 1, myocardial blood flow during basal conditions was essentially uniform across the left ventricular wall from epicardium to endocardium.

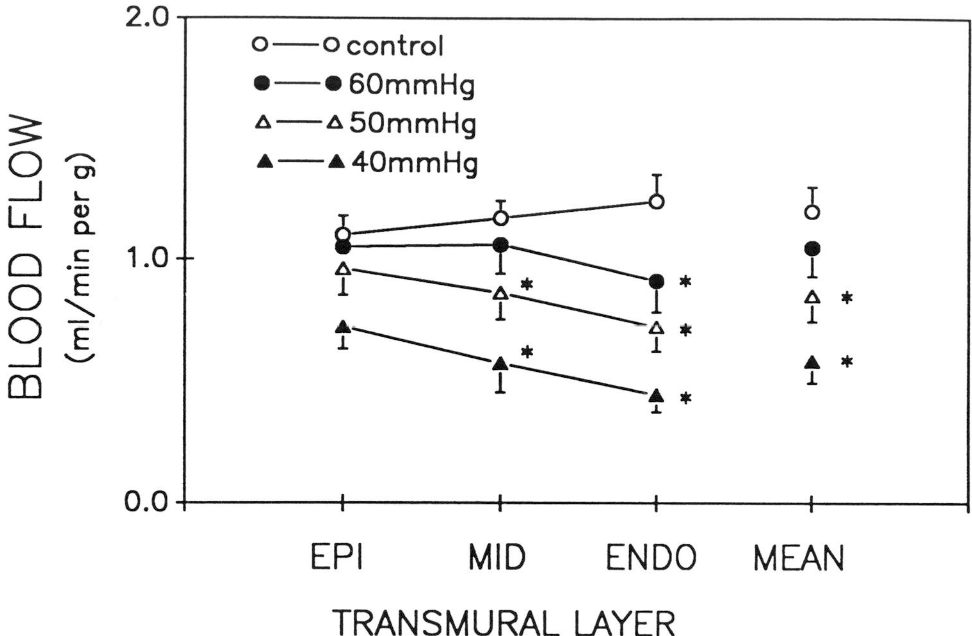

FIGURE 1. *Blood flow to the subepicardium (EPI), midmyocardium (MID), and subendocardium (ENDO) during control conditions and with coronary stenoses that reduced distal perfusion pressure to 60, 50, or 40 mm Hg. The presence of a coronary stenosis resulted in hypoperfusion that was most severe in the subendocardium. Reprinted from References 7 and 8 with permission.*

Reducing coronary pressure to 60 mm Hg caused a modest decrease in blood flow to the subendocardium, with no significant change in flow to the midwall or subepicardium, and no change in mean blood flow. Further reductions of coronary pressure caused progressive transmural redistribution of perfusion with absolute reductions in blood flow to the midwall and subendocardium, and preferential underperfusion of the subendocardium at each perfusion pressure.

Figure 2 illustrates the relationship between systolic segment shortening and myocardial blood flow in the subendocardium. Systolic function remained essentially normal until subendocardial blood flow fell below approximately 0.75 ml/min per gram of myocardium; reductions of flow below this level resulted in parallel reductions of systolic shortening so that subendocardial flow rates <0.5 ml/min per gram were almost always associated with akinesis or dyskinesis. In contrast to the close, predictable relationship between subendocardial blood flow and mechanical function, subepicardial blood flow had no predictable relationship with mechanical function. These findings are in agreement with previously reported data examining the relationship between perfusion and contractile performance during progressive myocardial hypoperfusion in both open-chest and chronically instrumented awake animals.[10,11]

Figure 3 demonstrates ^{31}P NMR spectra obtained from a representative animal during control conditions and in response to progressively increasing degrees of coronary stenosis. During control conditions the resonances corresponding to PCr

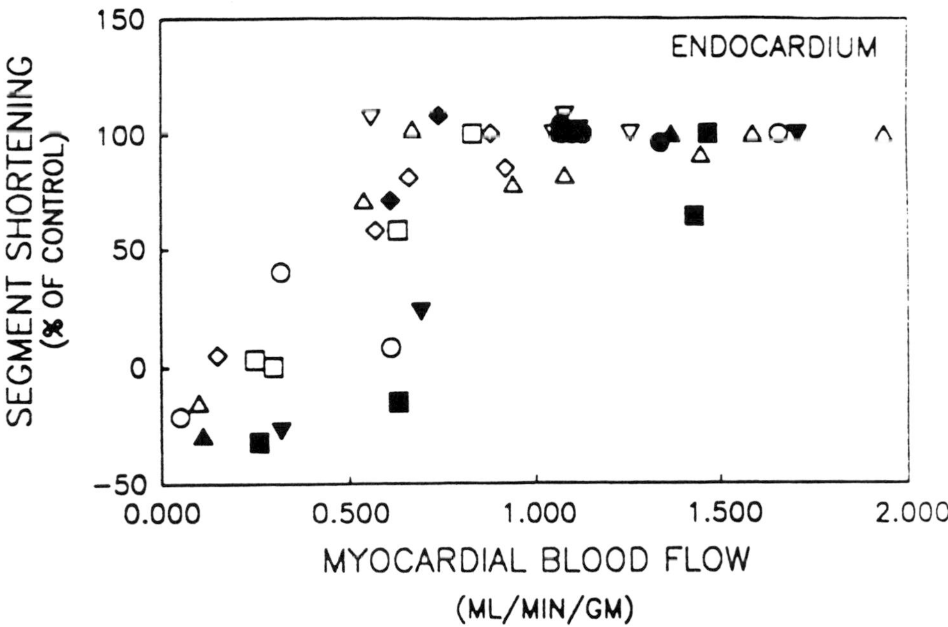

FIGURE 2. *Systolic segment shortening measured with ultrasonic microcrystals implanted in the subendocardium of the anterior left ventricular wall plotted against subendocardial blood flow measured with microspheres. Each individual animal is represented by a different symbol. Measurements were obtained during control conditions and with progressively increasing degrees of coronary stenosis. Systolic function remained essentially normal until subendocardial blood flow fell below approximately 0.75 ml/min per gram; reductions of flow below this level resulted in parallel reductions of systolic segment shortening. Reprinted from Reference 8 with permission.*

and the three phosphates of ATP are clearly seen in all transmural layers, whereas P_i is not detectable. Application of a coronary stenosis to reduce coronary pressure to 60 mm Hg caused reductions of PCr and appearance of P_i that were most prominent in the subendocardium and extended to the midwall, whereas subepicardial spectra were unchanged. As progressively worsening degrees of coronary stenosis were applied the appearance of P_i and depletion of PCr became more prominent and moved as a wave front toward the epicardium, so that during the most severe degree of stenosis, changes were apparent in all voxels, although changes were most marked in the deeper layers.

The relationships between blood flow and PCr in three transmural layers for all animals are shown in Figure 4. In the subendocardium PCr was generally unchanged until blood flow fell below approximately 0.7 ml/min per gram and then decreased precipitously with further flow reduction. A similar but less close relationship was seen in the midwall of the left ventricle. In contrast, there was little correlation between perfusion and PCr in the subepicardium. Of interest was the finding that in several cases subepicardial PCr levels decreased substantially with no change in blood

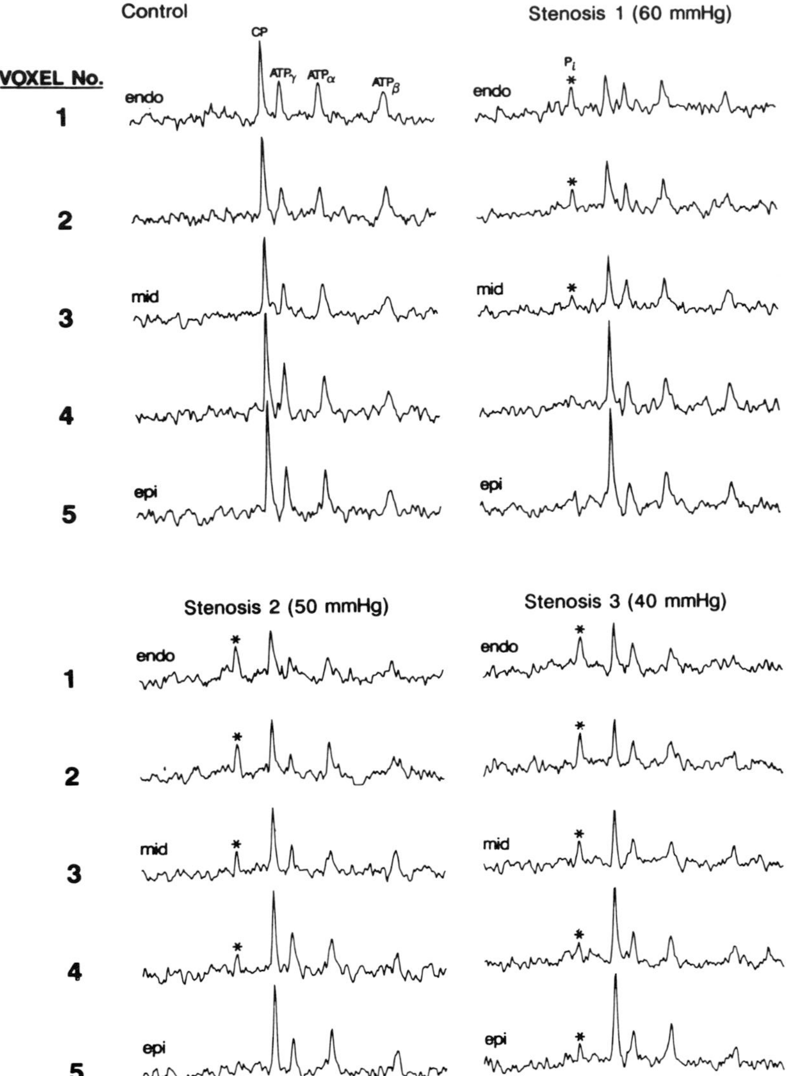

FIGURE 3. *Transmural response of phosphorylated metabolites detected by ^{31}P nuclear magnetic resonance during graded, sustained coronary stenosis in a typical animal. Spectra were obtained during control conditions and at coronary pressures of 60, 50, and 40 mm Hg. Each transmural set consists of a stack of five spectra corresponding to the 45°, 60°, 90°, 120°, and 135° voxels, respectively. Voxels 1 and 5 are the most distant and the most proximal voxels, respectively, relative to the coil. (*, inorganic phosphate [P_i] resonances; CP, phosphocreatine; ENDO, subendocardial voxel; MID, midmyocardial voxel; EPI, subepicardial voxel.) Reprinted from Reference 7 with permission.*

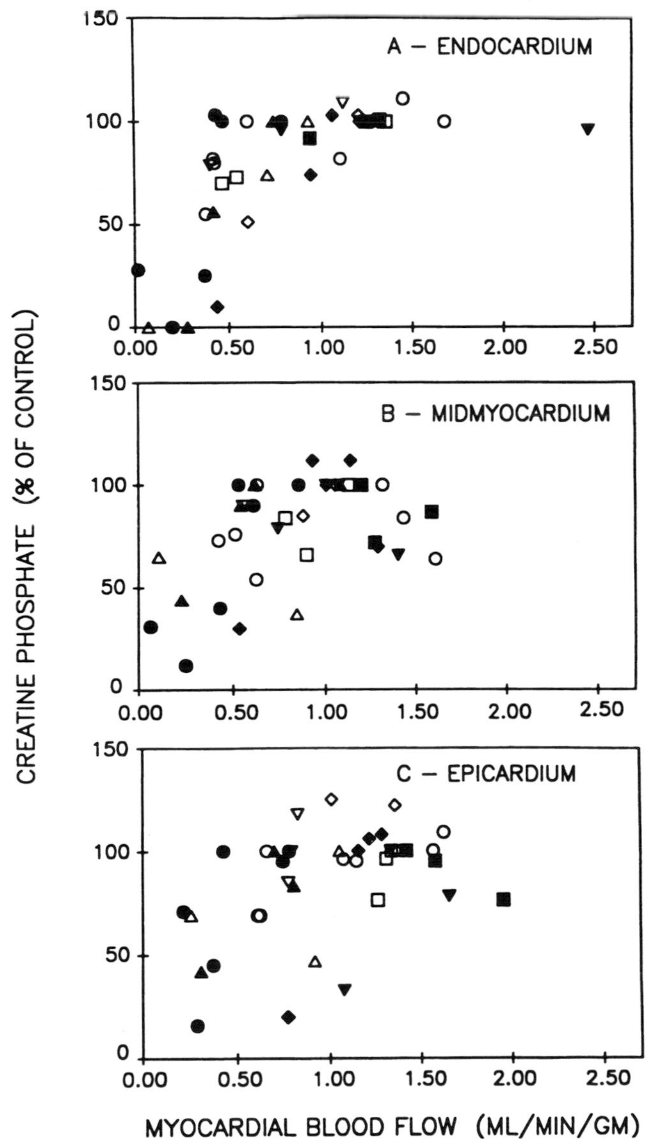

FIGURE 4. *Creatine phosphate content of the subendocardial (A), midmyocardial (B), and subepicardial regions (C) as a function of myocardial blood flow. Different symbols represent individual cases. Reprinted from Reference 8 with permission.*

flow to this layer. This finding always occurred at a degree of stenosis that had caused a considerable reduction of blood flow in the subendocardium. This suggested that ischemia in the subendocardium caused selective loss of subendocardial contractile function, thereby displacing a greater load onto the subepicardial fibers. The resultant increase in systolic load on the subepicardium could result in ischemic changes in the region despite a normal blood flow rate. To assess this possibility, PCr in the subepicardium was plotted against subendocardial PCr in cases in which the stenosis had caused a decrease in subendocardial blood flow with less than a 10% change in subepicardial blood flow. As shown in Figure 5, a significant correlation was found between subepicardial PCr and subendocardial PCr when subepicardial blood flow was unchanged. This finding supports the hypothesis that ischemic metabolic changes can occur in the subepicardium with no reduction of perfusion as the result of ischemia in the subendocardium.

Adenosine triphosphate values did not decrease until hypoperfusion was severe, with ATP levels decreasing with absolute flow rates below 0.5 ml/min per gram of myocardium. Unlike PCr, the relationship between flow and ATP was similar in all transmural layers. However, since blood flow rates were most depressed in the subendocardium, ATP values were least in this region. In contrast to the rapid recovery of PCr with reperfusion, when ATP levels decreased during hypoperfusion (generally only with the most severe stenosis), reperfusion did not result in recovery of ATP values to normal.

The relationship between PCr and systolic segment shortening is shown in Figure 6. In the subendocardium, segment shortening was closely correlated with PCr

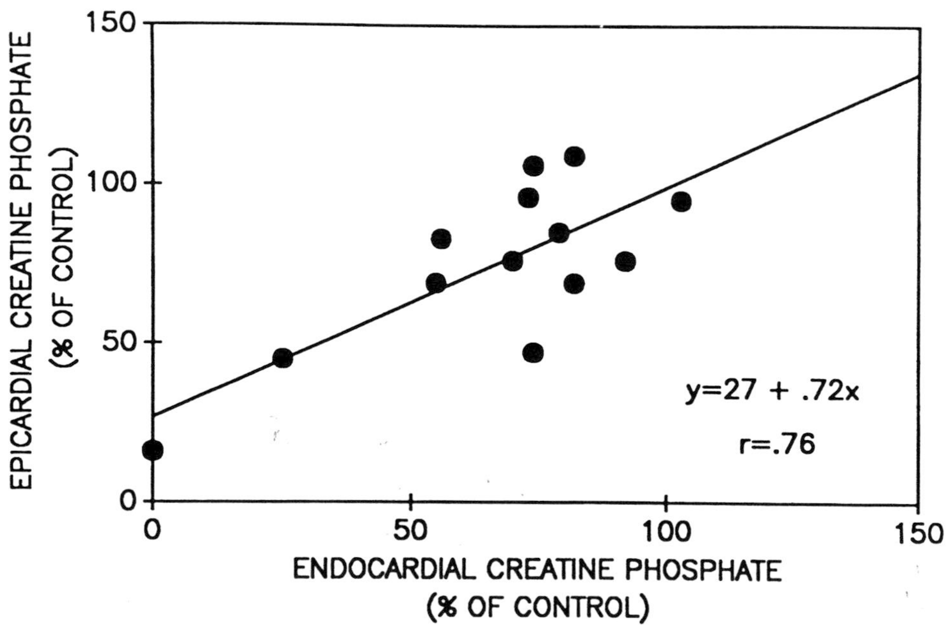

FIGURE 5. *Subepicardial versus subendocardial creatine phosphate levels in cases in which subepicardial blood flow was normal or was increased or decreased by <10% of the baseline flow. Reprinted from Reference 7 with permission.*

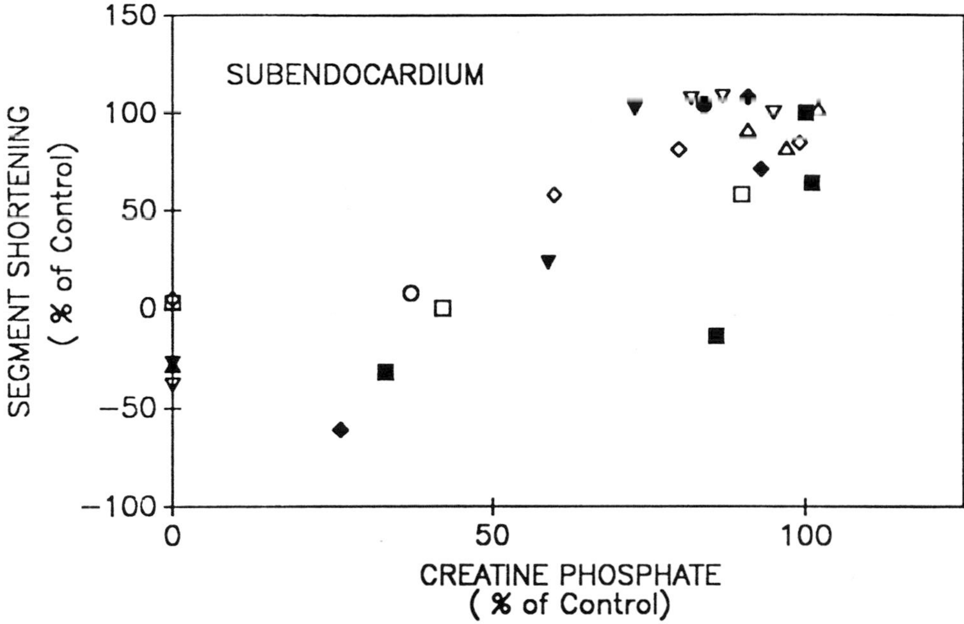

FIGURE 6. *Systolic segment shortening measured in the subendocardium plotted as a function of subendocardial phosphocreatine. Different symbols represent individual cases. When subendocardial phosphocreatine was reduced to <70% of control, systolic segment shortening was always abnormal. Reprinted from Reference 8 with permission.*

levels, so that when PCr was reduced to <70% of control, segment shortening was almost always abnormal. Reductions of PCr below 50% of normal were associated with akinesis or hypokinesis. In contrast, substantial reductions of systolic segment shortening occurred with no reduction of subepicardial PCr. This probably occurred because of transmural tethering within the left ventricular wall; because the subendocardial fibers normally contribute most to wall motion, loss of contractile function in this layer could cause decreased function of the entire wall, including the most superficial layers, where perfusion was not decreased.

Myocardial Stunning

Total coronary artery occlusions >20 minutes in duration generally result in myocardial infarction that begins first in the subendocardial muscle and then moves from the subendocardium toward the epicardium as a time-dependent wave front.[12] Total coronary occlusions of <20 minutes, duration or subtotal occlusions of longer duration do not produce infarct, but may result in contractile dysfunction that can persist for hours to days, with gradual progressive complete recovery of function.[13] This phenomenon of reversible ischemic dysfunction of viable myocardium has been termed "stunning." Previous studies in which chemical assay of high-energy phosphate compounds was performed have demonstrated that ATP levels are decreased in stunned myocardium and gradually recover roughly in parallel with recovery of contractile function.[14] Despite the temporal correspondence between recovery of mechanical function and myocardial ATP levels, loss of ATP during ischemia does not appear to play a causal role, since acceleration of ATP repletion by supplying precursors for ATP synthesis does not expedite recovery of contractile function.[15]

Because of its nondestructive nature, NMR spectroscopy is an ideal technique for longitudinal study of recovery of myocardial ATP following nonlethal ischemic injury. To allow study over a sufficient period of time to characterize complete recovery of myocardial ATP, we performed studies in chronically instrumented canines with a surface coil implanted on the anterior left ventricular wall in the region perfused by the left anterior descending coronary artery. Catheters were implanted for measurement of left ventricular and aortic pressures, and a left atrial catheter allowed administration of radioactive microspheres for measurement of regional blood flow. A pneumatic occluder was implanted around the proximal left anterior descending coronary artery.

Spectra from a typical animal are shown in Figure 7. After obtaining measurements during control conditions, stunning was produced with three successive 10-minute occlusions of the left anterior descending coronary artery; a 10-minute period of reperfusion was allowed between each occlusion. During occlusion the spectra showed depletion of PCr and ATP with accumulation of P_i; these abnormalities extended across the entire left ventricular wall but were most severe in the subendocardial layers. Following reperfusion, PCr rapidly recovered to normal or supranormal levels and P_i promptly disappeared, but, ATP remained depressed. Spectra recorded 24 hours after the ischemic insult showed little recovery of ATP, while at 48 hours

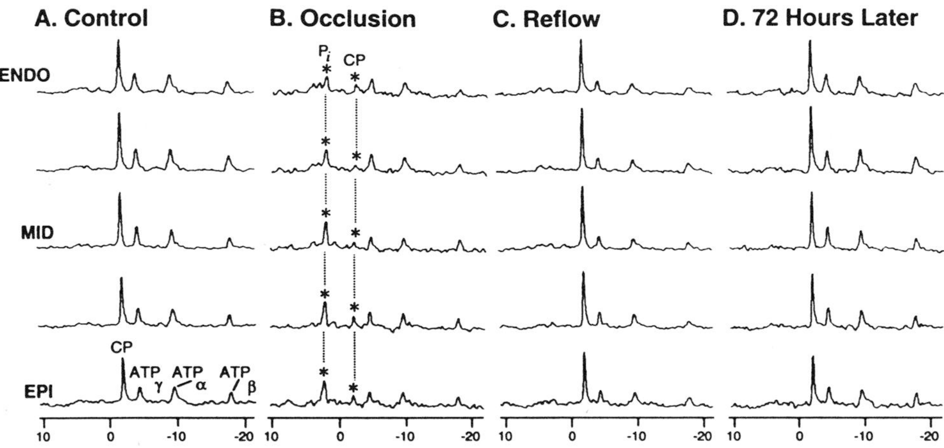

FIGURE 7. *Transmural response of phosphorylated metabolites detected by ^{31}P nuclear magnetic resonance during myocardial stunning. Spectra are shown during control conditions, during coronary occlusion, and at 1 and 72 hours after myocardial stunning produced by three successive 10-minute occlusions of the left anterior descending coronary artery.*

substantial recovery of ATP had occurred. Spectra obtained 72 hours after the ischemic insult showed return of ATP levels to the preischemic control level.

The results of this study are in agreement with previous reports in which high-energy phosphate compounds were measured in myocardial biopsy specimens.[14] However, the present study demonstrates the unique advantage of NMR technology for obtaining repetitive nondestructive transmurally localized measurements within the same region of the heart over a prolonged period of time in intact closed chest animals. Because of its invasive and destructive nature, the biopsy technique is unable to provide similar longitudinal data within the same animal over a prolonged period of time.

Summary

^{31}P NMR spectroscopy provides an ideal methodology for longitudinal study of the behavior of myocardial high-energy phosphate content in the ischemic and postischemic heart. Because of its nondestructive nature, multiple measurements over time can be performed. With proper gating techniques and attention to signal isolation between electronic measurement devices, these NMR observations can be correlated with simultaneous measurements of blood flow and systolic wall motion to fully characterize perfusion, high-energy phosphates, and contractile function of the myocardium.

References

1. Weiss HH, Neubauer JD, Lipp JD, Sinha AK: Quantitative determination of regional oxygen consumption in the dog heart. *Circ Res* 1978;42:394–401.
2. Moir TW, Debra DW: Effect of left ventricular hypertension, ischemia and vasoactive drugs on the myocardial distribution of coronary flow. *Circ Res* 1967;21:65–74.
3. Ball RM, Bache RJ: Distribution of the myocardial blood flow in the exercising dog with restricted coronary artery inflow. *Circ Res* 1976;38:60–66.
4. Ingwall JS: Phosphorus nuclear magnetic resonance spectroscopy of cardiac and skeletal muscles. *Am J Physiol* 1982;242:H729–H744.
5. Robitaille PM, Merkle H, Sublett E, et al: Spectroscopic imaging and spatial localization using adiabatic pulses and applications to detect transmural metabolite distribution in the canine heart. *Magn Reson Med* 1989;10:14–37.
6. Robitaille PM, Lew B, Merkle H, et al: Transmural metabolite distribution in regional myocardial ischemia as studied with ^{31}P NMR. *Magn Reson Med* 1989;10:108–118.
7. Path G, Robitaille PM, Merkle H, et al: Correlation between transmural high energy phosphate levels and myocardial blood flow in the presence of graded coronary stenosis. *Circ Res* 1990;67:660–673.
8. Path G, Tristani M, Zhang J, et al: Effects of a coronary stenosis on transmural myocardial high energy phosphates and systolic function (abstract). *Circulation* 1990;82(suppl III):III-65.
9. Robitaille PM, Lew B, Merkle H, et al: Transmural high energy phosphate distribution and response to alterations in workload in the normal canine myocardium as studied with spatially localized ^{31}P NMR spectroscopy. *Magn Reson Med* 1990;16:91–116.
10. Gallagher KP, Kumada T, Koziol JA, et al: Significance of regional wall thickening abnormalities relative to transmural myocardial perfusion in anesthetized dogs. *Circulation* 1980;62:1266–1274.
11. Gallagher KP, Matsuzaki M, Osakada G, et al: Effect of exercise on the relationship

between myocardial blood flow and systolic wall thickening in dogs with acute coronary stenosis. *Circ Res* 1983;52:716–729.

12. Reimer KA, Jennings RB: The "wavefront phenomenon" of myocardial ischemic cell death. II. Transmural progression of necrosis within the framework of ischemic bed size (myocardium at risk) and collateral flow. *Lab Invest* 1979;40:633–644.
13. Heyndrickx GR, Baig H, Nellens D, et al: Depression of regional blood flow and wall thickening after brief coronary occlusion. *Am J Physiol* 1978;234:H653–H659.
14. Reimer KA, Hill ML, Jennings RB: Prolonged depletion of ATP and of the adenine nucleotide pool due to delayed resynthesis of adenine nucleotides following reversible myocardial ischemic injury in dogs. *J Mol Cell Cardiol* 1981;13:229–239.
15. Ambrosio G, Jacobus WE, Mitchell MC, et al: Effects of ATP precursors on ATP and free ADP content and functional recovery of postischemic hearts. *Am J Physiol* 1989;256(Pt 2):H560–H566.

Chapter 26

Clinical Spectroscopy in Ischemic Heart Disease

Saul Schaefer, MD

Magnetic resonance spectroscopy (MRS) has the potential to increase our understanding of human ischemic heart disease by examining the metabolic changes in the myocardium due to either acute or chronic reductions in myocardial blood flow. Studies in humans to date have measured high-energy phosphates following myocardial infarction, during induced myocardial ischemia, and in patients with both ischemic and nonischemic cardiomyopathies. However, in order to understand the role of MRS in human ischemic heart disease, it is important to examine the findings of pertinent animal studies and the technical issues facing the investigator.

Animal Studies of Myocardial Ischemia

Perfused heart studies and large animal experiments have studied both acute total and partial ischemia, as well as conditions of prolonged ischemia, conditions parallel to those found in patients with coronary artery disease. Studies of acute total ischemia have found rapid changes in high-energy phosphates and pH that reverse when flow is reestablished within a few minutes,[1] but that persist and worsen when severe ischemia is maintained,[2] leading to myocardial infarction. Specifically, these changes include a rapid fall in phosphocreatine (PCr) and pH, an increase in inorganic phosphate (P_i), and a slower fall in the tissue content of adenosine triphosphate (ATP).[3]

Mild to moderate reductions of blood flow result in less severe metabolic abnormalities. Conditions of graded ischemia in pigs and canines studied with MRS, in conjunction with measurements of hemodynamics, function, and blood flow, have shown that metabolic changes closely parallel the reductions in blood flow and segment shortening during regional ischemia.[4,5] Specifically, whereas PCr is normal until subendocardial blood flow is reduced to approximately 50% of normal, the ratio of PCr/Pi is reduced when subendocardial blood flow is reduced by only 20%, and

Supported by grants from the National Institutes of Health (K08-HL-02131) and the California Affiliate of the American Heart Association.
From Pohost GM (ed.), *Cardiovascular Applications of Magnetic Resonance.* Mount Kisco, NY, Futura Publishing Co., Inc., © 1993.

therefore the PCr/P_i ratio is a sensitive metabolic indicator of ischemia (Figure 1). Furthermore, the changes in subendocardial blood flow, segment shortening, and PCr/Pi are all closely correlated, implying a regulatory role for these metabolites and indicating that these measures (ie, PCr/Pi and segment shortening) may be of equivalent efficacy in the diagnosis of regional myocardial ischemia. The decreased sensitivity of both PCr and ATP to mild reductions in blood flow indicate that these metabolites have a more limited role as diagnostic measures, and that measurement of Pi is important to maintain the sensitivity of the examination to reductions in myocardial blood flow.

Characterization of these acute changes in blood flow is important in order to understand mechanisms and develop diagnostic tests for inducible myocardial isch emia. However, many patients with coronary artery disease have intermittent ischemia, with periods of reduced flow interspersed with periods of relatively normal blood flow ("staccato ischemia").[6] This condition results in myocardial dysfunction in the presence of persistently reduced blood flow ("hibernating myocardium")[7] and/or myocardial dysfunction following an ischemic period with restoration of normal blood

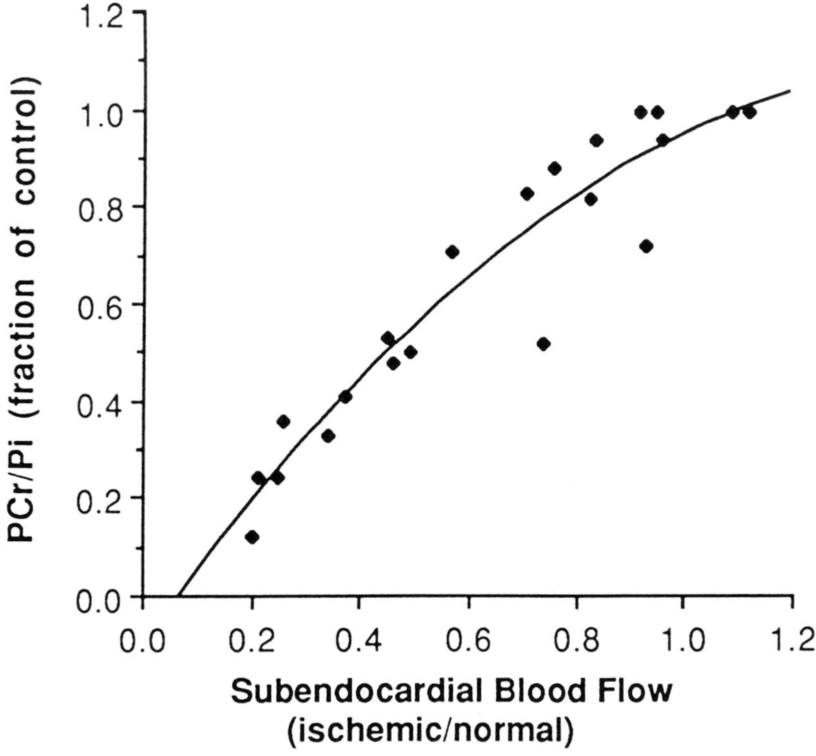

FIGURE 1. *The response of PCr/Pi to graded reduction of subendocardial blood flow in the open-chest pig. PCr/Pi is significantly reduced with only mild reductions in blood flow (on the order of 20% reduction), whereas concurrent measurements of PCr/ATP remain near control values until blood flow is reduced by 50%. PCr/Pi is also closely correlated to segment shortening, thus indicating that it is a sensitive marker of ischemia. Reprinted from Reference 4 with permission.*

flow ("stunned myocardium").[8] Myocardial energy metabolism has been studied under these conditions in animal models to increase our understanding of the relationship of these functional and metabolic events and, potentially, to apply this understanding to the human condition.

Stunned myocardium has been studied extensively in models of acute ischemia and reperfusion and appears to result from decreased myofilament sensitivity to calcium in the face of normal levels of high-energy phosphates, thus resulting in decreased efficiency of ATP utilization.[9] Hibernating myocardium has been less well characterized, since this chronic condition is poorly characterized in humans and is difficult to develop in an animal model. However, several animal studies of prolonged mild ischemia lasting 1 to 3 hours have resulted in evidence of functional and metabolic adaptation and recovery that appear to allow cell viability in the face of persistent ischemia.[10–12] Specifically, these studies have found recovery of the tissue content of PCr when the ischemia is mild, but persistence of PCr depression when the ischemia is more severe. Similarly, lactate production declines after an initial increase at the onset of ischemia, signifying a decrease in anaerobic glycolysis during ischemia (Figure 2).[11] These studies suggest that simple measurement of high-energy phosphates in patients with a spectrum of ischemic heart disease may be complex, but also may lead to more precise characterization of their metabolic status.

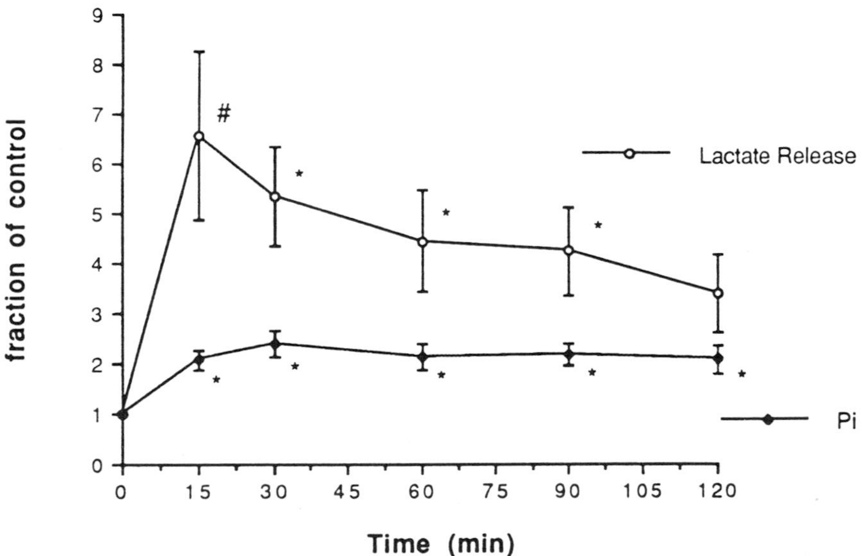

FIGURE 2. *The response of lactate production (measured using isotopic techniques) and inorganic phosphate (P_i) (measured using magnetic resonance spectroscopy) from the ischemic anterior region of the left ventricle during 2 hours of prolonged ischemia. Lactate production increased early during ischemia, but then fell toward control levels after 2 hours. In contrast, P_i remained significantly elevated during this period. Phosphocreatine (not shown) similarly remained depressed during ischemia. Reprinted from Reference 11 with permission.*

Methodologic Considerations

While animal studies have generally used a surface coil directly on the heart, human studies have been limited to surface coil acquisition from the chest wall. These efforts have primarily focused on surface coil localization techniques, such as depth-resolved surface coil spectroscopy (DRESS),[13] ISIS,[14,15] rotating frame,[16] and chemical shift imaging (CSI),[17] and each of these techniques has been used to acquire spectra from humans. An example of a spectrum obtained at 1.5 T using ISIS for localization and proton decoupling to enhance resolution is shown in Figure 3. This spectrum shows the typical resonances of PCr and ATP as well as a small resonance from intramyocardial P_i. The two resonances of 2,3-diphosphoglycerate (2,3-DPG) of chamber and myocardial blood are also shown, although in most spectra acquired from humans, the P_i resonance cannot be distinguished from the 2,3-DPG resonance.

Since localization is such an important issue in the accuracy of human cardiac spectroscopy, several investigators have used techniques to separate the myocardial signal from other tissue containing significant amounts of either PCr or ATP. One technique uses the slight (0.5 ppm) chemical shift of PCr between skeletal muscle and myocardium to identify cardiac spectra,[18] an effect thought due to differences in bulk susceptibility. Another technique to counter the potential contamination from side lobes of the phase encoding gradient waveform is to define a column perpendicular to

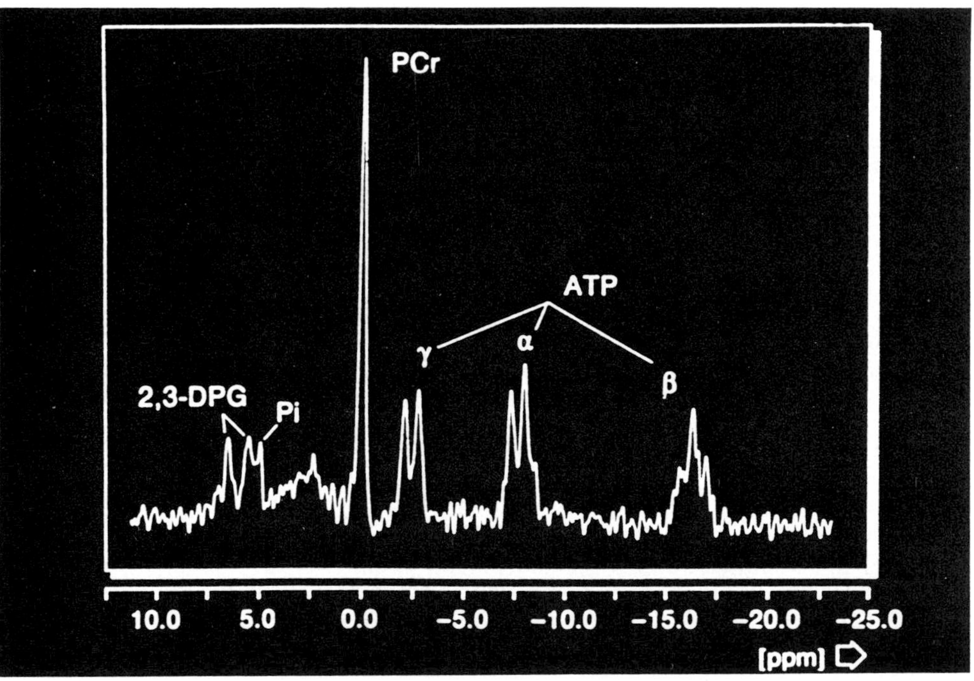

FIGURE 3. *A spectrum from the human heart obtained at 1.5 T using ISIS and proton decoupling. The spectrum shows the resonances of PCr, ATP, 2,3-diphosphoglycerate (2,3-DPG), as well as a small resonance from inorganic phosphate (P_i). Reprinted from Reference 14 with permission.*

the surface coil, using either two-dimensional ISIS or spiral pulses.[19] Using these latter techniques, contamination from nuclei outside the rectangular or round column is eliminated. Finally, spectral localization using phase-modulated rotating frame techniques allows visualization of a suite of spectra so that one can identify those spectra in which the PCr resonance is different from that of skeletal muscle.[20] However, since localization is defined by the B_1 field of the surface coil, there still exists lateral contamination from the curvilinear radiofrequency field of the coil.

A significant limitation to the accurate measurement of high-energy phosphates in the human heart has been the various sources of error involved in a human study. These sources include coil design and placement to minimize contribution from skeletal muscle; the localization technique used, with its resultant spatial selectivity; and the conditions of the experiment, such as the pulse width and the TR. Due to time considerations, all human cardiac studies have been performed under partially saturated conditions with TRs on the order of 1–2 seconds. Thus, investigators have used various methods in order to correct for these partial saturation effects. These methods include acquiring spectra from the entire sensitive volume of the coil under saturated and nonsaturated conditions,[21] a process that yields relatively similar T_1 for PCr and ATP, implying that correction factors are not necessary in human cardiac spectroscopy when calculating PCr/ATP. Similar findings were obtained by Neubauer et al.,[22] who calculated the T_1 of human cardiac PCr as 6.1 seconds, and ATP as 5.8 seconds, yielding a correction factor for PCr/ATP of 1.14 with a TR of 2 seconds. In contrast, van Dobbenburgh et al.[23] calculated the T_1 of PCr at 4.1 seconds and ATP at 2.7 seconds, yielding a saturation factor of 1.3 with a TR of 2.4 seconds. Thus, at this time, the precise values of human cardiac T_1 is not settled, but the prevailing weight of the data suggests that correction for partial saturation should be in the range of 1.1 to 1.3. Therefore, the most likely value for the actual ratio of PCr/ATP in the human heart is approximately 1.7.

Chemical Shift Imaging

Recently, CSI has emerged as the predominant localization technique because it allows acquisition of spectra from multiple locations and the generation of metabolic maps of organs, similar to the proton maps we read as images in magnetic resonance imaging (MRI). In this technique, varying magnetic field gradients are used to spatially encode the spectral information in one to three dimensions. Usually, two-dimensional images of the distribution of PCr or ATP, for example, are reconstructed from a number of slices through an organ, although the three-dimensional data set can theoretically be displayed in its entirety. Recent demonstration of the feasibility of three-dimensional metabolic imaging was achieved by Meyerhoff et al.[24] In this technique, a 14-cm surface coil was placed on the chest of a supine subject in a 2-T spectrometer. After proton imaging to define the location of the coil with respect to the heart, a three-dimensional data set was acquired using 10 phase encoding steps in each direction. Reconstruction of the images with interpolation of the 2-cm^3 voxels demonstrated the metabolite levels in the myocardium and the chest wall (Figure 4). Combined with software to provide simultaneous viewing of the proton images, phosphorus images in multiple planes, and spectra from any point, this technique is capable of providing spatial metabolic informa-

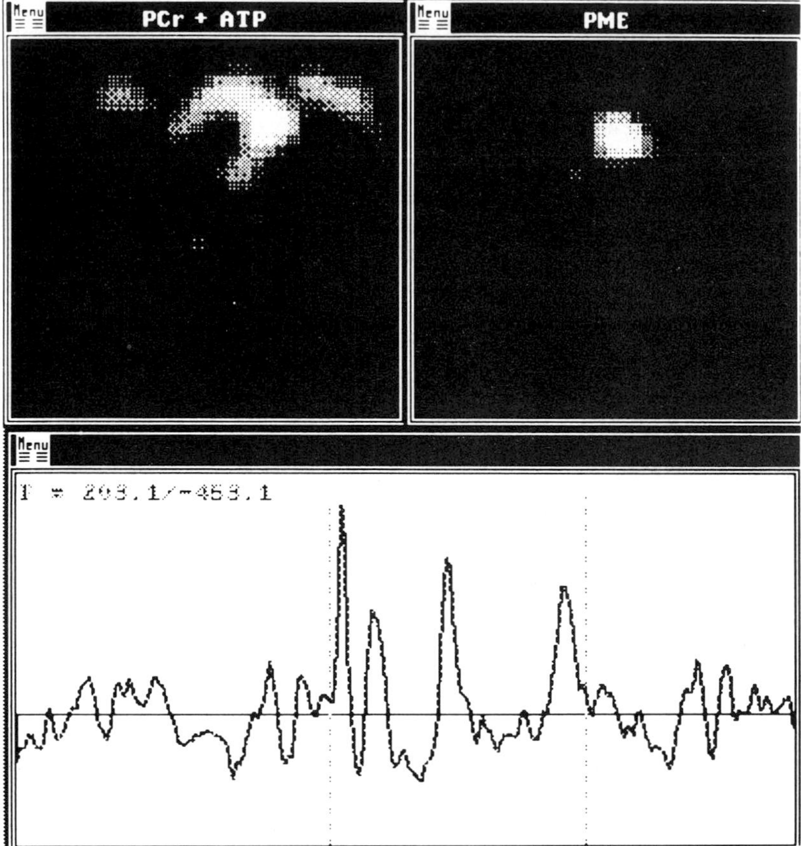

FIGURE 4. *Metabolite images of the human heart acquired with chemical shift imaging (CSI) at 2 T. CSI allows visualization of the spectrum from any selected voxel as well as the reconstruction of a metabolic image. The images have an in-plane resolution of approximately 2 cm² and demonstrate the relative concentrations of PCr and ATP (upper left) and 2,3-diphosphoglycerate in chamber blood (upper right). A spectrum from a selected myocardial voxel is shown at the bottom. Adapted from Reference 24 with permission.*

tion that is accessible as a visual image. Thus, spatial variations in metabolites can be more easily seen, and heterogeneity of tissues and localized abnormalities can be localized. In this manner, spectroscopy is moving more closely to conventional MRI. Despite these advances, the inherently poor sensitivity of the phosphorus nucleus limits the spatial resolution of this technique in reasonable imaging times.

Human Studies

Human studies of ischemic heart disease have addressed myocardial infarction and inducible myocardial ischemia. Studies of patients following myocardial infarction have demonstrated elevations of Pi and reductions of PCr, with some suggestion that subendocardial versus transmural abnormalities could be detected. Inducible ischemia has been studied using both isometric handgrip and dobutamine infusion. Weiss et al.[25] have demonstrated alterations in high-energy phosphates with handgrip exercise that raised rate pressure product approximately 15–20% (Figure 5). This study used one-dimensional CSI with a large transmit coil and a small receive coil. Patients were placed prone in a 1.5-T spectrometer and performed handgrip exercise after baseline spectroscopy. In those patients with severe proximal coronary artery disease, the ratio of PCr/ATP decreased from 1.45±0.31 at rest to 0.91±0.24 during exercise ($p<0.001$), and 2 minutes after exercise recovered to 1.27±0.38. Repeat testing of five patients who underwent revascularization demonstrated the resolution of the abnormal metabolic response to isometric handgrip. In addition to these studies of isometric hand exercise, the feasibility of performing aerobic leg exercise in a magnet has previously been demonstrated,[26] along with recent acquisition of spectra during exercise.[27]

In our laboratory, dobutamine has been used to elicit myocardial ischemia, with abnormalities in high-energy phosphates noted in a patient studied with one-

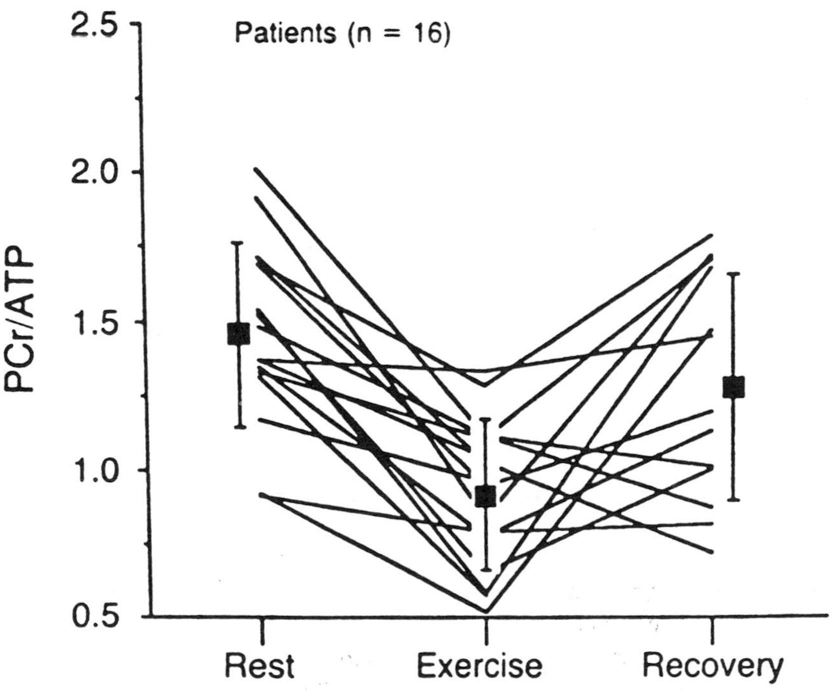

FIGURE 5. *The change in PCr/ATP in patients with severe coronary artery disease. Spectra were acquired at 1.5 T using one-dimensional chemical shift imaging. PCr/ATP fell significantly during isometric handgrip exercise and returned to control levels during recovery. The scatter in baseline levels of PCr/ATP is large, thus limiting the potential usefulness of resting measurements as a diagnostic tool. Reprinted from Reference 25 with permission.*

dimensional spectroscopic imaging. This patient, without a previous clinical myocardial infarction and with normal wall motion on angiography, had a totally occluded left anterior descending coronary artery with collateral filling of the artery from the right coronary. Spectroscopy was performed with the patient supine and continuous electrocardiographic, blood pressure, and visual monitoring. Following control hemodynamic and spectroscopic measurements, the patient was removed from the magnet isocenter while remaining in the same position on the spectrometer table. The dobutamine infusion was started at 2 μg/kg per minute and increased by 2 μg/kg per minute every 4 minutes, then titrated to a hemodynamic response and/or the development of chest pain and ECG changes. At the appropriate dose of dobutamine (16 μg/kg per minute in this instance), the patient was reinserted into the magnet and spectra were acquired in 7 minutes. The dobutamine infusion was then stopped and the patient was removed from the magnet. Analysis of the spectra demonstrated a marked reduction in PCr during the infusion of dobutamine, suggesting the regional myocardial blood flow in the anterior wall had fallen substantially below 50% of normal.

While no single technique is clearly superior in eliciting ischemic changes during spectroscopy, dobutamine infusion allows titration and maintenance of the stress for a sufficient period of time. It is also independent of patient motivation and strength, does not induce patient motion that can degrade the spectral signal, and can be rapidly stopped, with a half-life of only a few minutes. However, dobutamine can be arrhythmogenic and its effects persist longer than those induced by exercise alone. The importance of these combined studies is that MRS has been performed under a variety of stress conditions and has been able to detect stress-induced metabolic abnormalities in patients with coronary artery disease. In comparison with indirect measures of ischemia (such as perfusion abnormalities with radionuclide methods), MRS directly measures the metabolic consequences of ischemia. As noted earlier, MRS may be able to differentiate conditions in which perfusion is abnormal, yet there is no significant evidence of ischemia (such as in chronically ischemic ["hibernating"] myocardium). Although preliminary, these data suggest a role for MRS in the detection of myocardial ischemia. Further evolution of MRS localization techniques and stress methodologies will improve the efficacy of MRS in this setting.

Cardiac Transplantation

Although generally not due to epicardial coronary artery disease, rejection following transplantation has metabolic parallels to ischemic heart disease and is a promising area for the application of human MRS. Animal models of cardiac transplantation have demonstrated abnormalities of high-energy phosphates that paralleled the course of rejection.[28] An important question is whether, in humans, these changes can be detected and possibly provide earlier, or at least equivalent, information to endomyocardial biopsy. Herfkens et al.[29] showed that changes in high-energy phosphates paralleled, and in one instance preceded, histologic changes on biopsy. Recently, evidence from Evanochko et al.[30] supported these earlier findings, with moderately rejecting patients having a lower PCr/ATP ratio than nonrejecting or mildly rejecting patients. Furthermore, metabolic evidence of rejection was found in some patients with initially normal biopsies that subsequently became abnormal. In contrast, two studies examining the differences in PCr/ATP between groups with different degrees of rejection failed to distinguish between these groups, although the spectra were different from normal hearts (Figure 6).[31,32] Thus, there is a suggestion that noninvasive MRS may equal or supplant endomyocardial biopsy for the monitoring of transplant rejection, but only in instances in which patients can be serially studied over time.

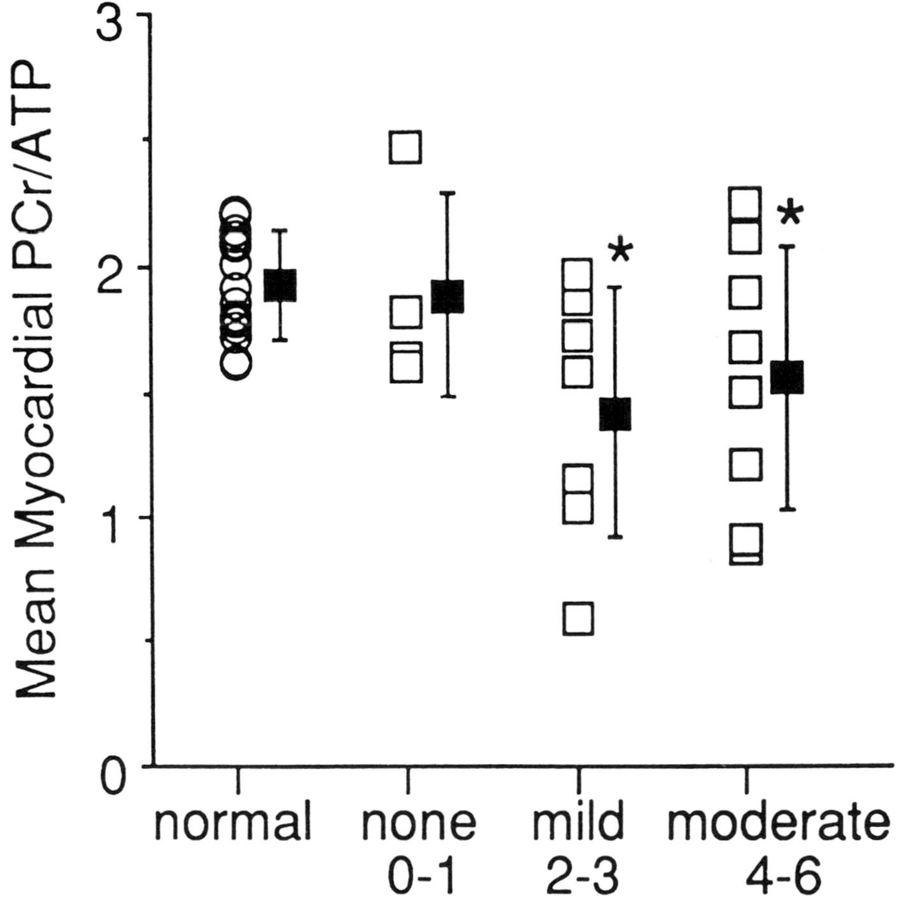

FIGURE 6. *The ratio of PCr/ATP in normal subjects and in patients after cardiac transplantation. While the ratio is significantly depressed in patients with either mild or moderate rejection, the overlap in the data make it difficult to separate these groups or to reliably differentiate individual abnormal measurements from the normal subjects. In contrast, studies serially following patients have suggested that MRS is sensitive to the degree of rejection. Reprinted from Reference 32 with permission.*

Summary

Magnetic resonance spectroscopy of the human heart is the only method that directly and noninvasively defines changes in myocardial high-energy phosphate metabolism. As noted above and by other authors, MRS has been successfully applied to investigate human ischemic heart disease, transplant rejection, and cardiomyopathies. Preliminary data indicate that metabolic abnormalities are a sensitive marker of regional ischemia and that reproducible data can be acquired from humans. Further investigations will define the role of MRS in the spectrum of diagnostic tests for cardiac disease in humans.

References

1. Schwartz GG, Schaefer S, Gober JG, et al: Myocardial high energy phosphate metabolism during brief coronary occlusion and reactive hyperemia in the pig. *Am J Physiol* 1990;259:H1190–H1196.
2. Neill WA, Ingwall JS: Stabilization of a derangement in adenosine triphosphate metabolism during sustained, partial ischemia in the dog heart. *J Am Coll Cardiol* 1986;8:894–900.
3. Camacho SA, Lanzer P, Toy BJ, et al: In vivo alterations of high energy phosphates and intracellular pH during reversible regional ischemia: a ^{31}P magnetic resonance spectroscopy study. *Am Heart J* 1988;116:701–708.
4. Schaefer S, Schwartz GG, Gober JR, et al: Relationship between myocardial metabolites and contractile abnormalities during graded regional ischemia: ^{31}P NMR studies of porcine myocardium in vivo. *J Clin Invest* 1990;85:706–713.
5. Path G, Robitaille PM, Merkle H, et al: Correlation between transmural high energy phosphate levels and myocardial blood flow in the presence of graded coronary stenosis. *Circ Res* 1990;67:660–673.
6. Ross J Jr: Myocardial perfusion-contraction matching: implications for coronary heart disease and hibernation. *Circulation* 1991;83:1076–1083.
7. Rahimtoola SH: The hibernating myocardium. *Am Heart J* 1989;117:211–221.
8. Kloner RA, DeBoer LWV, Darsee JR, et al: Recovery from prolonged abnormalities of canine myocardium salvaged from ischemic necrosis by coronary reperfusion. *Proc Natl Acad Sci U S A* 1981;78:7152–7156.
9. Sako EY, Kingsley-Hickman PB, From HL, et al: ATP synthesis kinetics and mitochondrial function in the postischemic myocardium as studied by ^{31}P NMR. *J Biol Chem* 1988;263:10600–10607.
10. Pantely GA, Malone SA, Rhen WS, et al: Regeneration of myocardial phosphocreatine in pigs despite continued moderate ischemia. *Circ Res* 1990;67:1481–1493.
11. Schaefer S, Schwartz GG, Wisneski JA, et al: Response of high-energy phosphates and lactate release during prolonged regional ischemia in vivo. *Circulation* 1992;85:342–349.
12. Zhang J, Yoshiyama M, Garwood M, et al: Transmural high energy phosphate distribution and response to coronary hyperperfusion (abstract). In: Proceedings of the Society of Magnetic Resonance in Medicine Ninth Annual Meeting. 1990:862.
13. Bottomley PA, Foster TH, Darrow RD: Depth resolved surface coil spectroscopy (DRESS) for in vivo ^{1}H, ^{31}P, and ^{13}C NMR. *J Magn Reson* 1984;59:338–342.
14. Luyten PR, Bruntink G, Sloff FM, et al: Broadband proton decoupling in human ^{31}P NMR spectroscopy. *NMR Biomed* 1989;1:177–183.
15. Matson GB, Twieg DB, Karczmar GS, et al: Image-guided surface coil ^{31}P MRS of human liver, heart, and kidney. *Radiology* 1988;169:541–547.
16. Blackledge MJ, Rajagopalan B, Oberhaensli RD, et al: Quantitative studies of human cardiac metabolism by ^{31}P rotating-frame NMR. *Proc Natl Acad Sci U S A* 1987;84:4283–4287.

17. Twieg DB, Meyerhoff DJ, Hubesch B, et al: Localized phosphorus-31 magnetic resonance spectroscopy in humans by spectroscopic imaging: localized spectroscopy and metabolic imaging. *Magn Reson Med* 1989;12:291–305.
18. Luyten PR, den Hollander JA, Marien AJH, et al: H 1 decoupled P 31 MR spectroscopy of the human heart: acquisition and quantification in controls and patients (abstract). *Magn Reson Imaging* 1991;1:167.
19. Hardy CJ, Bottomley PA: ^{31}P spectroscopic localization using pinwheel NMR excitation pulses. *Magn Reson Med* 1991;17:315–327.
20. Conway MA, Allis J, Ouwerkerk R, et al: Detection of low phosphocreatine to ATP ratio in failing hypertrophied human myocardium by ^{31}P magnetic resonance spectroscopy. *Lancet* 1991;338:973–976.
21. Bottomley PA, Hardy CJ, Weiss RG: Saturation factors for high energy phosphate ratios in human heart are homogeneous in normal and disease states. A practical solution for correcting partial saturation (abstract). In: Proceedings of the Society of Magnetic Resonance in Medicine Tenth Annual Meeting. 1991:578.
22. Neubauer S, Krahe T, Schindler R, et al: Direct measurement of spin-lattice relaxation times of phosphorus metabolites in human myocardium. *Magn Res Med* 1992;26:300–307.
23. van Dobbenburgh JO, Lekkerkerk C, van Echteld CJA: Saturation effects in human heart and chest wall muscle measured by ^{31}P 1-D spectroscopic imaging (abstract). In: Proceedings of the Society of Magnetic Resonance in Medicine Tenth Annual Meeting. 1991:988.
24. Meyerhoff DJ, Maudsley A, Schaefer S, Weiner MW: Phosphorus-31 magnetic resonance metabolite imaging in the human body. *Magn Reson Imaging* 1992;10:245–256.
25. Weiss RG, Bottomley PA, Hardy CJ, Gerstenblith G: Regional myocardial metabolism of high-energy phosphates during isometric exercise in patients with coronary artery disease. *N Engl J Med* 1990;323:1593–1600.
26. Schaefer S, Peshock RM, Parkey RW, Willerson JT: A new device for exercise magnetic resonance imaging. *AJR* 1986;147:1289–1290.
27. von Smekal A, Weiner MW: ^{31}P spectroscopic imaging of the human heart during isotonic leg exercise (abstract). In: Proceedings of the Society of Magnetic Resonance in Medicine Ninth Annual Meeting. 1990:930.
28. Canby RC, Evanochko WT, Barrett LV, et al: Monitoring the bioenergetics of cardiac allograft rejection using in vivo P-31 nuclear magnetic resonance spectroscopy. *J Am Coll Cardiol* 1987;9:1067–1074.
29. Herfkens RJ, Charles HC, Negro-Vilar R, Van Trigt P: In vivo P-31 NMR spectroscopy of human heart transplants. (abstract) *Radiology* 1988;169:179.
30. Evanochko WT, Bouchard A, Kirklin JK, et al: Detection of cardiac transplant rejection in patients by ^{31}P NMR spectroscopy (abstract). In: Proceedings of the Society of Magnetic Resonance in Medicine Ninth Annual Meeting. 1990:246.
31. Wolfe CL, Caputo G, Chew W, et al: Detection of cardiac transplant rejection by magnetic resonance imaging and spectroscopy (abstract). In: Proceedings of the Society of Magnetic Resonance in Medicine Tenth Annual Meeting 1991; 574.
32. Bottomley PA, Weiss RG, Hardy CJ, Baumgartner WA: Myocardial high energy phosphate metabolism and allograft rejection in patients with heart transplants. *Radiology* 1991;181:67-75.

Chapter 27

^{31}P Magnetic Resonance Spectroscopy in Hypertrophy and Heart Failure

Michael A. Conway, MB, MSc,
Ronald Ouwerkerk, PhD,
and George K. Radda, DPhil

The development of chronic congestive cardiac failure in patients with valvular heart disease is avoidable if surgery is performed at the correct time. Currently available techniques for determining the optimal timing of aortic and mitral valve replacement are inadequate. ^{31}P magnetic resonance spectroscopy (MRS) is a technique for measuring high-energy phosphate concentrations in heart muscle and, being noninvasive, is potentially a valuable clinical investigation for the serial monitoring of cardiac metabolism. The deterioration in cardiac function with myocardial hypertrophy in aortic stenosis is thought to involve alterations in phosphorus energetics.[1] Abnormalities in metabolism have been demonstrated from biopsy studies of the hypertrophied heart of both humans and animals[2,3] and some patients with myocardial hypertrophy have low creatine kinase activity on cardiac biopsy.[4] In order to determine whether ^{31}P MRS has a role in the evaluation of valvular heart disease we used the technique in patients with aortic stenosis and aortic incompetence to characterize metabolism in those with and without symptoms.

Patients and Methods

We studied 14 patients (age: 51 ± 20 years; mean $\pm$ SD) with free wall left ventricular hypertrophy due to aortic stenosis (six patients) or aortic incompetence (eight patients). The mean aortic valve area on Doppler or Gorlin formula in aortic

---

Supported by the British Heart Foundation, Medical Research Council, and the National Institutes of Health.
From Pohost GM (ed.), *Cardiovascular Applications of Magnetic Resonance.* Mount Kisco, NY, Futura Publishing Co., Inc., © 1993.

stenosis was 0.6 ± 0.3 cm^2 and the mean gradient across the aortic valve was 59 ± 34 mm Hg. The severity of aortic incompetence was grade 3–4 and the end-diastolic dimension in those with aortic stenosis (4.6 ± 0.8 cm) was significantly different from that in the patients with aortic incompetence (6.2 ± 0.8 cm; $p<0.005$). All patients were clinically assessed by electrocardiography, Doppler, and cross-sectional echocardiography and 10 underwent cardiac catheterization. One patient with aortic incompetence and four patients with aortic stenosis had coronary artery disease that was mild in all except one patient with aortic stenosis who had significant stenoses of the left anterior descending and diagonal coronary arteries. Myocardial hypertrophy was diagnosed on the electrocardiograph from Lepeschkin voltage criteria[5] and the Sokolow index.[6] The range of the electrocardiographic and echocardiographic values for hypertrophy were similar to those reported elsewhere[7]; $V_1S + V_5/6R$: 44 ± 9 mm (aortic stenosis) and 50 ± 13 mm (aortic incompetence) (NS) and posterior wall thickness: 1.4 ± 0.5 cm (aortic stenosis) and 1.2 ± 0.2 cm (aortic incompetence) (NS). The patients were compared with a group of 13 age-matched clinically normal controls.

Magnetic resonance spectroscopy was performed using a 1.9-T, 60-cm bore whole-body magnet and the phase-modulated rotating frame imaging technique.[8] Recordings were made from the apical region and left ventricular free wall of the heart with the subject lying prone over a double concentric surface coil (transmitter diameter 15 cm, receiver diameter 6.5 cm). The depth of the data to approximately 6.5 cm was calibrated from experiments on multicompartment samples.[9] Spectra were analyzed by triangulation of the peaks of phosphocreatine (PCr) and γ adenosine triphosphate (ATP). (The γATP peak was used because of off-resonance effects in the region of the βATP resonance). The size of the γATP peak in the nonhypertrophied heart is enlarged due to contamination with ATP from blood. An adjustment for this was made by subtracting an area from the ATP peak that was proportional to the area of the 2,3-diphosphoglycerate peak that is only present in blood (ratio = 5:1; from 19 ex vivo human blood samples). Individual cardiac spectra were identified using stacked plots (Figure 1). The depth in centimeters of each spectral row in the stacked plot was known from studies on the multicompartment samples and this was related to the depth in centimeters of the cardiac structures measured from the echocardiograms. All subjects gave informed consent for the study that was approved by the local ethics committee. All data are expressed as mean $\pm$ SD and statistical analysis was performed using unpaired Student's *t* test.

Results

Magnetic Resonance Spectroscopy in Left Ventricular Hypertrophy

A stacked plot from a patient with myocardial hypertrophy due to aortic stenosis is shown in Figure 1 in which the signals from the chest wall muscle, blood, and cardiac muscle can be identified. The signal from PCr in the heart is seen as the deeper PCr. The individual spectra from the middle of the rows of heart signal in a control and two patients are displayed in Figure 2.

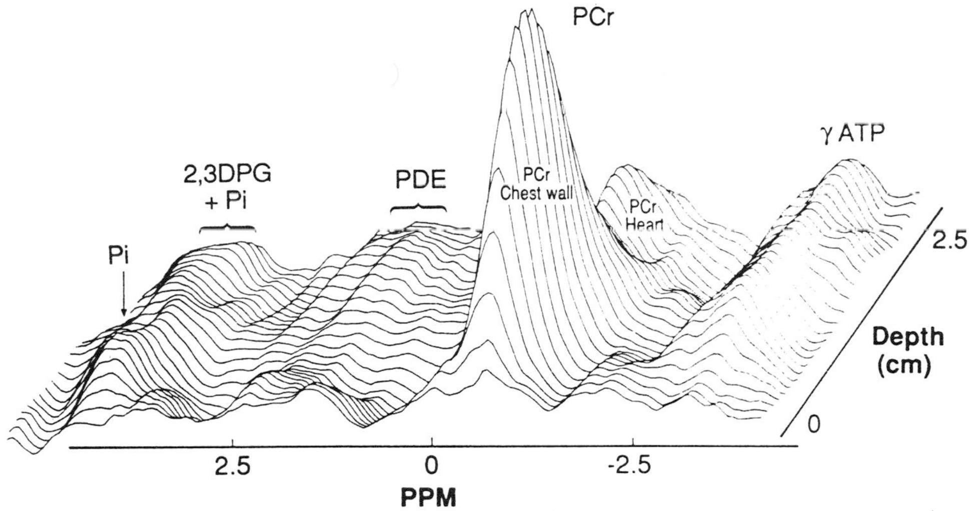

FIGURE 1. *Stacked plot of data sampled using a 6.5-cm surface coil. The stacked plot is constructed of 28 adjacent individual spectra with the spectra from the surface at the front. The portion of the data set with the peaks from α and β adenosine triphosphate (ATP) is left out for clarity. The prominent peak is phosphocreatine (PCr), which is largest in chest wall muscle and steps down to a plateau in the region of the heart. The inorganic phosphate (Pi) peak in skeletal muscle is clear.*

Nine patients had normal PCr:ATP ratios (1.58 ± 0.15 versus 1.5 ± 0.2 in controls; NS) and in five patients the PCr:ATP was 1.0 ± 0.15 ($p<0.001$).

Six of the patients (aortic stenosis, three; aortic incompetence, three) had been started on treatment for heart failure and were classified as NYHA Class II–III on the basis of the severity of dyspnea. All were on diuretics except for one patient who was on frequent dialysis and nitrates. The left ventricular end-diastolic pressure in four of these patients was 24 ± 10 mm Hg compared with 11 ± 7 mm Hg in five of the asymptomatic group. The fractional shortening was not significantly lower in the symptomatic patients ($33\% \pm 6\%$ versus $39\% \pm 12\%$ in the asymptomatic group), but the PCr:ATP ratio (1.1 ± 0.32) was significantly lower compared with the ratio in the group without dyspnea (1.56 ± 0.15; $p<0.004$). The latter ratio was not significantly different from control.

Discussion

In this study, the phase-modulated rotating frame imaging technique was used to measure the myocardial PCr:ATP ratio in a group of patients with hypertrophy of the free wall and apex of the left ventricle. The PCr:ATP was lower in the patients who were on diuretics and other therapies for symptoms of heart failure. Patients in this group also tended to have higher left ventricular end-diastolic pressures. These findings are consistent with previous reports of low PCr and decreased creatine kinase activity in hypertrophied muscle.[1,4,10]

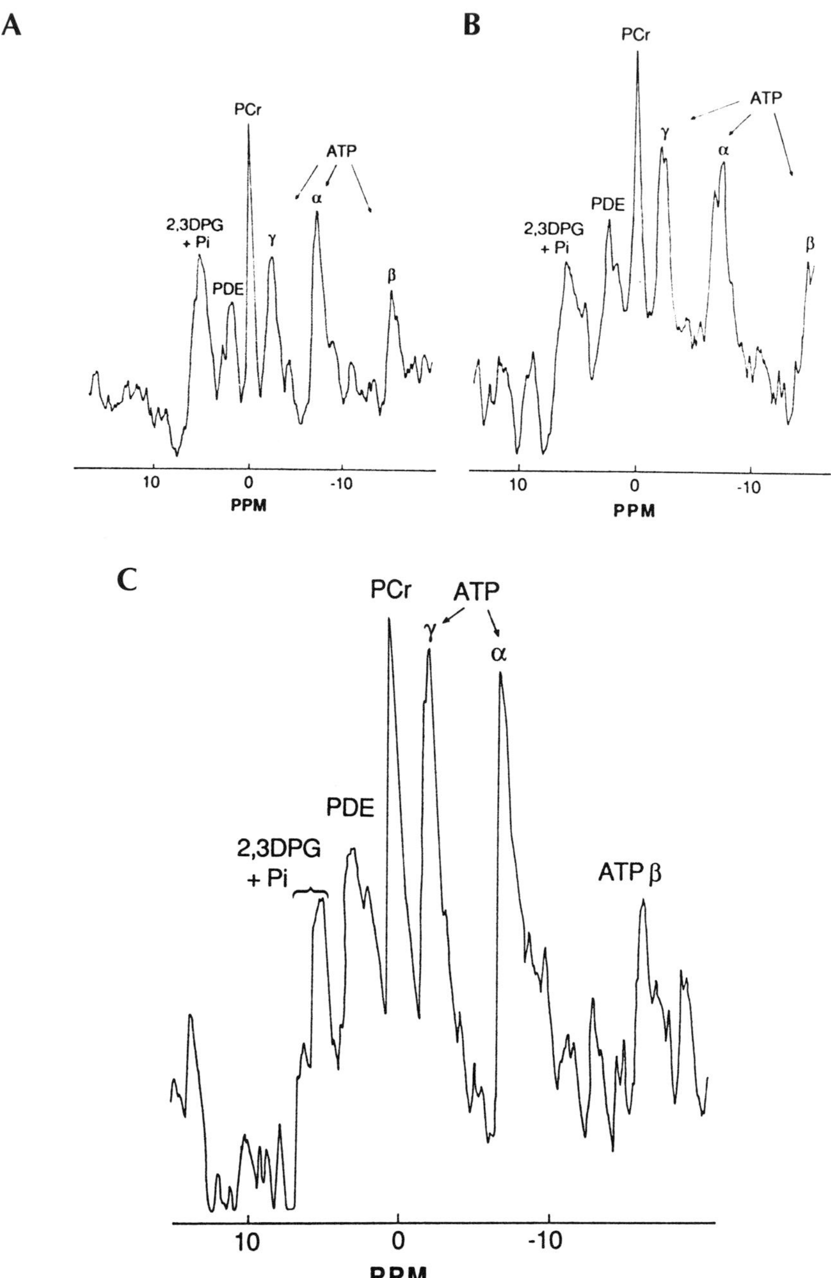

FIGURE 2. *Individual spectra from a control* **(A)** *and two patients with myocardial hypertrophy* **(B and C)**.

Some of the patients in the study had high PCr:ATP ratios despite an increase in muscle mass due to aortic stenosis or aortic incompetence. Normal high-energy phosphorus metabolism in hypertrophied hearts has been observed in animal models.[11–13] Others have reported normal metabolites in the subepicardium of the canine model of aortic stenosis and low PCr and ATP in the endocardium.[2] Similar endocardial and subepicardial changes in biopsy specimens have been observed in humans.[3] The possibility that there is a lower ratio in the endocardial layers in the patients in the current study cannot be ruled out because the PCr is the mean of the signal from all layers of the ventricular wall.

Few studies have been performed to characterize high-energy phosphorus metabolism in the failing human myocardium but recently, Ingwall et al.[14] suggested that there is evidence of impaired high-energy phosphorus metabolism in patients with heart failure due to severe dilated cardiomyopathy. Studies by this group in the spontaneously hypertensive rat in transition to heart failure were consistent with the low PCr detected in the failing hypertrophied heart in previously reported animal studies.[1,10,15]

The mechanism of the changes in the PCr:ATP ratio may relate to alterations in creatine kinase or a decrease in the total creatine content of the muscle.[4] The latter investigators suggested that the changes in myocardial hypertrophy are an adaptive response. The findings in the current group of patients suggest that the changes in PCr:ATP in myocardial hypertrophy due to aortic valve disease reflect the decompensating state rather than the adaptive phase of the disorder.

It is unlikely that the changes in the symptomatic patients are due to the effects of therapy and indeed the changes in the PCr:ATP might be more extreme in the absence of diuretics and vasodilators. Furthermore, in studies of high-energy phosphorus metabolism of resting skeletal muscle no abnormalities were found in those on diuretics for moderate heart failure.[16]

The results of the current study may be relevant to a frequently encountered clinical decision. This is the question of the optimal timing for surgery, particularly in patients with aortic valve disease. The ability to detect impairment noninvasively of myocardial metabolism would be a valuable asset in the management of patients with surgically treatable myocardial hypertrophy. The avoidance of "overt congestive heart failure"[17] by sensitive detection of impending metabolic failure is the goal of many of the previously reported studies in this area. Measurement of in vivo cardiac biochemistry would help separate those with cardiac exertional dyspnea from those with symptoms due to age and physical capacity. This would add to the clinical judgment based on risk factors[18] and echocardiographic measurements[19] and lead to more accurate identification of the at-risk group. Such noninvasive measurements are likely to be more useful than morphometric measurements on preoperative biopsies.[20]

Further examination of the relationship between indexes such as the ejection fraction at rest and during exercise, the end-systolic and end-diastolic dimensions, the phase analysis of wall motion[21] and the MRS findings both at rest and during exercise[22] is required, particularly in patients with aortic incompetence. The use of the technique in conjunction with such indexes would allow more accurate timing of surgery and in patients who are only minimally symptomatic the finding of low PCr:ATP ratios might be an indication not to procrastinate.

Acknowledgments

The authors would like to thank Dr. Bheesha Rajagopalan, Dr. Jonathan Allis, Dr. Tadashi Niioka, Prof. Peter Sleight, Dr. Colin Forfar, Mr. Anthony Prothero, and Dr. Peter Styles.

References

1. Furchgott RF, Lees KS: High energy phosphates and the force of contraction of cardiac muscle. *Circulation* 1961;24:416–432.
2. Attarian DE, Jones RN, Currie WD, et al: Characteristics of chronic left ventricular hypertrophy induced by subcoronary valvular aortic stenosis. *J Thorac Cardiovasc Surg* 1981;81:382–388.
3. Swain JL, Sabina RL, Peyton RB, et al: Derangements in myocardial purine and pyramidine nucleotide metabolism in patients with coronary artery disease and left ventricular hypertrophy. *Proc Natl Acad Sci U S A* 1982;79:655–659.
4. Ingwall JS, Kramer MF, Fifer MA, et al: The creatine kinase system in normal and diseased human myocardium. *N Engl J Med* 1985;313:1050–1054.
5. Clementy J, Bergere P, Bricaud H: Electrocardiography and vectorcardiography in the evaluation of left ventricular hypertrophy due to pressure overload. *Eur Heart J* 1982;3(suppl A):37–47.
6. Sokolow M, Lyon TP: The ventricular complex in left ventricular hypertrophy as obtained by unipolar precordial and limb leads. *Am Heart J* 1949;37:161–186.
7. Carroll JD, Gaasch WH, Naimi S, et al: Regression of myocardial hypertrophy: electrocardiographic-echocardiographic correlations after aortic valve replacement in patients with chronic aortic regurgitation. *Circulation* 1982;65:980–987.
8. Blacklege MJ, Rajagopalan B, Oberhaensli R, et al: Quantitative studies of human cardiac metabolism by ^{31}P rotating frame NMR. *Proc Natl Acad Sci U S A* 1987;84:4283–4287.
9. Cadoux-Hudson TAD, Wade D, Taylor DJ, et al: Persistent metabolic sequelae of severe head injury in humans in vivo. *Acta Neurochir* 1990;104:1–7.
10. Pool PE, Spann JF, Sonneblick EH, Braunwald E: Myocardial high energy phosphate stores in cardiac hypertrophy and heart failure. *Circ Res* 1967;21:365–373.
11. Aufferman W, Wu ST, Derugin N, et al: ^{31}P magnetic resonance spectroscopy of pressure overload hypertrophy in rats: effect of reduced perfusion pressure. *Cardiovasc Res* 1990;24:57–64.
12. Buser PT, Wagner S, Shao T, et al: Verapamil preserves myocardial performance and energy metabolism in left ventricular hypertrophy following ischemia and reperfusion. *Circulation* 1989;80:1837–1845.
13. Tubau JF, Wikman-Coffelt J, Massie BM, et al: Improved myocardial efficiency in the working perfused heart of the SHR. *Hypertension* 1987;10:396–403.
14. Ingwall JS, Atkinson DE, Clarke K, et al: Energetic correlates of cardiac failure: changes in the creatine kinase system in the failing myocardium. *Eur Heart J* 1990;11(suppl B):108–115.
15. Coleman HN, Taylor RR, Pool PE, et al: Congestive heart failure following tachycardia. *Am Heart J* 1971;81:790–798.
16. Massie B, Conway M, Yonge R, et al: Skeletal muscle metabolism in patients with congestive heart failure: relation to clinical severity and blood flow. *Circulation* 1987;76:1009–1019.
17. Hancock EW: Timing of valve replacement for aortic stenosis. *Circulation* 1990;82:310–312.
18. Lund O: Preoperative risk evaluation and stratification of long-term survival after valve replacement for aortic stenosis. *Circulation* 1990;82:124–139.
19. Henry WL, Bonow RO, Borer JS, et al: Observations on the optimum time for operative

intervention for aortic regurgitation. I. Evaluation of the results of aortic valve replacement in symptomatic patients. *Circulation* 1980;61:471–483.

20. Krayenbuehl HP, Hess OM, Monrad ES, et al: Left ventricular myocardial structure in aortic valve disease before, intermediate, and late after aortic valve replacement. *Circulation* 1989;79:744–755.
21. Ormerod OJM, Barber RW, Stone DL, et al: Radionuclide evaluation of aortic regurgitation: assessment of ventricular function by Fourier phase analysis. *Eur Heart J* 1987;8:702–709.
22. Conway MA, Bristow JD, Blackledge MJ, et al: Cardiac metabolism during exercise in normal volunteers measured by ^{31}P magnetic resonance spectroscopy. *Br Heart J* 1991;65:25–30.

Chapter 28

Quantitative Phosphorus Nuclear Magnetic Resonance Spectroscopy of the Human Heart

Paul A. Bottomley, PhD,
Christopher J. Hardy, PhD,
and Robert G. Weiss, MD

The body has been said to produce approximately 35 kg of adenosine triphosphate (ATP) per day. If this amount of ATP were present at any given time, there would be no sensitivity problem for human phosphorus (^{31}P) nuclear magnetic resonance (NMR) spectroscopy studies! The detection of high-energy phosphates at millimole per kilogram levels in tissue at any given time with ^{31}P NMR spectroscopy represents a severe challenge to the sensitivity of the technique, requiring compromises that typically affect spatial resolution and reliability.

The reliable and reproducible measurement of myocardial high-energy phosphate metabolism among normal and patient populations demands robust clinical protocols. There are four key requirements: 1) accurate identification of the myocardial anatomy; 2) accurate localization and prescription of the localized volumes examined by spectroscopy relative to the anatomy; 3) the achievement of useful signal-to-noise ratios within tolerable time limits; and 4) the establishment of protocols for reproducible adjustment of NMR acquisition parameters and methods for correcting for experimentally induced spectral distortions. The incorporation of new technologies in clinical examinations makes sense only if the technologies offer significant improvements in one or more of these or if they provide access to new moieties of physiologic or medical interest.

Some approaches to spatial localization and protocols for correcting spectral distortions that have been found useful are discussed here as well as clinical results and a review of progress in applying new technologies to human ^{31}P cardiac spectroscopy.

From Pohost GM (ed.), *Cardiovascular Applications of Magnetic Resonance.* Mount Kisco, NY, Futura Publishing Co., Inc., © 1993.

Spatial Localization

Spectra can be spatially localized to a single volume or voxel at a time, or alternatively can be spatially encoded and acquired from multiple voxels simultaneously. For studies of transient ischemia or focal abnormalities that are not readily distinguishable by anatomical imaging modalities or for dynamic studies, multiple voxel techniques are essential. For example, in stress testing for regional ischemia, when the precise location of the ischemic region is unknown a priori,[1] incorrect placement of a voxel localized with a single voxel technique will result in missed opportunities for detecting abnormal metabolism. Therefore, we now use multiple voxel techniques for all of our patient studies.

One of three multiple voxel techniques that have been successfully implemented is selected according to the particular requirements and limitations posed by the clinical investigation being undertaken. Nuclear magnetic resonance pulse and magnetic field gradient sequences corresponding to the three methods are depicted in Figure 1. The simplest uses a one-dimensional phase encoding gradient applied along the cylindrical axis of a flat circular ^{31}P NMR surface coil positioned on the chest

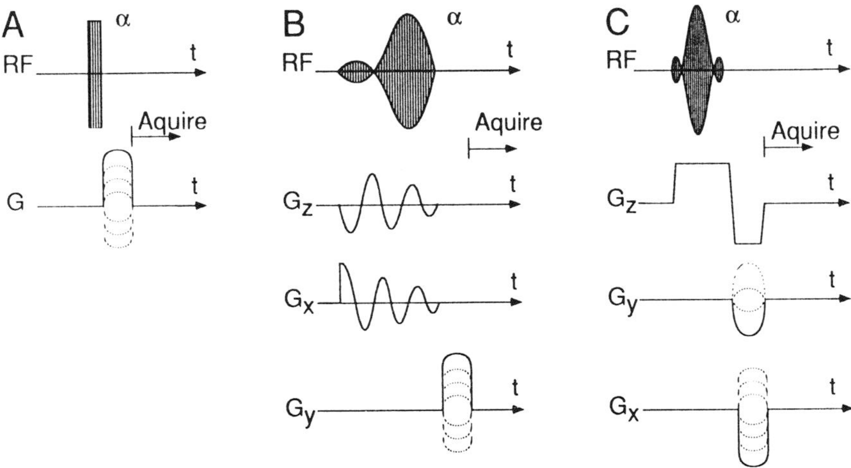

FIGURE 1. A: *NMR and magnetic field gradient pulse sequence for performing one-dimensional phase encoded spectroscopy. A hard α° (≤90°) NMR pulse excites the sample, and the NMR signal is spatially encoded by a magnetic field gradient pulse (G), whose amplitude is incremented in subsequent applications of the sequence. The direction of the gradient field is usually normal to the plane of the surface detection coil.* **B:** *Localized spectroscopy sequence incorporating "pinwheel" two-dimensional selective excitation.*[2] *This sequence provides full three-dimensional control of the size of localized voxels by replacing the hard α° pulse by a two-dimensional pinwheel pulse that selects a cylinder, which is subsequently encoded in the third dimension as in (A).* **C:** *Three-dimensional slice-selective spectroscopy imaging sequence with gradient encoding in the two dimensions of the slice selected by applying a gradient G_2 during the NMR pulse.*[5]

anterior to the heart. A series of spectra from slices parallel to the coil as a function of depth through the chest and heart is generated. Spatial localization of signals in the other two dimensions within the planes is afforded crudely by the inhomogeneous sensitivity profile of the surface coil. Advantages of this technique are that it is fast because it has the least number of spatial encoding steps, and it delivers the maximum signal-to-noise ratio of the three methods because of the extended voxel volume parallel to the coil. This renders it most suitable for cardiac stress testing.[1] A disadvantage is the requirement that the coil be carefully positioned relative to the heart and chest in order to substantially eliminate possible chest muscle contamination from the intersection of encoded planes with the chest.

A typical data set of ^{31}P spectra through the chest and heart and a conventional surface coil proton (^{1}H) NMR anatomical image obtained with this technique are shown in Figure 2. Because the principles of image localization for ^{1}H NMR imaging and spectroscopy are the same, there is a direct correspondence between the image and spectra. The ratio of phosphocreatine (PCr) to ATP decreases from approximately 5:1 in chest muscle to approximately 2:1 in myocardium and is consistent with animal studies.

The second localization method uses a two-dimensional spatially selective NMR pulse to restrict and control the spatial sensitivity in the two dimensions parallel to the surface coil by selectively exciting a cylinder coaxial with the surface coil's axis.[2] These pulses use a modulated radiofrequency excitation pulse that is applied in the

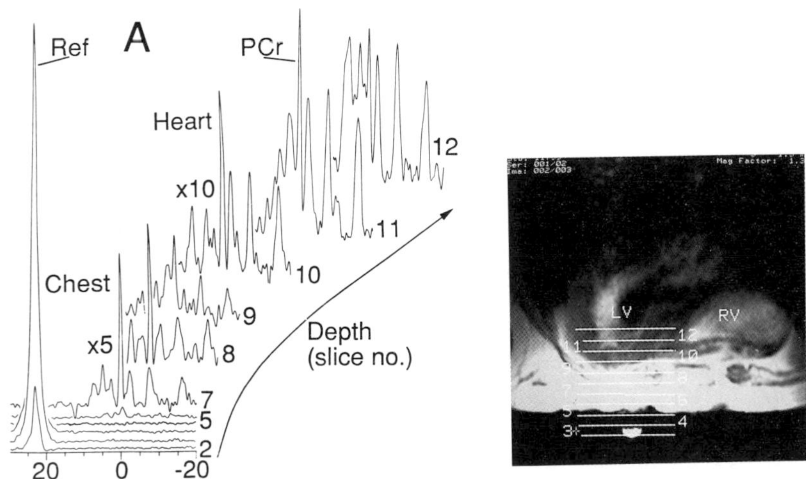

FIGURE 2. A: *A typical set of cardiac gated (TR=0.80 seconds) ^{31}P spectra acquired with a one-dimensional phase encoding gradient localization sequence in 12 minutes through the chest and heart of a female patient with anterior coronary artery disease.[7] Spectra derived from 6-mm thick coronal sections (spectra 10, 11, and 12) were derived from the anterior myocardium. The reference peak* **(Ref)** *is from a vial of phosphonitrilic chloride trimer embedded in the ^{31}P surface coil.* **B:** *Annotated ^{1}H NMR image acquired from the same subject showing the location of the spectra in (A). The image was obtained with a coaxial ^{1}H surface coil without disturbing the patient. The bright spot in slice 3 is the reference vial.*

presence of a magnetic field gradient that is reoriented through the two dimensions.[3] Because two-dimensional spatially selective pulses have an inherently smaller excitation bandwidth than one-dimensional selective pulses for a given gradient strength and slew rate, the pulse is broken into eight shorter components. In each of these eight components, the gradient traverses different arms of a "pinwheel" trajectory. The pulses are applied in eight consecutive applications of the sequence to ensure complete excitation of the ^{31}P spectral bandwidth.[2] The signals from each excitation are added to provide full localization in the two dimensions. The depth dimension is encoded with a one-dimensional phase encoding gradient as above, slicing the cylinder into disks.

The gradient and radiofrequency pulse waveforms for one arm of a two-dimensional pinwheel pulse are depicted in Figures 3A and 3B. The combination of both gradients results in a spiral trajectory for each arm of the pinwheel, as is evident in images acquired at different stages of the sequence cycle (Figure 3C). Figure 4A shows a ^{31}P data set from the chest and heart of a normal volunteer produced by this technique.[2] The advantages of this method are that it provides full three-dimensional localization, it is relatively insensitive to radiofrequency field inhomogeneity, it can be used with small pulse flip angles or at the Ernst angle to minimize saturation effects, and is about half as sensitive to motion artifact compared with techniques that use subtraction of large signals acquired with selective inversion followed by non-selective excitation to restrict sensitivity in the two dimensions parallel to the surface coil.[4]

The third technique uses phase encoding gradients in two dimensions and one-dimensional selective excitation in the third dimension.[5] The sequence is shown

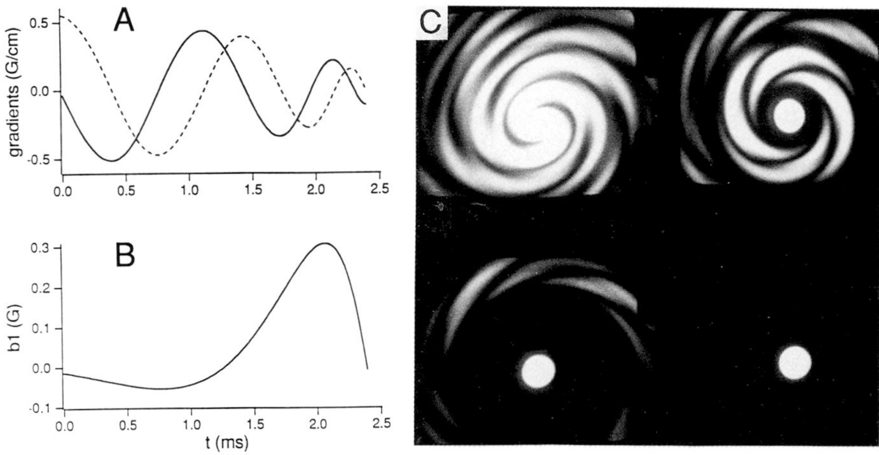

FIGURE 3. *The gradient* **(A)** *and radiofrequency pulse modulation* **(B)** *waveforms for a two-dimensional pinwheel pulse.[2] For subsequent applications of the pulse, the gradient waveforms are mixed with different phase angles. The combination of both gradients results in a gradient with a spiral trajectory, as is evident in ^{1}H NMR images produced from a uniform sample of water and reconstructed after 1, 2, 4, and all 8 arms of an 8-arm sequence cycle* **(C)**.

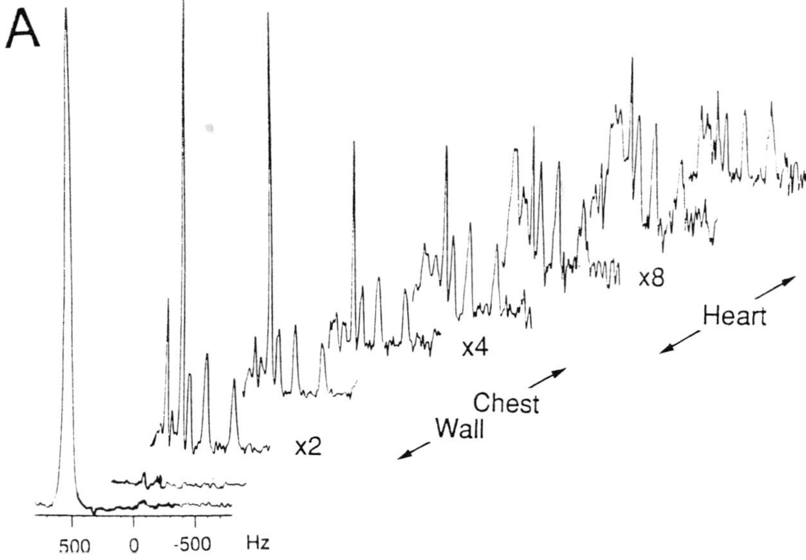

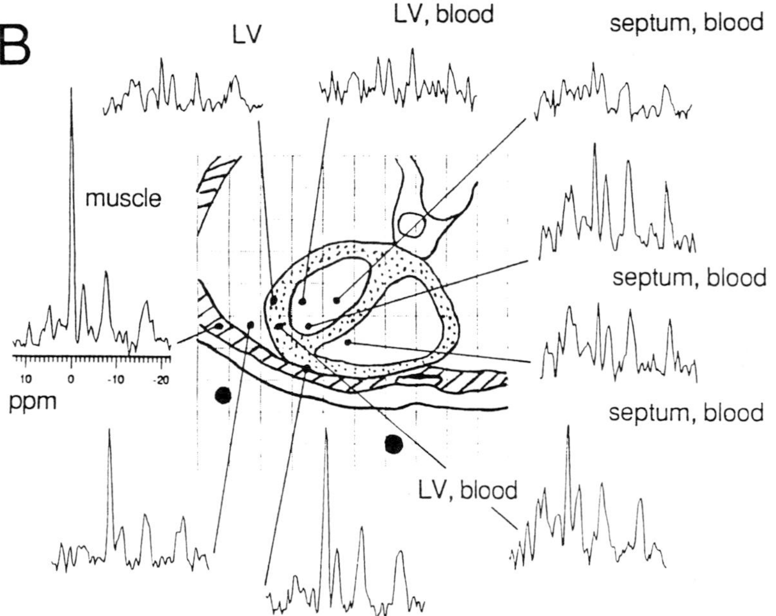

FIGURE 4. A: *Cardiac-gated (TR = 0.7 seconds) ^{31}P data set from the chest and heart of a normal volunteer produced with the pinwheel localization sequence technique in 12 minutes.*[2] *Each spectrum derives from a 1-cm thick disk, 10 cm in diameter.* B: *Cardiac-gated ^{31}P spectra from the chest and heart of a normal volunteer produced with the spatial localization sequence depicted in Figure 1C. Voxels are 2 × 2 cm² in a 4-cm thick axial plane, acquired with a phased array surface coil set in about 15 minutes in a 1.5-T imaging/spectroscopy system.*[6] *A sketch of the heart derived from the corresponding ^{1}H NMR image indicates relative locations of the spectroscopy voxels.*

in Figure 1C, and an example with 2×2 cm^2 voxels is shown in Figure 4B.[6] The advantages are the full three-dimensional spatial resolution and insensitivity to patient positioning, which is achieved without sacrificing signal-to-noise ratio per unit volume. The main disadvantages are that the adjustment of scan time is limited by the need to acquire at least one complete set of phase encoded data, the number of phase encoding steps required now being quite large, and that the technique will typically generate much superfluous and some data with automated spectral processing.

Robust Protocols and Spectral Distortion

The values of PCr/ATP measured by ^{31}P NMR in the human heart are invariably distorted to some extent by instrumental artifacts or by compromises inherent in the acquisition protocol. These distortions, when not properly accounted for, frustrate inter- and intralaboratory comparisons of results, with deleterious effects on the apparent reproducibility of clinical findings from different sites. Four common sources of distortion of the PCr/ATP ratio are: 1) partial saturation resulting from the use of NMR pulse sequence repetition periods, TR, that are less than or comparable to the spin lattice-relaxation times (T_1) of PCr or ATP because $T_1(PCr) > T_1(ATP)$[7]; 2) the presence of or variations in the acquisition delay between excitation and detection; eg, depending on the particular localization sequence used[5]; 3) contamination of myocardial metabolite signals with ATP signal from blood or PCr and ATP signals from chest muscle (with different PCr/ATP ratios); and 4) differences in spectral processing, especially in how overlapping resonances are handled.

The partial saturation distortion is exacerbated by the use of nonuniform NMR excitation fields. This is because nonuniform excitation introduces a spatially-dependent NMR flip angle, which in turn produces spatially-dependent partial saturation whose magnitude in the heart will vary as the location of the heart relative to the excitation coil varies from patient to patient. Therefore, we use a uniform excitation field, supplied by a very large (0.4×0.4 m^2) ^{31}P surface coil, to generate a field uniform to within approximately $\pm 5\%$ over the sensitive volume of a 6-cm diameter circular surface coil used for ^{31}P detection. The detection coil is located near the center of the large excitation coil, as shown in Figure 5.[8,9] The NMR flip angle is adjusted in each patient examination to maximize the PCr signal in localized surface coil spectra, which are gated to the heart with TR equal to the heart rate. This maximum signal occurs at the Ernst angle ($\cos \alpha = \exp[-TR/T_1]$).[7]

The protocol results in a standardized, uniform, NMR flip angle, even for cardiac gated studies in which the flip angle may vary with heart rate from patient to patient. To correct measurements of cardiac metabolites for partial saturation in such spectra acquired from patients, a measurement of their saturation factors is required because the T_1 values are not reliably documented at present.[7] We measure saturation factors on every subject by acquiring nonlocalized spectra from the chest and heart with the 6-cm coil at the same value of TR as used for the localized experiment, and again at a TR of 15 seconds, which is assumed to produce an unsaturated spectrum.[7] The saturation factor F(PCr/ATP) is given by the ratio of the ratios of PCr/ATP measured

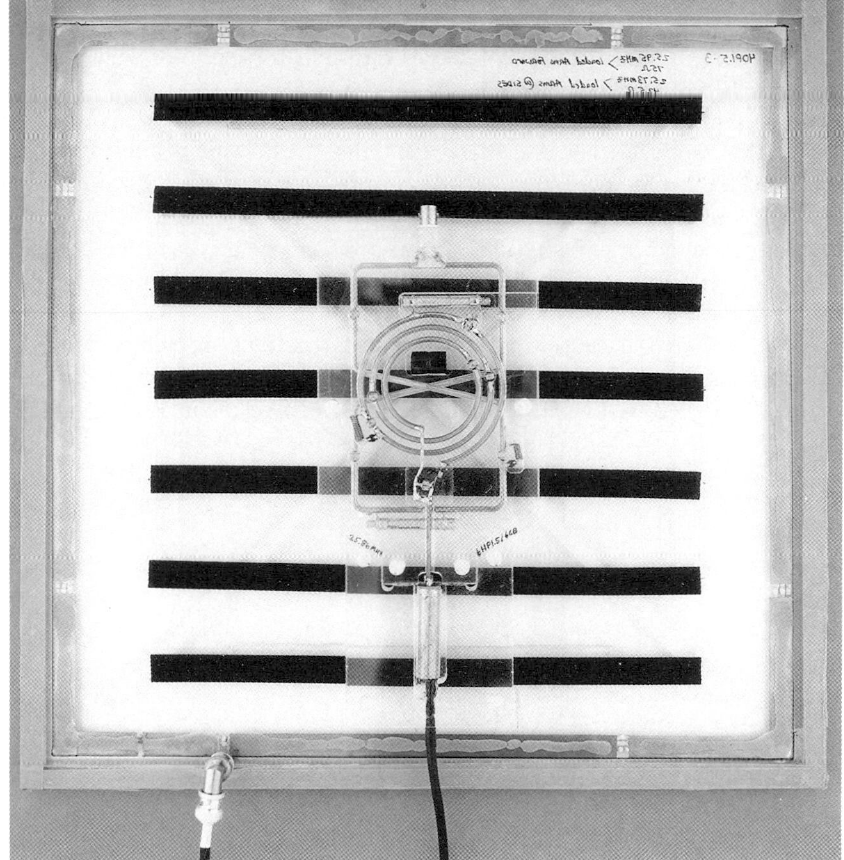

FIGURE 5. *Photograph of our coplanar three-coil set for human cardiac ^{31}P spectroscopy studies. The coil near the perimeter is a 40 × 40 cm^2 ^{31}P transmitter; the figure-of-eight–shaped coil is a ^1H receiver for imaging and shimming the magnetic field homogeneity; and the central three-turn spiral is a 6.5-cm ^{31}P receiver coil. All coils are tuned with distributed capacitors, and the coil set is cushioned with foam in clinical studies. Black Velcro strips permit eccentric placement of the central receiver coils.*

at the two TR values. This protocol step lasts 6 minutes or less (approximately 1.5–4.0 minutes for each acquisition) of the total patient examination time.

The use of nonlocalized measurements of saturation factors in this manner depends on the assumption that the relative T_1 values of PCr and ATP are the same in the skeletal and heart muscle tissues that generate the signals in the 6-cm coil [T_1(PCr)/T_1(ATP)]. This assumption has been tested theoretically and empirically using data from 82 subjects including normal controls and patients with heart transplants, coronary artery disease, and cardiomyopathy. No significant variation in either the measured saturation factors or the saturation-corrected myocardial PCr/

ATP was found, as the relative amount of chest muscle in the nonlocalized spectrum varied from 0% to 70%. In addition, the saturation factors did not vary with disease state. Some of the empirical data are plotted in Figure 6.[7]

Blood contamination can distort myocardial PCr/ATP measurements in voxels intersecting the ventricles because blood contains ATP but does not contain PCr. Because blood is characterized by a 2,3-diphosphoglycerate (DPG) "doublet" in its ^{31}P spectrum and [ATP]/[DPG]$\approx$0.3 in human blood, the PCr/ATP ratio can be substantially corrected by subtracting 15% of the DPG signal (which contains two phosphate moieties) from the signal in the appropriate ATP phosphates prior to the PCr/ATP calculation.[9]

The effect of partial saturation and blood corrections on some of our human myocardial PCr/ATP data is shown in Table 1. Metabolite measurements are based on integrals of curve-fitted (Gaussian and Lorentzian) resonances of corresponding

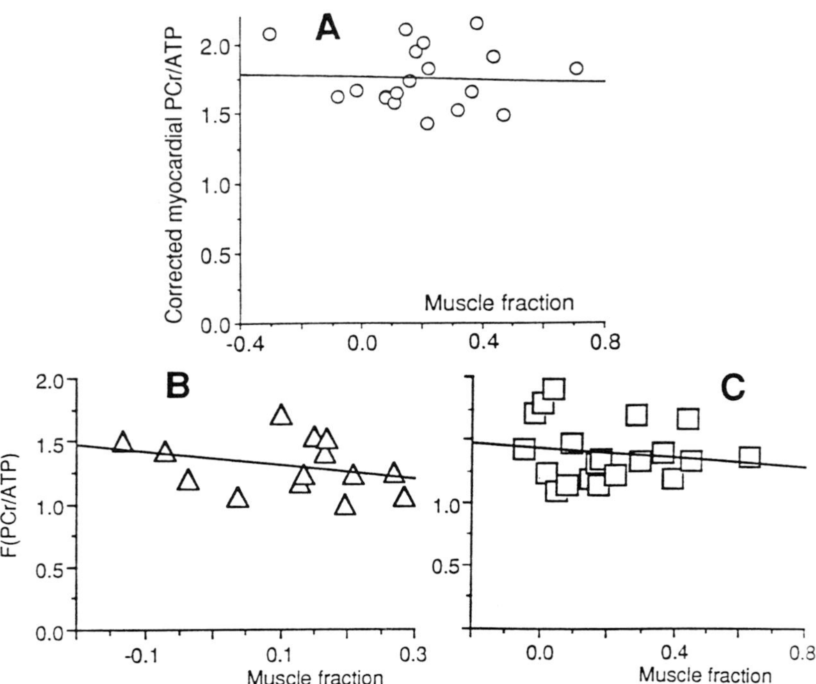

FIGURE 6. A: *Localized saturation-corrected myocardial PCr/ATP ratio in 19 normal volunteers as a function of the fraction of skeletal muscle contributing to the nonlocalized surface coil spectra used for deriving saturation factors.*[7] **B:** *Measured saturation factors for the PCr/ATP ratio, F(PCr/ATP), plotted as a function of the fraction of skeletal muscle contributing to the nonlocalized surface coil spectra used for deriving saturation factors in 16 patients with coronary artery disease and 20 patients with dilated cardiomyopathy* **(C)**.[7] *Negative values of skeletal muscle fraction reflect scatter in subjects with insignificant contributions from chest muscle (eg, due to atrophy).*[7] *Lines are least-squares fits with nonsignificant correlations throughout* (r^2<0.07).

TABLE 1. Effect of Partial Saturation and Blood Corrections on Myocardial PCr/ATP Measurements

PCr/ATP				
Raw	Saturation corrected	Blood ATP corrected	Localization method	Reference
1.3±0.4	(~1.6)		DRESS	16
1.6±0.4*	1.6±0.4*		DRESS	17
1.3	1.7±0.2		3-D CSI	5
		1.72±0.15	1-D CSI	1
1.14	1.64	1.8±0.2	1-D CSI	9
1.22	1.76	1.9±0.2	1-D CSI	10

*Adjusted for "minimum" saturation.
DRESS: depth resolved surface coil spectroscopy; CSI: chemical shift imaging (1-D CSI, Figure 1A; 3-DSCI, Figure 1C).

moieties. The partial saturation correction increases PCr/ATP values by about 30%, whereas the blood correction results in an increase of about 10%.

Clinical Studies

Several exploratory studies of high-energy phosphate metabolism in patients with dilated cardiomyopathy,[9] heart transplants,[10] and coronary artery disease[1] were completed at Johns Hopkins University (Baltimore, MD). The results from a group of 20 patients with dilated cardiomyopathy of idiopathic origin or with accompanying coronary artery disease, a group of 14 heart transplant recipients studied 39–2,021 days after surgery, and a group of 16 patients with severe stenoses of the anterior coronary arteries and myocardial ischemia are summarized in Tables 2–5.[1,9,10]

TABLE 2. Summary of Myocardial ^{31}P NMR Results in Dilated Cardiomyopathy[9]

Group	*n*	Age	EF%	PCr/ATP	PD/ATP
Normal	12	39±14	(>60)	1.80(0.06)	1.76(0.22)
	Without blood ATP correction			1.64(0.08)	
All DCM	20		22±8	1.46(0.07)**	
	Without blood ATP correction			1.24(0.07)**	
DCM, CAD	9	61±18	21±7	1.53(0.07)*	1.79(0.5)
DCM no CAD	11	45±18	25±8	1.41(0.12)*	1.72(0.4)

Note: errors are ±SD, or SE in brackets; EF: ejection fraction; *n:* number of subjects; PD: phosphodiesters; DCM: dilated cardiomyopathy; CAD: coronary artery disease. *p<0.01 versus normal; **p<0.001 versus normal.

TABLE 3. Summary of Myocardial ^{31}P NMR Results in Heart Transplant Patients[10]

Study group	Number of exams	PCr/ATP	PCr/Pi	PD/ATP
Normal	19	1.93±0.21	5.6±5.6 (n=7)	2.4±1.9
Patients	19	1.57±0.50	3.5±4.4 (n=17)	2.3±2.0
Patients needing treatment§	8	1.55±0.52†	3.1±3.7 (n=7)	3.3±2.5
No treatment	11	1.58±0.51†	2.2±1.6 (n=9)	1.5±1.1
Patients needing treatment next§	7	1.49±0.37*	1.7±0.9 (n=5)	2.6±2.2
No treatment	11	1.65±0.59	2.2±1.5 (n=10)	2.1±2.0

Note: errors are ±SD; P_i: inorganic phosphate; PD: phosphodiesters; n: number of exams in which Pi was detectable and a PCr/Pi measurement could be made. §Patients needing intervention to manage rejection detected by biopsy taken on the day of the NMR exam or the next biopsy thereafter (next). *$p<0.01$ compared with normal group. †$p<0.05$ compared with normal group.

TABLE 4. Predictive Value of Myocardial PCr/ATP in Detecting Heart Transplant Rejection Requiring Intervention by ^{31}P NMR[10]

				Predictive value of a:	
	Threshold range	Sensitivity	Specificity	Positive test	Positive or negative test
Test based on average anterior PCr/ATP	1.51–1.58	50%	73%	57%	63%
Test based on minimum anterior PCr/ATP	1.26–1.38	88%	55%	58%	68%

In dilated cardiomyopathy, significant reductions (~19%, $p<0.001$) in myocardial PCr/ATP ratios relative to 12 controls were observed, suggesting that some impairment of energy metabolism is implicated in the pathophysiology of the disorder (Table 2). In the heart transplant patients, significantly lower myocardial PCr/ATP ratios were also observed (Table 3). However, this index did not correlate well with endomyocardial biopsy scores for rejection, nor did it predict rejection sufficiently to warrant augmented immunosuppressive therapy, as detected by biopsies taken either on the day of the NMR examination or at the next scheduled biopsy (10–140 days after the NMR examination) (Table 4). At the University of Alabama at Birmingham, Evanochko and associates[11] have reported good predictability in a group of transplant patients studied in the acute phase of care following transplantation and with a more frequent biopsy interval.

The group of patients with coronary artery disease was studied with localized ^{31}P

TABLE 5. Isometric Hand-Grip Exercise Stress Testing of Patients With Anterior Coronary Artery Disease[1]

	Normal controls $n=11$	Noncoronary disease $n=9$	Coronary disease $n=16$
Heart rate–blood pressure products			
Rest	9600±2800	10200±3300	9900±2800
Exercise	12600±3700	13400±3700	13500±3800
% change	+31%	+31%	+36%
Anterior myocardial PCr/ATP ratios			
Rest	1.72±0.15	1.57±0.27	1.45±0.31
Exercise	1.74±0.17	1.55±0.24	0.91±0.25*
Recovery	1.77±0.16	1.54±0.28	1.27±0.38
% change	ns	ns	−37%

Note: errors are ±1 SD; ns: no significant change. *$p<0.001$ by a Bonferroni-corrected *t* test.

NMR spectroscopy before, during, and after an isometric handgrip exercise at 30% of their maximum effort.[1] The exercise was performed while the subject was lying prone in the magnet. An approximate 30% increase in the heart rate–blood pressure product was observed. During exercise, significant reductions (~37%, $p<0.001$) occurred in the anterior myocardial PCr/ATP of these patients. This was followed by a substantial recovery in PCr/ATP during the postexercise phase of the study. Control groups composed of 11 normal volunteers free of heart disease and 9 patients with nonischemic heart disease (valvular disease and cardiomyopathy) showed no change in myocardial PCr/ATP during exercise with the same protocol. Successful revascularization therapy correlated with improved myocardial PCr/ATP ratios[1] upon repeat testing performed after the therapy in five of the patients with coronary artery disease.

New Technologies

Several technological developments may be beneficial to ^{31}P cardiac spectroscopy. One is the advent of 4-T whole-body systems[12,13] that offer improved scan times, which permit extra experiments; eg, the measurement of creatine kinase metabolic reaction rates, in tolerable examination times. An example of a 4-T one-dimensional phase encoded ^{31}P data set from the chest and heart is shown in Figure 7.[13]

At 1.5 T, the application of phased-array detection coils[14] to ^{31}P cardiac spectroscopy provides greatly increased field-of-view relative to the single-surface detection coil without sacrificing sensitivity.[6] The range of spectroscopy experiments is thus extended and the need for careful coil placement thereby reduced.

Irradiating protons during the ^{31}P experiment provide significant signal enhancement via the nuclear Overhauser enhancement (nOe).[15] The nOe values of 0.6±0.3 SD for PCr and γ-ATP, and 0.3±0.2 for β-ATP in the heart at 1.5 T have been measured. However, the nOe distorts the myocardial PCr/ATP ratios, necessitating accurate corrections to fully realize the benefits of increased reliability in PCr/ATP measurements that the enhancement potentially offers. An example of the nOe effect on some heart spectra is shown in Figure 8.

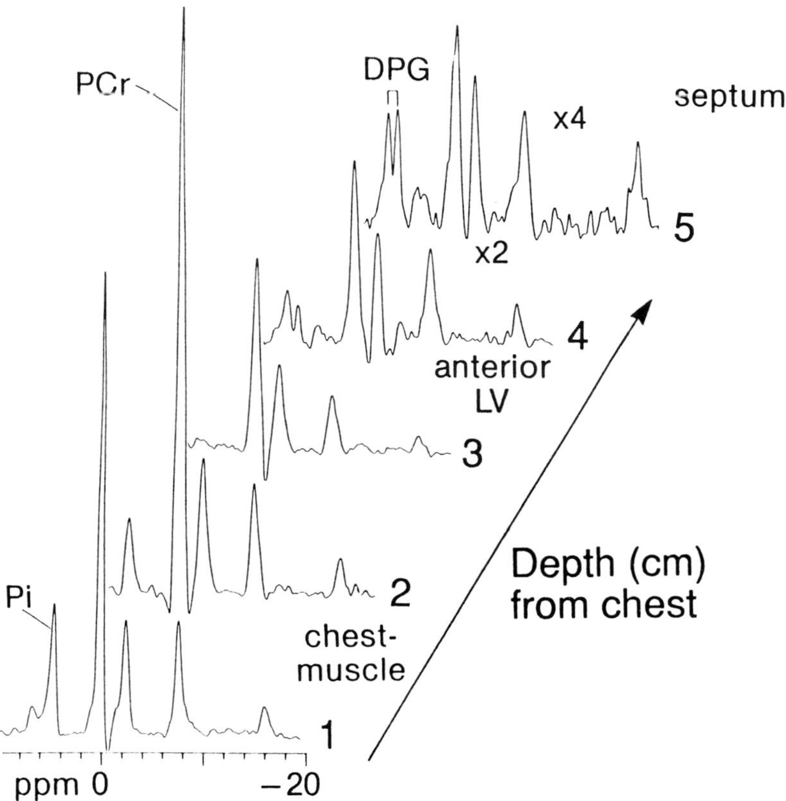

FIGURE 7. *Cardiac-gated ^{31}P spectra acquired in under 5 minutes at a field strength of 4 T from 1-cm thick slices through the chest and heart of a normal volunteer with a 32-step one-dimensional phase encoding gradient sequence (Figure 1A) and a 6.5-cm diameter surface detection coil with a uniform excitation field.[13] The ATP resonance at −16.3 ppm is artificially attenuated by the limited bandwidth of our transmitter (whose power must be increased to cover the larger frequency dispersion at higher fields).*

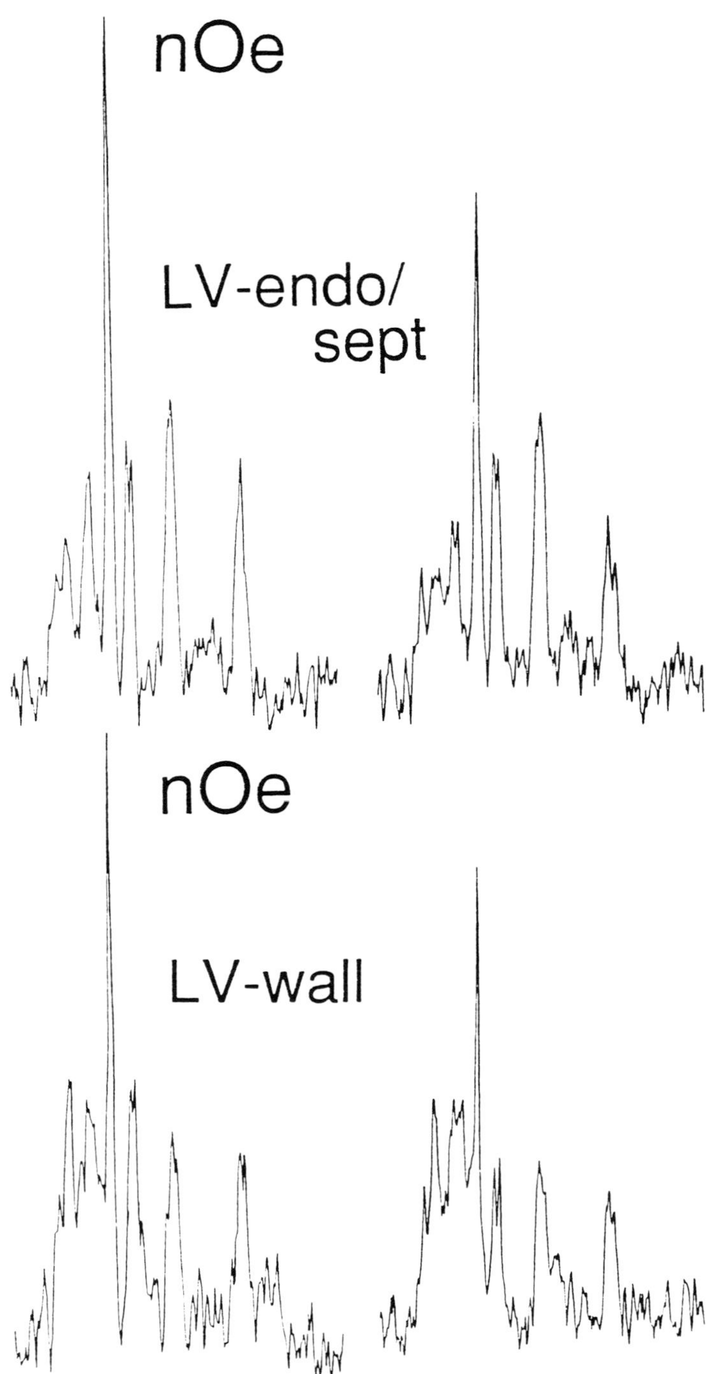

FIGURE 8. *Cardiac-gated ^{31}P spectra acquired from 1-cm thick coronal sections through the left ventricular (LV) wall of a normal volunteer using the one-dimensional encoding sequence of Figure 1A, with (left) and without (right) ^{1}H nuclear Overhauser enhancement (nOe).[15] The enhancement was produced by continuous irradiation of the H_2O resonance, gated off during acquisition, and applied with the figure-of-eight–shaped coil in Figure 5. The scan time was 10 minutes at 1.5 T. (endo/sept, endocardial/septal).*

References

1. Weiss RG, Bottomley PA, Hardy CJ, Gerstenblith G: Regional myocardial metabolism of high-energy phosphates during isometric exercise in patients with coronary artery disease. *N Engl J Med* 1990;323:1593–1600.
2. Hardy CJ, Bottomley PA: ^{31}P spectroscopic localization using pinwheel NMR excitation pulses. *Magn Reson Med* 1991;17:315–327.
3. Bottomley PA, Hardy CJ: Two-dimensional spatially selective spin inversion and spin-echo refocusing with a single nuclear magnetic resonance pulse. *J Appl Phys* 1987;62:4284–4290.
4. van Dobbenburgh JO, Lekkerkerk C, van Echteld CJA: Saturation effects in human heart and chest wall muscle measured by ^{31}P 1.D spectroscopic imaging (abstract). In: Proceedings of the Society of Magnetic Resonance in Medicine Tenth Annual Meeting. 1991:988.
5. Bottomley PA, Hardy CJ, Roemer PB: Phosphate metabolite imaging and concentration measurements in human heart by nuclear magnetic resonance. *Magn Reson Med* 1990;14:425–434.
6. Hardy CJ, Bottomley PA, Rohling KW, Roemer PB: An NMR phased array for human cardiac ^{31}P spectroscopy. *Magn Reson Med* 1992;28:54–64.
7. Bottomley PA, Hardy CJ: Correcting human heart ^{31}P NMR spectra for partial saturation. Evidence that saturation factors for PCr/ATP are homogeneous in normal and disease states. *J Magn Reson* 1991;95:341–355.
8. Bottomley PA, Hardy CJ: Strategies and protocols for clinical ^{31}P research in the heart and brain. *Phil Trans R Soc Lond A Math Phys Sci* 1990;333:531–544.
9. Hardy CJ, Weiss RG, Bottomley PA, Gerstenblith G: Altered myocardial high-energy phosphate metabolites in patients with dilated cardiomyopathy. *Am Heart J* 1991;122:795.
10. Bottomley PA, Weiss RG, Hardy CJ, Baumgartner WA: Myocardial high-energy phosphate metabolism and allograft rejection in patients with heart transplants. *Radiology* 1991;181:67-75.
11. Evanochko WT, Bouchard A, Kirklin JK, et al: Detection of cardiac transplant rejection in patients by ^{31}P NMR spectroscopy (abstract). In: Proceedings of the Society of Magnetic Resonance in Medicine Ninth Annual Meeting. 1990;1:246.
12. Hardy CJ, Bottomley PA, Roemer PB, Redington RW: Rapid ^{31}P spectroscopy on a 4 tesla whole-body system. *Magn Reson Med* 1988;8:104–109.
13. Bottomley PA, Hardy CJ: Mapping creatine kinase reaction rates in human brain and heart with 4 Tesla saturation transfer ^{31}P NMR. *J Magn Reson* 1992;99:443–448.
14. Roemer PB, Edelstein WA, Hayes CE, et al: The NMR phased array. *Magn Reson Med* 1990;16:192–225.
15. Bottomley PA, Hardy CJ: Proton Overhauser enhancements in human cardiac phosphorus NMR spectroscopy at 1.5-T. *Magn Reson Med* 1992;24:384–390.
16. Bottomley PA: Noninvasive study of high-energy phosphate metabolism in human heart by depth-resolved ^{31}P NMR spectroscopy. *Science* 1985;229:769–772.
17. Bottomley PA, Herfkens RJ, Smith LS, Bashore TM: Altered phosphate metabolism in myocardial infarction: P-31 MR spectroscopy. *Radiology* 1987;165:703–707.

Chapter 29

Clinical Phosphorus-31 Magnetic Resonance Spectroscopy in Cardiomyopathy

Albert de Roos, MD, Peter R. Luyten, PhD,
Joost Doornbos, PhD,
Arnoud van der Laarse, PhD,
and Ernst E. van der Wall, MD

Phosphorus-31 (^{31}P) magnetic resonance spectroscopy (MRS) is a noninvasive tool for the investigation of high-energy phosphate metabolism of the heart.[1,2] Three-dimensionally localized P-31 spectra can be obtained from the myocardium using a surface coil placed on the chest over the cardiac apex. The spectrum provides quantifiable information on the concentration of multiple metabolic high-energy phosphate compounds. Cardiac ^{31}P spectra disclose metabolites such as inorganic phosphate, phosphomonoesters, phosphodiesters, phosphocreatine, and three peaks from adenosine triphosphate (ATP) (Figure 1). The phosphomonoester region often includes 2,3-diphosphoglycerate contained in the blood pool of cardiac chambers and myocardium, overlapping the inorganic phosphate peak. Furthermore, technically it is difficult to separate myocardial signal from that of chest wall muscle and that of the nearby blood pool. However, when the inorganic phosphate peak is resolved, the intracellular pH of the myocardium can be estimated from the distance between the peaks of inorganic phosphate and phosphocreatine. The ratio between phosphocreatine and inorganic phosphate is an indicator of the energy reserve of the heart and this ratio will promptly change when ischemia develops. With reduction of myocardial blood flow, myocardial contraction of the affected segment will cease, accompanied by a rapid fall in phosphocreatine and rise in inorganic phosphate resulting in a fall in tissue pH, whereas the ATP levels are maintained until phosphocreatine is depleted. Phosphorus-31 spectroscopy can detect myocardial ischemia and infarction by profound changes in high-energy phosphate compounds.

From Pohost GM (ed.), *Cardiovascular Applications of Magnetic Resonance*. Mount Kisco, NY, Futura Publishing Co., Inc., © 1993.

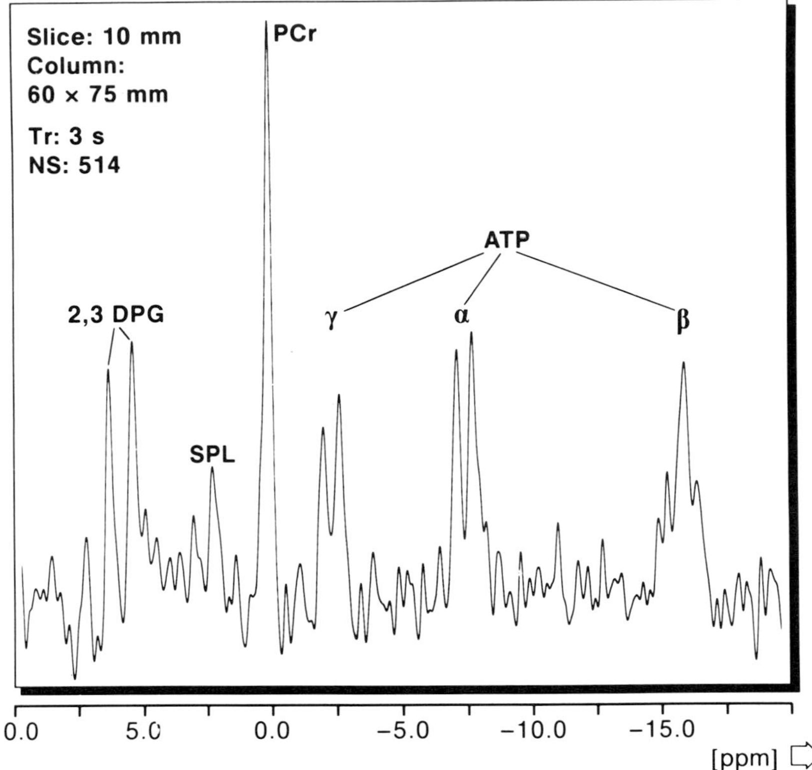

FIGURE 1. *Phosphorus-31 (^{31}P) spectrum from the human heart obtained with proton-decoupled ^{31}P spectroscopy using image selected in vivo spectroscopy (ISIS) at 1.5 T (Philips Gyroscan S15, Best, The Netherlands). Note resonances from 2,3-diphosphoglycerate (DPG) contained in blood, blood phospholipids (SPL), phosphocreatine (PCr), and the three peaks from adenosine triphosphate (ATP). Reprinted from Reference 2 with permission.*

Phosphorus-31 heart spectroscopy has been applied in various forms of cardiomyopathy to study alterations of normal cardiac biochemistry. Cardiomyopathic heart disease may disclose alterations in high-energy phosphate metabolism probably depending on the severity of the disease process. Both normal and decreased phosphocreatine-to-ATP ratios have been reported in dilated cardiomyopathy.

The phosphocreatine-to-ATP ratio may also be decreased in patients with hypertrophic cardiomyopathy. In this chapter the value of ^{31}P heart spectroscopy in cardiomyopathy is discussed based on the recent literature and the experience of our group.

Myocardial Energy Metabolism

Cardiac contraction and maintenance of cellular functions require the availability of energy. The energy present in food is made available for cardiac function in the form of ATP by oxidative metabolism of free fatty acids and carbohydrates like glucose and lactate. Under normal physiologic circumstances, free fatty acids (in particular, palmitate) provide most of the ATP used by the heart, whereas glucose is an important alternative fuel for ATP production.[3] Before entering the citric acid cycle (also known as Krebs cycle or tricarboxylic acid cycle), free fatty acids and glucose have to be converted to acetyl-coenzyme A.

After uptake of the glucose molecule into the cell, glucose is converted to two molecules of pyruvate by the process of glycolysis. The next stage in the degradation of glucose is conversion of pyruvate molecules into acetyl-coenzyme A, which then can enter the citric acid cycle. Free fatty acids are converted to acetyl-coenzyme A by β-oxidation.

The citric acid cycle yields a large number of hydrogen atoms that enter the electron transport chain. The final ATP is formed in the mitochondria during subsequent oxidation of the released hydrogen atoms by the process of oxidative phosphorylation.

As part of the process of energy conservation, the high-energy phosphate group of ATP is transferred to phosphocreatine catalyzed by the mitochondrial creatine kinase. Cytosolic creatine kinase splits phosphocreatine to form ATP and creatine. Then, energy consumption will occur by hydrolysis of ATP at the myofilaments to enable contraction.

Clinical Studies in Cardiomyopathy

Altered Myocardial Energy Metabolism in Cardiac Hypertrophy

Phosphorus-31 spectroscopy may be helpful in assessing high-energy phosphate metabolism in patients with cardiac hypertrophy and may be useful for planning treatment options.

A decreased phosphocreatine-to-ATP ratio has been identified in a patient with hypertrophic cardiomyopathy associated with heart failure.[4] However, in the absence of concomitant heart failure, normal phosphocreatine-to-ATP ratios have been noted in patients with ventricular hypertrophy.[5] A case of congenital cardiomyopathy revealed a decreased phosphocreatine-to-inorganic phosphate ratio that improved to normal values after intravenous glucose administration.[6] These initial studies were limited to a few patients, but were valuable in demonstrating the potential value of this new methodology.

Several reports from our group have discussed alterations in the phosphocreatine-with-ATP ratio in patients with dilated and hypertrophic cardiomyopathy as compared with a control group.[7–10] Furthermore, preliminary reports have also discussed the assessment of intracellular myocardial pH using proton-decoupled ^{31}P heart spectroscopy in normal volunteers and patients with hypertrophic cardiomyopathy.[9,10]

Sakuma et al.[11] identified a decreased phosphocreatine-to-ATP ratio in a series of 13 patients with hypertrophic cardiomyopathy. Interestingly, the spectroscopic alterations appeared to correlate with myocardial contrast enhancement with the use of gadolinium-DTPA. In a later conference report, Sakuma et al.[12] showed a significantly lower phosphocreatine-to-ATP ratio in a series of 19 patients with hypertrophic cardiomyopathy after correcting the phosphocreatine-to-ATP ratio for blood contamination.

Recently, Conway et al.[13] reported a significantly lower phosphocreatine-to-ATP ratio in six patients who received treatment for heart failure in left ventricular hypertrophy due to aortic valve disease. The authors concluded that measurement of the phosphocreatine-to-ATP ratio could eventually have a role in helping to determine the optimum timing for aortic valve replacement.

Altered Myocardial Energy Metabolism in Dilated Cardiomyopathy

Several clinical studies have reported metabolic alterations in dilated cardiomyopathy assessed by ^{31}P heart spectroscopy. A significant elevation of the phosphodiester level has been observed in ^{31}P spectra obtained from patients suffering from dilated cardiomyopathy.[5,14] This spectroscopic finding has been attributed to breakdown products of phospholipid catabolism in myocardial muscle, more specifically to glycerophosphorylcholine and glycerophosphorylethanolamine. Schaefer et al.[5] discussed the possibility that the greater inclusion of chamber blood signal in the spectra of patients with dilated cardiomyopathy may have artificially elevated the area of the phosphodiester peak in those patients. Auffermann et al.[14] concluded that myocardial phosphodiesters may be a marker for diseased myocardium, but that further study is needed to assess the sensitivity and specificity of this finding. Of note, these studies did not include correction for possible contributions from blood pool signal. Recently, several reports have addressed the significance of correcting cardiac ^{31}P spectra for blood contamination.[8,10,12,15] Blood contamination of cardiac ^{31}P spectra can alter the observed phosphocreatine-to-ATP ratio because blood contains ATP but no phosphocreatine. Therefore, the blood correction might be expected to reduce observed differences between patient groups in phosphocreatine-to-ATP ratios due to greater contributions from chamber blood, especially with thin-walled ventricles in patients with dilated cardiomyopathy. Hardy et al.[15] reported abnormal cardiac biochemistry in a series of 20 patients with dilated cardiomyopathy of either ischemic ($n=9$) or idiopathic ($n=11$) etiology after correction for partial saturation and contamination of the spectra by blood metabolites. This study demonstrated reduced myocardial phosphocreatine-to-ATP ratios under resting conditions in both ischemic and idiopathic dilated cardiomyopathy. No significant correlation was found between the myocardial phosphocreatine-to-ATP ratio and left ventricular ejection fraction in patients with dilated cardiomyopathy. Of note, all patients included in this study had symptoms of congestive heart failure. Apparently, the presence of concomitant heart failure in patients with dilated cardiomyopathy contributes to the observed alterations in cardiac metabolism.

Proton-Decoupled Phosphorus-31 Spectroscopy in Cardiomyopathy

We have studied cardiac metabolism using proton-decoupled ^{31}P heart spectroscopy in normal volunteers ($n = 10$) and in patients with idiopathic dilated cardiomyopathy ($n = 9$), hypertrophic cardiomyopathy ($n = 9$), and in patients suffering from systemic sclerosis ($n = 6$). Preliminary results of this work have been reported at several scientific meetings.[7–10] Low myocardial phosphocreatine-to-ATP ratios may be found in the various forms of cardiomyopathy.

Spectroscopic Technique

The spectroscopic experiments were performed on a 1.5-T whole-body magnetic resonance system (Gyroscan; Philips Medical Systems, Best, The Netherlands). A 10-cm diameter transmit/receive single tuned P-31 surface coil was applied over the cardiac apex to acquire the spectra. The localization technique combined one-dimensional phase encoding and two-dimensional selective image selected in vivo MRS (ISIS). Proton decoupling was applied during acquisition of the ^{31}P signal using the body coil for transmission.[16]

Spectral Quantification

Quantification of the information present in in vivo ^{31}P magnetic resonance spectra is not a straightforward process due to limiting factors such as peak overlap and relatively low signal-to-noise ratios. Methods for spectral quantification and their respective advantages and drawbacks were recently discussed by Bottomley.[17] Generally speaking, spectra can be quantified by either processing of the data in the frequency domain or by analysis of the time domain data from the free induction decay (FID). Frequency domain processing involves peak area approximation that is usually done by curve fitting of the data with a spectrum built up of theoretical line shapes. Overlapping peaks pose a serious problem to this method.

In our work we use a method based on time domain analysis[18] that involves iterative curve fitting of the time domain data with a calculated FID containing the expected resonances. Prior knowledge is used as starting parameters in the curve fitting process and as constraints on some spectral characteristics. In our analysis of ^{31}P magnetic resonance spectra of the myocardium we applied a combination of free and constrained parameters, including the J coupling patterns, the amplitude ratios, and the line width ratios, within which each moiety of the ATP signal were fixed. The chemical shift (relative to phosphocreatine) of the glycerophosphorylcholine and the serum phospholipid (SPL) diester signals were kept constant. The line widths of glycerophosphorylcholine, SPLs, inorganic phosphate, and 2,3-diphosphoglycerate were constrained at fixed ratios of the line width of the phosphocreatine peak, which was analyzed without constraints.

The time domain fitting routine allows evaluation of the accuracy of the quantification by using the Cramér-Rao method. The Cramér-Rao method has the advantage of providing standard deviations for each spectrum and thus indicating the signal-to-noise ratio of individual spectra. Taking into account the individual Cramér-Rao standard deviations helps to improve the validity of intergroup differences, because the mean metabolite ratio for the group is a weighted average based on individual variations in spectral quality.

Correction for Blood and Partial Saturation

The ATP level observed in ^{31}P heart spectra should be corrected for the ATP contribution from blood contained in the myocardium and cardiac chambers. Especially in patients with dilated cardiomyopathy that is characterized by a variable degree of wall thinning, a possible reduction of the phosphocreatine-to-ATP ratio might be caused by the greater inclusion of chamber blood in the volume of interest. The blood contains ATP but no phosphocreatine and therefore might artificially lower the phosphocreatine-to-ATP ratio. Partial saturation effects may occur due to the use of relatively short TR. However, correction for partial saturation will systematically affect all measurements and therefore will not change intergroup differences.

Discussion

As discussed in recent articles and conference reports, ^{31}P heart spectroscopy is capable of defining alterations in cardiac metabolism in groups of patients with various forms of cardiomyopathy. Patients with either dilated or hypertrophic cardiomyopathy may be characterized by low phosphocreatine-to-ATP ratios, probably depending on the severity of the disease process. Furthermore, attention to technical details of the spectroscopic technique improves assessment of alterations in cardiac biochemistry using localized ^{31}P spectroscopy. For example, correction of ^{31}P heart spectra for blood contamination is essential to reveal true metabolic changes in the myocardium.

The mechanism of the alterations in the phosphocreatine-to-ATP ratio in failing hypertrophied hearts may relate to changes in creatine kinase activity or a fall in the total creatine content of cardiac muscle.[13] Ingwall et al.[19] studied changes in the creatine kinase system in hypertrophied human myocardium. Creatine kinase regulates the synthesis, transport, and utilization of ATP and phosphocreatine in heart muscle. That study showed that myocardium from patients with left ventricular hypertrophy contains less total creatine than normal myocardium.[19] The calculated phosphocreatine content in tissue with left ventricular hypertrophy was several times lower than in normal myocardium. Furthermore, Ingwall et al.[19] speculated that the primary stimulus for altered creatine kinase activity in severely hypertrophied myocardium is hypoxia. Indeed, one of the earliest biochemical consequences of hypoxia is reduced phosphocreatine content in the myocardium.

In cardiac hypertrophy decreased rates of oxidative metabolism and increased anaerobic metabolism have been demonstrated. Anaerobic glycolysis can partly compensate for impaired oxidative metabolism. However, enhanced anaerobic glycolytic metabolism results in the accumulation of glycolytic catabolites (in particular, lactate), which may be responsible for increased ischemic injury in hypertrophied hearts. In general, cardiac hypertrophy contributes to enhanced susceptibility of the myocardium to ischemic damage, resulting in greater mortality and more rapidly developing and larger infarcts.

Currently, myocardial hypertrophy is considered to be a phenomenon of adaption and is associated with alterations in intermediate myocardial metabolism (increased glycolytic capacity), energy conservation (impaired regulation of mitochondrial oxygen consumption by creatine kinase flux), energy consumption at the level of the contractile units, and adrenoceptor-mediated regulatory mechanisms of cardiac performance.

Several studies have demonstrated that hypertrophied myocardium has relatively higher glycolytic capacity. Smith et al.[20] demonstrated increased lactate dehydrogenase activity in hypertrophied myocardium, indicating a relatively higher glycolytic capacity of the myocardium. In addition, this effect may be further enhanced in the presence of high blood pressure. Anderson et al.[21] found that hypertrophied hearts have a greater potential for glycolytic metabolism, resulting in an increased accumulation of by-products of anaerobic glycolytic metabolism (lactate, NADH, or H^+) during ischemia, which may be responsible for the increased susceptibility of hypertrophied hearts to ischemic injury. As further evidence for enhanced glycolytic activity in hypertrophied myocardium, Kagaya et al.[22] reported increased uptake of labeled glucose in hypertrophied myocardium, whereas the extraction of labeled free fatty acids was decreased.

In conclusion, P-31 spectroscopy is a promising technique to evaluate normal and abnormal myocardial energy metabolism. Specific derangements in myocardial metabolism may be detected in patients with various forms of cardiomyopathy. The most informative situations (rest, exercise) to distinguish metabolic alterations and cardiac function are issues of continuing research. It is expected that cardiac P-31 spectroscopy in humans, of which a clinical evaluation has just started, has great potential in future diagnosis and therapy of patients with cardiomyopathy.

References

1. Schaefer S: Clinical nuclear magnetic resonance spectroscopy: insight into metabolism. *Am J Cardiol* 1990;66:45F–50F.
2. de Roos A, van der Wall EE: Magnetic resonance imaging and spectroscopy of the heart. *Curr Opin Cardiol* 1991;6:946–952.
3. Brown JJ, Mirowitz SA, Sandstrom JC, Perman WH: MR spectroscopy of the heart. *AJR* 1990;155:1–11.
4. Rajagopalan B, Blackledge MJ, McKenna WJ, et al: Measurement of phosphocreatine to ATP ratio in normal and diseased human heart by P-31 NMR using the rotating frame-depth selection technique. *Ann N Y Acad Sci* 1987;508:321–332.
5. Schaefer S, Gober JR, Schwartz GG, et al: In vivo phosphorus-31 spectroscopic imaging in patients with global myocardial disease. *Am J Cardiol* 1990;65:1154–1161.
6. Whitman GJR, Chance B, Bode H, et al: Diagnosis and therapeutic evaluation of a pediatric case of cardiomyopathy using phosphorus-31 nuclear magnetic resonance spectroscopy. *J Am Coll Cardiol* 1985;5:745–749.
7. Mariën AJH, Doornbos J, De Roos A, et al: ^1H decoupled 31-P NMR spectroscopy of the normal human heart at 1.5 T: a reassessment of metabolite ratios and bulk susceptibility effects (abstract). In: Proceedings of the Society of Magnetic Resonance in Medicine. 1990:249.

8. Luyten PR, Den Hollander JA, Mariën AJH, et al: H-1 decoupled P-31 MR spectroscopy of the human heart: acquisition and quantification in controls and patients. *J Magn Reson Med* 1991;2:167.
9. Luyten PR, de Roos A, Oosterwaal LJMJ, et al: PCr/ATP ratio changes and pH values in dilated and hypertrophic cardiomyopathy patients determined by 31 P NMR heart spectroscopy. (abstract). In: Proceedings of the Society of Magnetic Resonance in Medicine. 1991:74.
10. de Roos A, Luyten PR, Mariën AJH, et al: Metabolite ratios in normal human myocardium and cardiomyopathy: quantification by 31-P spectroscopy. *J Am Coll Cardiol* 1991;17:77A.
11. Sakuma H, Takeda K, Yamakado K, et al: P-31 NMR spectroscopy in patients with hypertrophic cardiomyopathy (abstract). In: Proceedings of the Society of Magnetic Resonance in Medicine. 1990:248.
12. Sakuma H, Takeda K, Tagami T, et al: P-31 MR spectroscopy in hypertrophic cardiomyopathy with correction of blood contamination: comparison with Tl-201 myocardial perfusion imaging (abstract). In: Proceedings of the Society of Magnetic Resonance in Medicine. 1991:75.
13. Conway MA, Allis J, Ouwerkerk R, et al: Detection of low phosphocreatine to ATP ratio in failing hypertrophied human myocardium by 31P magnetic resonance spectroscopy. *Lancet* 1991;338:973–976.
14. Auffermann W, Chew WM, Wolfe CL, et al: Normal and diffusely abnormal myocardium in humans: functional and metabolic characterization with P-31 MR spectroscopy and cine MR imaging. *Radiology* 1991;179:253–259.
15. Hardy CJ, Weiss RG, Bottomley PA, Gerstenblith G: Altered myocardial high-energy phosphate metabolites in patients with dilated cardiomyopathy. *Am Heart J* 1991;122:795–801.
16. Luyten PR, Bruntink G, Sloff FM, et al: Broadband proton decoupling in human P31 NMR spectroscopy. *NMR Biomed* 1989;1:177–183.
17. Bottomley PA: The trouble with spectroscopy papers. *Radiology* 1991;181:344–350.
18. Van der Veen JWC, De Beer R, Luyten PR, Van Ormondt D: Accurate quantification of in vivo 31-P NMR signals using the variable projection method and prior knowledge. *Magn Reson Med* 1988;6:92–98.
19. Ingwall JS, Kramer MF, Fifer MA, et al: The creatine kinase system in normal and diseased human myocardium. *N Engl J Med* 1985;313:1050–1054.
20. Smith SH, Kramer MF, Reis I, et al: Regional changes in creatine kinase and myocyte size in hypertensive and nonhypertensive cardiac hypertrophy. *Circ Res* 1990;67:1334–1344.
21. Anderson PG, Allard MF, Thomas GD, et al: Increased ischemic injury but decreased hypoxic injury in hypertrophied rat hearts. *Circ Res* 1990;67:948–959.
22. Kagaya Y, Kanno Y, Takeyama D, et al: Effects of long-term pressure overload on regional myocardial glucose and free fatty acid uptake in rats. A quantitative autoradiographic study. *Circulation* 1990;81:1353–1361.

Chapter 30

Shift Reagent-Aided ^{23}Na Nuclear Magnetic Resonance Spectroscopy

Gabriel A. Elgavish, PhD

Nondestructive observation of intracellular sodium (Na_i) levels is of utmost clinical and biochemical importance. In viable cells, a 10- to 20-fold concentration gradient between Na_i and extracellular sodium (Na_o) is maintained. Deviation from this gradient is an important indicator of detrimental processes. Therefore, it may be a valuable parameter for the assessment of cell viability and reversibility of normal function following damage, eg, an ischemic insult.

Via the various sodium transport mechanisms (Na^+-H^+ anti-port, Na^+-Ca^{2+} exchange, Na^+-K^+ ATPase, and others), sodium levels and fluxes have an important role in the regulation of intracellular pH, of intracellular calcium levels, and therefore, of cellular function. In muscle cells, eg, in the myocardium, changes in Na_i levels are coupled with contractile function. Real-time, nondestructive monitoring of Na_i, therefore, would be a powerful research tool that could enhance our biochemical understanding of cellular processes in health and disease. Once development of the methodology reached the stage of safe human application, its use in the clinical context could offer a sensitive in vivo marker of localized variations in tissue viability.

^{23}Na is a quadripolar nuclide with spin 3/2, 100% natural abundance, nuclear magnetic resonance (NMR) receptivity of 9.27 (relative to 100 for ^{1}H), and an average concentration of 44 mM in the human body. Therefore, it is a relatively sensitive (50% more sensitive than ^{31}P) NMR-observable nuclide, and thus the goals stated previously should be approachable by ^{23}Na NMR. Unfortunately, however, no chemical shift difference exists between Na_i and Na_o. Taken together with a total tissue quantity of Na_o, which is much larger than that of Na_i, NMR observation of Na_i was precluded until Degani and Elgavish[1] demonstrated that anionic paramagnetic complexes of gadolinium, used as relaxation reagents, could be used to differentiate the sodium signals from the two compartments. This was followed in 1982 with the introduction of paramagnetic dysprosium complexes as shift reagents for metal cations.[2,3] Combined with the intrinsic features of NMR spectroscopy, the ability

Partial support by NHLBI (P50 HL17667) is gratefully acknowledged.
From Pohost GM (ed.), *Cardiovascular Applications of Magnetic Resonance*. Mount Kisco, NY, Futura Publishing Co., Inc., © 1993.

of an aqueous shift reagent to differentiate signals from intracellular and extracellular spaces provided a nondestructive, continuous method to monitor intracellular cation concentration. Subsequently, ^{23}Na NMR studies of various biologic systems quickly followed.

Theory

The Lanthanide-Induced Shift

Nuclei of ligands in paramagnetic complexes are magnetically coupled to the unpaired electronic spin of the central ion by the electron nuclear hyperfine interaction. One of the consequences of this interaction is large chemical shifts (relative to the same system not coupled to a paramagnetic lanthanide ion) in the NMR spectra of the ligands. There are two major independent mechanisms of hyperfine interaction. The contact interaction results from a finite probability of finding an unpaired electronic spin on an atomic s orbital. In lanthanides, this occurs via spin polarization, and the contact shift (in frequency units) can be expressed as:

$$\delta_{hc} = A \cdot < S_z > \qquad [1]$$

where $_{hc}$ is the hyperfine contact, A is the hyperfine coupling constant (in frequency units), and $<S_z>$ is the projection of the total electron spin magnetization of the lanthanide on the direction of the external magnetic field.

The dipolar interaction takes place via space and causes shifts only if the magnetic susceptibility of the central ion is anisotropic, otherwise it is effectively averaged out and no dipolar shifts are observed. The latter case, eg, with S-state ions such as Gd^{3+}, occurs when the only paramagnetic shifts are of contact and of bulk magnetic susceptibility (BMS) origin. A concise theory of dipolar shifts in lanthanide complexes in solution has been presented by Bleaney.[4] The core of this theory is a second-order approximation of the population of the energy sublevels split by the ligand field. This approximation yields a T^{-1}-dependent population distribution. These population values then serve as weighting factors in calculating the average magnetic moment. The latter, combined with Curie's law, results in an anisotropic, T^{-2}-dependent susceptibility. This second-order anisotropic susceptibility is the source of the dipolar nuclear resonance shifts in lanthanide complexes.

In axially symmetrical systems it is convenient to express the dipolar shift as follows:

$$\delta_{i,hd} = D \cdot G_i \qquad [2]$$

where $G_i = (3\cos^2\epsilon_i - 1)/r_i^3$ is the geometrical function specific for ligand nucleus i, and D is a temperature-dependent factor characteristic of the lanthanide. Thus, excluding BMS, the net paramagnetic shift, Δ_p, is the sum of the hyperfine contact (δ_{hc}) and the hyperfine dipolar (δ_{hd}) contributions:

$$\delta_p = \delta_{hc} + \delta_{hd} \qquad [3]$$

Induced Relaxation

Nuclear relaxation is generated by the time-dependent terms of the nuclear spin Hamiltonian. The magnitude of the relaxation effect in paramagnetic lanthanide complexes is predominantly dipolar in origin and is governed by the intensity of the electron-nuclear interaction and by the rate at which this interaction is interrupted. Thus, the relaxation rates of ligand nuclei are determined by the molecular structure and by the molecular dynamics in solution and may in turn be used for studying these factors.

The electron spin relaxation time, T_{1e}, in the lanthanide cations is of the order of 10^{-13} seconds (except Gd^{+3}). Thus, T_{1e} is always much shorter than any rotational reorientation time, τ_r. Consequently the electron nuclear dipolar interaction in a small molecular weight lanthanide complex (except Gd^{3+}) will contribute to the nuclear relaxation rate of a given ligand nucleus according to Equation 4[5]:

$$1/T_{1M} = 1/T_{2M} = (20/15)\gamma_N^2 \cdot g_N^2 \cdot \beta^2 \cdot J(J+1) \cdot r^{-6} \cdot T_{1e} \qquad [4]$$

where T_{1M} and T_{2M}, respectively, are the intrinsic longitudinal and transverse relaxation times of a given ligand nucleus in its lanthanide-bound state, γ_N is the nuclear magnetogyric ratio, r is the nucleus -Ln^{+3} distance, g_N is the nuclear g-factor, J is the resultant electronic spin angular momentum (in units of $h/2\pi$), and β is the Bohr magneton.

In relatively large molecular weight complexes, a so-called "susceptibility term"[6,7] becomes an additional, significant contribution to an extent that depends on molecular size, as manifested in the molecular rotational time, τ_r. The contribution of the contact interaction to the nuclear relaxation in lanthanide complexes is usually negligible.

In the case of Gd^{3+}, whose T_{1e} is relatively long, more than one dynamic mechanism contributes to the overall correlation time, τ_c. Thus, the approximations that lead to the relatively simple formula in Equation 4 cannot be applied, and the full correlation function should be used, yielding:

$$1/T_{1M} = 2 \cdot C\left(\frac{3\tau_c}{1+\omega_N^2\tau_c^2} + \frac{7\tau_c}{1+\omega_e^2\tau_c^2}\right), \quad 1/T_{2M} = C\left(4\tau_c + \frac{3\tau_c}{1+\omega_N^2\tau_c^2} + \frac{13\tau_c}{1+\omega_e^2\tau_c^2}\right) \qquad [5]$$

where

$$C = \frac{1}{15}\gamma_N^2 \cdot g_N^2 \cdot \beta^2 \cdot J\,(J+1)\,r^{-6} \qquad 1/\tau_c = 1/T_{1e} + 1/\tau_r + 1/\tau_M$$

and ω_N and ω_θ are the resonance frequencies of the observed nucleus and of the unpaired electron, respectively, at the operating external magnetic field, and τ_M is the lifetime of the observed ligand nucleus in the gadolinium coordination sphere.

Experimental Methods

Mechanism of Shift Reagent Action

The method of induced differentiation in the NMR spectra of aqueous cationic species by either paramagnetic lanthanide shift reagents or by the corresponding gadolinium complex that acts as a relaxation reagent was introduced by Elgavish and Reuben.[8] The shift method was first applied by Gupta and Gupta[2] to the problem of the separation of the ^{23}Na NMR signals of Na_i and Na_o in cells and tissues. This is currently the method used most frequently for observation of the Na_i signal. The Na_i and Na_o signals can be separated in the ^{23}Na NMR spectrum using a lanthanide shift reagent. These reagents do not cross the cell membrane and thus, interacting only with the extracellular ions, cause a paramagnetic shift in the frequency position of the Na_o signal moving it away from the unshifted position of Na_i.

The discrimination between the ^{23}Na NMR resonances in the two compartments, extracellular and intracellular, is enabled by the fact that the appropriate shift reagents are membrane impermeable, so that only the extracellular resonance is affected by the paramagnetic chelate. The magnetically important moiety in a paramagnetic chelate, serving as a shift reagent, is the lanthanide metal ion. The lanthanides are the 15 elements in the periodic table between atomic numbers 57 and 71. Their trivalent cations display a calcium-like chemistry and form multidentate complexes—*chelates*—with a large number of polyvalent organic and inorganic anions that serve as ligands. Thirteen of the lanthanide ions possess unpaired electrons in their inner (4*f*) electron shell. This property gives rise to the unique magnetic behavior called paramagneticity. This paramagneticity consists of creating a local magnetic field around the lanthanide ion. The effective strength of this field is quite large, and sometimes comparable to that of the external field generated by the magnet of the NMR instrument. Unlike the latter, however, the paramagnetic effect of the lanthanide ion decays within very short distances, typically becoming negligible beyond about 1 nM. Consequently, for an NMR-observed nucleus to be significantly affected, this nucleus has to be within such a short distance from the paramagnetic center. In the case of the positively charged sodium ion, this most likely necessitates the formation of ion pairs with negatively charged functional groups of a ligand complexed to the lanthanide ion (Figure 1).

During the time an individual sodium ion resides in the proximity of the lanthanide metal ion, its NMR spectral parameters will be strongly affected (see above under *Theory*). The intrinsic chemical shift position of the bound sodium is shifted by up to hundreds of parts per million in the ^{23}Na NMR spectrum, its T_1 and T_2 relaxation times are shortened, and its linewidth is extensively increased. Shift reagents, however, are used at a concentration typically 10- to 30-fold lower (4–12 mM/l) than the concentration of Na_o^+ (140 mM). Consequently, the effect of the shift reagent on all the sodium ions is mediated by a constant exchange between the ions bound to the reagent and the much larger pool of ions free in the aqueous solution. Since the rate at which this exchange occurs is fast compared with the relevant NMR time scale, averaging of all NMR parameters takes place between the two pools of sodium ions, the bound and the free. The resulting observed values of chemical shift and relaxation rates then become the weighted averages of the corresponding intrinsic values in the two pools, and the mole fractions of sodium in these pools are the weighting factors. Nevertheless, although the mole fraction of the bound ions is typically quite small, because of the large magnitude of the paramagnetic effect its contribution is still significantly reflected in the weighted average values observed in the actual spectrum.

Because of the short-range effect of lanthanide paramagneticity, sodium ions that have no immediate access to the chelate, and are also in slow exchange with both the

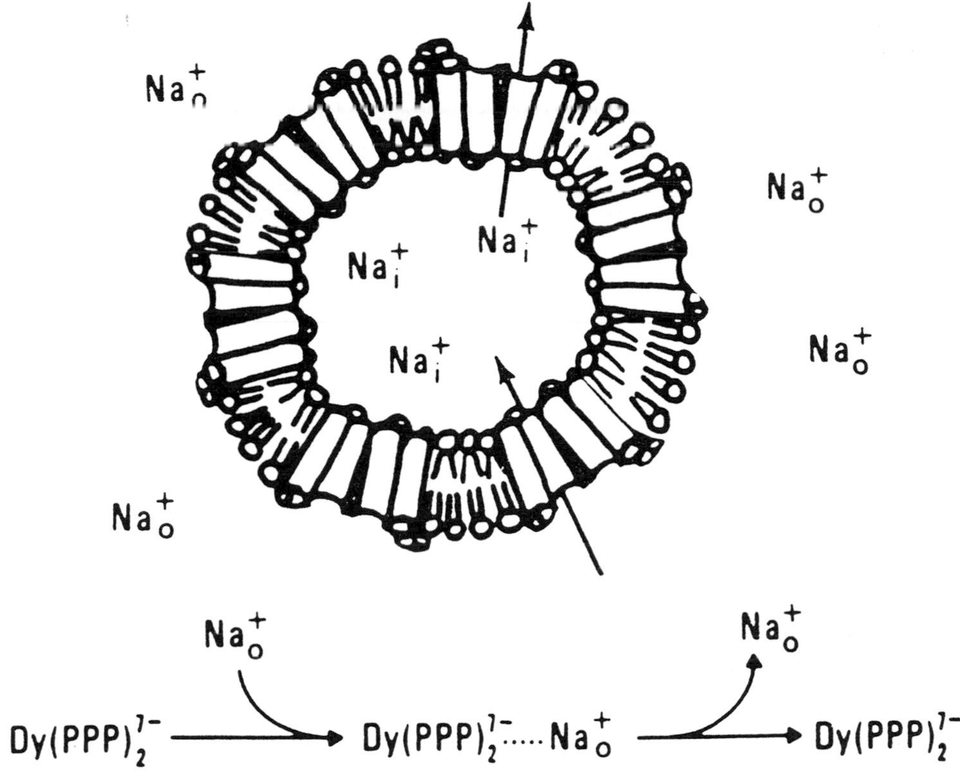

FIGURE 1. *The exchange of sodium ions between intracellular (Na_i^+), free extracellular (Na_O^+), and extracellular shift-reagent bound pools. Reprinted from Elgavish GA: Invest Radiol 1989;24:1028–1033 with permission.*

bound as well as the free extracellular pools, are not affected by the presence of a shift reagent. Such is the case with Na_i when the shift reagent is restricted to the extracellular compartment. The result in the NMR spectrum is the separation of the sodium signal into two resolved resonances: one, arising from Na_o, which is shifted from the original position, and a second resonance, arising from the intracellular pool, which remains unshifted. If there are several compartments that contain sodium ions in slow exchange with the extracellular, shift reagent-affected sodium pool, they all give rise to one superimposed resonance in the unshifted position. Therefore, the method of shift reagent-aided spectroscopy does not differentiate, in principle, among the various possible intracellular pools of sodium ions.

Shift Reagents

Paramagnetic lanthanide metal ions with non–S-state electronic configuration, eg, Dy^{3+}, can affect the chemical shift position of nuclei in their immediate proximity. Furthermore, the lanthanide ion can be chelated to ligands that will preferentially interact with a particular nucleus, such as the triphosphate (PPP) ligand, which binds

Na^+. Also, the choice of ligand can affect the properties of the complex that determine its clinical toxicity, such as a tendency to bind Ca^{2+}. Although a variety of lanthanide chelates have been offered as aqueous shift reagents for cationic NMR, reagents typically used are $Dy(PPP)_2$, Dy(TTHA), where TTHA is triethylenetetramine-hexaacetic acid, and more recently Dy(DOTP) and Tm(DOTP), where DOTP is tetraazacyclododecane-*N, N', N'', N'''*-tetramethylenephosphonate. Recently, polyoxa tetraaza macrocyclic complexes of dysprosium have been synthesized and characterized to serve as calcium inert shift reagents for ^{23}Na NMR.[9] One of them produces a dysprosium complex that is indeed more calcium inert than any other existing reagent, but its small induced shift makes it impractical as a shift reagent for most purposes.

Dy(PPP)₂

Dysprosium chelated to two equivalents of the PPP ligand gives the largest shift known to date, but has a tendency to bind Ca^{2+} and in the presence of 4–6 mM of this reagent only low concentrations (0.1–0.7 mM) of free Ca^{2+} can be routinely attained. Even to attain these levels of free Ca^{2+}, approximately 6–8 mM of $CaCl_2$ need to be added.

Lanthanide complexes containing PPP can be troublesome to use in buffer solutions because they bind Ca^{2+} and may precipitate. Therefore, a balance between added $CaCl_2$ and an acceptable shift must be obtained. The exact manner in which complexes are prepared can have a direct effect on the stability of the buffer solution. Our group has had success with preparing $Dy(PPP)_2$ using a modified procedure of Burstein and Fossel.[10] Two solutions of $Na_5P_3O_{10}$ (PPP) are prepared: the first, a 550-mM solution, is prepared to ensure complete dissolution by adjusting pH between 7 to 8; the second, a 250-mM solution, is prepared without pH adjustment. Dysprosium chloride ($DyCl_3{\cdot}6H_2O$) is dissolved to a concentration of about 250 mM with a pH of 4.8. The exact concentration is determined by colorimetric techniques. The dysprosium stock solution and the 550-mM PPP solution are then mixed in a 1:2 ratio, respectively. A precipitate forms from this mixture. The 250-mM PPP solution is added to this mixture until the precipitate dissolves. The pH is then adjusted to 7.0. We use the $Dy(PPP)_2$ stock in buffer solutions, eg, HEPES, that contain no carbonates. Because of the relatively low solubility of lanthanide carbonates, carbonate ions would cause sequestration and precipitation of lanthanide metal ions from the shift reagent chelate. In some studies, eg, in perfused hearts, extra Ca^{2+} must be added to increase the free Ca^{2+} concentration. This causes some precipitation, and therefore, the final solution is filtered through a micropore filter after the precipitate has settled.

The major problem with $Dy(PPP)_2$ is its high affinity for calcium and the upper limit of about 0.5–0.7 mM it sets to the free Ca^{2+} concentration. This in turn is particularly deleterious in perfused heart experiments because of the direct correlation between the extracellular free calcium concentration (Ca_o^{2+}) and developed contractile force (DF). Nevertheless, this limitation is not as severe as would be expected on the basis of typical DF versus Ca_o^{2+} curves. In isolated perfused rat hearts we have routinely obtained systolic pressures in the range of 50–80 mm Hg, and occasionally 100–120 mm Hg, whereas on the basis of the Ca_o^{2+} concentration as measured by a calcium-specific electrode only about 10–20 mm Hg should be obtained. It seems that calcium is bound to the $Dy(PPP)_2$ chelate and that this bound calcium, not detected by the calcium-specific electrode, serves as "contractile calcium" in addition to Ca_o^{2+}. Indeed, approximately one equivalent of calcium ions has been found bound to $Dy(PPP)_2$ in our buffers prepared for heart perfusion (Chu and Elgavish, unpublished). Unfortunately, however, it seems that some yet unknown and thus experimentally uncontrolled mechanism, possibly an equilibrium between two different structures of the $Dy(PPP)_2{\cdot}Ca$ complex, makes the routine preparation of perfusates that retain contractile function at the level of preshift reagent control difficult despite frequent, but random, success. The existence of such $Dy(PPP)_2{\cdot}Ca$ complexes, most probably with stoichiometries of 1:1 and 2:1, has been shown by ^{43}Ca NMR.[11]

Despite the disadvantages discussed above, $Dy(PPP)_2$ has two major advantages: its large induced shift, which produces excellent spectral resolution, and its simple spectrum, ie, two resonances, which produces a truly unshifted Na_i and an upfield-shifted Na_o signal. Figure 2 shows spectra from a rat heart perfused with $Dy(PPP)_2$ (5.5 mM). A 5.0-ppm shift of the Na_o peak is evident, exposing the Na_i resonance. The Na_o resonance probably contains the contributions of all extracellular compartments, mainly interstitium, vasculature, and the bath surrounding the heart. This seems to indicate that $Dy(PPP)_2$ distributes quickly and homogeneously in all these compartments without creating concentration gradients and complex BMS effects.

Dy(TTHA)

Dy(TTHA) can tolerate large concentrations of Ca^{2+} with the addition of $CaCl_2$ to overcome calcium buffering by the reagent, but the shift is small and the signals are relatively broad and thus Na_i is poorly resolved from the extracellular resonances. Furthermore, Na NMR spectra in organs in the presence of Dy(TTHA) display more signals than with other shift reagents. While sodium spectra of isolated hearts perfused with $Dy(PPP)_2$ consist of only two signals, a relatively sharp unshifted Na_i resonance and a somewhat broadened and upfield-shifted Na_o resonance, spectra of hearts perfused with Dy(TTHA) have seven or eight poorly resolved peaks, with the one assigned as "unshifted" Na_i being in fact shifted 0.5–0.6 ppm downfield.[12,13] A valiant effort was carried out by Kohler et al.[12] to resolve this problem. Through a series of modeling experiments and ischemia and reflow experiments in perfused hearts of various species, they identified the contributions to the sodium spectrum, in the presence of Dy(TTHA), of the four physical compartments in the perfused heart. They also concluded that the Dy(TTHA)-aided Na NMR spectrum is sensitive to effects of BMS and concentration gradients, and thus to heart geometry and positioning and to differences in animal species.

Although their work led to a better understanding of the reasons for the complexity of the Dy(TTHA)-aided ^{23}Na NMR spectrum, the complexity and the typically poor spectral resolution induced by this reagent remain and still hamper reliable Na_i quantitation. Furthermore, several questions remain unanswered. Why is Dy(TTHA) uniquely sensitive to the above mentioned effects, in contrast with other dysprosium chelates? BMS effects, being dependent on the magnetic moment and concentration of the paramagnetic metal ion, should be similar for all dysprosium

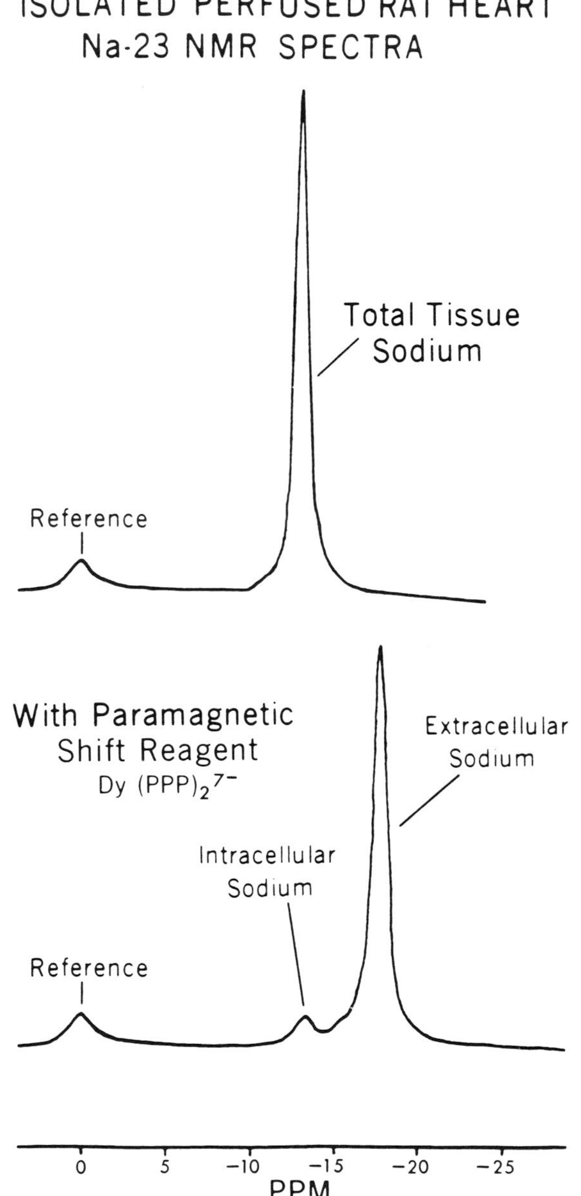

FIGURE 2. *^{23}Na NMR spectra of an isolated perfused rat heart in the absence* **(top)** *and presence* **(bottom)** *of the paramagnetic shift reagent Dy(PPP)$_2$. Reprinted from Elgavish GA: Invest Radiol 1989;24:1028–1033 with permission.*

chelates at similar concentrations. Is it possible that unlike other shift reagents, Dy(TTHA) distributes, and is retained in tissue with a pattern that results in unique compartmentalization and in local concentration gradients? Answers to these questions may be interesting, but these possibilities are hardly an encouragement for the use of this particular shift reagent.

The TTHA ligand is commercially available and forms a stable complex with Dy^{3+}. A slight excess of TTHA (1.1:1) should be coordinated with Dy^{3+} since free Dy^{3+} is quite toxic.[14] The free Ca^{2+} concentration can be adjusted to a high (3 mM) level without precipitation problems. The Dy(TTHA) shift is unaffected by addition of Ca^{2+} and therefore can be used with higher free Ca^{2+} concentrations.

Dy(DOTP) and Tm(DOTP)

A new, stable ^{23}Na shift reagent, $Dy(DOTP)^{5-}$ DOTP is 1,4,7,10-tetraazacyclododecane-N, N′, N″, N‴-tetramethylenephosphonate, has been offered by Sherry et al.[15] With human erythrocytes, it yielded a shift close in magnitude to that generated by $Dy(PPP)_2$, but allowed a somewhat higher free Ca^{2+} concentration in the perfusate.

Several recent studies used Tm(DOTP), a reagent developed by Sherry et al.[15] as a shift reagent for ^{23}Na spectroscopy. Tm(DOTP) produces a slightly larger shift than Dy(TTHA), but not as large as $Dy(PPP)_2$, and can tolerate free Ca^{2+} levels of up to approximately 1.0 mM.[16] Also, Tm(DOTP) does not produce as much line broadening as Dy(TTHA), so even a smaller shift would be sufficient for good resolution between Na_i and Na_o. Tm(DOTP) binds Ca^{2+}, but is stable with added Ca^{2+} up to approximately 1 mM free Ca^{2+}, above which precipitation occurs. Bulk magnetic susceptibility effects and hyperfine shifts were determined for Tm(DOTP) and compared with Dy(TTHA). It was found that Tm(DOTP) has low BMS to hyperfine shift ratios, indicating a dominance of the hyperfine interaction even in the presence of Ca^{2+}, and is comparable to $Dy(PPP)_2$.[17] The DOTP ligand can be synthesized from the HBr salts of the corresponding cyclic amines via a Mannich-type reaction.[15]

In in vivo studies, slightly better resolution of Na_i is achieved with Tm(DOTP) than with Dy(TTHA) but complete resolution of Na_i is not achieved and larger doses appear to be acutely toxic to the rat.[18] The large affinity for Ca^{2+}, the high osmolarity at concentrations required for in vivo experiments, and the instability at high concentrations render Tm(DOTP) difficult, but effective, to use. Several studies with Tm(DOTP) in the heart have been recently presented[17,19] as well as in the eye[20] and in in vivo spectroscopy of the rat head.[18]

Relaxation Methods

Degani and Elgavish[1] first showed that the Na_i and Na_o resonances could be distinguished by paramagnetically modifying the T_1 of the Na_o signal. A relaxation agent, gadolinium ethylenediaminetetraacetic acid [Gd(EDTA)], was devised and added to a suspension of phosphatidylcholine vesicles that had been prepared to contain both intra- and extravesicular Na^+. The Gd(EDTA) complex did not cross

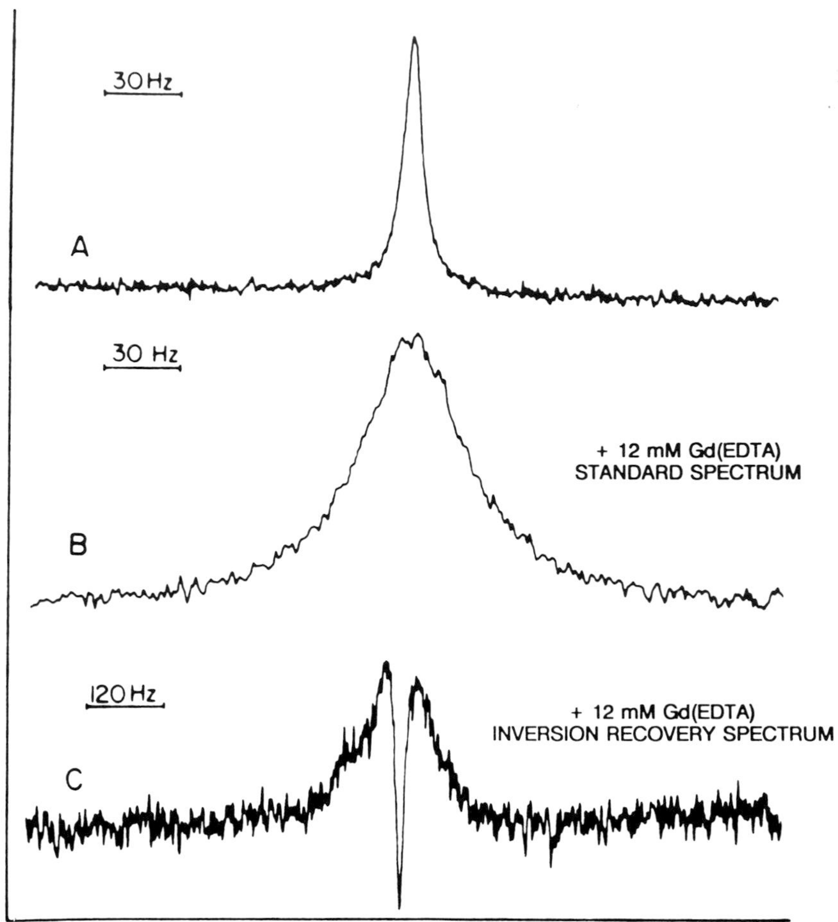

FIGURE 3. *^{23}Na NMR spectra of:* **(A)** *150 mM NaCl dissolved in phosphatidylcholine vesicle suspension P^{2}H 9.2 at 28°C;* **(B)** *the same as (A) after addition of 11.6 mM Gd(EDTA);* **(C)** *the same as (B) using a 180°-τ-90° pulse sequence in order to separate the signal due to the ions trapped in the inner vesicular medium. Forty transients were accumulated in (A) and (B) and 4,800 transients with τ = 4 msec in (C), with a recycle time of 1.1 seconds. Reprinted from Reference 1 with permission.*

the vesicular membrane, and thus only Na_o was appreciably affected by the paramagnetic chelate, shortening its T_1 predominantly by a hyperfine dipolar interaction, but also partly by enhancing its quadripolar relaxation rate.[21] ^{23}Na NMR spectra of the vesicular suspension were acquired using an inversion recovery pulse sequence with an interpulse delay time selected such that the sequence would null the Na_o signal. Since the T_1 of the Na_o signal was paramagnetically shortened, it would also null at a shorter delay time than would the Na_i signal with its now longer T_1. The Na_i signal would now lag in recovery and remain inverted (Figure 3). Since the gadolinium chelate did not introduce any appreciable shift in the chemical shift position, the nulled

Na_o signal and the inverted Na_i signal remained superimposed. This fact has somewhat hindered accurate quantitation of the area of the Na_i signal using this method.

Renshaw et al.[22] exploited alteration of the T_2 value between the Na_o and Na_i. They used dextran-magnetite as a relaxation enhancer because it has the effect of broadening the ^{23}Na signal and is too large to cross the cell membrane. The ^{23}Na resonance in saline has a linewidth of approximately 20 Hz, whereas in the presence of dextran-magnetite in this study it displayed a linewidth of 6,900 Hz. In in vivo measurements where dextran-magnetite was infused into a rat reaching a circulatory concentration of 0.1 μM, the following percent reduction in Na_o was observed: hind leg (14±4), liver (19±2), kidney (47±4), and heart (53±4). This is not the best method for Na_i quantitation because Na_i is not well resolved.

Shift Relaxation Method

The shift relaxation method, developed in the isolated perfused heart system,[23] is a combination of the relaxation method and of the shift method. A similar approach using the relaxation enhancement induced by a shift reagent was shown in solution, and a combined method proffered.[24] Miller et al.[23] used a lanthanide agent such as $Ln(PPP)_2$, in which lanthanide represents both a shift-inducing lanthanide ion, eg, Dy^{3+}, and a lanthanide ion that strongly affects the relaxation rates, ie, Gd^{3+}. As long as these lanthanide chelates do not cross the cell membrane, only the Na_o resonance will experience the shift and relaxation effects.

The ^{23}Na spectra should be acquired using an inversion recovery pulse sequence that consists of a 180° pulse, followed by a delay time τ, followed by a 90° pulse for acquisition. The signal intensity obtained using this pulse sequence is a function of T_1 and τ:

$$M_\tau = M_o(1 - 2e^{-\tau/T_1}) \qquad [6]$$

Based on the difference between the T_1 of the Na_i and the Na_o it is possible to select a τ value that minimizes or nulls the shifted Na_o signal, leaving an Na_i signal that is a constant fraction of its original intensity as long as its T_1 remains constant. To illustrate the differential behavior of the Na_i and Na_o signal intensities induced by this method, the simulated signal intensities of these two resonances generated with an inversion recovery sequence, is shown in Figure 4 as a function of the delay time selected. Using parameters typical for a perfused heart experiment, it is evident that optimal reduction of Na_o would be obtained with τ = 6.2 msec. Actual spectra obtained with 100 scans from a rat heart perfused and submerged in $Dy(PPP)_2$:$Gd(PPP)_2$ at 2.5 mM:2.0 mM concentration are shown in Figure 5. Good resolution was obtained with a 2.5-ppm shift between the Na_i and Na_o resonances. When the spectrum was acquired using an inversion recovery pulse sequence (with τ = 5.5 msec) the Na_o signal was reduced to 6.4%±2.0% of its original intensity, whereas 62%±7% of the equilibrium intensity of Na_i was retained. Since in this method the residual intensity of Na_i is a function of T_1, it is important that the latter remain constant during any experimental perturbations applied.

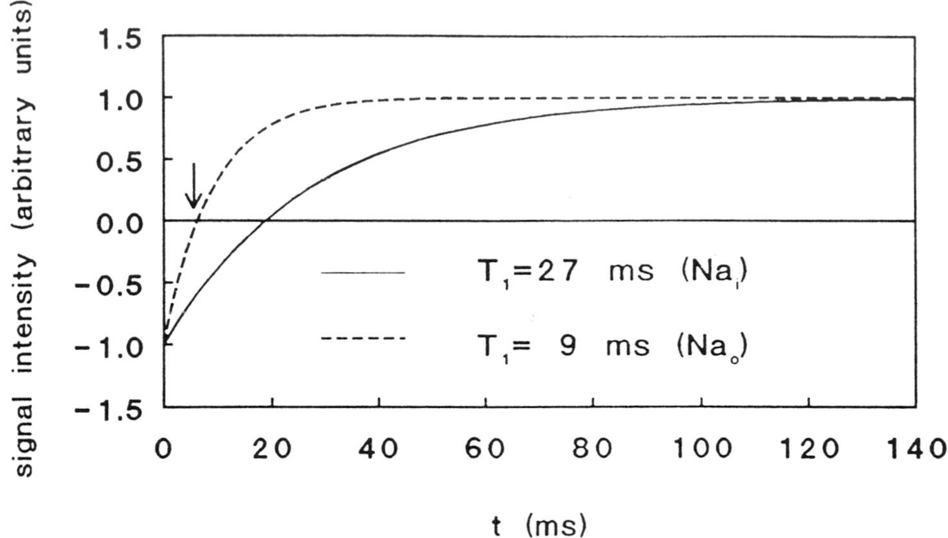

FIGURE 4. *A simulation of signal intensity versus the delay time (τ) using an inversion recovery pulse sequence. Intensities were calculated with $I = I_O(1-2\exp[-\tau/T_1])$, $T_1 = 9$ msec, or $T_1 = 27$ msec, values that represent the T_1 of Na_O in a $Dy(PPP)_2$:$Gd(PPP)_2$ (4 mM:2 mM) perfusate, and the T_1 of Na_I in rat hearts, respectively. Reprinted from Reference 23 with permission.*

Selective Inversion Recovery Method

A disadvantage of the shift relaxation method discussed above is a reduction in the intensity of Na_i resulting from the nonselectivity of the inversion pulse. We have recently developed a selective inversion recovery (SIR) method to minimize the Na_o signal without affecting the intensity of the Na_i resonance and have demonstrated its application in the isolated-perfused rat heart model.[25]

^{23}Na spectra were obtained on a Bruker AM 360 wide-bore NMR spectrometer (8.5 T) equipped with a broadband probe accepting 20-mm sample tubes. The SIR pulse sequence consisted of a "soft" 180° preparation pulse followed by a delay time (τ), followed by a nonselective "hard" 90° sampling pulse and data acquisition. In spectra acquired by this manner, quantitation of Na_i could be carried out with good spectral resolution even in the presence of relatively small shifts (~ 2.5 ppm) between the Na_i and Na_o signals. The ability to improve resolution with such small shifts should allow quantitation of Na_i with calcium-tolerant agents [eg, Dy(TTHA)] that induce relatively small shifts or should allow a reduction in the concentration of $Dy(PPP)_2$. Either way, the deleterious impact of these agents on contractile function can be substantially reduced.

In perfused hearts, to obtain a ^{23}Na NMR spectrum with good resolution using conventional single-pulse acquisition, a shift of at least 5.5 ppm is necessary. This usually requires the use of $Dy(PPP)_2$, which, due to its limiting effect on free Ca^{2+} concentration, depresses (typically to about 50 mm Hg) the left ventricular developed pressure (LVDP). Using a lower concentration of this shift reagent (3.5 mM) or using

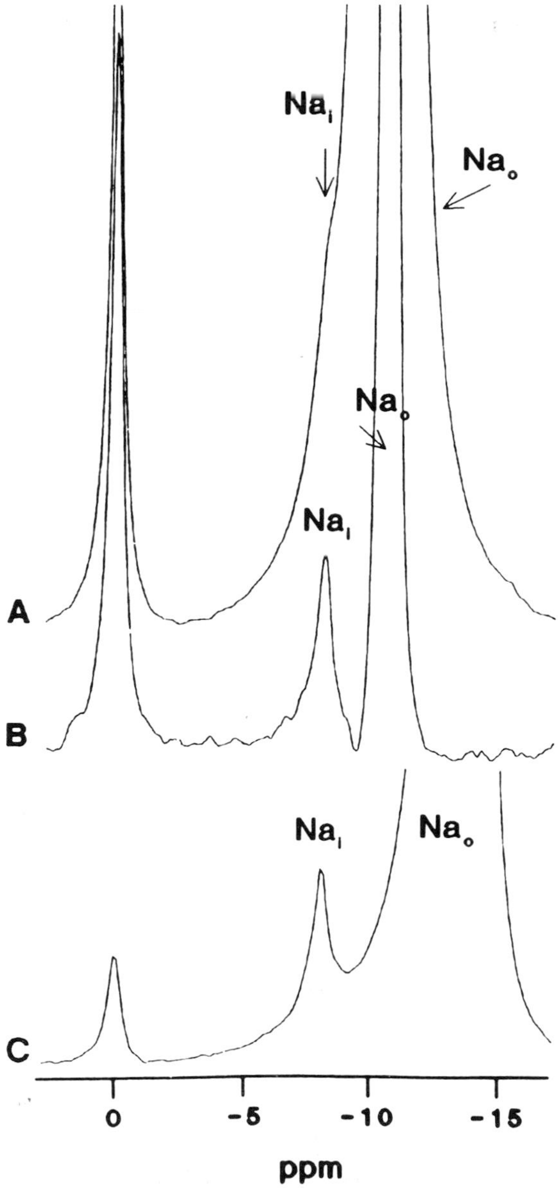

FIGURE 5. *^{23}Na NMR (95.132 MHz) spectra of a rat heart submerged in perfusate, and perfused with* **(A)** *HEPES plus the "shift relaxation" reagent Dy(PPP)$_2$:Gd(PPP)$_2$ (2 mM:2.5 mM) using a 90° one-pulse experiment;* **(B)** *the same perfusate as in (A) with data acquisition by an inversion recovery pulse sequence and phased upright with the scale adjusted such that the reference signal is of the same height as in spectrum (A); and (C) HEPES plus shift reagent Dy(PPP)$_2$ (4.5 mM) using a 90° one-pulse experiment with the scale adjusted such that the Na$_I$ is similar in height to (B). Spectra were acquired with 100 scans, 4,000 data points, and a 1-kHz spectral window. Note the good resolution between Na$_I$ and Na$_O$ in (B) in contrast to only partial resolution in (C). Reprinted from Reference 23 with permission.*

10 mM Dy(TTHA) improves LVDP (to 70–90 mm Hg). The disadvantage, however, is a shift reduced to about 2.5–3 ppm. Presaturating the Na_o resonance in $Dy(PPP)_2$-aided spectra improves resolution, but may affect the Na_i intensity due to saturation transfer.

Figure 6 (I) displays ^{23}Na NMR spectra that were acquired using 10 mM Dy(TTHA). Left ventricular developed pressure was 108% of preshift-reagent control, and induced shift was 2.45 ppm. Spectrum A was acquired by a one-pulse and was filtered by exponential multiplication. In B the same spectrum is shown after Gaussian filtering. Using either of these methods, the typically poor resolution of Na_i obtained with Dy(TTHA) is evident. Spectrum C was obtained with the SIR method. Reasonable resolution allowing quantitative analysis of Na_i was demonstrated.

Figure 6 (II) shows ^{23}Na NMR spectra of isolated rat hearts perfused with HEPES buffer solution containing high (6 mM) (A) or low (3.5 mM) (B, C)

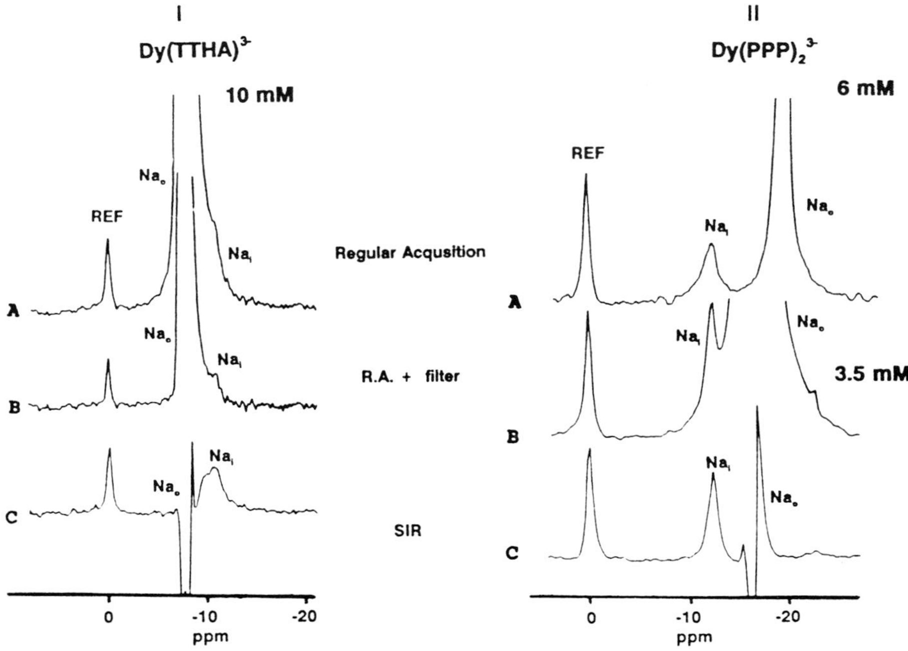

FIGURE 6. *^{23}Na NMR spectra of isolated rat hearts perfused with HEPES buffer containing as shift reagent either Dy(TTHA) (I) or $Dy(PPP)_2$ (II). Spectra **A** and **B** were acquired by one-pulse and were filtered by either exponential multiplication (A) or Gaussian filtering (B). In **(I)**, 10 mM Dy(TTHA) induced a 2.45-ppm downfield shift of Na_O from Na_I; using either of the two filters, the typically poor resolution of Na_I obtained with 10 mM Dy(TTHA) is evident. In **(II,A)**, with 6 mM $Dy(PPP)_2$ Na_I is shifted approximately 6.5 ppm upfield, and the spectrum is well resolved. At the lower $Dy(PPP)_2$ concentration of 3.5 mM heart function is increased, spectral resolution, however, is reduced below Na_I quantifiability. Spectra **C** were obtained with the SIR method. Reasonable resolution allowing quantitative analysis of Na_I is demonstrated both for 10 mM Dy(TTHA) (I, C) and for 3.5 mM $Dy(PPP)_2$ (II, C). Reprinted from Reference 25 with permission.*

concentrations of $Dy(PPP)_2$, respectively. Left ventricular developed pressure in A and B was 50% and 80% of preshift reagent control, respectively. Spectra A and B were obtained with one pulse acquisition. Spectrum B differentiates between Na_o and Na_i, but total separation is not achieved. Spectrum C was obtained with the SIR method. Good spectral resolution is evident, allowing reliable quantitative analysis of Na_i.

Applications

Since the inception of the method of paramagnetic NMR differentiation of Na_i in 1978,[1] an increasing amount of research in biologic systems using ^{23}Na NMR spectroscopy has been carried out by numerous investigators. A comprehensive review of methodology and research using shift reagent-aided ^{23}Na NMR spectroscopy in the heart and other systems is presented in a chapter dedicated to this subject.[26] Therefore, only some recent work from our laboratory is presented here.

In our laboratory, we have used the isolated perfused rat heart model in ^{23}Na NMR experiments using the shift reagent $Dy(PPP)_2$ for monitoring Na_i, specifically in the study of the effects of hypoxia and ischemia, ouabain and amiloride action, and the "staircase" effect induced by increased pacing rate.

Changes in levels of Na_i and high-energy phosphates were monitored during varying durations of hypoxia (<25 mm Hg pO_2) or global ischemia, and upon subsequent 10 minutes of reoxygenation or reflow, in the isolated perfused rat heart to determine possible correlations between Na_i and reversibility of function.[27] All hearts subjected to 20 minutes of hypoxia and three of the six hearts subjected to 30 minutes of hypoxia recovered left ventricular function upon reoxygenation. These hearts also displayed no increase in Na_i during hypoxia. Three of the six hearts subjected to 30 minutes of hypoxia and all hearts subjected to 40 minutes of hypoxia failed to recover function upon reoxygenation. In all nonrecovering hearts, a significant increase in Na_i was detected 27 minutes into hypoxia, and this increased level remained elevated throughout reoxygenation. In hearts subjected to ischemia of 30 minutes or longer, a correlation was found between probability of recovery upon reflow, the extent of Na_i elevation, and duration of ischemia (Figure 7). Contrary to Na_i, high-energy phosphate levels, measured by ^{31}P NMR interleaved with ^{23}Na NMR, were not found to be a predictor of reversibility of left ventricular function in hypoxic or ischemic hearts.

The increase in the level of Na_i, secondary to inhibition of the Na^+-K^+ ATPase by cardiac glycosides, is known to increase calcium influx via Na^+-Ca^{2+} exchange, and therefore lead to an increase in contractile function. This increase in Ca_i^{2+} has been related to the development of intracellular acidification and activation of Na^+-H^+ exchange as a measure to prevent further acidification. Thus, the efflux of intracellular H^+ results in an additional increase in Na_i. This may subsequently lead to an increased rate of Ca^{2+} influx and therefore to the potentiation of the effects of cardiac glycosides. To assess the role of Na^+-H^+ exchange in the mechanism of ouabain action, amiloride, a known inhibitor of the Na^+-H^+ exchanger, was used in a $Dy(PPP)_2$-aided ^{23}Na NMR and ^{31}P NMR study in isolated perfused rat hearts.[28,29]

The results obtained in this study suggested that Na^+-H^+ exchange played a role in ouabain-induced intracellular acidification, that amiloride displayed inhibitory

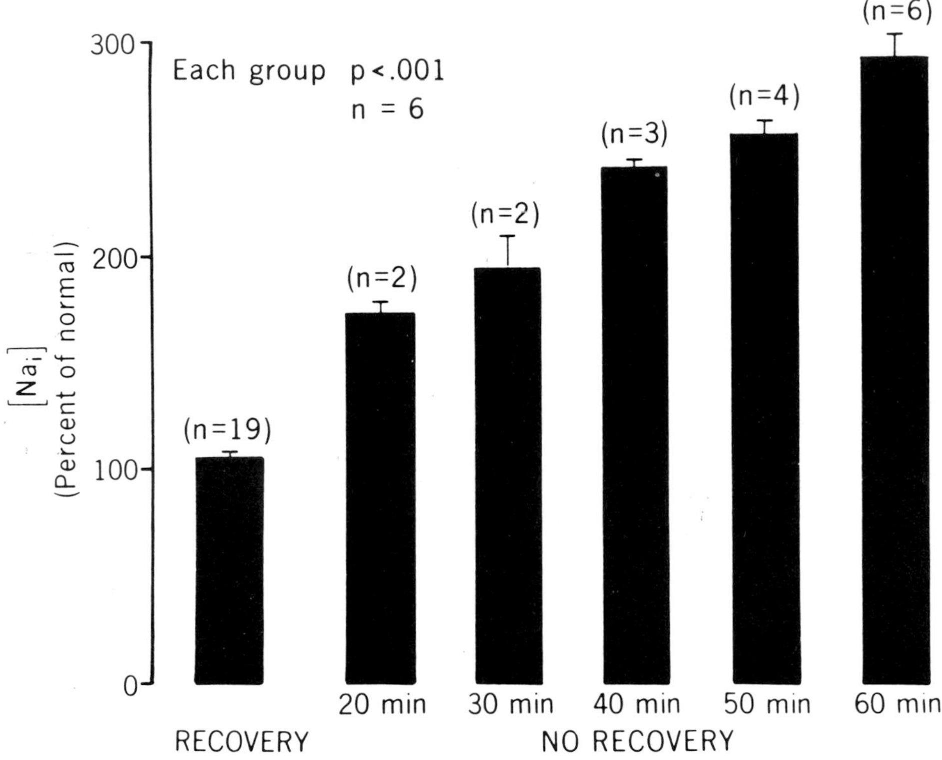

FIGURE 7. *Levels of* Na_i *determined by* ^{23}Na *NMR in the presence of 6 mM* $Dy(PPP)_2$ *in isolated perfused rat hearts after varying durations of total global ischemia and 10 minutes of reperfusion. Five groups of hearts (six hearts in each) were studied, each with either 20, 30, 40, 50, or 60 minutes of ischemia achieved by cross clamping the aortic perfusion line. The mean* Na_i *level in hearts from all groups that recovered at least 90% of preischemic function following 10 minutes of reperfusion* (n = 13) *is shown by the leftmost bar (labeled* Recovery*). The mean* Na_i *levels in nonrecovering hearts are shown by separate bars (labeled* No Recovery*) for each of the five groups with the duration of the ischemic period shown under the bars and the numbers of nonrecovering hearts indicated above the bars. Reprinted from Reference 27 with permission.*

effects beyond its effects on the Na^+-H^+ exchanger, and that the arrhythmogenic effects of cardiac glycosides might be related to the rate of Na_i rise.

The staircase (treppe) phenomenon, or the positive interval-strength relationship, is the increase in myocardial force development resulting from an increase in stimulation frequency. It had been suggested that a rise in Na_i, attributed to a "sodium pump lag," may be the primary cause for the observed changes in developed force. ^{23}Na and ^{31}P NMR spectroscopy, with $Dy(PPP)_2$, were used to assess the relationship between stimulation frequency, level of Na_i, high-energy phosphate stores, intracellular pH, and left ventricular pressure in the isolated perfused rat heart.[30] An increase in the level of Na_i, consistent with the Na^+-K^+ pump lag theory, was found with increasing stimulation frequency (Figure 8). The ultimate pressure response, however, represented a delicate balance between this positive inotropic effect and a negative inotropic effect possibly resulting from the shortening of the time interval between beats (restitution effect).

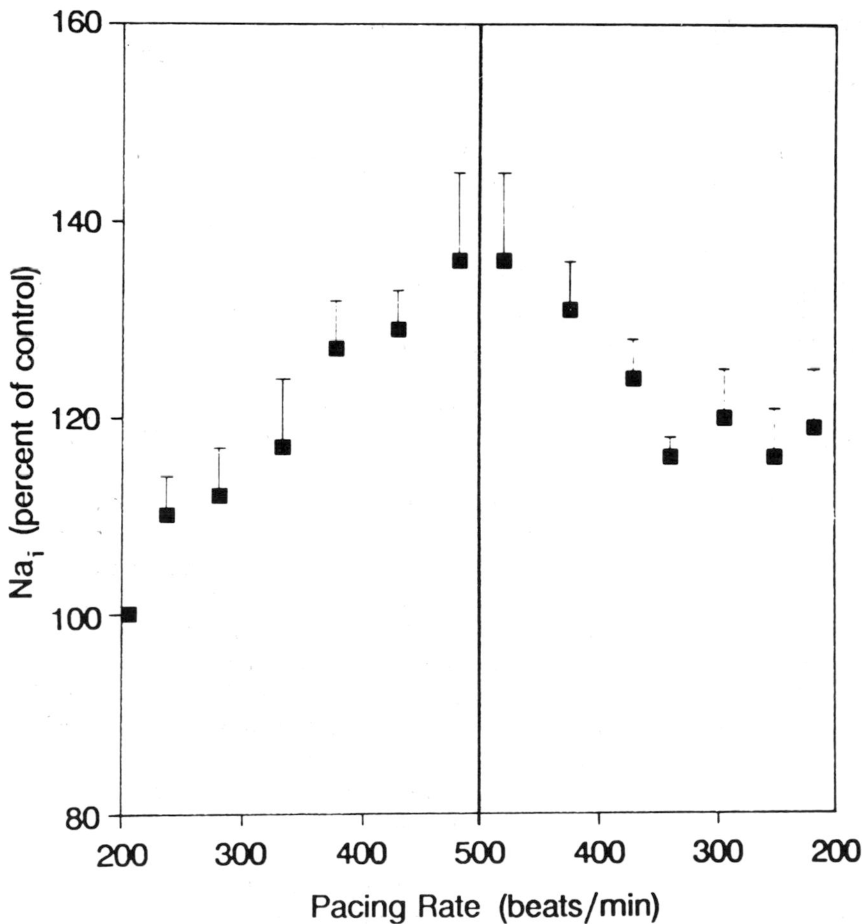

FIGURE 8. *Na_i versus pacing rate (beats per minute) for all hearts (n = 7). Levels of Na_i were determined from the area under the Na_i resonance in ^{23}Na NMR spectra, normalized to the area under the reference signal in the spectrum. Na_i values for each heart were expressed as percent of Na_i level in unpaced control and then averaged for all seven hearts for each pacing rate. Vertical bars denote SEM. Note the almost linear increase of Na_i with upward pacing. A single heart, paced up to 500 beats per minute, displayed an even higher Na_i of 154% (datum not shown). The decline of Na_i with downward pacing is slightly slower, and it does not fully return to control upon termination of pacing. Reprinted from Reference 30 with permission.*

Our group[31] has studied the effect of mild hypoxia on isolated perfused rat hearts externally paced at a constant stimulation frequency of 260 beats per minute. The hearts were perfused with a HEPES buffer that contained 6 mM $Dy(PPP)_2$. In this model of mild hypoxia, oxygen tension was maintained at $pO_2 \sim 100$ mm Hg for 60 minutes followed by 60 minutes of normoxic perfusion. In comparison with the nonrecovery group in the model of severe hypoxia of 30-minute duration and no external pacing (see above and Elgavish et al.[27]), these hearts displayed more limited Na_i accumulation. It seems, therefore, that Na_i increase, and to a larger extent contractile function, seem to be sensitive to the extent of oxygen deprivation, in a manner that a threshold level for possible post-hypoxic recovery seems to exist below 100 mm Hg of pO_2 during hypoxia. The role of controlled stimulation frequency in determining cardiac response to hypoxic conditions, however, requires further clarification.

We also studied the effect of 30 minutes of hypoxia ($pO_2 \sim 25$ mm Hg) followed by 60 minutes of reoxygenation on the T_1 of the Na_i resonance in isolated perfused rat hearts.[32] The Na_i signal was differentiated by 6 mM $Dy(PPP)_2$, and T_1 was measured by an inversion recovery sequence every 5 minutes. Prehypoxic control T_1 of Na_i was found to be 27 ± 1 msec ($n = 8$). Although during hypoxia the level of Na_i increased approximately 50% above prehypoxic control, no significant change in T_1 was found. No such change occurred during reoxygenation, and the overall mean T_1 for Na_i over the entire 120-minute duration of perfusion was determined (27.7 ± 1.8 msec). This observed constancy of T_1 in spite of the increase in the level of Na_i was explained on the basis of the relatively low association constant for the binding of Na^+ to intracellular polyelectrolytes.

Changes in membrane permeability of the Na^+ ion are an important parameter in the action potential and thus in the cardiac cycle. Thus, a shift reagent-aided ^{23}Na NMR spectroscopic approach that enabled the monitoring of the cycle-dependent level of Na_i in the isolated perfused heart would be desirable. We have developed such a method and demonstrated its application to the isolated perfused rat heart paced at a constant rate of 250 beats per minute by means of an external pacemaker.[33] ^{23}Na spectra were obtained on a Bruker AM 360 wide-bore NMR spectrometer. Prior to acquisition, a selective presaturation of 40-msec duration was applied to reduce the intensity of the Na_o signal. "In memory" signal acquisition and the acquisition pulse program shown in Figure 9 (I) were used, allowing a time resolution of FID acquisition every 80 msec. Three hundred scans were averaged to obtain a spectrum for each of the six 40-msec intervals. Three consecutive cardiac cycles were used to provide one scan for each of six different intervals, denoted A through F, of the full cardiac cycle. The first two of each three-cycle set is shown in Figure 9 (I). In the third cycle in each set, only interval A is used for NMR data collection. Each set of six spectra was collected from a total of 900 cardiac cycles, ie, a total of 3.6 minutes per set.

The area under the Na_i peak was determined for each spectrum and expressed as a percent of the Na_i level of the last 40-msec interval of the cardiac cycle (interval F in Figure 9 [I]). Figure 9 (II) depicts the mean ($n = 5$) of the Na_i levels during each of the six intervals. An increase of 14% in Na_i is evident during intervals A and B, which roughly correspond to the depolarization phase of the cardiac cycle. This Na_i level is significantly ($p < 0.05$) higher than those of intervals C–F. Thus, we have developed a

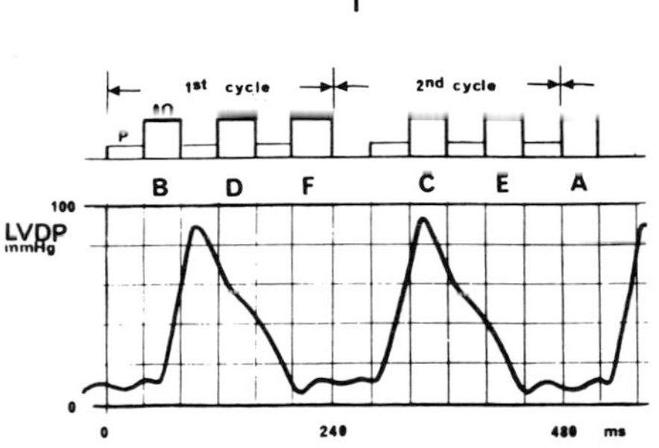

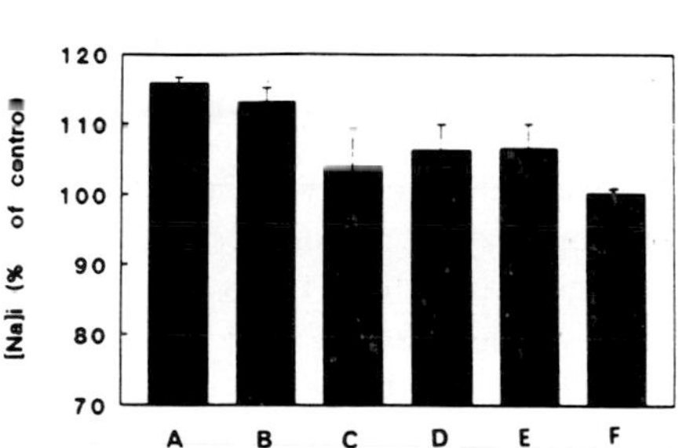

FIGURE 9. (I): *The acquisition pulse program for monitoring by ^{23}Na NMR the heart cycle-dependent level of Na_i.* **(II):** *A shift reagent-aided ^{23}Na NMR spectroscopic monitoring of the cycle-dependent level of Na_i in isolated perfused rat hearts paced at a constant rate of 250 beats per minute by means of an external pacemaker. ^{23}Na spectra were obtained on a Bruker AM 360 wide-bore NMR spectrometer. Prior to acquisition (AQ) a selective presaturation (P) of 40-msec duration was applied to reduce the intensity of the Na_o signal. "In memory" signal acquisition and the acquisition pulse program shown in (I) were used, allowing a time resolution of fixed-interval delay acquisition every 80 msec. Three hundred scans were averaged to obtain a spectrum for each of the six 40-msec intervals. Three consecutive cardiac cycles were used to provide one scan for each of six different intervals, denoted A through F, of the full cardiac cycle. The first two of each three-cycle set is shown in Figure 9 (I). In the third cycle in each set, only interval A is used for NMR data collection. Each set of six spectra was collected from a total of 900 cardiac cycles, ie, a total of 3.6 minutes per set. The area under the Na_i peak was determined for each spectrum and expressed as percent of the Na_i level of the last 40-msec interval of the cardiac cycle (interval F). The mean (n=5) of the Na_i levels during each of the six cycle intervals is depicted. An increase of 14% in Na_i is evident during intervals A and B, which roughly correspond to the depolarization phase of the cardiac cycle. This Na_i level is significantly ($p<0.05$) higher than those of intervals C–F.*

method to obtain Na NMR spectra with a differentiated Na_i resonance at every 40-msec interval in the cardiac cycle. The levels of Na_i during each of six such intervals of the entire cycle show that a significant increase in Na_i takes place during the first 80 msec, as would be anticipated on the basis of the role of Na^+ in the cardiac depolarization phase.

Conclusions

Each of the three major shift reagents currently used suffer from some weakness, either in providing insufficient spectral resolution, thus hampering quantitation, doubts about our full understanding of its compartmental distribution, or because of physiologically deleterious interaction with calcium ions. Furthermore, the validity of conclusions with regard to absolute Na_i concentrations needs to be cautiously scrutinized in light of questions about spectral visibility and limitations of methodology.[26]

Nevertheless, while bearing in mind the limitations, useful work has been carried out during the last decade using shift reagent-aided ^{23}Na NMR spectroscopy in a wide array of biologic systems in general, and in the heart in particular.[26] To date, it seems that there is no single shift reagent and spectral technique that are best for all experimental systems, but rather, optimal results can be achieved by selecting the appropriate agent and spectral technique for the particular experimental conditions. For instance, when good spectral resolution is required in a relatively short time, eg, in heart cycle studies, and medium levels of calcium concentrations are tolerable, $Dy(PPP)_2$ would be the reagent of choice. Ultimately, a calcium-tolerant, nontoxic reagent, which also induces reasonably large shifts (4–5 ppm) at relatively low concentrations (3–4 mM), and whose compartmental distribution is well understood, should emerge for shift reagent-aided ^{23}Na NMR spectroscopy to become a standard in vivo research technique, and eventually a useful clinical tool.

References

1. Degani H, Elgavish GA: ^{23}Na and ^{7}Li NMR studies of ion transport across the membrane of phosphatidylcholine vesicles. *FEBS Lett* 1978;90:357–360.
2. Gupta RJ, Gupta P: Direct observations of resolved resonances from intra- and extracellular sodium-23 ions in NMR studies of intact cells and tissues using dysprosium (III) tripolyphosphate as paramagnetic shift reagent. *J Magn Reson* 1982;47:344-350.
3. Pike MM, Springer CS Jr: Aqueous shift reagents for high resolution cationic nuclear magnetic resonance. *J Magn Reson* 1982;46:348.
4. Bleaney B: Nuclear magnetic resonance shifts in solution due to lanthanide ions. *J Magn Reson* 1972;8:91.
5. Reuben J, Fiat D: Nuclear magnetic resonance studies of solutions of the rare earth ions and their complex. IV. Concentration and temperature dependence of the oxygen-17 transverse relaxation in aqueous solutions. *J Chem Phys* 1969;51:4918.
6. Gueron M: Nuclear relaxation in macromolecules by paramagnetic ions: A novel mechanism. *J Magn Reson* 1975;19:58.
7. Vega AJ, Fiat D: Nuclear relaxation processes of paramagnetic complexes. The slow motion case. *Mol Physiol* 1976;11:347.
8. Elgavish GA, Reuben J: Aqueous lanthanide shift reagents. III. Interaction of the EDTA chelates with substituted ammonium cations. *J Am Chem Soc* 1977;99:1762–1765.
9. Sink RM, Buster DC, Sherry AD: Synthesis and characterization of a series of macrocyclic chelates containing O-donors and N-donors. Prospects for alkali-metal cations. *Inorg Chem* 1990;29:3645.
10. Burstein D, Fossel ET: Nuclear magnetic resonance studies of intracellular ions in perfused frog hearts. *Am J Physiol* 1987;252:H1138-H1146.
11. Vogel HJ, Braunlin WH: Shift reagents for calcium-43 NMR studies of calcium-binding proteins. *J Magn Reson* 1985;62:42–53.
12. Kohler SJ, Perry SB, Stuart LC, et al: Analysis of ^{23}Na NMR spectra from isolated perfused hearts. *Magn Reson Med* 1991;18:15–27.
13. Pike MM, Frazier JC, Dedrick DF, et al: ^{23}Na and ^{39}K NMR studies of perfused, beating, rat hearts: discrimination of intra- and extracellular ions using a shift reagent. *Biophys J* 1985;48:159–173.
14. Evans CH: *Biochemistry of the Lanthanides*. New York: Plenum Press; 1990:339–380.
15. Sherry AD, Malloy CR, Jeffrey FMH, et al: $Dy(DOTP)^{5-}$: a new stable ^{23}Na shift reagent. *J Magn Reson* 1988;76:528–533.
16. Buster DC, Castro MMCA, Geraldes CFGC, et al: $Tm(DOTP)^{5-}$ a $^{23}Na^{+}$ shift agent for perfused rat hearts. *Magn Reson Med* 1990;15:25–32.
17. Kohler SJ, Ingwall JS, Kolodny NH: Evaluation of $TmDOPT^{5-}$ as a shift reagent for

^{23}Na spectroscopy and ^{23}Na chemical shift imaging (abstract). In: Proceedings of the 9th Annual Meeting of the Society of Magnetic Resonance in Medicine. 1990;39.

18. Albert MS, Lee J-H, Springer CS Jr: The use of $TmDOTP^{5-}$ as a ^{23}Na shift reagent in living rat studies at 9.4 T (abstract). In: Proceedings of the 9th Annual Meeting of the Society of Magnetic Resonance in Medicine. 1990:1269.
19. Pike MM, Clark D, Kitakaze Madden M, et al: ^{23}Na and ^{39}K nuclear magnetic resonance studies of perfused rat hearts (abstract). In: Proceedings of the 9th Annual Meeting of the Society of Magnetic Resonance in Medicine. 1990:40.
20. Kolodny NH, Kohler S, Weinberg D, et al: Dynamic three-dimensional ^{23}Na chemical shift imaging as a probe of ocular processes (abstract). In: Proceedings of the 9th Annual Meeting of the Society of Magnetic Resonance in Medicine. 1990:666.
21. Elgavish GA: The interaction of 1:1 and 1:2 lanthanide EDTA chelates with alkali cations. Aqueous relaxation reagents for metal nuclide NMR. In: McCarthy GJ, Silber HB, Rhyne JJ (eds) *The Rare Earth in Modern Science and Technology*. New York: Plenum Press; 1982:193–198.
22. Renshaw PF, Blum H, Leigh JS Jr: Applications of dextran-magnetite as a sodium relaxation enhancer in biological systems. *J Magn Reson* 1986;69:523–526.
23. Miller SK, Chu WJ, Pohost GM, Elgavish GA: Improvement of spectral resolution in shift-reagent-aided ^{23}NMR spectroscopy in the isolated perfused rat heart system. *Magn Reson Med* 1991;20:184–195.
24. Brown MA, Stenzel TT, Ribeiro AA, et al: NMR studies of combined lanthanide shift and relaxation agents for differential characterization of ^{23}Na in a two-compartment model system. *Magn Reson Med* 1986;3:289–295.
25. Simor T, Kim SK, Chu WJ, et al: A selective inversion recovery method for the improvement of ^{23}Na NMR spectral resolution in isolated perfused rat hearts (abstract). In: Proceedings of the 10th Annual Meeting of the Society of Magnetic Resonance in Medicine. 1991:1189.
26. Miller SK, Elgavish GA: Shift-reagent-aided ^{23}Na NMR spectroscopy in cellular, tissue and whole-organ systems. In: Berliner LJ, Reuben J (eds) *Biological Magnetic Resonance*. Volume 11. New York: Plenum Press; 1992:159–240.
27. Elgavish GA, Foster RE, Canby RC, Pohost GM: Prediction of reversibility of function in the hypoxic or ischemic isolated perfused heart using sodium-23 and phosphorus-31 NMR (abstract). In: Proceedings of the 6th Annual Meeting of the Society of Magnetic Resonance in Medicine. 1987:512.
28. Lotan C, Miller SK, Pohost GM, Elgavish GA: The role of Na-H exchange in ouabain induced intracellular acidification. A ^{23}Na and ^{31}P NMR study in isolated, perfused rat hearts (abstract). In: Proceedings of the 7th Annual Meeting of the Society of Magnetic Resonance in Medicine. 1988:37.
29. Lotan C, Miller SK, Pohost GM, Elgavish GA: Amiloride in ouabain-induced acidification, inotropy and arrhythmia: ^{23}Na and ^{31}P NMR in perfused hearts. *J Mol Cell Cardiol* 1992;24:243–257.
30. Miller SK, Lotan C, Hefner LL, et al: Real-time ^{23}Na NMR measurement of intracellular sodium level in isolated perfused rat hearts during stepped pacing: evidence supporting the Na pump lag theory (abstract). In: Proceedings of the 8th Annual Meeting of the Society of Magnetic Resonance in Medicine. 1989:497.
31. Chu WJ, Kim SK, Pohost GM, Elgavish GA: Correlation between intracellular sodium levels and heart function in hypoxic, isolated, perfused rat hearts: a ^{23}Na-NMR study (abstract). In: Proceedings of the 9th Annual Meeting of the Society of Magnetic Resonance in Medicine. 1990:916.
32. Prince LS, Miller SK, Pohost GM, Elgavish GA: The longitudinal relaxation time (T_1) of the intracellular ^{23}Na NMR signal in the isolated perfused rat heart during hypoxia and reoxygenation. *Magn Reson Med* 1992;23:376–382.
33. Elgavish GA, Simor T, Kim SK, et al: Cardiac cycle dependence of the level of intracellular Na in isolated perfused rat hearts: a gated ^{23}Na NMR spectroscopy study. Fifteenth International Congress on Biochemistry. Jerusalem, Israel, August 4–8, 1991, pp. 192.

Chapter 31

Measurement of Intracellular Ca^{2+} in Intact Perfused Hearts by ^{19}F Nuclear Magnetic Resonance

Hideo Kusuoka, MD, PhD, V.P. Chacko, PhD, and Eduardo Marban, MD, PhD

Intracellular Ca^{2+} is both vital to the function of the heart (as the activator of contraction) and potentially lethal (as a mediator of cellular injury in ischemia and reperfusion).[1] Until recently, little direct information has been available regarding the regulation of the intracellular free Ca^{2+} concentration ($[Ca^{2+}]_i$) in intact perfused hearts. Most of our understanding of $[Ca^{2+}]_i$ in myocardium was derived from superfused papillary muscles[2,3] or single cells.[4] The extrapolation of measurements of $[Ca^{2+}]_i$ from such preparations to the intact heart requires a number of untested assumptions. This restricts the potential for understanding the consequences of altered coronary flow, because such a situation can only be mimicked in superfused preparations. Direct measurements of $[Ca^{2+}]_i$ in perfused hearts are clearly desirable.

Three strategies have recently been used to estimate $[Ca^{2+}]_i$ in perfused hearts. One uses the fluorescent Ca^{2+} indicators quin-2 or indo-1.[5,6] When narrow-band ultraviolet (UV) light is focused on hearts loaded with these indicators, the resultant fluorescent emission from epicardium varies as a function of $[Ca^{2+}]_i$. In a second strategy, the bioluminescent calcium indicator aequorin is used. Aequorin is loaded into subepicardial myocytes by microinjection[7] or by extracellular macroinjection.[8] Aequorin emits light as a complex but direct function of $[Ca^{2+}]_i$. Both optical techniques potentially have rapid time resolution, but are limited by several problems as discussed later.

The third strategy uses a fundamentally different principle: nuclear magnetic resonance (NMR) spectroscopy is used to measure a Ca^{2+}-sensitive chemical change. Smith et al.[9] have developed ^{19}F NMR-detectable Ca^{2+} indicators by fluorinating the Ca^{2+} chelator BAPTA [1,2-bis(o-aminophenoxy) ethane-*N,N,N′,N′*-tetraacetic acid]. The derivative that appears best suited for measuring physiologic levels of $[Ca^{2+}]_i$ and that has been applied most extensively is 5,5′-F_2-BAPTA (5F-BAPTA), the structure of which is depicted in Figure 1A.

This study was supported by the National Institutes of Health (Specialized Center of Research Grant number HL17655) and R01 HL44065.
From Pohost GM (ed.), *Cardiovascular Applications of Magnetic Resonance*. Mount Kisco, NY, Futura Publishing Co., Inc., © 1993.

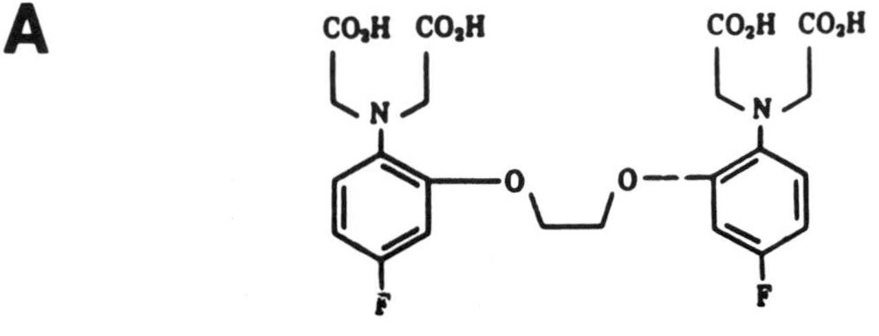

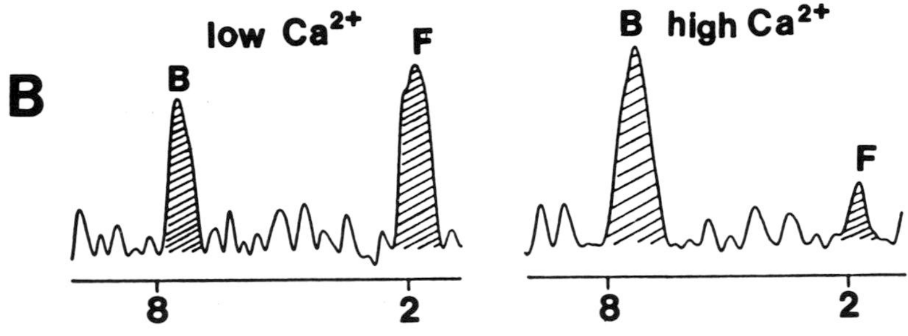

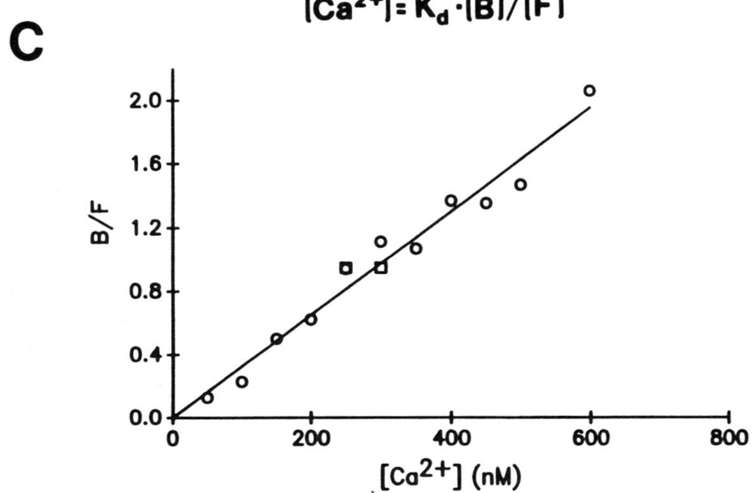

FIGURE 1. **A:** *Molecular structure of 5F-BAPTA.* **B:** *^{19}F NMR spectra obtained from a heart loaded with 5F-BAPTA. B and F indicate the peaks for calcium-bound 5F-BAPTA and calcium-free 5F-BAPTA, respectively. Note that the right spectrum shows a larger peak for B and a smaller peak for F than the left one, indicating that* $[Ca^{2+}]_i$ *in the right is higher than the left.* **C:** *Calibration curve of 5F-BAPTA at 30°C. Ratio of the bound-to-free 5F-BAPTA concentration in the cytoplasm (B/F) is plotted as a function of* $[Ca^{2+}]$ *in each solution at pH 7.2 (circles). The line is a least-squares fit to all data points, constrained to pass through the origin. The two square symbols represent samples at pH 6.4, not included in regressing the line.*

In this chapter, we describe the measurement of $[Ca^{2+}]_i$ in intact perfused hearts using ^{19}F NMR with 5F-BAPTA and discuss the characteristics of the $[Ca^{2+}]_i$ measurements by the three different techniques.

Measurements of $[Ca^{2+}]_i$ by ^{19}F Nuclear Magnetic Resonance

Perfused Heart Preparation

We chose ferret hearts for most of our experiments, primarily because measurements of $[Ca^{2+}]_i$ are plentiful in isolated ventricular muscle from this species,[2,3] facilitating direct comparison with our results. Ferret hearts are also quite hardy and are conveniently sized for experiments in high-field wide-bore magnets. This technique has also been successfully applied to rat[10,11] and rabbit hearts.[12]

The method for the perfusion of isolated hearts has been described in detail.[13–15] Briefly, hearts are excised from male ferrets (10–14 weeks of age) that are anesthetized with sodium pentobarbital and heparinized. The hearts are Langendorff-perfused at 30°C with a modified Tyrode's solution of the following composition (in millimoles): NaCl 108, KCl 5, $MgCl_2$ 1, HEPES 5, $CaCl_2$ 2, glucose 10, and sodium acetate 20 (pH adjusted to 7.4 by titration with NaOH). The perfusate is bubbled continuously with 100% oxygen. A thin latex balloon tied to the end of a polyethylene tube is inserted into the left ventricle through the mitral valve and is connected to a pressure transducer (Statham P23ID, Gould, Oxford, CA) to monitor left ventricular contractility. The balloon is filled with 1 mM 6-fluorotryptophan (6F-Trp) as a standard for the calcium measurements by ^{19}F NMR spectroscopy. The balloon volume is generally set to achieve an initial end-diastolic pressure of 8–12 mm Hg, then kept isovolumic throughout each experiment. Left ventricular pressure and perfusion pressure are recorded on a chart recorder. After 10–20 minutes of stabilization, coronary flow rate, controlled by a peristaltic pump, is adjusted such that perfusion pressure equals 80–90 mm Hg. The heart rate is controlled by right ventricular pacing with an agar wick soaked in saturated KCl, encased in polyethylene tubing, and connected to a stimulator.

^{19}F Nuclear Magnetic Resonance Measurements of Time-Averaged $[Ca^{2+}]_i$

To obtain the NMR signals, the preparation is lowered into a 25-mm diameter NMR tube and placed into the wide-bore superconducting magnet of a 360-MHz spectrometer (8.5 T) (Bruker Intruments, Billerica, MA).

As previously described,[14,16] the Ca^{2+} indicator 5F-BAPTA (Figure 1A) is loaded into cells by perfusion with its tetraacetoxymethyl ester derivative (5F-BAPTA-AM). We add 12.5 μM 5F-BAPTA-AM (Molecular Probes, Eugene, OR) to the perfusate for 15–17 minutes to achieve a favorable signal-to-noise ratio in a ^{19}F NMR spectrum. The perfusate is then switched to modified Tyrode's solution and supplemented with 1 mM probenecid (Sigma, St. Louis, MO) to minimize the time-dependent extrusion of 5F-BAPTA from myocardial cells.[16] In some experiments, extracellular calcium concentration ($[Ca]_o$) is increased to 8 mM to partially antagonize the substantial negative inotropic effect of the calcium buffering induced by 5F-BAPTA.[14]

^{19}F NMR spectra are obtained on a 25-mm broad-band probe, the ^{1}H decoupling coil of which was tuned to the ^{19}F resonance frequency (338.86 MHz). The free induction decays from the hearts are accumulated with 1,000-kHz data points at a spectral width of about 5 kHz using 70° pulses delivered at repetition intervals of 0.4 seconds. All chemical shifts are referenced with respect to the signal of 6F-Trp, which is conventionally assigned a value of 0 ppm.

Temperature can be maintained at the desired value (±1°C) by appropriate prewarming of the perfusate, supplemented with a thermostatically controlled air jacket around the NMR tube.

Determination of $[Ca^{2+}]_i$ from Nuclear Magnetic Resonance Spectra

As shown in Figure 1B, the fluorine NMR spectra from a heart loaded with 5F-BAPTA consist of two signals, one from the free ligand at ≈2 ppm (F in Figure 1B), and another at ≈8 ppm for the calcium-bound species (B in Figure 1B). Because the area under each peak is proportional to the concentration of each species, and the calcium binding reaction exhibits 1:1 stoichiometry, $[Ca^{2+}]_i$ can be calculated as follows:

$$[Ca^{2+}]_i = k_d\,([B]/[F]),$$

where k_d is the dissociation constant of calcium 5F-BAPTA, [B] is the area under the Ca-5F-BAPTA peak, and [F] is the area under the calcium free 5F-BAPTA peak. [B] and [F] were obtained by planimetry using a digitizer.

Calibration of 5F-BAPTA

The value of the K_d for calcium binding to 5F-BAPTA remains controversial. Values of 635 nM[17] and 710 nM[9] at 37°C have been previously reported, but the method to control $[Ca^{2+}]$ in both reports is problematic.[15] In contrast, we previously found a K_d of 285 nM at 30°C and pH 7.2 with a more direct method to control $[Ca^{2+}]$.[14]

Because of the discrepancy among the various reported values, we have rechecked the K_d using a somewhat different strategy.[15] Fluorine NMR spectra were acquired from solutions of 5F-BAPTA (200 μM) in which the desired $[Ca^{2+}]$ was achieved by varying the calcium added to a fixed amount of EGTA buffer (20 mM). Figure 1C shows the results of such a calibration for 5F-BAPTA, in which [B]/[F] is plotted as a function of $[Ca^{2+}]_i$. The data are well fit by a line passing through the origin; linear regression ($r = 0.984$) yields a K_d (1/slope) of 308±26 nM (mean±SD). Our previous value of 285 nM falls within one standard deviation of the newer estimate;

since this difference is certainly within the range of experimental error, we have chosen to continue to use the older value for the sake of consistency.

The close agreement between the present and the former K_d determinations, performed with and without 1 mM magnesium, respectively, confirms the claim[9] that magnesium has little effect on the calcium affinity of 5F-BAPTA. We also checked whether the K_d might be changed at acid pH comparable with that reached in cells during ischemia. As the two data points plotted as squares in Figure 1C show, the values for $[Ca^{2+}]$ versus [B]/[F] at pH 6.4 agree quite well with those at pH 7.2. Thus, it is unlikely that the changes in pH_i or $[Mg^{2+}]_i$ expected during ischemia will require substantial modification of the K_d used to calculate $[Ca^{2+}]_i$.

^{19}F Nuclear Magnetic Resonance Measurements of Calcium Transients

Our low values for the k_d of calcium 5F-BAPTA are entirely consistent with its well-described ability to buffer intracellular Ca^{2+} and thereby to blunt contractile force development. Given that the cytoplasmic concentration of 5F-BAPTA must be minimized in order to preserve at least moderate contractility, the signal-to-noise ratio under optimal recording conditions at 8.5 T necessitates at least 1 minute of data acquisition per spectrum (eg, Koretsune and Marban[18]); 5 minutes is a more typical value for the time required to obtain each measurement. For investigation of excitation-contraction coupling in the heart, temporal resolution must be rapid relative to the known duration of the transient rise in $[Ca^{2+}]_i$ during each heartbeat (the "Ca^{2+} transient," which lasts only 100–200 msec).[19]

To satisfy the desire for temporal resolution despite the need for signal averaging, we gated the spectra with respect to each cardiac cycle. The methods have been described in detail previously.[16] The excitatory radiofrequency pulses and the subsequent NMR data acquisition were gated according to a programmable delay from the time of the pacing stimulus. Two pacemakers were used for gating. The first, which set the overall cycle length, supplied a synchronization signal to the pulse programmer controlling the spectrometer and to a second pacemaker that stimulated the heart with no delay.

For gated NMR data acquisition, one pulse was applied during each cycle. At each point in the cardiac cycle, 300–800 consecutive gated scans were averaged to achieve an acceptable signal-to-noise ratio. Figure 2 (middle row) shows ^{19}F NMR spectra obtained at the two times during the cardiac cycle indicated on the pressure record (top): a, 10 msec before the stimulus and b, 75 msec after the stimulus. At time a, just before the pacing stimulus, the bound peak (B) at 8 ppm is smaller than the free peak (F) at 2 ppm ([B]/[F] = 0.62), corresponding to a diastolic $[Ca^{2+}]_i$ of 177 nM. Just 75 msec after the stimulus (b), however, the spectrum changes dramatically: the bound peak now exceeds the free ([B]/[F] = 2.9), yielding a $[Ca^{2+}]_i$ of nearly 1 μM. By obtaining ^{19}F NMR spectra at various delay settings during the cardiac cycle, we can map out the change in $[Ca^{2+}]_i$ during each contraction (the Ca^{2+} transients; Figure 2, bottom). This method has provided useful measurements of Ca^{2+} transients in whole hearts under various steady-state conditions.[15,16,18,20–22]

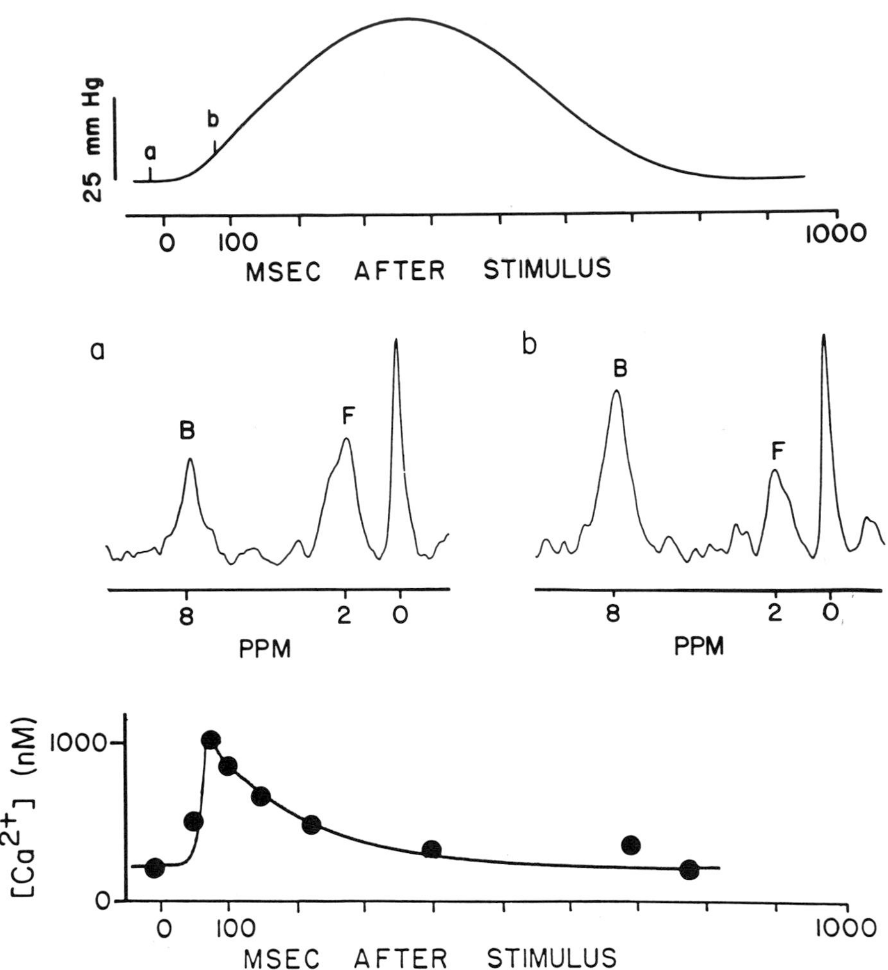

FIGURE 2. *Changes in gated NMR spectra during the cardiac cycle and the Ca^{2+} transient derived from such spectra.* **Top panel:** *Isovolumic left ventricular pressure in a ferret heart paced at 0.99 Hz in 8 mM $[Ca]_O$. Nuclear magnetic resonance (NMR) spectra were acquired at the two times indicated on the pressure record:* **a:** *10 msec prior to stimulation;* **b:** *75 msec after stimulation. Middle panel shows gated ^{19}F NMR spectra (each from acquisition of 800 free induction delays) recorded at a and b, as indicated. The bound (B) and free (F) peaks of 5F-BAPTA exhibit distinct chemical shifts at ≈8 and ≈2 ppm, respectively, downfield from a standard of 1 mM 6F-Trp at 0 ppm.* **Bottom panel** *shows a Ca^{2+} transient obtained with ^{19}F NMR by sampling at various times throughout the cardiac cycle.*

Characterization of $[Ca^{2+}]_i$ Measurements Using ^{19}F Nuclear Magnetic Resonance

Stability of Intracellular [5F-BAPTA]

The presence of 6F-Trp occupying a known volume in the ventricular balloon allows us to estimate the myocardial concentration of 5F-BAPTA (see Kusuoka et al.[13]). Intracellular [5F-BAPTA] remains quite stable after washout of 5F-BAPTA-AM when working at 30°C,[14] but less so at 37°C. The progressive decrease in [5F-BAPTA] at 37°C may reflect a slow loss of the indicator from cells, which also occurs with quin-2.[5] For this reason, and also because most measurements of $[Ca^{2+}]_i$ in isolated ferret ventricular muscle have been performed at 30°C, we favored the lower temperature.

Such stability of intracellular [5F-BAPTA] at 30°C was observed not only during well-oxygenated control conditions, but also during ischemia and reperfusion. Intracellular [5F-BAPTA] did not change significantly during 50 minutes of ischemia[23] at 30°C or during 30-minute reperfusion after 20-minute ischemia at 30°C.[14,15]

Compartmentalization of 5F-BAPTA

One of the major problems that has plagued the use of fluorescent Ca^{2+} indicators loaded by the acetoxymethyl ester method is compartmentalization, both intracellular and intercellular.

Intracellular compartmentalization is due to the preferential uptake of the AM form of Ca^{2+} indicators by mitochondria.[24] The common signs of such a problem are small Ca^{2+} transients and falsely low estimates for $[Ca^{2+}]_i$. Our estimates of Ca^{2+} transients in perfused hearts show no hint of such problems: during each cardiac cycle, $[Ca^{2+}]_i$ changes rapidly (in <100 msec) by an order of magnitude consistent with estimates from the cytoplasmic Ca^{2+} indicator aequorin.[19] Furthermore, the mitochondrial fraction isolated from the hearts that had been loaded with 5F-BAPTA in the usual manner generally contained no measurable ^{19}F.[15] Thus, these data indicate that essentially all the NMR visible 5F-BAPTA is confined to the cytosol.

Intercellular compartmentalization is due to the accumulation of the Ca^{2+} indicators by endothelial cells. Lorell and co-workers[25] have recently demonstrated that bradykinin, at concentrations that raise endothelial (but not myocardial) $[Ca^{2+}]_i$, causes a pronounced increase in 'diastolic' fluorescence in hearts loaded with indo-1 by the AM method. Epifluorescence microscopy of slices from such hearts additionally verifies the idea that indo-1 is particularly concentrated within endothelial cells. In contrast to indo-1, this is not the case for 5F-BAPTA; $[Ca^{2+}]_i$ at end diastole measured by gated ^{19}F NMR with 5F-BAPTA showed no changes with bradykinin.[15] Thus, the measurements of $[Ca^{2+}]_i$ using ^{19}F NMR with 5F-BAPTA are fortunately free from the intracellular or intercellular compartmentalization problems that complicate the measurement of $[Ca^{2+}]_i$ by fluorescent indicators.

Strengths and Limitations of the 5F-BAPTA and Nuclear Magnetic Resonance Methods

A number of observations support the validity of our estimates of $[Ca^{2+}]_i$ from 5F-BAPTA. First, intracellular [5F-BAPTA] at 30°C is quite stable: no bleaching (unlike fluorescent dyes) and no consumption (unlike aequorin). Second, the calibration of 5F-BAPTA is relatively insensitive to changes in Mg^{2+} or pH; acidosis or increases in $[Mg^{2+}]$ significantly reduce light emission of aequorin.[26] Third, compartmentalization into organelles is negligible. Fourth, the absence of a response to bradykinin implies that signals from endothelial cells do not dominate the measured spectra. Fifth, de-esterification of 5F-BAPTA-AM appears to be prompt and complete.[15] Sixth, the extent of the errors in quantification introduced by time averaging are small relative to changes recorded during ischemia.[15] Under steady-state conditions, gating can be used to achieve millisecond temporal resolution. Finally, hearts loaded with 5F-BAPTA have normal high-energy phosphate concentrations, and their metabolic response to ischemia closely resembles that of hearts not containing the indicator.[15] Indeed, the ability to measure not only the ^{19}F in the indicator but also the endogenous ^{31}P signals represents a major and unique advantage of the NMR approach, particularly in studies of ischemia.

The third, fourth, and fifth points represent additional distinct advantages of 5F-BAPTA over fluorescent indicators loaded by the AM method.[24,25] Furthermore, 5F-BAPTA does not require subtraction of an endogenous signal, in contrast to the autofluorescence that complicates fluorescent measurements. The lack of movement artifacts is another favorable property of the 5F-BAPTA method, especially in a contracting organ.

The major limitations of 5F-BAPTA (calcium buffering and limited temporal resolution) have been acknowledged.[10,11,14,16] The fact that the K_d of calcium-bound 5F-BAPTA is within the physiologic range makes it a sensitive indicator for both systolic and diastolic $[Ca^{2+}]_i$, but the same property leads to substantial calcium buffering at useful concentrations of the indicator. Although we can partially offset the buffering by working in high $[Ca]_o$, it is important to ascertain in any given protocol that the phenomena under investigation are not importantly altered by such a strategy. Further advances in the investigation of Ca^{2+} metabolism during pathologic conditions will be facilitated by comparison with the results of entirely complementary methods and by the development of new NMR-detectable indicators with more favorable properties.

References

1. Kusuoka H, Porterfield JK, Weisman HF, et al: Pathophysiology and pathogenesis of stunned myocardium. Depressed Ca^{2+} activation of contraction as a consequence of reperfusion-induced cellular calcium overload in ferret hearts. *J Clin Invest* 1987;79:950–960.
2. Marban E, Rink TJ, Tsien RW, et al: Free calcium in heart muscle at rest and during contraction measured with calcium-sensitive microelectrodes. *Nature* 1980;286:845–850.
3. Allen DG, Kurihara S: Calcium transients in mammalian ventricular muscle. *Eur Heart J* 1980;1(suppl A):5–15.

4. Wier WG, Cannell M, Berlin J, et al: Fura-2 fluorescence imaging reveals cellular and sub-cellular heterogeneity of $[Ca^{2+}]_i$ in single heart cells. *Science* 1987;235:325–328.
5. Lattanzio FA Jr, Pressman BC: Alterations in intracellular calcium activity and contractility of isolated perfused rabbit hearts by ionophores and adrenergic agents. *Biochem Biophys Res Commun* 1986;139:816–821.
6. Lee HC, Mohabir R, Smith N, et al: Effect of ischemia on calcium-dependent fluorescence transients in rabbit hearts containing indo 1. *Circulation* 1988;78:1047–1059.
7. Guarnieri T: Direct measurement of $[Ca^{2+}]_i$ in early and late reperfused myocardium. (abstract) *Circulation* 1989;80(suppl II):II-241.
8. Kihara Y, Grossman W, Morgan JP: Direct measurement of changes in intracellular calcium transients during hypoxia, ischemia, and reperfusion of the intact mammalian heart. *Circ Res* 1989;65:1029–1044.
9. Smith GA, Hesketh RT, Metcalfe JC, et al: Intracellular calcium measurements by ^{19}F NMR of fluorine-labelled chelators. *Proc Natl Acad Sci U S A* 1983;80:7178–7182.
10. Steenbergen C, Murphy E, Levy L, et al: Elevation in cytosolic free calcium concentration early in myocardial ischemia in perfused rat heart. *Circ Res* 1987;60:700–707.
11. Metcalfe JC, Hesketh TR, Smith GA: Free cytosolic Ca^{2+} measurements with fluorine labelled indicators using ^{19}F NMR. *Cell Calcium* 1985;6:183–195.
12. Corretti MC, Koretsune Y, Kusuoka H, et al: Glycolytic inhibition and calcium overload as consequences of exogenously generated free radicals in rabbit hearts. *J Clin Invest* 1991;88:1014 1025.
13. Kusuoka H, Weisfeldt ML, Jacobus WE, et al: Mechanism of early contractile failure during hypoxia in intact ferret heart: evidence for modulation of maximal Ca^{2+}-activated force by inorganic phosphate. *Circ Res* 1986;59:270–282.
14. Marban E, Kitakaze M, Kusuoka H, et al: Intracellular free calcium concentration measured with ^{19}F NMR spectroscopy in intact ferret hearts. *Proc Natl Acad Sci U S A* 1987;84:6005–6009.
15. Marban E, Kitakaze M, Koretsune Y, et al: Quantification of $[Ca^{2+}]_i$ in perfused hearts: critical evaluation of the 5F-BAPTA/NMR method as applied to the study of ischemia and reperfusion. *Circ Res* 1990;66:1255–1267.
16. Marban E, Kitakaze M, Chacko VP, et al: Ca^{2+} transients in perfused hearts revealed by gated ^{19}F NMR spectroscopy. *Circ Res* 1988;63:673–678.
17. Levy LA, Murphy E, London RE: Synthesis and characterization of ^{19}F NMR chelators for measurement of cytosolic free Ca. *Am J Physiol* 1987;252:C441–C449.
18. Koretsune Y, Marban E: Cell calcium in the pathophysiology of ventricular fibrillation and in the pathogenesis of postarrhythmic contractile dysfunction. *Circulation* 1989;80:369–379.
19. Blinks JR, Wier WG, Hess P, et al: Measurement of Ca^{2+} concentration in living cells. *Prog Biophys Mol Biol* 1982;40:1–114.
20. Koretsune Y, Marban E: Relative roles of Ca^{2+}-dependent and Ca^{2+}-independent mechanisms in hypoxic contractile dysfunction. *Circulation* 1990;82:528–535.
21. Kitakaze M, Marban M: Cellular mechanism of the modulation of contractile function by coronary perfusion pressure in ferret hearts. *J Physiol* 1989;414:455–472.
22. Kusuoka H, Koretsune Y, Chacko VP, et al: Excitation-contraction coupling in post-ischemic myocardium. Does failure of activator Ca^{2+} transients underlie stunning? *Circ Res* 1990;66:1268–1276.
23. Koretsune Y, Marban E: Mechanism of ischemic contracture in ferret hearts: relative roles of $[Ca^{2+}]_i$ elevation and ATP depletion. *Am J Physiol* 1990;258:H9–H16.
24. Steinberg SF, Bilezikian JP, Al-Awquate Q: Fura-2 fluorescence is localized to mitochondria in endothelial cells. *Am J Physiol* 1987;253:C744–C747.
25. Lorell BH, Apstein CS, Cunningham MJ, et al: Contribution of endothelial cells to calcium-dependent fluorescence transients in rabbit hearts loaded with indo 1. *Circ Res* 1990;67:415–425.
26. Allen DG, Lee JA, Smith GL: The consequences of simulated ischaemia on intracellular Ca^{2+} and tension in isolated ferret ventricular muscle. *J Physiol (Lond)* 1989;410:297–323.

Chapter 32

Practical Aspects of In Vivo ^{31}P Nuclear Magnetic Resonance Spectroscopy of the Human Myocardium

Jan A. den Hollander, PhD,
Albert de Roos, MD, Joost Doornbos, PhD,
Lambère J.M.P. Oosterwaal, MS,
and Peter R. Luyten, PhD

While the measurement of in vivo ^{31}P nuclear magnetic resonance (NMR) spectra of different human tissues and organs has become fairly routine, the ^{31}P NMR examination of the human heart remains a difficult proposition. The heart presents a moving target, and one needs to apply cardiac triggering to sychronize data acquisition to the cardiac cycle. Even then, spectroscopic localization techniques used to acquire in vivo NMR spectra tend to be sensitive to motion, which may lead to signal loss or localization errors. Also, irregularities in heart rate may cause variations between acquisitions. Because all in vivo shimming techniques depend upon the reproducible measurement of localized ^{1}H NMR signals over the area of interest it also remains difficult to obtain a good shimming of the magnetic field over the heart, leading to poor spectra resolution.

The sensitivity to motion of the spectroscopic localization techniques can cause ^{31}P NMR spectra of the myocardium to suffer from spurious signal contributions from chest muscle. In addition, one may also get muscle contributions if the sensitive volume included some skeletal muscle, which can occur when the profile of the sensitive volume is poorly defined. This is exacerbated by the fact that there is no obvious way to recognize contaminating signals from overlying skeletal muscle. For ^{31}P spectra of the liver the appearance of a signal from phosphocreatine signal provides a readily available clue to whether signal contributions are present from skeletal

From Pohost GM (ed.), *Cardiovascular Applications of Magnetic Resonance*. Mount Kisco, NY, Futura Publishing Co., Inc., © 1993.

muscle. For the heart, this is much more difficult to recognize, because the ^{31}P NMR spectrum of heart and skeletal muscle exhibit the same metabolite signals, albeit with different concentrations.

Yet over the past several years steady progress has been made with ^{31}P spectroscopy of the human heart. Here we will present and discuss a number of advances that have been made recently, leading to significant improvements in spectral resolution, signal-to-noise ratio, localization, and quantitation.

Magnetic Field Homogeneity

Optimization of the magnetic field over the human heart is a particularly difficult problem, both because of motion and because of the heterogeneity of the heart. It is common practice to monitor the ^{1}H NMR signal of the water resonance from the region of interest and then optimize the magnetic field on the basis of that signal. The most straightforward way to obtain ^{1}H NMR signals is by means of a surface coil. When applied to the heart, one has to face the fact that with surface coils one observes mainly the signal from the chest, and when using that for optimizing the magnetic field one may actually deteriorate the magnetic field homogeneity over the heart rather than improve it.

The alternative is to use localization techniques applied through the surface coil to obtain a water signal localized from the heart. The problem with this approach is that it is difficult to obtain a reproducible localized signal from the heart in a single experiment because the inhomogeneous B_1 field generated by the surface coil exacerbates the motion sensitivity of the spectroscopic localization scheme.

The technique that works well in practice uses the imaging body coil for sending/receiving the ^{1}H signal. By using the PRESS sequence[1,2] it has been possible to obtain reasonably reproducible localized ^{1}H NMR signals from the heart in single acquisitions. The PRESS sequence has the advantage that it is relatively insensitive to motion, in particular for short TE ($\leq$36 msec). Thus the method used involves selection of a large volume of interest (typically $80 \times 80 \times 60$ mm) centered on the left ventricle and monitoring the ^{1}H NMR water signal from that volume using single shot localization.[3] The time domain signal obtained over that volume is optimized by adjusting the linear and second-order field corrections. In our approach we have used an automatic shimming algorithm that maximizes the modulus of the time domain signal,[4] but once one is able to obtain a reproducible ^{1}H NMR signal of the myocardium it should be possible to use other shimming strategies as well. At the magnetic field strength of clinical magnetic resonance instruments (1.5 T) the line width of the water signal can be optimized to about 0.1–0.2 ppm over the entire left ventricle using the procedure outlined here.

Obtaining Localized ^{31}P Nuclear Magnetic Resonance Spectra of the Human Myocardium

For the ^{31}P NMR examination of the human heart at 1.5 T, the subject is in a supine position, with a 10-cm diameter surface coil placed on the chest over the heart.

The surface coil, tuned to the ^{31}P frequency, is equipped with a reference sample located at its center. The examination starts with ^{1}H magnetic resonance imaging (MRI), using the standard body coil to verify the position of the surface coil, with the reference sample as a marker.

Once the surface coil is properly positioned over the anterior wall of the left ventricle, a large volume of interest is selected (typically $80 \times 80 \times 60$ mm) to cover the entire left ventricle; then the magnetic field is shimmed over that volume, using the procedure outlined in the previous paragraph.

To obtain localized spectra of the human myocardium we have been using two different procedures. In the first procedure a smaller volume of interest is selected from the anterior wall of the left ventricle (typical size $50 \times 70 \times 40$ mm), and the ISIS sequence[5] is used to obtain a ^{31}P NMR spectrum localized to that selected volume. The 10-cm surface coil is used both for radiofrequency transmission and detection. By using radiofrequency inversion and detection pulses the performance of the ISIS sequence has been rendered independent of variations in the B_1 field such that the sequence can be used with a single transmit/receive coil.[6] The B_1 radiofrequency transmit field is adjusted to give a 20-μsec 90° block pulse at the center of the surface coil, which enables the frequency modulation pulses to provide optimal excitation to up to 10 cm away from the surface coil. We have used a recycle delay of 3 seconds while triggering the next acquisition at 200 msec after the R wave as shown by electrocardiogram. This long recycle delay is needed to obtain an optimal signal-to-noise ratio with the long T_1 characteristic for in vivo ^{31}P NMR spectroscopy. The single-volume procedure is particularly suitable to obtain high signal-to-noise spectra from a relatively large sensitive volume. The main drawback of the method is that one needs to be very careful about selecting the sensitive volume. On one hand, one likes to select a volume close to the chest wall in the most sensitive region of the surface coil to obtain a spectrum of high signal-to-noise. On the other hand, one needs to be careful to not include some section of the chest muscle in the sensitive volume. Even a small contribution from chest muscle may significantly alter the phosphocreatine:adenosine triphosphate (PCr:ATP) ratio of the resultant ^{31}P NMR spectrum, and it is difficult to correct for or even verify such a muscle contamination once one has obtained the single-volume spectrum.

The alternative approach we have used is based upon a combination of volume selection by ISIS and spectroscopic imaging using gradient phase encoding.[7] In this approach, the ISIS sequence is used to select a bar-shaped volume, which can be achieved by using two mutually orthogonal slice-selective inversion pulses, rather than the three inversion pulses used for conventional volume selection by ISIS. The bar-shaped volume is angulated perpendicular to the chest wall to minimize overlap between chest muscle and myocardium. Typical dimensions of the bar-shaped volume are 50×70 mm, to include most of the left ventricle. Then one-dimensional gradient phase encoding is applied along the direction of the selected bar to obtain a one-dimensional spectroscopic imaging data set. Usually, 32 phase encoding steps are used with a field of view of 320 mm, leading to 10-mm thick slices. For the zero-order profile, 32 acquisitions were acquired; for the higher order profiles, that number was reduced following a $\cos^2$ window. This procedure reduces finite sampling artifacts and the total acquisition time by a factor of two. A schematic of the whole pulse sequence is shown in Figure 1. After appropriate windowing and two-dimensional Fourier

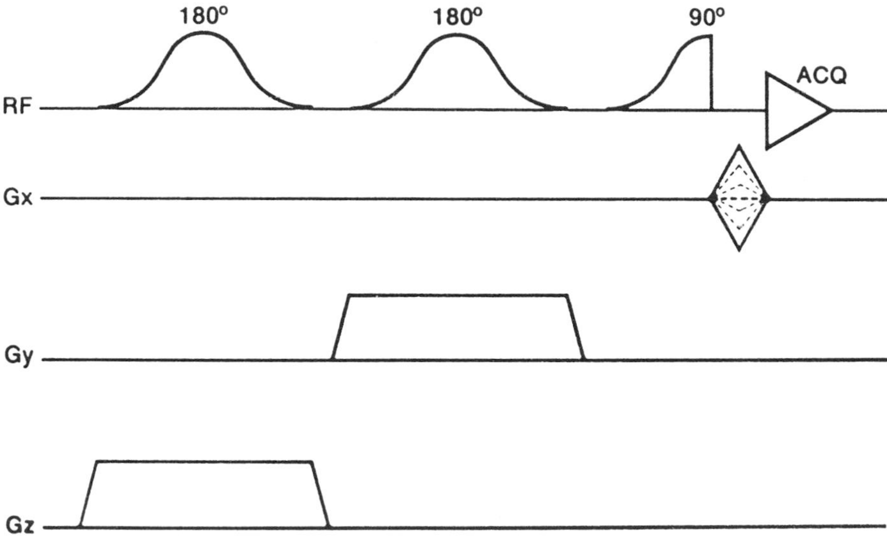

FIGURE 1. *Pulse sequence used to obtain a stack of ^{31}P NMR spectra. The two slice-selective frequency modulation inversion pulses are cycled through four on/off combinations to select a bar-shaped region of interest while gradient phase encoding along G_X is applied. After appropriate processing this gives rise to a stack of spectra originating from within the selected bar.*

transform, this yields a stack of spectra that originates from consecutive slices along the selected bar.

The stack of spectra thus obtained contains spectra coming from chest muscle as well as from the myocardium. Figure 2 shows an axial magnetic resonance image through the chest of a normal volunteer with the selected bar superimposed upon it. A major advantage of this approach is that it is possible to retrospectively inspect the data set and select spectra that are substantially free of contamination from chest muscle. One may also add several spectra that originate from the myocardium to obtain a spectrum with a higher signal-to-noise ratio.

^{1}H-Decoupled ^{31}P Nuclear Magnetic Resonance Spectroscopy of the Human Heart

The three-bond ^{1}H-^{31}P coupling constant in phosphomonoesters is typically in the range of 5–10 Hz. Although these coupling constants can be resolved in high-resolution spectra of extracts or solutions of pure compounds, they usually remain unresolved in in vivo ^{31}P NMR spectra. However, at the relatively low field of clinical MRI instruments (1.5 T) long-range isotropic ^{1}H-^{31}P couplings can make a significant contribution to the line width observed in in vivo ^{31}P NMR spectra. At these low

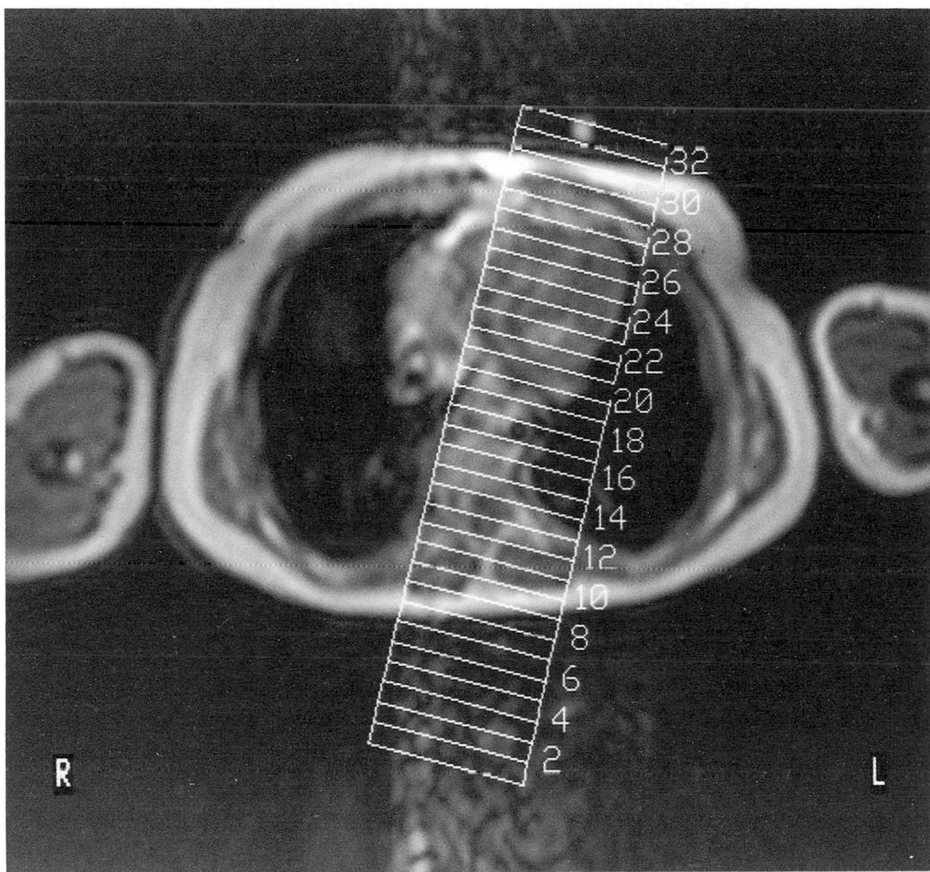

FIGURE 2. *Axial image through the chest of a normal volunteer, with the selected bar superimposed. The reference sample in the center of the surface coil is visible as a bright spot. After processing of the data set obtained by applying the sequence of Figure 1, a stack of spectra is obtained corresponding to the sections indicated on the selected bar.*

fields a broadening of 10 Hz amounts to 0.3 ppm, while according to our experience, the magnetic field can be shimmed to achieve a line width ranging from 0.1–0.2 ppm over the left ventricle.

For in vivo ^{31}P NMR spectra of the heart, the most significant phosphate compound exhibiting long-range ^{1}H-^{31}P couplings is 2,3-diphosphoglycerate (2,3-DPG). This compound is more abundant in blood than in myocardium, but with the large sensitive volumes required at 1.5 T for ^{31}P NMR spectroscopy of the human heart a significant signal contribution is often included from blood within the ventricle. Figure 3 shows a typical ^{31}P NMR spectrum obtained from a sensitive volume selected from the left ventricle of a healthy volunteer using the ISIS localization sequence. The spectrum shows the familiar signals from ATP and phosphocreatine. In addition, in the range of 5–6 ppm downfield from phosphocreatine a broad

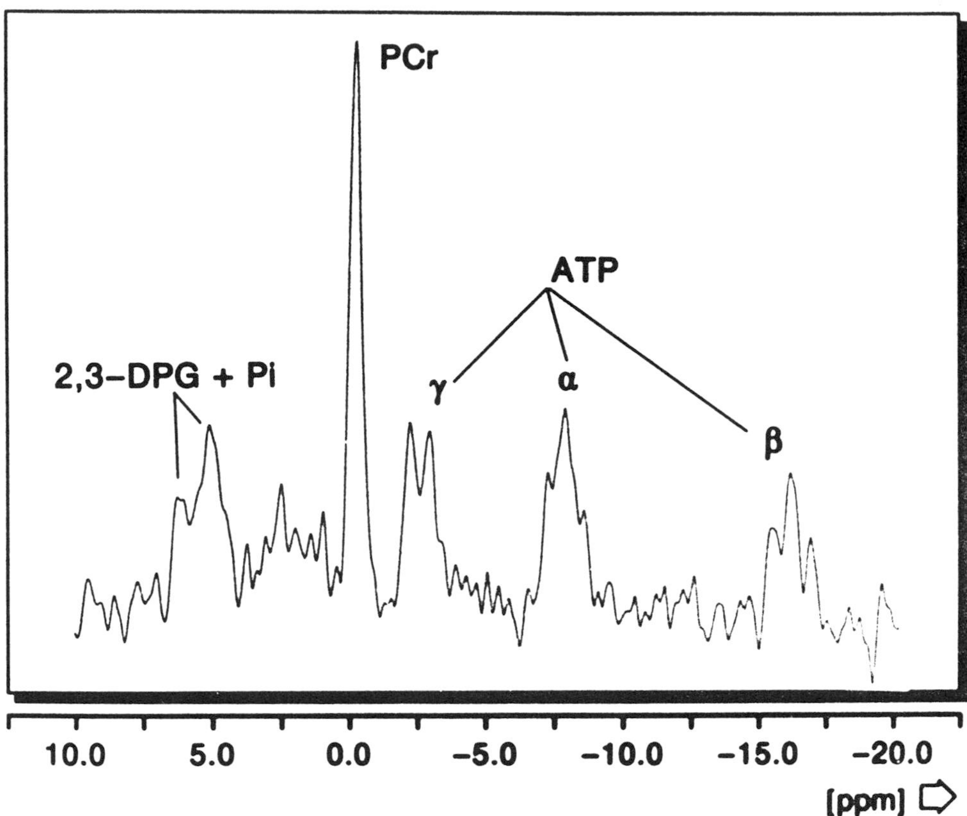

FIGURE 3. *Single-volume 1.5-T ^{31}P NMR spectrum of the human heart with no ^{1}H decoupling applied. The low-field region of the spectrum is characterized by a broad resonance containing contributions from 2,3-DPG and P_i.*

structure is observed, which consists of the 2- and the 3-phosphate of 2,3-DPG overlapping with the inorganic phosphate (P_i) signal. The overlap between the signals of 2,3-DPG and the P_i signal is particularly unfortunate because the concentration of P_i and tissue pH that can be derived from its chemical shift are particularly important markers of abnormal metabolism. In order to resolve the P_i signal from 2,3-DPG, further improvement in spectral resolution is needed.

It is possible to collapse the splittings due to the ^{1}H-^{31}P couplings by using ^{1}H decoupling techniques.[8] This can be achieved by radiofrequency irradiation of the ^{1}H resonances during acquisition of the ^{31}P NMR signal. Figure 4 shows a ^{1}H-decoupled ^{31}P NMR spectrum of the normal human myocardium obtained at 1.5 T. Due to the

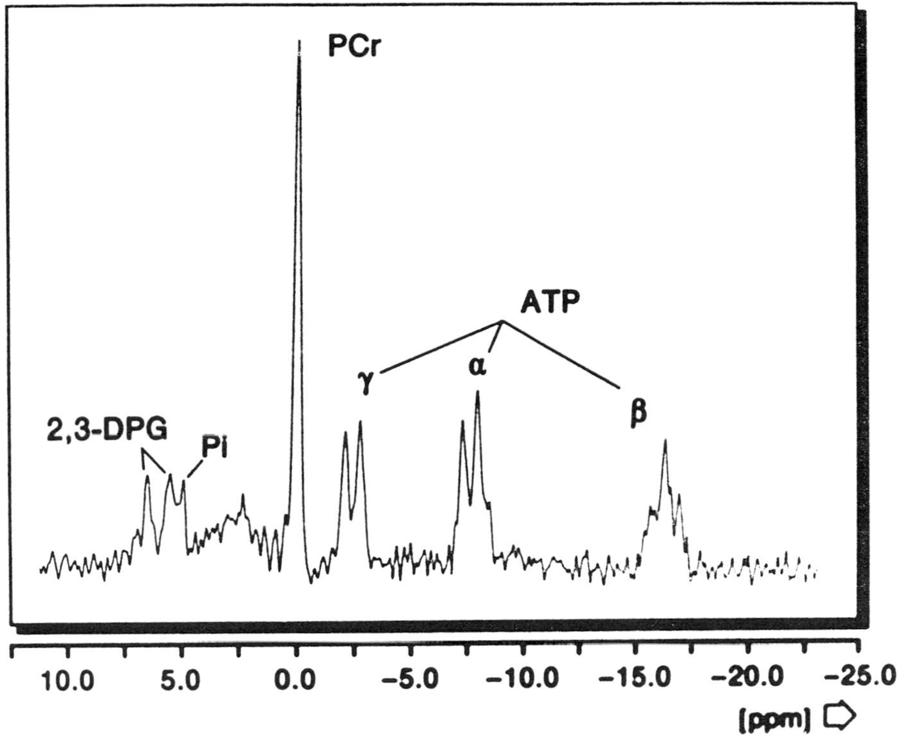

FIGURE 4. *^{1}H-decoupled 1.5-T ^{31}P NMR spectrum of the human heart. The P_i is resolved from the 2,3-DPG signal by collapsing the unresolved long-range ^{1}H-^{31}P couplings.*

reduction of the line widths of the 2,3-DPG signals by ^{1}H decoupling, the myocardial P_i signal has been uncovered. As a result, from this spectrum we are able to determine the P_i:phosphocreatine (PCr) ratio, as well as the myocardial pH. The most convenient way to perform ^{1}H decoupling is by using the ^{1}H body coil for transmission. Since the long-range coupling constants are small (typically 5–10 Hz), and also because the $-CHOP$ and $-CH_2OP$ protons that are responsible for these couplings resonate in a narrow range of the ^{1}H NMR spectrum, it is possible to achieve adequate decoupling using a ^{1}H decoupling bandwidth of no more than 100 Hz. This can be easily achieved within the Food and Drug Administration (FDA) safety guidelines for radiofrequency heating if at least the duty cycle for decoupling is kept below 20%. In view of the long T_1 encountered in in vivo ^{31}P NMR spectroscopy, this does not impose any added limitation to the recycle delay used in the spectroscopic measurement.

Data Processing of ^{31}P Nuclear Magnetic Resonance Spectra of the Myocardium

Usually one is interested in obtaining spectral parameters, such as PCr:ATP ratios, pH, or P_i:PCr ratios from the measured spectra. We have used a fully automated time domain fitting procedure to extract these parameters using prior knowledge to improve the accuracy of the remaining parameters, and to improve the stability of the fitting process.[9] The fully automated approach not only saves valuable time for the user, but more importantly it is free from any user bias that could conceivably be introduced by interactive phase correction and baseline correction.

The time domain fitting program used here includes optimization of the zero-order phase as well as the zero time offset (which is equivalent to the first-order phase in the frequency domain) along with resonance frequencies, line widths, and amplitudes. With this approach it is only necessary to provide a first estimate of the phase factors, which can be provided by an automated procedure. A first estimate of resonance frequencies, line widths, and amplitudes is provided by a representative model spectrum. The prior knowledge taken into account[10] in the fitting process includes information about the ATP splitting patterns (ie, the frequency separation within the multiplets are fixed, the relative intensities within the multiplets are maintained, and the line widths within the multiplets are kept equal). For 2,3-DPG the relative intensity and the chemical shift difference between the 2- and the 3-phosphate are kept constant, while in the nondecoupled spectra the splitting patterns are taken into account as well.

Standard deviations of the spectral parameters obtained by the fitting procedure can be predicted from the spectral noise by using the Cramér-Rao theory. This is particularly important because it helps to determine whether observed differences between spectra obtained from a control population and spectra from individual patient examinations are statistically significant.

^{31}P Nuclear Magnetic Resonance Results Obtained from Volunteers and Patients

Figure 5 shows a stack of ^{1}H-decoupled ^{31}P NMR spectra obtained from a healthy volunteer using the bar selection/phase encoding technique.[7] The lower two spectra contain signals that originate from the chest wall; signal ratios observed in these spectra are typical for those of skeletal muscle. The upper two spectra originate from the myocardium; these spectra show the much lower PCr:ATP ratio characteristic of the myocardium. The middle spectrum contains contributions both from skeletal muscle and from myocardium. These spectra were analyzed by the time fitting procedure previously described. Simulated spectra produced on the basis of spectral parameters obtained by the fitting procedure are shown in Figure 6. The PCr:ATP ratios for the upper two spectra determined by the time domain analysis approach were 0.86 and 0.90, respectively. These values are not corrected for contributions from blood or for partial saturation effects.

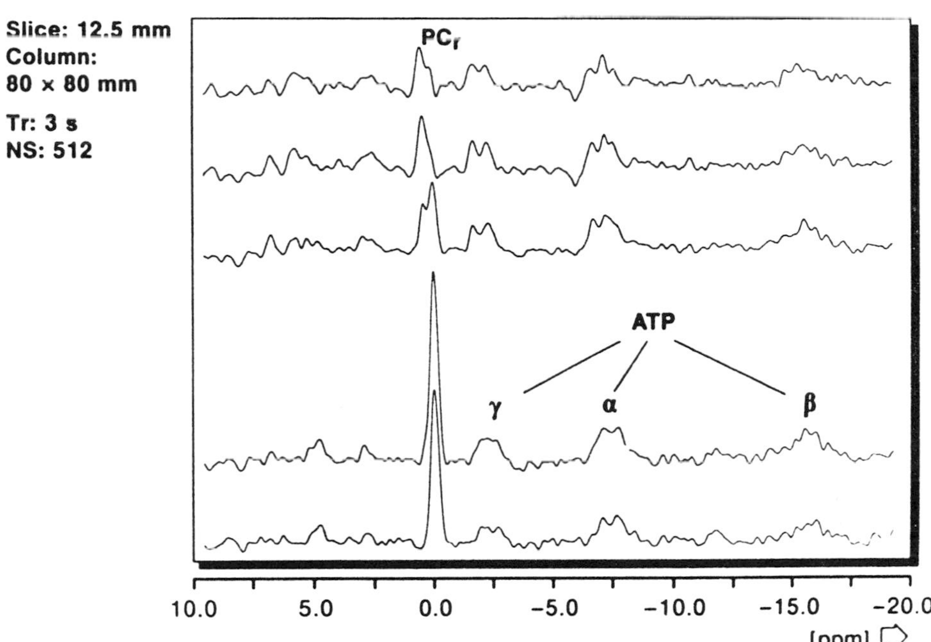

FIGURE 5. *Stack of ^{1}H-decoupled ^{31}P NMR spectra of the human chest obtained by means of the bar select/phase encoding technique. The lower two spectra come from chest muscle, while the upper two traces originate from the heart. The middle trace contains contributions from both. The phosphocreatine signal shows a downfield shift when proceeding from chest muscle to the heart.*

From the 2,3-DPG signals it is possible to estimate the contribution of blood ATP to these spectra. To perform this correction we have measured the ATP:2,3-DPG ratio to be 0.36 ± 0.06. From the 3-second recycle delay used in these measurements and measured T_1 values we estimate a correction factor of 1.53 for the PCr:ATP ratio. With these two corrections applied we have determined for a group of nine healthy volunteers an average PCr:ATP ratio of 1.58 ± 0.14. In four of the normal subjects the P_i signal could be resolved from the 2,3-DPG signals in these ^{1}H-decoupled ^{31}P NMR spectra; for these four normal volunteers we determined an average myocardial pH value of 7.13 ± 0.02.

When measuring the position of the phosphocreatine peak, one observes a shift in the downfield direction when proceeding from skeletal muscle to myocardium; in Figure 5, this downfield shift amounts to 12 Hz (or 0.46 ppm). Such a downfield shift of the myocardial phosphocreatine signal relative to that of skeletal muscle has been observed consistently in ^{31}P NMR examinations of the heart, although there is considerable variation in the magnitude of the effect; the average value observed for this shift was 0.44 ± 0.15 for a group of nine volunteers. The most likely explanation

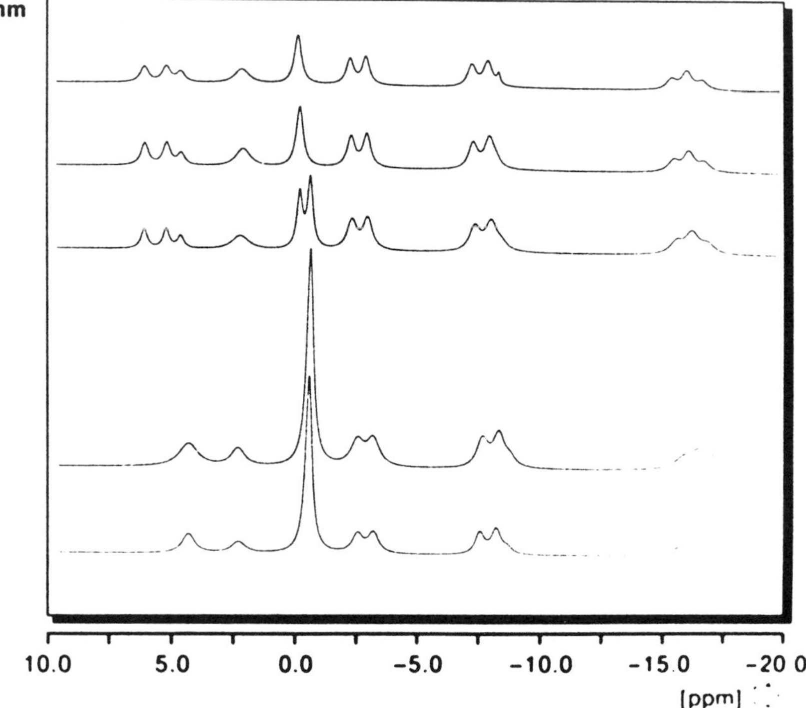

FIGURE 6. *Simulated spectra reconstructed from the parameters obtained by time domain analysis of the experimental spectra shown in Figure 5.*

for this shift is that it is caused by bulk susceptibility effects between skeletal muscle and the heart. The split phosphocreatine signal observed in the middle spectrum of Figure 5 indicates that this spectrum contains contributions from skeletal muscle as well as from the myocardium. In this way the shift in phosphocreatine helps in identifying the transition between skeletal muscle and myocardium and whether a particular spectrum from the stack of spectra is free from contributions from skeletal muscle.

Figure 7 shows a stack of ^{31}P NMR spectra from a patient who suffered from dilated myocardiomyopathy.[11] In this stack, the upper two traces represent spectra coming from chest muscle, while the lower two come from myocardium. Once again we observe the abrupt transition in PCr:ATP ratio between the spectra from skeletal muscle and myocardium.

By adding spectra originating from the myocardium, both for the volunteer and the patient with dilated cardiomyopathy, we obtain the two spectra shown in Figure 8. This direct comparison between the normal volunteer and the patient reveals two obvious differences. First, the 2,3-DPG:ATP ratio is higher in the spectrum obtained from the patient than the spectrum from the volunteer. Also, the phospholipid signal

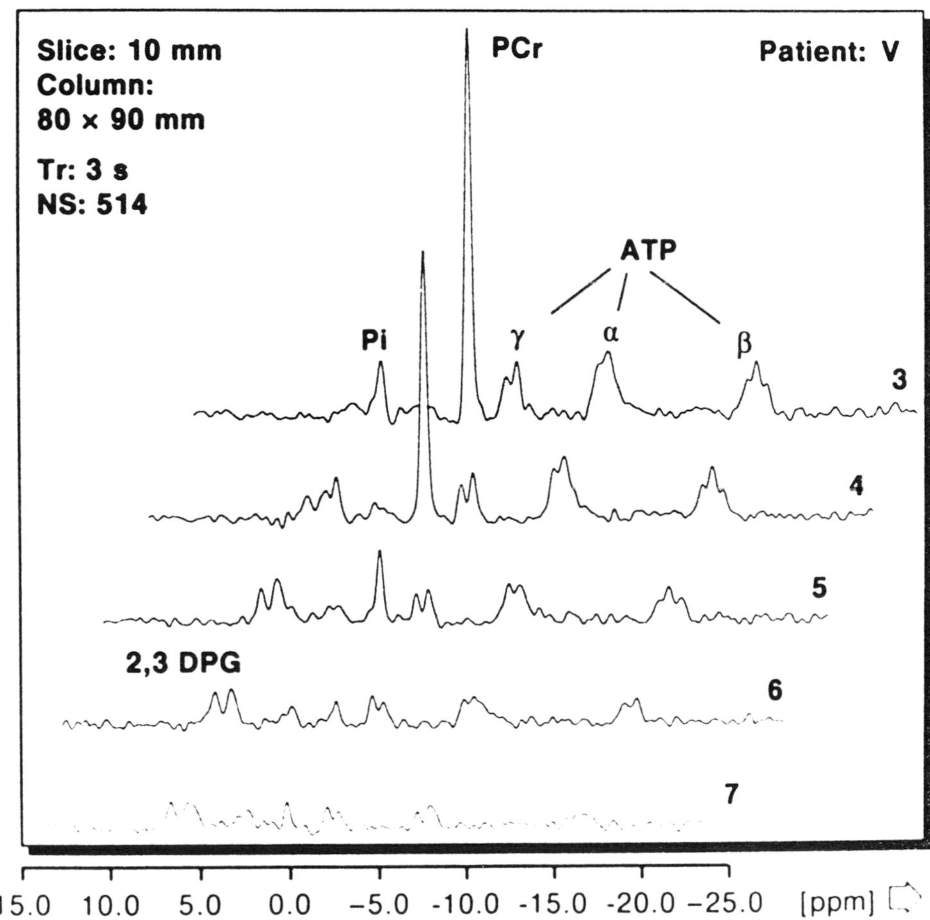

Figure 7. *Stack of ^{1}H-decoupled ^{31}P NMR spectra from the chest of a patient suffering from dilated cardiomyopathy. The upper two spectra arise from chest muscle, while the lower two spectra come from the heart. The spectrum at the middle contains contributions from muscle and heart.*

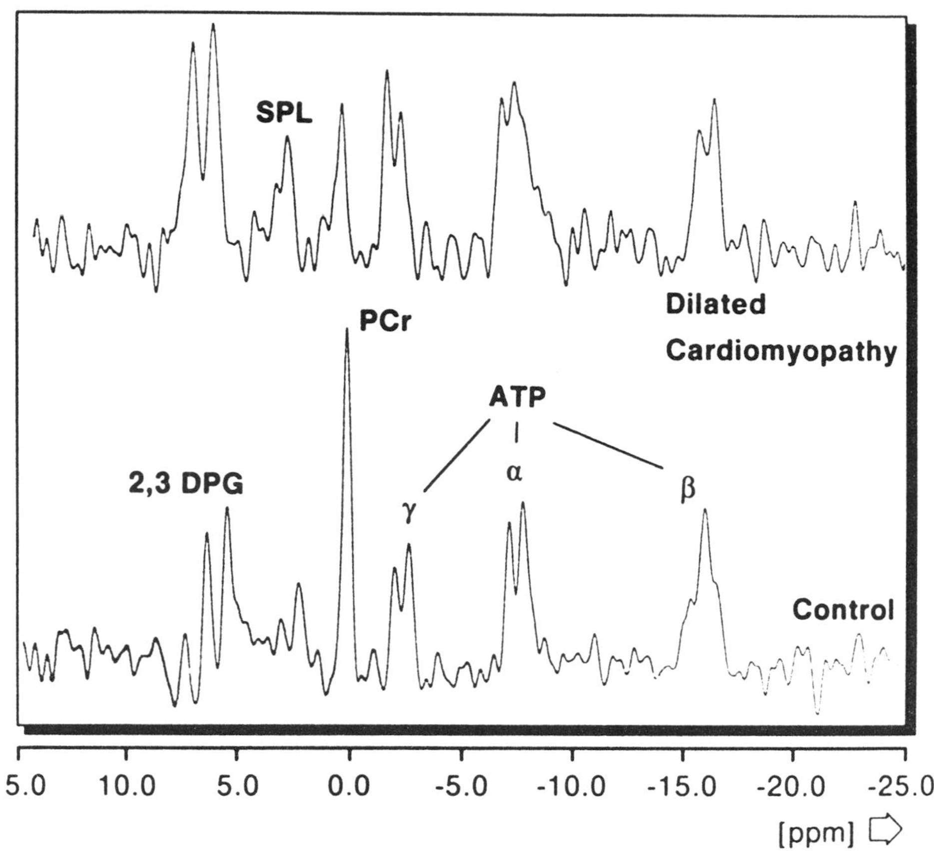

FIGURE 8. *Comparison of ^{1}H-decoupled ^{31}P NMR heart spectra of the normal volunteer (lower trace) and the patient with dilated cardiomyopathy. Note the higher 2,3-DPG and blood phospholipid (SPL) signals and the lower phosphocreatine signal in the spectrum of the dilated cardiomyopathy patient.*

labeled SPL is higher in the spectrum from the patient. The rather trivial explanation for this difference is that in the examination of the patient we have included a larger contribution from blood from the enlarged left ventricle, because both the 2,3-DPG and the SPL signal originate from the blood.

The difference observed in PCr:ATP ratios between the volunteer and the patient is statistically significant, even when corrected for the contribution from blood and for partial saturation effects. Using the time domain analysis procedure described above we determined uncorrected PCr:ATP ratios of 1.15 ± 0.24 for the volunteer and 0.28 ± 0.08 for the dilated cardiomyopathy patient; after correction for blood contribution, the PCr:ATP ratios are 2.02 and 0.56, respectively. In a series of examinations we observed that in spectra obtained from some dilated cardiomyopathy patients there is a significant reduction in PCr:ATP compared with a normal control group. However, for most dilated cardiomyopathy patients the difference is not statistically significant.

Conclusion

With the improvements in experimental techniques and examination protocols as well as data analysis methods it has been possible to reproducibly acquire ^{31}P NMR spectra of the human myocardium. The values of the PCr:ATP ratio determined for a group of normal volunteers were all within a range of two times the standard deviation predicted by the Cramér-Rao theory from the spectral noise. That means that within a group of normal volunteers any possible biologic variations in PCr:ATP are smaller than the uncertainties caused by spectral noise.

The blood-corrected and saturation-corrected PCr:ATP ratio reported here for a group of normal volunteers (1.58 ± 0.14) is somewhat lower than has been reported previously. This difference may be caused by a number of factors. In the analysis of the data obtained by bar selection/phase encoding, any spectra suspected of containing some muscle contribution were disregarded. By doing so some signal-to-noise has been sacrificed in the spectra analyzed, leading to higher standard deviations of the spectral parameters. Another possible reason for the lower PCr:ATP ratios reported could conceivably be related to the use of different measurement and/or data analysis techniques.

The introduction of ^{1}H decoupling has allowed us to resolve the P_i signal in 4 of 9 ^{31}P NMR spectra obtained from normal volunteers. From this a normal myocardial pH was derived of 7.13 ± 0.02. It has not been possible to resolve the P_i signal in spectra obtained from patients with dilated cardiomyopathy because of the large 2,3-DPG signal from blood. On the other hand, preliminary ^{31}P NMR spectra obtained from patients with hypertrophic cardiomyopathy have consistently shown well-resolved P_i signals. The average myocardial pH found for four hypertrophic cardiomyopathy patients was found to be 7.07 ± 0.02; this is significantly lower than the value obtained for normal volunteers (7.13 ± 0.02). This particular example serves to illustrate the important information that may be gained by the spectroscopic improvements described here.

References

1. Ordidge RJ, Bendall MR, Gordon RE, Connelly A: Volume selection for in vivo biological spectroscopy. In: Govil G, Khetrapal CL, Saran A, eds. *Magnetic Resonance in Biology and Medicine*. New Delhi: Tata McGraw Hill; 1985;387–397.
2. Bottomley PA: Spatial localization in NMR Spectroscopy in vivo. *Ann N Y Acad Sci* 1987;508:333–348.
3. Luyten PR, Mariën AJH, den Hollander JA: Acquisition and quantitation in proton spectroscopy. *NMR Biomed* 1991;4:64-69.
4. Vermeulen JWAH, den Hollander JA, Mariën AJH: Automatic shimming for localized human NMR spectroscopy (abstract). In: Proceedings of the 8th Annual Meeting of the Society of Magnetic Resonance in Medicine. 1989:626.
5. Ordidge RJ, Connelly A, Lohman JAB: *J Magn Reson* 1986;66;283.
6. Luyten PR, Groen JP, Vermeulen JWAH, den Hollander JA: Experimental approaches to image localized human ^{31}P NMR spectroscopy. *Magn Reson Med* 1989;11:1–21.

7. Mariën AJH, Doornbos J, de Roos A, et al: ^{1}H decoupled ^{31}P NMR spectroscopy of the normal human heart at 1.5 T: a reassessment of metabolite ratios and bulk susceptibility effects (abstract). In: Proceedings of the 9th Annual Meeting of the Society of Magnetic Resonance in Medicine. 1990:249.
8. Luyten PR, Bruntink G, Sloff FM, et al: Broadband proton decoupling in human ^{31}P NMR spectroscopy. *NMR Biomed* 1989;1:177–283.
9. den Hollander JA, Mariën AJH, Luyten PR, et al: Automated time-domain quantification of in vivo ^{31}P NMR spectra (abstract). In: Proceedings of the 10th Annual Meeting of the Society of Magnetic Resonance in Medicine. 1991:761.
10. de Beer R, van Ormondt D, Mariën AJH, et al: Improved quantitative time domain analysis of in vivo ^{31}P NMR by invoking prior knowledge on ATP (abstract). In: Proceedings of 8th Annual Meeting of the Society of Magnetic Resonance in Medicine. 1989:604.
11. Luyten PR, de Roos, Oosterwaal LJMP, et al: PCr/ATP ratio changes and pH values in dilated and hypertrophic cardiomyopathy patients determined by ^{31}P NMR heart spectroscopy (abstract). In: Proceedings of the 10th Annual Meeting of the Society of Magnetic Resonance in Medicine. 1991:74.

Chapter 33

Nuclear Overhauser Enhancement and Proton Decoupling in Phosphorus Chemical Shift Imaging of the Human Heart

Heinrich Kolem, PhD, Rolf Sauter, PhD,
Matthias Friedrich, MD,
Monika Schneider, MS,
and Karsten Wicklow, MS

Various spectroscopic localization techniques have been successfully applied to achieve localized phosphorus (^{31}P) spectra of the human heart.[1–6] However, the evaluation of ^{31}P heart spectra obtained under clinical conditions is often limited by poor signal-to-noise ratios, compromised spatial resolution, or poor spectral resolution. The application of ^{31}P-^{1}H double-resonance techniques is one possibility that is expected to provide a significant improvement for both sensitivity and specificity of ^{31}P heart spectra. It has been reported that proton decoupling results in improved spectral resolution,[4] while exploitation of the nuclear Overhauser effect (NOE) provides a significant increase in the signal-to-noise ratio in in vivo ^{31}P spectroscopy[7] that can be translated into improved spatial or temporal resolution. Both ^{31}P-^{1}H double-resonance techniques can be successfully combined with chemical shift imaging (CSI) techniques for localized ^{31}P spectroscopy.[8]

It has been our goal to acquire localized spectra from different well-defined regions of the left ventricle. We have developed a ^{31}P-^{1}H double resonance three-dimensional CSI technique, taking advantage of the NOE, decoupling, and hard ^{31}P readout pulses. In contrast to other published three-dimensional techniques, we tilted the CSI grid in two angles to align the long axis of the $25 \times 25 \times 50$-mm volumes parallel to the long axis of the heart so that the tissue in each target volume would be supplied by one principle artery only. This technique meets the requirement of a

From Pohost GM (ed.), *Cardiovascular Applications of Magnetic Resonance.* Mount Kisco, NY, Futura Publishing Co., Inc., © 1993.

planned clinical study: clear spatial separation of the left ventricular anterior wall, lateral wall, and the septum yielding spectra of comparable quality and sufficient signal-to-noise ratios for the determination of reliable ratios of phosphocreatine (PCr) to adenosine triphosphate (ATP). Cardiac gating minimized motion artifacts. The angles for an oblique tilting of the CSI space lattice are chosen as in routine imaging. Postprocessing software allows the grids to be shifted in all directions to best match the anatomy.

Previous studies on human cardiac muscle have not reported on the effects of proton saturation; we therefore attempted to quantify the signal enhancement by NOE. This gain in sensitivity was then used to allow the examination of smaller volumes. We performed ^{31}P magnetic resonance spectroscopy (MRS) heart studies on healthy volunteers using this ECG-gated ^{31}P-^{1}H double-resonance three-dimensional CSI technique.

Due to the low sensitivity of ^{31}P MRS, we chose to use a surface coil. This restricts the application to the evaluation of ^{31}P metabolism in anterior regions and septum of the myocardium. Hence, regionally impaired ^{31}P energy metabolism may be detectable by localized ^{31}P MRS in patients with regional infarction of the left ventricular anterior wall and septum or in patients suffering from coronary artery disease.

Methods

Experiments were performed with a commercially available 1.5-T whole-body magnetic resonance imaging (MRI)/spectroscopy system (Magnetom, Siemens Medical Systems, Iselin, NJ) that was equipped with an experimental second radiofrequency transmit channel to allow the application of double-resonance techniques. We used a custom-built double-resonant surface coil system with coaxial arrangement of the ^{1}H transmit/receive coil (18-cm diameter) and the ^{31}P transmit/receive coil (10-cm diameter). In order to achieve a radiofrequency field that was homogeneous over the region of interest and to avoid the risk of hot spots on the patient's surface, the 18-cm ^{1}H coil was arranged 1 cm below the plane of the ^{31}P coil. This resulted in a minimum distance of about 3 cm between patient and ^{1}H coil. Fourteen healthy male volunteers (age 22–54 years) were examined. Informed consent was obtained in all volunteer studies. The volunteers were positioned prone, but rotated slightly to the left on the surface coil system. Prior shimming and localized ^{31}P spectroscopy, ^{1}H multislice, multiphase cardiac imaging (FISP, TE = 12 msec) was performed in coronal and transverse orientations using the 18-cm ^{1}H transmit/receive surface coil. Localized ^{31}P spectra were acquired using two-dimensional and three-dimensional CSI techniques, respectively. In the two-dimensional CSI sequence, a 640-μsec slice-selective radiofrequency pulse was used to excite a 40-mm slab; the in-plane resolution, as defined by the 8×8 increments of phase encoding gradients, was 30×30 mm. The delay time between end of excitation pulse and beginning of the data acquisition window was 1.4 msec. In the three-dimensional CSI sequence, the delay time between the end of the 300-μsec nonselective excitation pulse and the beginning of data acquisition was 1 msec. The spatial resolution, as defined by the $8 \times 8 \times 8$

increments of phase encoding gradients, was 25 × 25 × 50 mm. The space lattice, as defined by the three-dimensional CSI technique, was tilted in a double oblique manner in order to align the long axis of the CSI voxels with the long axis of the left ventricle. The two angles that define the double oblique orientation have been determined from the coronal and transverse heart images. Nuclear Overhauser enhancement was achieved by two nonselective ^{1}H radiofrequency saturation pulses preceding each ^{31}P scan. Proton decoupling was performed during the first 40 msec of ^{31}P data acquisition by application of a WALTZ-4 sequence using a basic 90° pulse length of 2 msec that corresponds to a decoupling bandwidth of ±120 Hz centered at the water resonance (Figure 1). The acquisition was triggered by every heartbeat. The ^{31}P and ^{1}H radiofrequency pulse amplitudes have been adjusted to give maximal ^{31}P signal and maximal nuclear Overhauser enhancement, respectively. Great care was taken in calculation of the total radiofrequency power as applied during the double-resonant pulse sequence. Typical values have been 2 W, which for the given coil geometry resulted in specific absorption rates that are well below the Food and Drug Administration (FDA) limits of 8 W/kg. To minimize motion artifacts, the 256-msec acquisition window (512 data points) was shifted into the diastolic cardiac phase. Typical total acquisition times have been 20 minutes, which corresponds to three or four accumulations in the three-dimensional CSI experiment and to 24 to 32 accumulations in the two-dimensional CSI experiment, respectively.

A 1.6-Hz Gaussian line broadening has been applied to all ^{31}P spectra. The spectra have been corrected by a sine function in the frequency domain for baseline distortion induced by the missing data points in the time domain signal.

In addition, fully relaxed ^{31}P spectra from the chest wall muscle were acquired

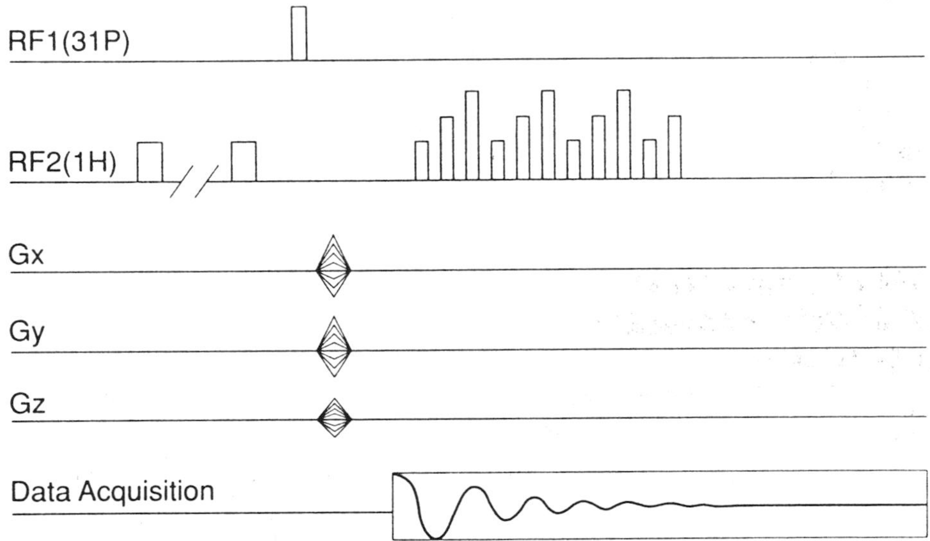

FIGURE 1. *Radiofrequency (RF) and gradient waveforms of the ^{31}P three-dimensional CSI sequence with ^{1}H saturation pulses for nuclear Overhauser enhancement and ^{1}H WALTZ-4 pulse sequence for ^{1}H decoupling.*

using a pulse sequence with low excitation angles. From these fully relaxed spectra and the spectra obtained from chest wall muscle by the ECG-triggered CSI examination, we calculated the saturation factors for the individual metabolites. Assuming similar relaxation parameters for chest wall and cardiac muscle, and neglecting the effects of spatial variation of flip angles, we used these saturation factors to correct the PCr:ATP ratios as obtained from the CSI spectra representing cardiac muscle. The PCr:ATP ratios were based on the peak areas of total ATP divided by 3 and the peak area of PCr. For quantitation, a least-square fit was applied to the baseline and phase-corrected real part spectra.

In order to quantify the nuclear Overhauser enhancement, in three volunteer studies the ^{31}P CSI scan was repeated without application of ^{1}H radiofrequency saturation pulses, keeping all other experimental parameters constant.

Results

Twenty-six MHz ^{31}P heart spectra acquired with the CSI technique enabled a clear spectral resolution of resonances from α-, β- and γATP, PCr, phosphodiesters (PDE), and the 2,3-diphosphoglycerate (2,3-DPG) from blood. Usually the achieved homogeneity was sufficient to resolve the J-splitting of the ATP resonances. All resonances revealed a significant nuclear Overhauser enhancement of 35% to 60% (Table 1). ^{1}H decoupling resulted in a line narrowing that was most prominent for the γ- and α-ATP resonances and for 2,3-DPG. Therefore, due to ^{1}H decoupling in some of the spectra, inorganic phosphate (P_i, 4.85 ± 0.1 ppm) could be identified on the shoulder of the downfield component of 2,3-DPG (5.25 ± 0.1 ppm) (Figure 2).

The nuclear Overhauser enhanced ^{1}H-decoupled ^{31}P heart spectrum shown in Figure 2 was acquired with the two-dimensional CSI technique and represents a $40 \times 30 \times 30$ mm-voxel of transverse orientation including left ventricular cardiac muscle and parts from the septum. A clear spatial resolution of left ventricular anterior wall, lateral wall, and septum requires a double oblique tilting of the space lattice defined by the CSI technique (Figure 3). As the correct definition of the excited slice turned out to be very difficult, all double oblique examinations were performed using three-dimensional CSI techniques, which retrospectively enabled an optimal adaption of the CSI voxel to the myocardium. Spectra representing left ventricular anterior wall

TABLE 1. Nuclear Overhauser Effect Enhancements for Chest Wall and Cardiac Muscle as Observed for the Given Experimental Parameters (refer to text).

	2,3-DPG	PCr	α-ATP	γ-ATP	β-ATP
Chest wall muscle	—	55 (10)%	35 (20)%	45 (20)%	40 (20)%
Cardiac muscle	40 (10)%	60 (10)%	35 (20)%	40 (20)%	40 (20)%

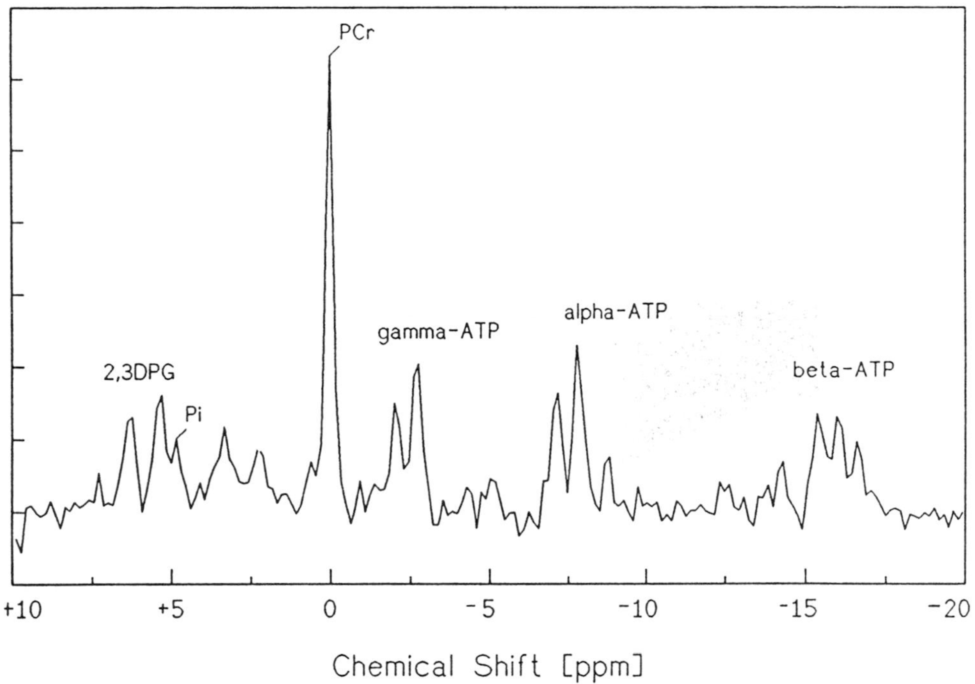

FIGURE 2. *Twenty-six–MHz nuclear Overhauser enhanced ^{1}H-decoupled ^{31}P two-dimensional CSI spectrum representing a 36-ml volume of the left ventricle including anterior wall and septum (transverse voxel). Total acquisition time, approximately 20 minutes.*

and septum could be obtained with comparable quality (Figure 4A) using the double oblique three-dimensional CSI technique. With the chosen orientation and geometry of the space lattice, spectra representing the left ventricular lateral wall could also be obtained from the same three-dimensional CSI data set (Figure 4B). However, due to the restricted sensitivity profile of the small ^{31}P coil used in our experiments, the signal-to-noise ratio achieved for the spectra from the left ventricular lateral wall was not sufficient for evaluation.

The PCr:ATP ratios determined from data sets acquired with the CSI technique in transverse and in double oblique orientations, respectively, reveal systematic differences: after correction for saturation effects, for the healthy cardiac muscle PCr:ATP ratios of 1.8 ± 0.2 ($n = 6$) and 1.0 ± 0.2 ($n = 8$) have been calculated from the transverse- and double oblique-oriented voxels within the myocardium, respectively. Table 2 summarizes the PCr:ATP ratios from 14 volunteer studies. Table 2 contains both the ratios as observed under the experimental conditions with the nuclear Overhauser enhanced ^{1}H-decoupled CSI technique and the corresponding ratios as obtained after correction for saturation.

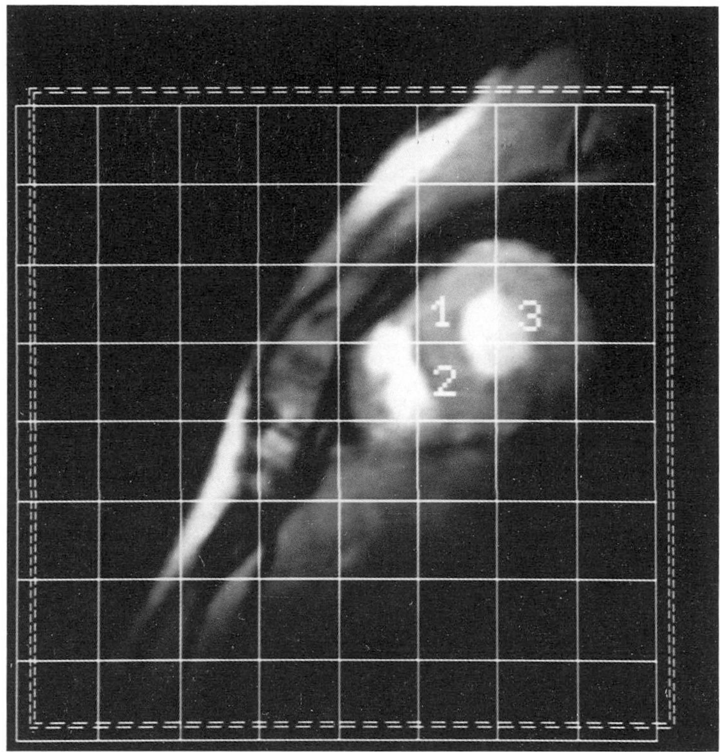

FIGURE 3. *[1]H image of the heart acquired with the 18-cm transmit/receive coil. The double oblique orientation of the space lattice used for the three-dimensional CSI experiment is indicated.*

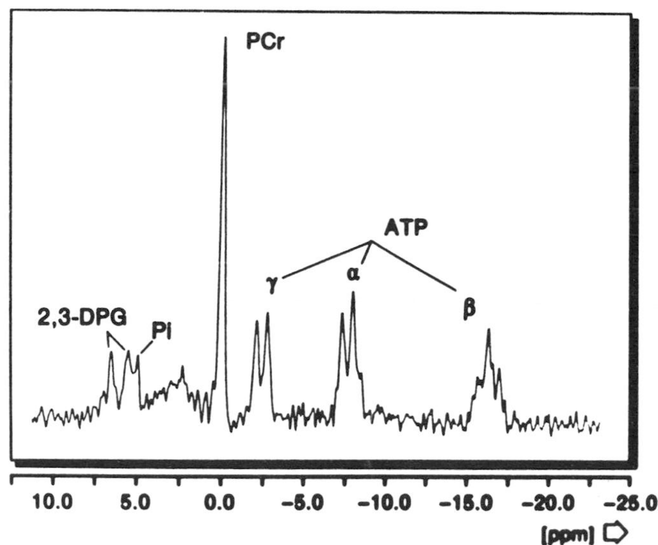

FIGURE 4A. *Double oblique ^{31}P-^{1}H double resonance three-dimensional-CSI MRS of the human heart: ^{31}P spectra representing left ventricular arterior wall (1) and septum (2), respectively (refer to Figure 3 for voxel position). Spatial resolution, 31 ml; total acquisition time approximately 20 minutes.*

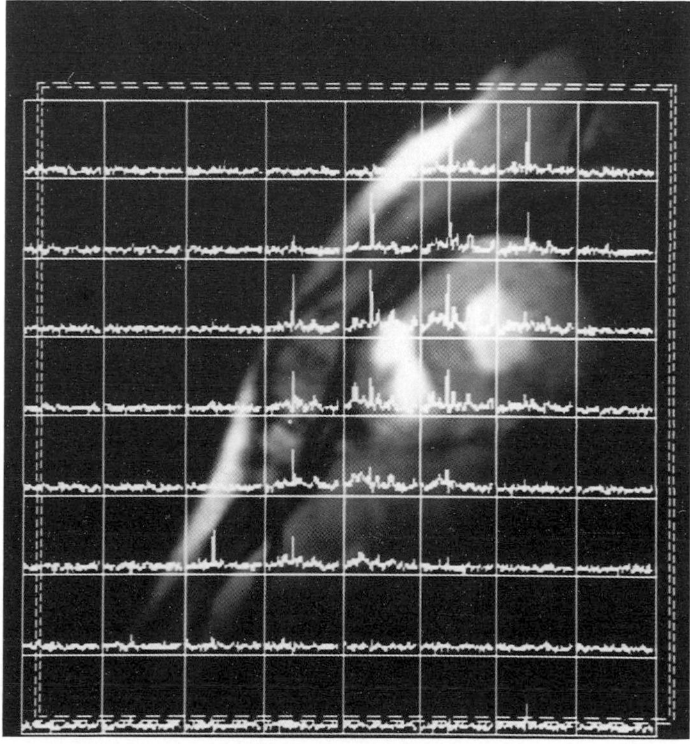

FIGURE 4B. *Double oblique ^{31}P-^{1}H double resonance three-dimensional-CSI MRS of the human heart: ^{1}H image with superimposed ^{31}P spectral map. Spatial resolution, 31 ml; total acquisition time approximately 20 minutes.*

TABLE 2.

					PCr/ATP (uncorr.)		PCr/ATP (corr.)
Volunteer	Acqu. T.	VOI [ccm]	Ori.	Age	Ch. M.	Myoc.	Myoc.
1	2D CSI	4 × 4 × 4	tra	40	2.4	1.3	1.7
2	2D CSI	4 × 4 × 4	tra	30	2.2	1.4	2.0
3	2D CSI	3 × 3 × 4	tra	22	2.1	1.2	1.8
4	2D CSI	3 × 3 × 4	tra	29	2.0	1.4	2.0
7	2D CSI	3 × 3 × 4	tra	23	2.3	.9	1.7
9	3D CSI	3 × 3 × 5	d.o.	26	2.7	1.0	1.1
12	3D CSI	2.5 × 2.5 × 5	d.o.	43	2.2	.9	1.1
14	3D CSI	2.5 × 2.5 × 5	d.o.	28	3.3	1.0	1.0
16	3D CSI	2.5 × 2.5 × 5	d.o.	46	1.7	.5	1.0
17	3D CSI	2.5 × 2.5 × 5	d.o.	28	2.7	.9	1.1
18	3D CSI	2.5 × 2.5 × 5	d.o.	51	3.7	.7	.7
19	3D CSI	2.5 × 2.5 × 5	d.o.	52	3.4	1.2	1.2
21	3D CSI	2.5 × 2.5 × 5	d.o.	54	2.6	.6	.7
22	3D CSI	2.5 × 2.5 × 5	tra	26	1.8	1.0	1.7

PCr:ATP ratios as observed for chest wall muscle (Ch. M.) and myocardium (Myoc.) with the given experimental parameters and after correction for saturation effects. The corrected PCr:ATP ratio for chest wall muscle is 3.3 ± 0.2. With exception of volunteer 22, the three-dimensional CSI technique was applied with double oblique (d.o.) orientation of the space lattice.

Discussion

With the application of ^{31}P-^{1}H double-resonance techniques, the sensitivity of human cardiac ^{31}P MRS studies can be improved by approximately 50%. This gain in signal-to-noise ratio is primarily due to signal enhancement by exploitation of the NOE. Line narrowing achieved by ^{1}H decoupling makes only minor contributions to the improvement in signal-to-noise ratio observed in the cardiac spectra. Although in some cases ^{1}H decoupling resulted in a better resolution of the resonance from P_i from the downfield component of 2,3-DPG, the achieved resolution of P_i was not sufficient for the calculation of reliable PCr:P_i ratios.

The PCr:ATP ratios obtained in this study with transverse orientation of the space lattice (1.8 ± 0.2) correspond well with values reported from other human heart studies using CSI techniques (1.72 ± 0.15)[9] and are close to values of approximately 2 found in various animal models.[10,11] However, in all our studies with double oblique space lattice, significantly lower PCr:ATP ratios (1.0 ± 0.2) were found. From our preliminary data, we are not able to explain this observation. Although the partial volume from blood and the spatial variation of the radiofrequency field will be different in the double oblique and in the transverse CSI voxels, it is not very likely that these effects (which we did not consider in our calculations) account for the observed differences in the PCr:ATP ratios of about 80%. The double oblique voxel 1 (Figure 3) represents a higher portion of the left ventricular inner wall, while the transverse voxels include the inner and outer wall. One could therefore speculate that our observations reflect transmural differences in metabolite concentrations as they have been reported in animal models.[12] It should also be mentioned that in a previous study of the human heart using the ISIS technique for localization, of low PCr:ATP ratios (0.83 ± 0.27)[13] have been observed.

For the given experimental parameters, similar nuclear Overhauser enhancement factors were observed for chest wall and cardiac muscle. This indicates that the 18-cm ^{1}H coil provides a homogeneous ^{1}H saturation over the sensitive volume of the 10-cm ^{31}P coil. The values observed in the CSI experiment (Table 1) are close to the maximum nuclear Overhauser enhancement factors for in vivo ^{31}P calf muscle spectra as derived from nonlocalized studies.[14]

For many potential clinical applications of cardiac ^{31}P MRS, either fast acquisition techniques are required to enable dynamic studies, eg, to study metabolic changes under stress induced by physical work or pharmaceutics, or high spatial resolution is desired, eg, to enable the evaluation of regional differences of the cardiac metabolism in patients with coronary artery disease. As it is of primary interest to compare different spectra obtained from the same individual, in these situations we consider the application of ^{31}P-^{1}H double-resonance techniques, although complicating the absolute quantification of metabolites in requiring an additional correction for the metabolite-specific nuclear Overhauser enhancement, indispensable to achieve maximal sensitivity and specificity in clinical cardiac ^{31}P MRS studies.

With the ^{31}P-^{1}H double-resonance CSI techniques, spectra from different well-defined regions of the myocardium could be obtained with comparable quality. In order to differentiate principle regions of coronary blood supply, the space lattice as defined by the three-dimensional CSI technique needs to be tilted in a double oblique way. In enabling a retrospective shift of the matrix of acquired data along all three spatial coordinates, the three-dimensional CSI technique provided the clear practical advantage over the two-dimensional CSI technique of minimizing contributions from blood and chest wall muscle by postprocessing of the CSI data. For the examination of patients with coronary heart disease in whom coronary angiography suggests a reduced blood supply to the left ventricular anterior wall, and for the examination of patients with regional infarction of the anterior wall, ideally CSI spectra from the anterior and lateral wall should be compared. With the coil configuration used in this volunteer study we have not been able to obtain spectra with sufficient signal-to-noise ratios from the lateral wall, spectra from the septum showed signal-to-noise ratios comparable to those from the anterior wall. In a clinical pilot study we therefore plan to examine whether spectra from the septum could serve as an internal reference in these patients. Apart from the question of the "true" value, the double oblique CSI technique seems to provide consistent PCr:ATP ratios that will have to be consolidated by further volunteer studies. We therefore expect to be able to characterize the status of energy metabolism in the affected regions of the myocardium of patients also relative to normal volunteers. As with the spectral resolution achieved in this volunteer study, we have not been able to evaluate P_i unambiguously. Both methods for the characterization of impaired cardiac metabolism, intraindividual as well as interindividual comparison, will have to be based on the evaluation of PCr:ATP ratios. Hence, the forthcoming clinical examinations will only be successful in characterization of cardiac metabolism if we can expect that regional ischemia affects the concentration of PCr significantly more than ATP concentrations.[9–11,15]

References

1. Bottomley PA: Noninvasive study of high-energy phosphate metabolism in human heart by depth-resolved ^{31}P NMR spectroscopy. *Science* 1985;229:769–772.
2. Blackledge MJ, Rajagopalan B, Oberhaensli RD, et al: Quantitative studies of human cardiac metabolism by ^{31}P rotating-frame NMR. *Proc Natl Acad Sci U S A* 1987;84:4283–4287.
3. Müller S, Sauter R, Weber H, et al: Multivolume selective spectroscopy. *J Magn Reson* 1988;76:155–161.
4. Luyten PR, Bruntink G, Sloff FM, et al: Broadband proton decoupling in human ^{31}P NMR spectroscopy. *NMR Biomed* 1989;1:177–183.
5. Sauter R, Kiefer B, Lewin JS, et al: MR imaging and MR spectroscopy of the heart: present and future possibilities and limitations. *Radiol Med* 1990;80:172–180.
6. Bottomley PA, Hardy CJ, Roemer PB: Phosphate metabolite imaging and concentration measurements in human heart by nuclear magnetic resonance. *Magn Reson Med* 1990;14:425–434.
7. Bachert-Baumann P, Ermark F, Zabel H-J, et al: In vivo nuclear Overhauser effect in ^{31}P-^{1}H double resonance experiments in a 1.5 T whole-body MR system. *Magn Reson Med* 1990;15:165–172.
8. Kolem H, Sauter R, Schneider M, et al: Decoupled and nuclear Overhauser enhanced localized phosphorus liver spectroscopy using the CSI technique (abstract). In: Proceedings of the Society of Magnetic Resonance in Medicine. 1991:318.
9. Weiss G, Bottomley PA, Hardy CJ, et al: Regional myocardial metabolism of high-energy phosphates during isometric exercise in patients with coronary artery disease. *N Engl J Med* 1990;323:1593–1600.
10. Robitaille P-M, Lew B, Merkle H, et al: Transmural metabolite distribution in regional myocardial ischemia as studied with ^{31}P NMR. *Magn Reson Med* 1989;10:108–118.
11. Gober JR, Schaefer S, Camacho SA, et al: Epicardial and endocardial localized ^{31}P magnetic resonance spectroscopy: evidence for metabolic heterogeneity during regional ischemia. *Magn Reson Med* 1990;13:204–215.
12. Robitaille P-M, Merkle H, Lew B, et al: Transmural high energy phosphate distribution and response to alterations in workload in the normal canine myocardium as studied with spatially localized ^{31}P NMR spectroscopy. *Magn Reson Med* 1990;16:91–116.
13. Friedrich M, Weikl A, Sauter R, et al: Lokalisierte ^{31}P-NMR-Spektroskopie des menschlichcn Herzens—Entwicklung einer Meβmethode und erste klinische Applikation. *Z Kardiol* 1991;80:266–271.
14. Kolem H, Schneider M, Wicklow K, et al: Fast in vivo phosphorus spectroscopy using nuclear Overhauser enhancement (abstract). In: Proceedings of the Society of Magnetic Resonance in Medicine. 1990:889.
15. Holt WW, Wendland MF, Derugin N, et al: Effect of repetitive brief episodes of cardiac ischemia on ^{31}P magnetic resonance spectroscopy in the cat. *Magn Reson Med* 1990;15:70–80.

Section 3

Safety Issues

Chapter 34

Safety Considerations of Cardiovascular Magnetic Resonance Studies

Frank G. Shellock, PhD
and Emanuel Kanal, MD

Magnetic resonance (MR) techniques expose the patient to three different forms of electromagnetic radiation: a static magnetic field; gradient magnetic fields; and radiofrequency (RF) electromagnetic fields. Each of these may cause significant bioeffects if applied at sufficiently high exposure levels.[1–6] In addition, there are several other areas of health concern for both the patient and health practitioner with respect to the clinical use of magnetic resonance imaging (MRI) and spectroscopy. Therefore, the purpose of this chapter is to discuss the bioeffects of static, gradient, and RF electromagnetic fields and to provide an overview of other safety considerations related to MRI and spectroscopy, with an emphasis on information that pertains to cardiovascular MR studies.

Static Magnetic Field Bioeffects

Temperature Effects

Conflicting statements exist in the literature regarding the effect of static magnetic fields on body and skin temperatures of humans and other mammals. For example, one report indicated that static magnetic fields either increase or decrease temperature, depending on the orientation of the organism in the static magnetic field.[7] A different report stated that a static magnetic field had no effect on skin and body temperatures of humans.[8] The study conducted to specifically determine if exposure to a 1.5-T static magnetic field of an MR scanner alters skin and body

Supported in part by PHS grant 1 R01 CA 44014-04 awarded by the National Cancer Institute, National Institutes of Health.
From Pohost GM (ed.), *Cardiovascular Applications of Magnetic Resonance*. Mount Kisco, NY, Futura Publishing Co., Inc., © 1993.

temperatures in humans was performed using a special fluoroptic thermometry system known to be unperturbed by high-intensity static magnetic fields.[8] Therefore, skin and body temperatures of human subjects are believed to be unaffected by exposure to static magnetic fields up to 1.5 T.

Cardiac and Electrical Induction Effects

A magnetohydrodynamic effect may be observed during exposure to static magnetic fields and is caused by blood, a conductive fluid, flowing through a static magnetic field.[6,9–12] The result is an induced biopotential that is exhibited by an augmentation of the T wave amplitude that is apparent on the electrocardiogram (ECG).[6,9–12] This phenomenon has been observed at static magnetic field strengths as low as 0.1 T.[6,9,12] The most marked effect on the T wave is believed to be caused when the blood flows through the thoracic aortic arch.[6,9,12] This T wave amplitude change can be significant enough to falsely trigger the RF excitation during cardiac gated MR studies. Other portions of the ECG may also be altered by the static magnetic field and this varies with the placement of the recording electrodes.[13] Alternate lead positions can be used to diminish the static magnetic field-induced electrocardiographic changes and facilitate obtaining a usable ECG signal for cardiac gating studies.[13]

Once the patient is no longer exposed to the static magnetic field, ECG voltage abnormalities revert to normal. There are no circulatory alterations that coincide with the static magnetic field-induced electrocardiographic changes. Therefore, no significant bioeffects are believed to be associated with the magnetohydrodynamic effect that occurs in conjunction with static magnetic field strengths up to 2.0 T.[6,9–12]

Theoretically, electrical impulse conduction in nerve tissue may also be affected by exposure to static magnetic fields.[1,6,14] However, this is another area in the bioeffects literature that contains contradictory information. Some studies have reported remarkable effects on both the function and structure of the central nervous system during exposure to static magnetic fields, whereas others have failed to show any significant changes.[1,2,6,14–19] Further investigations of potential unwanted bioeffects are needed because of the relative lack of clinical studies in this field that are directly applicable to MR procedures.

Presently, exposure to static magnetic fields up to 2.0 T do not appear to significantly influence bioelectric properties of neurons in human subjects.[6,10,11,20,21] However, as of 1991, there are at least four 4.0-T whole-body MR scanners operating at various research sites around the world. A preliminary study has indicated that workers and volunteer subjects exposed to a 4.0-T MRI system have experienced vertigo, nausea, headaches, a metallic taste in their mouths, and magnetophosphenes (visual flashes).[22] Therefore, additional research is required to study the mechanisms responsible for these bioeffects.

Gradient Magnetic Field Bioeffects

Magnetic resonance imaging procedures expose the human body to the transient application of magnetic field gradients during the imaging sequence. Gradient magnetic fields can induce electrical fields and currents in conductive media (including biological tissue) according to Faraday's law of induction.[4,10,11,21] The potential for interaction between gradient magnetic fields and biological tissue is inherently dependent on the fundamental field frequency, the maximum flux density, the average flux density, the presence of harmonic frequencies, the waveform characteristics of the signal, the polarity of the signal, the current distribution in the body, and the electrical properties and sensitivity of the particular cell membrane.[10,11,20,21]

Bioeffects of gradient magnetic fields can be due either to the power deposited by the induced currents (thermal effects) or to direct effects of the current (nonthermal effects). Thermal effects due to switched gradients used in MRI are negligible and, therefore, are not believed to be clinically significant.[10,11,20,21]

Possible nonthermal effects of induced currents are stimulation of nerve or muscle cells, induction of ventricular fibrillation, increased brain mannitol space, epileptogenic potential, and stimulation of visual flash sensations.[1,3,10,11,20,21,23–25] The threshold currents required for nerve stimulation and ventricular fibrillation are known to be much higher than the estimated current densities that will be induced under routine clinical MRI conditions.[10,21,22] To our knowledge there have been no reports of such effects during the application of conventional MR procedures performed at the levels recommended by the United States Food and Drug Administration (FDA).

The production of magnetophosphenes is considered to be one of the most sensitive physiologic responses to gradient magnetic fields.[10,11,20,21] Magnetophosphenes are presumed to be caused by electrical stimulation of the retina and are completely reversible with no associated health effects.[10,11,20,21] Although there have been no reported cases of magnetophosphenes for fields of 1.95 T or less, magnetophosphenes have been reported in volunteers working in and around a 4.0-T research system.[20] In addition, a metallic taste and symptoms of vertigo seem also to be reproducible and associated with rapid motion within the static magnetic field of these 4.0-T systems.[22]

One of the current recommendations issued by the FDA[26] for exposure to gradient magnetic fields during MR procedures is that the rate of change should not be sufficient to cause peripheral nerve stimulation by an adequate margin of safety (at least a factor of three). In the event that significant electrical currents are induced during MR, it is predicted that cutaneous nerves or peripheral skeletal muscle will be stimulated and, thus, give ample warning before the occurrence of a more deleterious response, such as cardiac arrhythmia or fibrillation.[10,11,20,21,26]

Although the current FDA guidelines are believed to provide a sufficient margin of safety with respect to exposure to gradient magnetic fields during MR studies, it is imperative to realize that the newer echo-planar techniques that require more rapid and complex applications of gradient magnetic fields may easily exceed the recommended levels and must be thoroughly evaluated for potential health hazards. Preliminary studies performed in human subjects have demonstrated that induced eddy currents have resulted in peripheral nerve stimulation producing muscle twitches or contractions in synchrony with field pulses.[23,24]

Radiofrequency Electromagnetic Field Bioeffects

Radiofrequency radiation is capable of generating heat in tissues as a result of resistive losses. Therefore, the main bioeffects associated with exposure to RF radiation are related to the thermogenic qualities of this electromagnetic field.[10,11,27–40] Exposure to RF radiation may also cause athermal, field-specific alterations in biological systems that are produced without a significant increase in temperature.[1,3–5] The athermal bioeffects of RF radiation are somewhat controversial due to assertions concerning the role of electromagnetic fields in producing cancer and developmental abnormalities, along with the concomitant ramifications of such effects.[1,3–5,41] A report from the U.S. Environmental Protection Agency claimed that the existing evidence on this issue is sufficient to demonstrate a relationship between low-level electromagnetic field exposures and the development of cancer.[41] To date, there have been no specific studies performed to study potential athermal bioeffects of MR procedures. Those interested in a thorough review of this topic, particularly as it pertains to MR studies, are referred to the extensive review article written by Beers.[3]

Regarding RF power deposition concerns, investigators have typically quantified exposure to RF radiation by means of determining the specific absorption rate (SAR).[4,5,28,29] The SAR is the mass normalized rate at which RF power is coupled to biological tissue and is commonly indicated in units of watts per kilogram (W/kg). Measurements or estimates of SAR are not trivial, particularly in human subjects, and there are several methods of determining this parameter for the purpose of RF energy dosimetry.[4,5,28,29]

The SAR that is produced during MR studies is a complex function of numerous variables, including the frequency (which, in turn, is determined by the strength of the static magnetic field), type of RF pulse (ie, 90° or 180°), TR time, pulse width, type of RF coil used, volume of tissue within the coil, resistivity of the tissue, configuration of the anatomical region imaged, as well as other factors.[4,5,28,29] The actual increase in tissue temperature caused by exposure to RF radiation is dependent on the subject's thermoregulatory system (eg, skin blood flow, skin surface area, sweat rate, etc.).[4,5,28,29]

The efficiency and absorption pattern of RF energy are mainly determined by the physical dimensions of the tissue in relation to the incident wavelength.[4,5,27–29] Therefore, if the tissue size is large relative to the wavelength, energy is predominantly absorbed on the surface; if it is small relative to the wavelength, there is little absorption of RF power.[4,5,27–29] Because of the above relationship between RF energy and physical dimensions, studies designed to investigate the effects of exposure to RF radiation during MR studies that are intended to be applicable to the clinical setting require tissue volumes and anatomical shapes comparable to that of human subjects. Of additional note is that there is no laboratory animal that sufficiently mimics or simulates the thermoregulatory system or responses of humans. For these reasons, results obtained in laboratory animal experiments cannot simply be scaled or extrapolated to human subjects.[11,28,29]

Several studies of RF power absorption during MR have been performed recently and have yielded useful information about tissue heating in human subjects.[30–40] During MR studies, tissue heating results primarily from magnetic induction with a negligible contribution from the electric fields, so that ohmic heating is greatest at the surface of the body and approaches zero at the center of the body. Predictive calculations and measurements obtained in phantoms and human subjects exposed to MR supports this pattern of temperature distribution.[27,30–40]

Although one study reported significant temperature rises in internal organs produced by MR procedures,[40] this study was conducted on anesthetized dogs and is unlikely to be applicable to conscious adult human subjects because of factors related to the physical dimensions and dissimilar thermoregulatory systems of these two species.[11,21] However, these data may have important implications for the use of MR in pediatric patients since this patient population is typically sedated or anesthetized for MR examinations.[11,21]

An investigation using fluoroptic thermometry probes that are unperturbed by electromagnetic fields[37] demonstrated that human subjects exposed to MR studies at SAR levels up to 4.0 W/kg (ie, 10 times higher than the level currently recommended by the FDA) have no statistically significant increases in body temperatures and elevations in skin temperatures that are believed to be clinically hazardous.[37] These results imply that the suggested exposure level of 0.4 W/kg for RF radiation during MR studies is too conservative for individuals with normal thermoregulatory function.[11,21,37] Additional studies are needed, however, to assess physiologic responses of patients with conditions that may impair thermoregulatory function (eg, elderly patients; patients with underlying health conditions such as fever, diabetes, cardiovascular disease, or obesity; and patients taking medications that affect thermoregulation such as calcium blockers, β-blockers, diuretics, vasodilators, etc.) before subjecting them to MR procedures that require high SARs.[11,21]

Temperature-Sensitive Organs

Certain human organs that have reduced capabilities for heat dissipation, such as the testis and eye, are particularly sensitive to elevated temperatures. Therefore, these are primary sites of potential harmful effects if RF radiation exposures during MR studies are excessive.

Laboratory investigations have demonstrated detrimental effects on testicular function (ie, a reduction or cessation of spermatogenesis, impaired sperm motility, degeneration of seminiferous tubules, etc.) caused by RF radiation-induced heating from exposures sufficient to raise scrotal and/or testicular tissue temperatures to 38°C to 42°C.[38] Scrotal skin temperatures (ie, an index of intratesticular temperature) were measured in volunteer subjects undergoing MRI at a whole-body averaged SAR of 1.1 W/kg.[38] The largest change in scrotal skin temperature was 2.1°C, and the highest scrotal skin temperature recorded was 34.2°C.[38] These temperature changes were below the threshold known to impair testicular function. Excessively heating the scrotum during MR studies could exacerbate certain preexisting disorders associated with increased scrotal/testicular temperatures (eg, acute febrile illnesses, varicocele, etc.) in patients who are already oligospermic and lead to possible temporary or permanent sterility.[38] Therefore, additional studies designed to investigate these issues are needed, particularly if patients are scanned at whole-body averaged SARs higher than those previously evaluated.

Dissipation of heat from the eye is a slow and inefficient process due to its relative lack of vascularization. Acute near-field exposures of RF radiation to the eyes or heads of laboratory animals have been demonstrated to be cataractogenic as a result of the thermal disruption of ocular tissues if the exposure is of a sufficient intensity and duration.[4,5] Corneal temperatures have been measured in patients undergoing MRI of the brain using a send/receive head coil at local SARs up to 3.1 W/kg.[35] The largest corneal temperature change was 1.8°C, and the highest temperature measured was 34.4°C.[35] Since the temperature threshold for RF radiation-induced cataractogenesis in animal models has been demonstrated to be between 41°C to 55°C for acute, near-field exposures, it does not appear that clinical MRI using a head coil has the potential to cause thermal damage in ocular tissue.[35] The effect of MR studies performed at higher SARs and the long-term effects of MR on ocular tissues remain to be determined.

Radiofrequency Radiation "Hot Spots"

Theoretically, RF radiation "hot spots" caused by an uneven distribution of RF power may arise whenever current concentrations are produced in association with restrictive conductive patterns.[11,21] There has been the suggestion that RF radiation hot spots may generate thermal hot spots under certain conditions during MR studies. Since RF radiation is mainly absorbed by peripheral tissues, thermography has been used to study the surface heating pattern associated with MR studies performed at high whole-body SARs.[31] This study demonstrated no evidence of surface thermal hot spots related to MRI of human subjects.[31] The thermoregulatory system apparently responds to the heat challenge by distributing the thermal load, producing a smearing effect of the surface temperatures. However, there is a possibility that internal thermal hot spots may develop from MRI.[11,21]

Future Studies of Radiofrequency Electromagnetic Field Bioeffects

Recent advances in the applications of MR have produced special pulse sequences (ie, RARE, fast spin-echo, etc.) that allow imaging to be performed up to 32 times faster than previously possible. This requires a substantial increase in RF power because of the frequent requirement for 180° RF pulses that is predicted in some cases to exceed a whole-body averaged SAR of 10.0 W/kg (D.J. Schaefer, personal communication, 1991). The clinical importance and cost-effective use of MR studies accomplished with these new pulse sequences is obvious. However, the safety of subjecting patients to RF energy at these potentially excessive levels is unknown. Therefore, studies are currently needed to investigate human thermoregulatory responses to SARs that are even higher than those that have been studied in recent years.

In addition, the 4.0-T whole-body MR scanners that are being used for a combination of imaging and spectroscopy on human subjects use approximately seven times as much RF energy as a 1.5-T MR scanner. Investigations evaluating thermal responses in human subjects will also need to be performed to assess the safety of these powerful devices.

The United States Food and Drug Administration Guidelines for Magnetic Resonance Devices

On July 28, 1988, MR diagnostic devices were reclassified from Class III, in which premarket approval is required, to Class II, which is regulated by performance standards.[26] Four primary areas relating to MR devices have been identified for which safety guidelines have been issued by the FDA. These include the static magnetic field, the gradient magnetic fields, the RF power of the examination, and the acoustical considerations. Selected excerpts from the wording of the FDA document are as follows:[26]

Static magnetic field: Static magnetic field strengths not exceeding 2.0 T are below the level of concern for the static magnetic field. Should the static magnetic field strength exceed 2.0 T, additional evidence of safety must be provided by the sponsor.

Gradient magnetic field: Limit patient exposure to gradient magnetic fields with strengths less than those required to produce peripheral nerve stimulation or other effects. There are three alternatives:

1. Demonstrate that the maximum dB/dt of the system is 6 T/sec or less.
2. Demonstrate that for axial gradients, dB/dt <20 T/sec for $\pi \geq 120$ μsec, or dB/dt $<(2{,}400/\pi)$ T/sec for 12 μsec $<\pi<120$ πsec, or dB/dt <200 T/sec for $\pi \leq 12$ πsec (π equals the width in microseconds of a retangular pulse or the half period of a sinusoidal dB/dt pulse). For transverse gradients, dB/dt is considered to be below the level of concern when it is less than three times the above limits for axial gradients.
3. Demonstrate with valid scientific evidence that the rate of change of magnetic field for the system is not sufficient to cause peripheral nerve stimulation by an adequate margin of safety (at least a factor of three).

RF power deposition: Options to control the risk of systemic thermal overload and local thermal injury caused by RF energy absorption are as follows:

1. If the specific absorption rate is 0.4 W/kg or less for the whole body and 8.0 W/kg or less spatial peak in any 1 gram of tissue, and if the specific absorption rate is 3.2 W/kg or less averaged over the head, then it is below the level of concern.
2. If exposure to RF magnetic fields is insufficient to produce a core temperature increase of 1°C and localized heating to no greater than 38°C in the head, 39°C in the trunk and 40°C in the extremities then it is considered to be below the level of concern.

The parameter RF heating must be below either of the two levels of concern by presentation of valid scientific measurement or calculational evidence sufficient to demonstrate that RF heating effects are of no concern.

Acoustic noise levels: The acoustic noise levels associated with the device must be shown to be below the level of concern established by pertinent federal regulatory or other recognized standards setting organizations. If the acoustic noise is not below the level of concern, the sponsor must recommend steps to reduce or alleviate the noise perceived by the patient.[26]

Magnetic Resonance Imaging and Acoustic Noise

The acoustic noise produced during MRI represents a potential risk to patients. Acoustic noise is associated with the activation and deactivation of electrical current that induces vibrations of the gradient coils.[10,20,21,42,43] This repetitive sound is enhanced by higher gradient duty cycles and sharper pulse transitions.[10,20,21,42,43] Acoustic noise is thus likely to increase with decreases in section thicknesses, decreased fields of view, TR, and TE.[10,20,21,42,43] Gradient-echo, partial flip angle pulse sequences, and echo-planar imaging techniques produce the most significant acoustic noise.

The safest and least expensive means of preventing problems associated with acoustic noise during clinical MRI is to encourage the routine use of disposable earplugs.[43,44] The use of hearing protection has been demonstrated to successfully avoid the potential temporary hearing loss that can be associated with clinical MRI examinations.[43,44] Magnetic resonance compatible headphones that significantly muffle acoustic noise are also commercially available.

Electrically, Magnetically, or Mechanically Activated Implants and Devices

The FDA requires labeling of MR scanners to indicate that the device is contraindicated for patients who have electrically, magnetically, or mechanically activated implants because electromagnetic fields produced by the MR device may interfere with the operation of these devices.[26] Therefore, patients with internal cardiac pacemakers, implantable cardiac defibrillators, cochlear implants, neurostimulators, bone growth stimulators, implantable electronic drug infusion pumps, and other similar devices that could be adversely effected by the electromagnetic fields used for MR should not be examined by this technique.[10,11,21,44–46] Prior ex vivo testing of certain of these implants and devices may indicate that they are, in fact, MRI compatible.

The associated risks of performing MR studies in patients with cardiac pacemakers are related to the possibility of movement, reed switch closures or damage, programming changes, inhibition, or reversion to an asynchronous mode of operation, electromagnetic interference, and induced currents in lead wires.[44,46] At least one patient with a pacemaker has been scanned by MRI without incident.[47] A letter-to-the-editor[47] recently indicated that a patient who was not pacemaker-dependent underwent MRI by having his pacemaker "disabled" during the procedure. Although this patient sustained no apparent discomfort and the pacemaker was not damaged, it is unadvisable to routinely perform this type of maneuver on patients with pacemakers because of the potential of encountering the aforementioned hazards. Of note is the fact that there has been at least one MRI-related death of a patient with a pacemaker.[48]

Of particular concern is the possibility that the pacemaker lead wire(s) or other similar intracardiac wire configuration could act as an antenna in which the gradient and/or RF electromagnetic fields may induce sufficient current to cause fibrillation, a burn, or other potentially dangerous events.[10,11,21,45] Because of this theoretically deleterious and unpredicted effect, patients referred to MR studies with residual external pacing wires, temporary pacing wires, Swan-Ganz thermodilution catheters, and/or any other type of internally or externally positioned conductive wire or similar device should not undergo MR because of the possible associated risks.[10,11,21,45,49,50]

Because there is a potential for demagnetizing implants that involve magnets (eg, dental implants, sphincters, stoma plugs, ocular prostheses, tissue expanders, etc.) that may necessitate surgery to replace the damaged implant, these should be removed from the patient prior to the MR study, if possible.[21,44,51,52] Otherwise, MR procedures should not be performed on a patient with a magnetically activated implant or device. A patient with any other similar electrically, magnetically, or mechanically activated implant or device should be excluded from examination by MR unless the particular implant or device has been previously demonstrated to be unaffected by the electromagnetic fields.[44]

Metallic Implants, Materials, and Foreign Bodies

Magnetic resonance imaging or spectroscopy is contraindicated for patients who have certain ferromagnetic implants, materials, or foreign bodies, primarily due to the possibility of movement or dislodgment of these objects. Other problems may also occur in patients with ferromagnetic implants, materials, or foreign bodies who undergo MRI or spectroscopy, including the induction of electric current in the object, excessive heating of the object, and for MRI, the misinterpretation of an artifact produced by the presence of the object as an abnormality.[21,53–65] However, these latter potentially hazardous situations are rarely encountered or are relatively minor in comparison with movement or dislodgment of a ferromagnetic object by the magnetic fields of the MR scanner.

Numerous studies have evaluated the ferromagnetic qualities of various different metallic implants, materials, or foreign bodies by measuring movement deflection forces found in association with the static magnetic fields of the MR scanner. A variety of factors require evaluation when establishing the relative risk of performing MRI in a patient with a ferromagnetic implant, material, device, or foreign body, such as the strength of the static and gradient magnetic fields, the relative degree of ferromagnetism of the object, the mass of the object, the geometry of the object, the location and orientation of the object in situ, and the length of time the object has been in place.[10,11,21] Each of these should be carefully considered before allowing a patient who has a ferromagnetic object to enter the electromagnetic environment of the MR scanner. Table 1 lists metallic implants, materials, and foreign bodies that are potential risks for patients undergoing MR studies. These evaluations were performed with MR scanners with static magnetic field strengths up to 2.35 T.[62]

With respect to metallic objects that have been tested and are of specific interest to those performing cardiovascular MR studies, the following should be noted:[21,62,63]

Aneurysm and hemostatic clips: Of the 32 different aneurysm ($n = 26$) and vascular clips ($n = 6$) studied and reported in the literature, 19 aneurysm clips and none of the vascular clips were found to be ferromagnetic. Therefore, only patients who definitely have nonferromagnetic aneurysm clips should be exposed to the magnetic fields used

TABLE 1. Metallic Implants, Materials, and Foreign Bodies that are Potential Risks for Patients Undergoing MR Studies

Aneurysm clips:
- Drake (DR14, DR 24), Edward Weck, Triangle Park, NJ
- Drake (DR16), Edward Weck
- Drake (301 SS), Edward Weck
- Downs multi-positional (17-7PH)
- Heifetz (17-7PH), Edward Weck
- Housepian
- Kapp (405 SS), V. Mueller
- Kapp curved (404 SS), V. Mueller
- Kapp straight (404 SS), V. Mueller
- Mayfield (301 SS), Codman, Randolph, MA
- Mayfield (304 SS), Codman
- McFadden (301 SS), Codman
- Pivot (17-7PH), V. Mueller
- Scoville (EN58J), Downs Surgical, Decatur, GA
- Sundt-Kees (301-SS), Downs Surgical
- Sundt-Kees Multi-Angle (17-7PH), Downs Surgical
- Vari-Angle (17-7PH), Codman
- Vari-Angle Micro (17-7PM SS), Codman
- Vari-Angle Spring (17-7PM SS), Codman

Cartoid artery vascular clamp:
- Poppen-Blaylock (SS), Codman

Dental devices and materials:
- +Palladium clad magnet, Parkell Products, Farmindale, NY
- +Titanium clad magnet, Parkell Products
- +Stainless steel clad magnet, Parkell Products

Heart valves:
- Starr-Edwards, Model Pre 6000, American Edwards, Irvine, CA

Intravascular coils, stents, and filters:
- *Gianturco embolization coil, Cook, Bloomington, ID
- *Gianturco bird nest IVC filter, Cook
- *Gianturco zig-zag stent, Cook
- *Gunther IVC filter, Cook
- *New retrievable IVC filter, Thomas Jefferson University, Philadelphia, PA
- *Palmaz endovascular stent, Ethicon, Sommerville, NJ

Ocular implants:
- +Fatio eyelid spring/wire
- Retinal tack (SS-martensitic), Western European

Otologic implants:
- Cochlear implant (3M/House)
- Cochlear implant (3M/Vienna)
- Cochlear implant, Nucleus Mini 22-channel, Cochlear, Engelwood, CO
- McGee piston stapes prothesis, (platinum/17Cr-4Ni SS), Richards Medical, Memphis, TN

Pellets, bullets, schrapnel, etc.:
- BBs, Daisy
- BBs Crosman
- Bullet, 7.62 × 39 mm (copper, steel), Norinco
- Bullet, 0.380 inch, (copper, nickel, lead), Geco
- Bullet 0.45 inch, (steel, lead), North American Ordinance
- Bullet, 9 mm, (copper, lead), Norma

Penile implants:
- +Penile Implant, OmniPhase, Dacomed Corp., Minneapolis, MN

Miscellaneous:
- Cerebral ventricular shunt tube, connector (type unknown)
- #Swan-Ganz Thermodilution Catheter, Thermodilution, American Edwards, Irvine, CA
- +Tissue expander with magnetic port, McGhan Medical, Santa Barbara, CA

*Ferromagnetic coils, filters, and stents typically become firmly incorporated into the vessel wall several weeks following placement, and therefore, it is unlikely that they will become dislodged by magnetic forces after a suitable period of time has passed.

+The potential for these metallic implants or devices to produce significant injury to the patient is minimal. However, performing an MR study in a patient with one of these devices may be uncomfortable for the individual and/or may result in damage to the implant.

#While there is no magnetic deflection associated with the Swan-Ganz thermodilution catheter, there has been a report of a catheter "melting" in a patient undergoing MR imaging. Therefore, this catheter is considered contraindicated for MR imaging.

The relative risks of performing MR studies in patients with pellets, bullets, or schrapnel are related to whether or not they are positioned near a vital structure.

Manufacturer information is provided if indicated in a previously published reference or if otherwise known.

SS, stainless steel.

for MR, while any patient with one of the previously tested hemostatic clips may safely undergo an MR study.

Carotid artery vascular clamps: Each of the five carotid artery vascular clamps evaluated for ferromagnetism exhibited deflection forces. However, only the Poppen-Blaylock clamp was considered to be contraindicated for patients undergoing MR studies because of the significant ferromagnetism shown by this object. The other carotid artery vascular clamps are believed to be safe for MR because of the minimal deflection forces relative to their use in an in vivo application (ie, the deflection forces are insignificant and, therefore, there is little possibility of significant movement or dislodgment of the implant in vivo).

Heart valves: Twenty-nine heart valve prostheses have been tested for ferromagnetism. Twenty-five of these displayed measurable deflection forces, however, the deflection forces were relatively insignificant compared with the force exerted by the beating heart. Therefore, patients with these heart valve prostheses may safely undergo MR studies. The only possible exception is that MR studies performed with a static magnetic field >0.35 T may be potentially hazardous for a patient who has a Starr-Edwards Pre 6000 valve if there is concern regarding the integrity of the annulus or the presence of valvular dehiscence.

Intravascular coils, filters, and stents: Five of the 14 different intravascular coils, filters, and stents tested were ferromagnetic.[62,64] These ferromagnetic devices are usually attached firmly to the vessel wall approximately 4 to 6 weeks following introduction.[64] Therefore, it is unlikely that any of them would become dislodged by attraction from magnetic forces presently used for MR studies. Patients with intravascular coils, filters, or stents in whom there is a possibility that the device is not properly positioned or held firmly in place should not undergo MR.

Pellets, bullets, shrapnel, etc.: Most of the pellets and bullets previously tested for ferromagnetism are composed of nonferromagnetic materials.[63,65] Ammunition found to be ferromagnetic typically came from foreign countries and/or was used by the military. Shrapnel usually contains various amounts of steel and, therefore, presents a potential hazard for MR studies. Furthermore, since pellets, bullets, and schrapnel may be contaminated with ferromagnetic materials, these objects represent relative contraindications for MR studies. Patients with these foreign bodies should be regarded on an individual basis with respect to whether the object is positioned near a vital neural, vascular, or soft tissue structure. This may be assessed by taking a careful history and using plain film radiography to determine the location of the foreign body.[44]

Vascular access ports: Of the 33 different vascular access ports tested for ferromagnetism, two showed measurable deflection forces, but the forces were felt to be insignificant relative to the in vivo application of these implants. Therefore, it is considered safe to perform MR studies in patients who may have these previously tested vascular access ports.

Miscellaneous: Various types of other metallic implants, materials, and foreign bodies have also been tested for ferromagnetism. Of these, the cerebral ventricular shunt tube connector (type unknown) and tissue expander that is magnetically activated exhibited deflection forces that may pose a risk to patients during MR studies. An "O-ring" washer used as a vascular marker also showed ferromagnetism, but the deflection force was determined to be minimal relative to the in vivo use of this device.

According to the *Policies, Guidelines, and Recommendations for MR Imaging Safety and Patient Management* information issued by the MR Safety Committee of the Society for Magnetic Resonance Imaging,[44] patients with electrically, magnetically, or mechanically activated or electrically conductive devices should be excluded from MR studies unless the particular device has been previously shown (ie, usually by ex vivo testing procedures) to be unaffected by the electromagnetic fields used for clinical MR and there is no possibility of injuring the patient. During the screening process for MR studies, patients with these objects should be identified before their examination and prior to being exposed to the electromagnetic fields used for MR. Many implants, materials, devices, or other foreign bodies that have yet to be evaluated for MR compatibility may be encountered in the clinical setting. Patients that have untested objects should not be allowed to undergo MR studies.

Screening Patients With Metallic Foreign Bodies

Patients referred for cardiovascular MR procedures may present with a history of metallic foreign bodies such as slivers, bullets, shrapnel, or other types of metallic fragments. The relative risk of scanning these patients is dependent upon the ferromagnetic properties of the object, the geometry and dimensions of the object, and the strength of the static and gradient magnetic fields of the MR scanner.[44] Also important is the force with which the metallic foreign body is fixed within the tissue and whether it is positioned in or adjacent to a potentially hazardous location of the body, such as a vital neural, vascular, or soft tissue structure.[21,44]

Plain film radiography is a sensitive and relatively inexpensive technique for identifying or excluding a metallic foreign body that may be a potential hazard to the patient undergoing MR studies.[21,44] For example, patients with a high suspicion of having an intraocular metallic foreign body (eg, a metal worker exposed to metallic slivers with a history of an eye injury) should have plain film radiographs of the orbits to rule out the presence of a metallic fragment prior to exposure to the static magnetic field of the MR scanner.[21,44]

Performing Magnetic Resonance Studies During Pregnancy

Although MRI and spectroscopy are not believed to be hazardous to the fetus, only a few investigations have examined the teratogenic potential of this imaging modality. This topic has been summarized in previous review papers.[10,11,21] By comparison, literally thousands of studies have been performed to examine the possible hazards of ultrasound during pregnancy and controversy still exists concerning the safe use of this nonionizing radiation imaging technique.

According to the MR Safety Committee of the Society for Magnetic Resonance Imaging,[44] MR studies are indicated for use in pregnant women if other nonionizing forms of diagnostic imaging are inadequate or if the examination provides important information that would otherwise require exposure to ionizing radiation (ie, x-ray, computed tomography, etc.). It is recommended to inform pregnant patients that, to date, there has been no indication that the use of clinical MR studies during pregnancy has produced deleterious effects. However, as noted by the FDA, the safety of MR during pregnancy has not been proved.[26]

Patients who are pregnant or suspect they are pregnant must be identified prior to undergoing MR studies in order to assess the risks versus the benefits of the examination. Since there is a high spontaneous abortion rate in the general population during the first trimester of pregnancy (ie, >30%), particular care should be exercised with the use of MR studies during the first trimester because of associated potential medicolegal implications relative to spontaneous abortions.

Monitoring Physiologic Parameters During Magnetic Resonance Studies

Because the typical MR scanner is constructed such that the patient is placed inside a cylindrical structure, routine observations and vital signs monitoring are not simple procedures. Conventional monitoring equipment was not designed to operate in the MR environment where static, gradient, and RF electromagnetic fields can adversely affect the operation of these devices.[66–69] Fortunately, MR-compatible monitors have been developed and are commonly used in inpatient and outpatient MR centers.[66–69]

Physiologic monitoring is required for the safe utilization of MR in patients who are sedated, anesthetized, comatose, critically ill, or otherwise unable to communicate with the MR operator.[66–69] All of the above categories of patients should be routinely monitored during MR and, considering the current availability of MR-compatible monitors, there is no reason to exclude these types of patients from clinical MR procedures.[21,66–69] Physiologic parameters that can be obtained using MR-compatible devices include heart rate, systemic blood pressure, end-tidal carbon dioxide, oxygen saturation, respiratory rate, skin blood flow, and temperature.[21,66–69] Table 2 lists examples of MR-compatible monitors that have been successfully tested and operated in MR scanners at static magnetic field strengths up to 1.5 T. In addition, there are now MR-compatible ventilators for patients who require ventilatory support.

A primary source of adverse MR scanner and physiologic monitor interactions has been the interface that is used between the patient and the equipment because this usually requires a conductive cable or other device.[49,50,70] The presence of a conductive material in the immediate MR scanner area is a safety concern because of the potential for monitor-related burns. There have been several reports of first-, second-, and third-degree burns involving sedated or anesthetized patients who were presumedly monitored inappropriately during MR studies. Investigations of these incidents typically revealed that the cables or leads leading from the monitors to the patients may have been looped during the MR procedures and the gradient and/or RF magnetic fields induced sufficient current to exorbitantly heat the conductive material, resulting in the burns.[49,50,70] Therefore, it is imperative that personnel be trained in the proper use and implementation of monitoring equipment before its utilization in the MR environment.[21,49,50,66–70]

TABLE 2. Examples of MR Compatible Monitors and Respirators*

Device and Manufacturer	Function
Omega 1400 In Vivo Research, Inc. Winter Park, FL	blood pressure heart rate
Fiber-Optic Pulse Oximeter Nonin Medical Plymouth, MN	oxygen saturation heart rate
525 Respiratory Rate Monitor Boiochem International Waukesha, WI	respiratory rate
MicroSpan Capnometer 8800 Biochem International Waukesha, WI	respiratory rate end-tidal carbon dioxide
Aneuroid Chest Bellows Coulbourn Instruments Allentown, PA	respiratory rate
Laserflow Blood Perfusion Monitor Vasomedics, Inc. St. Paul, MN	skin blood flow
Medpacific LD 5000 Laser-Doppler Perfusion Monitor Medpacific Corporation Seattle, WA	skin blood flow
Fluoroptic Thermometry System Model 3000 Luxtron Mountain View, CA	temperature
In Vivo Omni-Trak 3100 MRI Vital Signs Monitoring System In Vivo Research Inc. Winter Park, FL	heart rate blood pressure temperature oxygen saturation respiration
Omni-Vent, Series D Columbia Medical Marketing Topeka, KS	respirator
Ventilator, Model 225 Monaghan Medical Corporation Plattsburgh, PA	respirator

*Note that these devices may require modifications to make them MR compatible and none of them should be positioned closer than 8 feet from the entrance of the bore of a 1.5-T MR scanner. Also, monitors with metallic cables, leads, or probes will cause mild to moderate imaging artifacts if placed near the imaging area of interest. Consult manufacturers to determine compatibility with specific MR scanners and for additional safety information.

Acknowledgment

The authors wish to express their gratitude for the editorial assistance provided by Ms. Stacy M. Myers.

References

1. Adey WR: Tissue interactions with nonionizing electromagnetic fields. *Physiol Rev* 1981;61:435–514.
2. Barnothy MF: *Biological Effects of Magnetic Fields*. New York: Plenum Publishing Corp; 1964.
3. Beers J: Biological effects of weak electromagnetic fields from 0 Hz to 200 MHz: a survey of the literature with special emphasis on possible magnetic resonance effects. *Magn Reson Imaging* 1989;7:309–331.
4. Michaelson SM, Lin JV: *Biological Effects and Health Implications of Radiofrequency Radiation*. New York: Plenum Publishing Corp; 1987.
5. National Council on Radiation Protection and Measurements. Biological effects and exposure criteria for radiofrequency electromagnetic fields. Report No. 86. 1986.
6. Tenforde TS, ed: *Magnetic Field Effects on Biological Systems*. New York: Plenum Publishing Corp; 1979.
7. Sperber D, Oldenbourg R, Dransfeld K: Magnetic field induced temperature change in mice. *Naturwissenschaften* 1984;71:100–101.
8. Shellock FG, Schaefer DJ, Crues JV: Exposure to a 1.5 Tesla static magnetic field does not alter body and skin temperatures in man. *Magn Reson Med* 1989;11:371–375.
9. Beischer DE, Knepton J: Influence of strong magnetic fields on the electrocardiogram of squirrel monkey. *Aerospace Med* 1964;35:939–944.
10. Kanal E, Shellock FG, Talagala L: Safety considerations in MR imaging. *Radiology* 1990;176:593–606.
11. Shellock FG: Biological effects and safety aspects of magnetic resonance imaging. *Magn Reson Q* 1989;5:243–261.
12. Tenforde TS, Gaffey CT, Moyer BR, Budinger TF: Cardiovascular alterations in Macaca monkeys exposed to stationary magnetic fields. Experimental observations and theoretical analysis. *Bioelectromagnetics* 1983;4:1–9.
13. Dimick RN, Hedlund LW, Herfkens RJ, et al: Optimizing electrocardiographic electrode placement for cardiac-gated magnetic resonance imaging. *Invest Radiol* 1987;22:17–22.
14. Hong CZ: Static magnetic field influence on human nerve function. *Arch Phys Med Rehab* 1987;68:162–164.
15. Doherty JU, Whitman GJR, Robinson MD, et al: Changes in cardiac excitability and vulnerability in NMR fields. *Invest Radiol* 1985;20(2):129–135.
16. Hong CZ, Shellock FG: Short-term exposure to a 1.5 Tesla static magnetic field does not effect somato-sensory evoked potentials in man. *Magn Reson Imaging* 1990;8:65–69.
17. Jehenson P, Duboc D, Lavergne T, et al: Change in human cardiac rhythm by a 2 Tesla static magnetic field. *Radiology* 1988;166:227–230.
18. McRobbie D, Foster MA: Cardiac responses to pulsed magnetic fields with regard to safety in NMR imaging. *Phys Med Biol* 1985;30:695–702.
19. Yuh WTC, Ehrhardt JC, Fisher DJ, et al: Induced pain in an amputated arm by strong static magnetic field. *J Magn Reson Imaging* 1992;2:221–223.
20. Persson BR, Stahlberg F: *Health and Safety Clinical NMR Examinations*. Boca Raton, Fla: CRC Press, Inc; 1989.
21. Shellock FG, Litwer C, Kanal E: MRI bioeffects, safety, and patient management: a review. *Rev Magn Reson Imaging* 1992;4:21–63.
22. Redington RW, Dumoulin CL, Schenck JF, et al: MR imaging and bioeffects in a whole body 4.0 Tesla imaging system (abstract). In: Proceedings of the Society of Magnetic Resonance Imaging. 1988:20.

23. Cohen MS, Weiskoff R, Rzedzian R, Kantor H: Sensory stimulation by time-varying magnetic fields. *Magn Reson Med* 1990;14:409–414.
24. Fischer H: Physiological effects of fast oscillating magnetic field gradients. *Radiology* 1989;173:(P)382.
25. Reilly JP: Peripheral nerve stimulation by induced electric currents: exposure to time-varying magnetic fields. *Med Biol Eng Comput* 1989;27:101–112.
26. Food and Drug Administration: Magnetic resonance diagnostic device: panel recommendation and report on petitions for MR reclassification. *Federal Register* 1988;53:7575–7579.
27. Bottomley PA, Redington RW, Edelstein WA, Schenck JF: Estimating radiofrequency power deposition in body NMR imaging. *Magn Reson Med* 1985;2:336–349.
28. Gordon CJ: Thermal physiology. In *Biological Effects of Radiofrequency Radiation*. 1984; EPA-600/8–83-026A:414:28.
29. Gordon CJ: Normalizing the thermal effects of radiofrequency radiation: body mass versus total body surface area. *Bioelectromagnetics* 1987;8:111–118.
30. Shellock FG, Gordon CJ, Schaefer DJ: Thermoregulatory responses to clinical magnetic resonance imaging of the head at 1.5 Tesla: lack of evidence for direct effects on the hypothalamus. *Acta Radiol Suppl* 1986;369:512–513.
31. Shellock FG, Schaefer DJ, Grundfest W, Crues JV: Thermal effects of high-field (1.5 Tesla) magnetic resonance imaging of the spine: clinical experience above a specific absorption rate of 0.4 W/kg. *Acta Radiol Suppl* 1986;369:514–516.
32. Shellock FG, Crues JV: Alterations in cutaneous blood flow related to tissue heating during high-field magnetic resonance imaging. *Clin Res* 1986;34:344A.
33. Shellock FG, Crues JV: Temperature, heart rate, and blood pressure changes associated with clinical magnetic resonance imaging at 1.5 T. *Radiology* 1987;163:259–262.
34. Shellock FG, Crues JV: Temperature changes caused by clinical MR imaging of the brain at 1.5 Tesla using a head coil. *Am J Neuroradiol* 1988;9:287–291.
35. Shellock FG, Crues JV: Corneal temperature changes associated with high-field MR imaging of the brain with a head coil. *Radiology* 1988;167:809–811.
36. Shellock FG, Schaefer DJ, Crues JV: Evaluation of skin blood flow, body and skin temperature in man during MR imaging at high levels of RF energy. *J Magn Reson Imaging* 1989;7(suppl 1):P35.
37. Shellock FG, Schaefer DJ, Crues JV: Alterations in body and skin temperatures caused by MR imaging: is the recommended exposure for radiofrequency radiation too conservative? *Br J Radiol* 1989;62:904–909.
38. Shellock FG, Rothman B, Sarti D: Heating of the scrotum by high-field strength MR imaging. *AJR* 1990;154:1229–1232.
39. Shellock FG: Thermal responses in human subjects exposed to magnetic resonance imaging. In: *Biological Effects and Safety Aspects of Nuclear Magnetic Resonance Imaging and Spectroscopy*. New York: New York Academy of Sciences; 1992.
40. Shuman WP, Haynor DR, Guy AW, ef al: Superficial and deep-tissue increases in anesthetized dogs during exposure to high specific absorption rates in a 1.5-T MR imager. *Radiology* 1988;167:551–554.
41. Pool R: Electromagnetic fields: the biological evidence. *Science* 1990;249:1378–1381.
42. Goldman AM, Grossman WE, Friedlander PC: Reduction of sound levels with antinoise in MR imaging. *Radiology* 1989;173:549–550.
43. Brummett RE, Talbot JM, Charuhas P: Potential hearing loss resulting from MR imaging. *Radiology* 1988;169:539–540.
44. Shellock FG, Kanal E: Policies, guidelines, and recommendations for MR imaging safety and patient management. *J Magn Reson Imaging* 1991;1:97–101.
45. ECRI: A new MRI complication? *Health Devices Alert* 1988;27:1.
46. Hayes DL, Holmes DR, Gray JJE: Effect of a 1.5 Tesla nuclear magnetic resonance imaging scanner on implanted permanent pacemakers. *J Am Coll Cardiol* 1987;10:782–786.
47. Alagona P, Toole JC, Maniscalco BS, et al: Nuclear magnetic resonance imaging in a patient with a DDD pacemaker (letter to the editor). *PACE* 1989;12:619.

48. Gangarosa RE, Minnis JE, Nobbe J, et al: Operational safety aspects in MRI. *Magn Reson Imaging* 1987;5:287–292.
49. Kanal E, Shellock FG: Burns associated with clinical MR examinations. *Radiology* 1990;175:585.
50. Kanal E, Applegate GR: Thermal injuries/incidents associated with MR imaging devices in the U.S: a compilation and review of the presently available data (abstract). In: Proceedings of the Society for Magnetic Resonance Imaging. 1990: 274.
51. Shellock FG: Ex vivo assessment of deflection forces and artifacts associated with high-field MRI of "mini-magnet" dental prostheses. *Magn Reson Imaging* 1989;7(suppl 1):P38.
52. Yuh WTC, Hanigan MT, Nerad JA, et al: Extrusion of a magnetic eye implant after MR examination: a potential hazard to the enucleated eye. *J Magn Reson Imaging* 1992;1:351–352.
53. Davis PL, Crooks L, Arakawa M, et al: Heating effects of changing magnetic fields and RF fields on small metallic implants. *AJR* 1981;137:857–860.
54. Pusey E, Lufkin RB, Brown RKJ, et al: Magnetic resonance imaging artifacts: mechanism and clinical significance. *Radiographics* 1986;6:891–911.
55. Randall PA, Kohman LJ, Scalzetti EM, et al: Magnetic resonance imaging of prosthetic cardiac valves in vitro and in vivo. *Am J Cardiol* 1988;62:973–976.
56. Shellock FG, Crues JV: High-field MR imaging of metallic biomedical implants: an in vitro evaluation of deflection forces and temperature changes induced in large prostheses. *Radiology* 1987;165:150.
57. Shellock FG, Crues JV: High-field MR imaging of metallic biomedical implants: an ex vivo evaluation of deflection forces. *AJR* 1988;151:389–393.
58. Shellock FG, Schatz CJ, Shelton C, Brown B: Ex vivo evaluation of 9 different ocular and middle-ear implants exposed to a 1.5 Tesla MR scanner. *Radiology* 1990;177(P):271.
59. Shellock FG, Slimp G: Halo vest for cervical spine fixation during MR imaging. *AJR* 1990;154:631–632.
60. Shellock FG, Meeks T: Ex vivo evaluation of ferromagnetism and artifacts for implantable vascular access ports exposed to a 1.5 T MR scanner. *J Magn Reson Imaging* 1991;1:243.
61. Shellock FG, Schatz CJ: High-field strength MRI and otologic implants. *Am J Neuroradiol* 1991;12:279–281.
62. Shellock FG, Curtis JS: MR imaging and biomedical implants, materials, and devices: an updated review. *Radiology* 1991;180:541–550.
63. Shellock FG, Crues JV: Safety aspects of MRI in patients with metallic implants or foreign bodies: absolute and relative contraindications. *Appl Radiol* 1992:Nov:44–48.
64. Teitelbaum GP, Bradley WG, Klein BD: MR imaging artifacts ferromagnetism, and magnetic torque of intravascular filter stents, and coils. *Radiology* 1988;166:657–664.
65. Teitelbaum GP, Yee CA, Van Horn DD, et al: Metallic ballistic fragments: MR imaging safety and artifacts. *Radiology* 1990;175:855–859.
66. Holshouser BA, Hinshaw DB, Shellock FG: Sedation, anesthesia, and physiologic monitoring during MRI. In: Hasso AN, Stark DD, eds. *American Roentgen Ray Society, Categorical Course Syllabus, Spine and Body Magnetic Resonance Imaging. May 9–15, 1991.*
67. Shellock FG, Myers SM, Kimble K: Monitoring heart rate and oxygen saturation during MRI with a fiber-optic pulse oximeter. *AJR* 1992;158:663–664.
68. Shellock FG: Monitoring during MRI: an evaluation of the effect of high-field MRI on various patient monitors. *Med Electronics* 1986;100:93–97.
69. Shellock FG: Monitoring sedated pediatric patients during MRI. *Radiology* 1990;177:586.
70. Shellock FG, Slimp G: Severe burn of the finger caused by using a pulse oximeter during MRI. *AJR* 1989;153:1105.

Index